Aligner Techniques in Orthodontics

Aligner Techniques in Orthodontics

Susana Palma Moya
Javier Lozano Zafra

WILEY Blackwell

This edition first published 2021

Registered Office(s)
John Wiley & Sons, Inc., 111 River Street, Hoboken, NJ 07030, USA
John Wiley & Sons Ltd, The Atrium, Southern Gate, Chichester, West Sussex, PO19 8SQ, UK

Editorial Office
9600 Garsington Road, Oxford, OX4 2DQ, UK

For details of our global editorial offices, customer services, and more information about Wiley products visit us at www.wiley.com.

Wiley also publishes its books in a variety of electronic formats and by print-on-demand. Some content that appears in standard print versions of this book may not be available in other formats.

Library of Congress Cataloging-in-Publication Data

Names: Lozano Zafra, Javier, author. | Palma Moya, Susana, author.
Title: Aligner techniques in orthodontics / Javier Lozano Zafra, Dr Susana Palma Moya.
Description: Hoboken, NJ : Wiley-Blackwell, 2020.
Identifiers: LCCN 2020024180 (print) | LCCN 2020024181 (ebook) | ISBN 9781119607229 (paperback) | ISBN 9781119607212 (adobe pdf) | ISBN 9781119607236 (epub)
Subjects: MESH: Malocclusion–therapy | Orthodontics, Corrective–methods | Orthodontic Appliance Design–methods
Classification: LCC RK523 (print) | LCC RK523 (ebook) | NLM WU 440 | DDC 617.6/43–dc23
LC record available at https://lccn.loc.gov/2020024180
LC ebook record available at https://lccn.loc.gov/2020024181

Cover Design: Wiley
Cover Image: Courtesy of Javier Lozano Zafra

Set in 9.5/12.5pt STIXTwoText by SPi Global, Pondicherry, India
Printed and bound by CPI Group (UK) Ltd, Croydon, CR0 4YY
C9780470681619_120124

Contents

Preface

I started to work with aligners in 2001 and immediatly I realized that they had a huge potential. It was easy for me to get familiar with the whole idea because I used to work with dental positioners at that time. In contrast, most of my colleagues were quite skeptical and did not consider aligners as a real orthodontic system.

Reviewing the literature we can see how the possibilities of the aligners have increased over the years. In 2001, there were limited tools available to solve mild crowded Class I malocclusions; however, several years after, we started to speak about extraction cases, Class II malocclusions, and open bites, which were treated more successfully each time. This situation was due to two factors: on the one hand, the continuous feedback the manufacturers use to make constant improvements, and on the other hand, the tremendous effort by many orthdontists who have been trying to understand and explain what we call "*the plastic biomechanics*." Therefore, the perception of using the aligners as an effective orthodontic method is improving due to the irrefutable fact that the results are getting better and better and, in many cases, they overtake the outcomes achieved by conventional orthodontics.

We are only beginning to understand how the aligners move teeth, and the learning curve is slower than we thought. Those are the reasons why their effectiveness is indisputably attached to academic training and experience. The professionals with greater knowledge and greater number of treated cases will achieve better results. This is no surprise as this is what happens when a new technique is introduced.

For all these reasons, as professionals, we are the ones who still establish our treatment goals. Aesthetics and the patient's comfort should not conflict with the quality of the treatment results. This means that in quite a few situations, we need to use auxiliary techniques to complement the aligners deficiencies. It also means on the part of the practitioner a greater effort and dedication than usual to the occlusal and functional finishing treatment, and especially to training. I understand that leaving the comfort zone is not easy for those who have been treating patients the same way their *whole life*. This is where Dr Palma and Dr Lozano are absolutely exactly correct. This book fills a gap in our interpretation of the orthodontic movement with aligners. It offers a great number of essential keys to the understanding of the aligners biomechanics. It is the right publication at the right moment, with guides to treat different malocclusions with confidence, predictability and quality. Following their solid biomechanics knowledge and experience-based advice, the reader will be introduced to the treatment of more and more difficult cases, always keeping the traditional occlusal standards.

The book covers all the different malocclusions from the easiest mild crowding cases to the complex pre-prosthetic treatments. It is written like an atlas, with specific cases fully explained step by step. The reader will also find an innovative and attractive video format of each treatment. For all these reasons, this book is a wonderful and easy tool for references suitable for beginners, but also for orthodontists well trained in aligners. Moreover, for the skeptical ones, the book, at least, will peak their curiosity. Is it really possible to perform a good quality orthodontics with aligners? This book will provide answers, and without doubt, many arguments for discussion.

We are at the beginning of a new technique. Previous and complete case planification through a powerful software has radically changed the way we work. This means we have to go back to school, but we have never had so many possibilities to train ourselves like today. In this way, the professional is able to become as competent as he or she wishes. However, it seems that some things never change; and I do not just mean the huge reluctance to accept new concepts or techniques (that is really frequent in our profession), I also mean the small percentage of people such as Dr Palma and Dr Lozano, whose great desire for self-improvement and progress gives as a result the finding of new knowledge. The knowledge that they generously share serves as an example and guide for many people.

Dr Arturo Vela Hernandez

About the Authors

Dr Susana Palma Moya is an Orthodontist running a private practice in Ciudad Real, Spain. She obtained her postgraduate degree in Orthodontics and PhD in Dentofacial Orthopaedic and Orthodontics from the University of Madrid in 2002.

- Was among the first group of Spanish Invisalign Providers in 2001.
- International Invisalign Speaker since 2015.
- Assistant professor for the postgraduate's program in orthodontics at U.C.M University in Madrid from 2003 to 2007, and currently teaching orthodontics at Salamanca University.
- University degree in Orthodontics with Surfery from the International University of Cataluña UIC 2007
- University degree in lingual Orthodontics by Valencia University 2009- 2011
- Invisalign peer award 2015 (first International Award) and Invisalign peer award 2017 (second European Award).
- Member of the EMEA teen global group and member of Ortodoncis group in Spain
- Invisalign Diamond II practitioner since 2015 and lectured in Invisalign treatment throughout Spain and Europe.

Dr Javier Lozano Zafra is an Orthodontist running a private practice in Murcia, Spain. Degree in Dentistry, Murcia University

- PhD, Murcia University
- Postgraduate programme in Orthodontics, San Pablo CEU University
- Honorary lecturer, Seville University, Spain
- Invisalign International Speaker
- Invisalign Diamond Practitioner
- Honorary Member of the French Society of Aligners
- Member of the Invisalign TEEN global group and member of Ortodoncis group in Spain

Acknowledgements

My thanks must go first to my husband Paco who has worked just as much as I on the preparation of this book. He has worked tirelessly in gathering together the evidence from videos and other photographic material required. I also want to thank him for his love and understanding which have given me the inspiration and strength to write it.

To my children Marta and Paco for the time I have stolen from them and the continuous inspiration and strength they provide to enable me to get the best from myself: thank you.

To my parents, Mercedes and Paco, whose love and effort encouraged me to become an orthodontist and who have been pillars of strength throughout my life.

To Align Technology for believing in me and giving me the opportunity to share my orthodontic experience with other practitioners from 2015 onwards.

I also want to thank all my orthodontics team, because without them we could not get the results we see today, which we are able to demonstrate in the book.

I want to thank my good friend and partner, Dr Javier Lozano Zafra, not only because it has been a pleasure sharing our time working on making the book (and ultimately helping many students master the aligner technique in Aligners Academy), but also because his friendship has led to a tipping point in my life.

And finally, my thanks go to the entire Wiley team for their help in producing this book.

Dr Susana Palma Moya

To Susana and Paco,
You both take me to the 'next level' every day, inspire my work and my life.
I do not know where I will be in 10 or 20 years' time but, of this I am sure, our friendship will remain one of the most important pillars of life to me.

Thanks for trusting me, for taking care of me, for having me as a friend: I hope life brings you as much happiness as I think you deserve.

To Dani,
Your smile is the most important thing to me.

Dr Javier Lozano Zafra

About the Companion Website

This book is accompanied by a companion website:

Companion website: www.wiley.com/go/lozano-zafra/aligner-techniques

The website includes:

- ClinCheck videos of every treatment in the book. Watch them simultaneously to every chapter, in order to fully understand biomechanics and staging used in every treatment.
- Patient Cases

1

History, Present and Future of Aligners

1.1 History of Clear Aligners

1.1.1 Early Beginning

Recent advances in technology have allowed many inventions that were previously only thought of to become a reality. Such is the case with clear aligners whose history began at the start of the 20th century.

These early retainers were developed by Hawley and others and made from Vulcanite and gold.

Rubber was first used in 1924, when Orrin Remensnyder developed the 'Flex-o-Tite',[1] a device that was meant to stimulate gums through home use combined with toothpaste, and was therefore convenient for periodontally compromised patients.

1 Remensnyder, O. A gum-massaging appliance in the treatment of pyorrhea. *Dent Cosmos*. 1926; **48**: 381–384.

Aligner Techniques in Orthodontics, First Edition. Susana Palma Moya and Javier Lozano Zafra.

Companion website: www.wiley.com/go/lozano-zafra/aligner-techniques

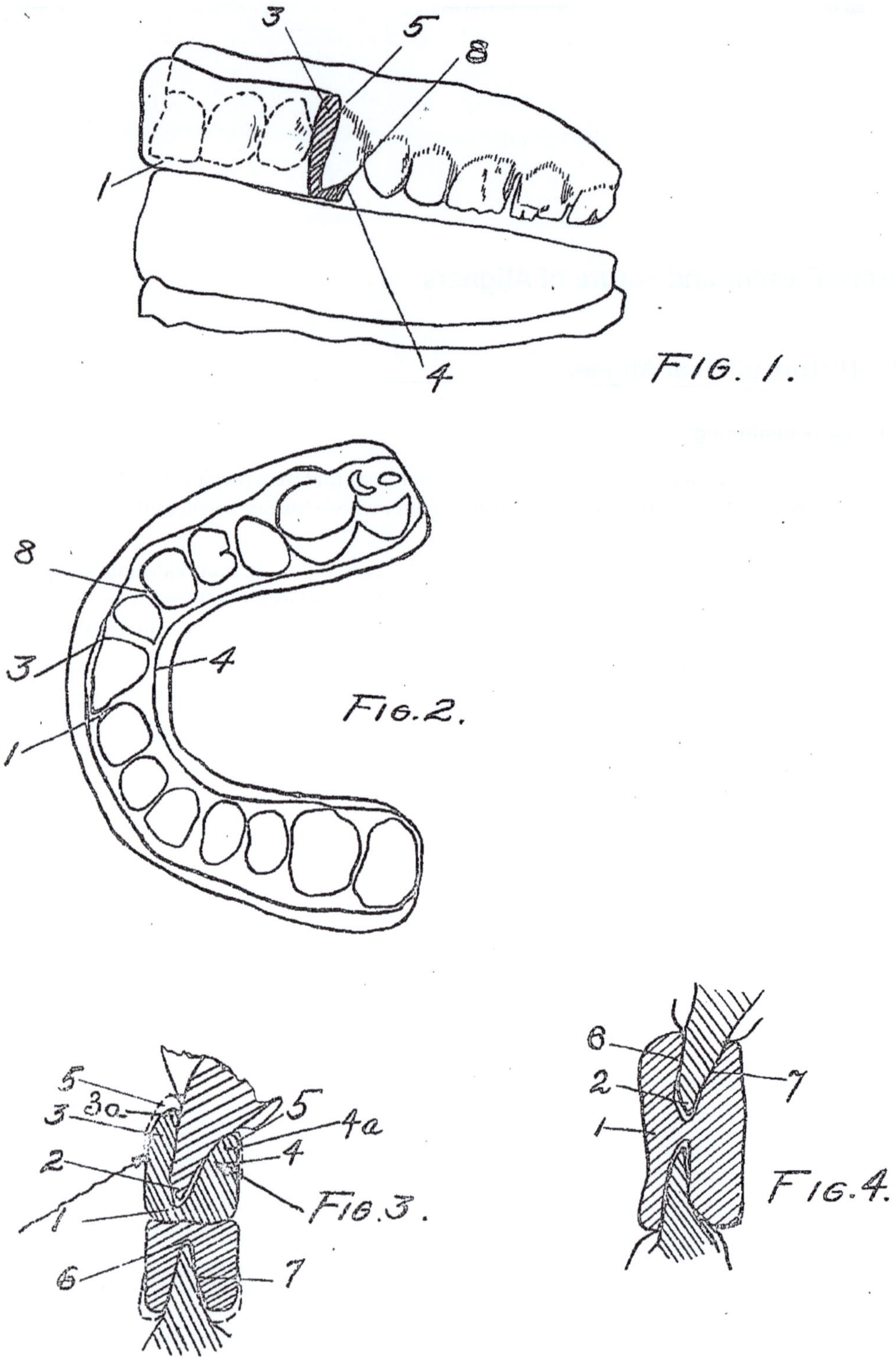

Fig. 1.1 Remensnyder patent file.

On approval of the patent, Remensnyder described that the device might cause small teeth movements, using the expression 'orthodontic appliance' to describe it on his second patent for the device.[2]

Twenty years later, in 1946, Harold Kesling was responsible for developing what he called the 'Tooth Positioner', a device made from Vulcanite meant to prevent relapse after orthodontic treatment.

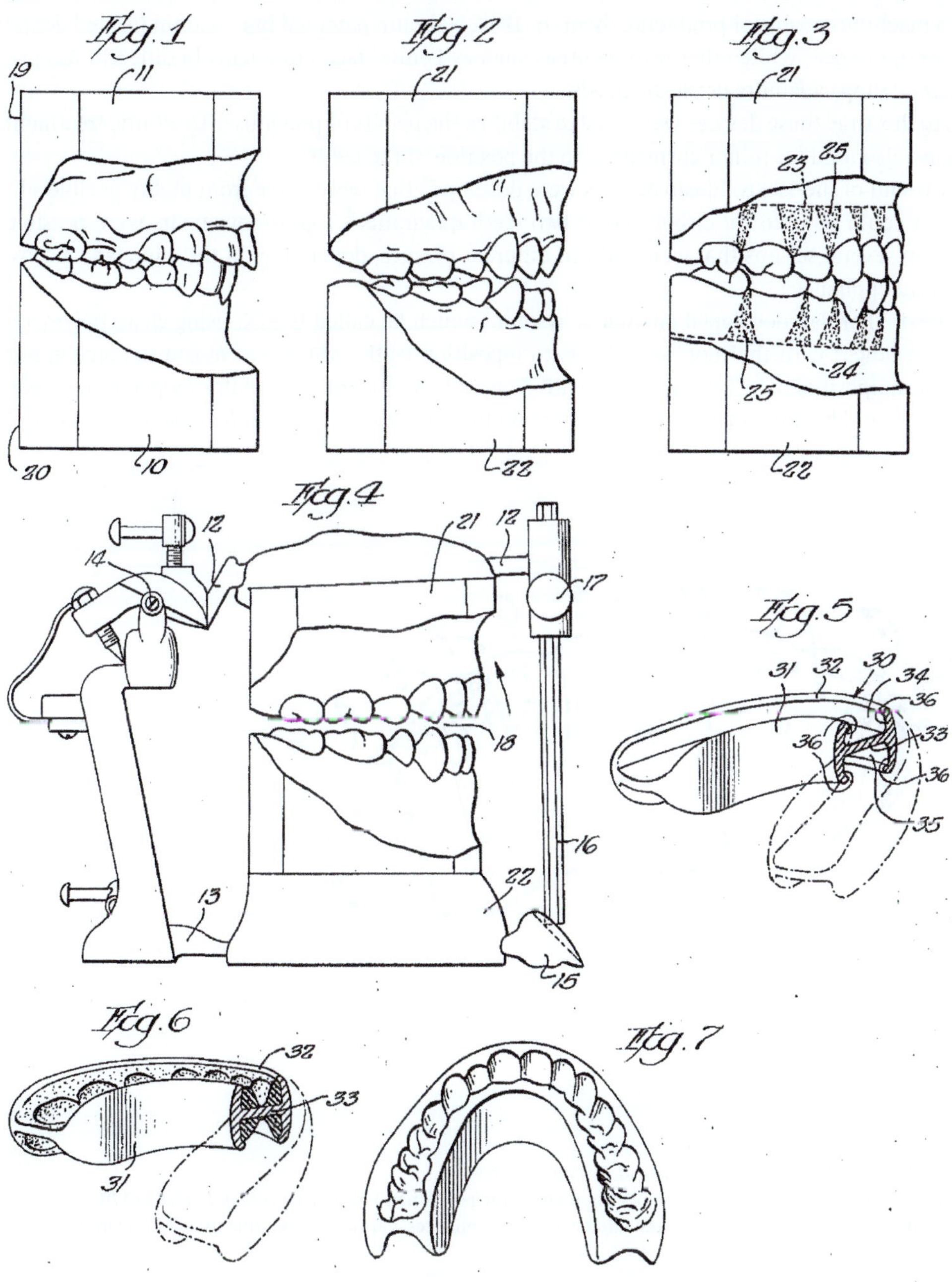

Fig. 1.2 Kesling patent file.

2 Remonsnyder, O. United States Patent 2,479,780, Orthodontic Appliance, Aug. 23, 1949.

This, alongside variations from other orthodontists, was considered a gold standard for several years, in which black vulcanite was the preferred option.

By using the tooth positioner, Kesling suggested 'major tooth movements could be accomplished with a series of positioners by changing the teeth on the setup slightly as treatment progresses. At present this type of treatment does not seem to be practical. It remains a possibility, however, and the technique for its practical application might be developed in the future'.

In 1963, Shanks developed a technique for producing mouth guard style transparent retainers, with a machine capable of producing them. In 1964, Nahoum patented his 'vacuum formed dental contour appliance', while other orthodontists such as Ponitz[3] faced problems in different designs such as heating capability or plastic needs.

Up to this time these devices were used to stabilize the results of previous orthodontic treatment but were also used for minor corrections to the position of the teeth.

At the end of the 1980s, Elasto devices were developed that were made from highly flexible silicon that could be used for either one or two teeth quadrants.[4] Tooth movements were possible thanks to several set-ups that were built in different plastics, depending on the clinician's needs, after fixed appliances.

In 1994, Sheridan developed an aligner system,[5] which he called ESSIX, using clear, polymeric shell appliances with thermoplastic divots to reposition teeth, which was meant to solve minor anterior malpositions. In 1997, together with Schwartz, they standardized this by patenting a system that would be implemented in many dental offices until now, an 'in-office' vacuum system.

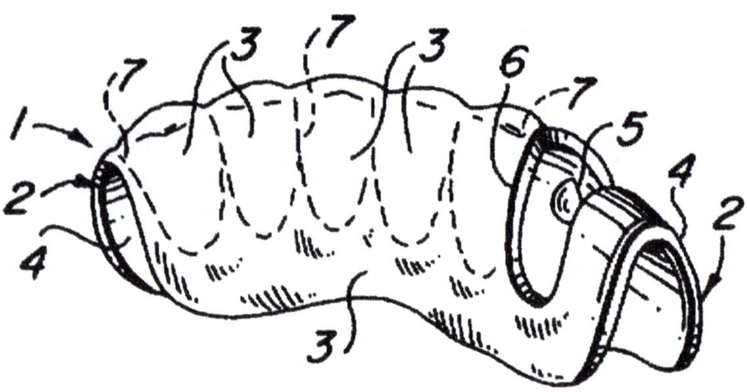

Fig. 1.3 Schwartz and Sheridan patent file.

3 Ponitz, R. Invisible retainers. *Am J Orthod.* 1971 59(3): 266–272.
4 Hinz R. Elasto-orthodontic system – a development of the positioner. *Prakt Kieferorthop.* 1991;5(3):179–88.
5 Sheridan JJ, McMinn R, LeDoux W. Essix thermosealed appliances: various orthodontic uses. *J Clin Orthod.* 1995;**29**(2):108–13.

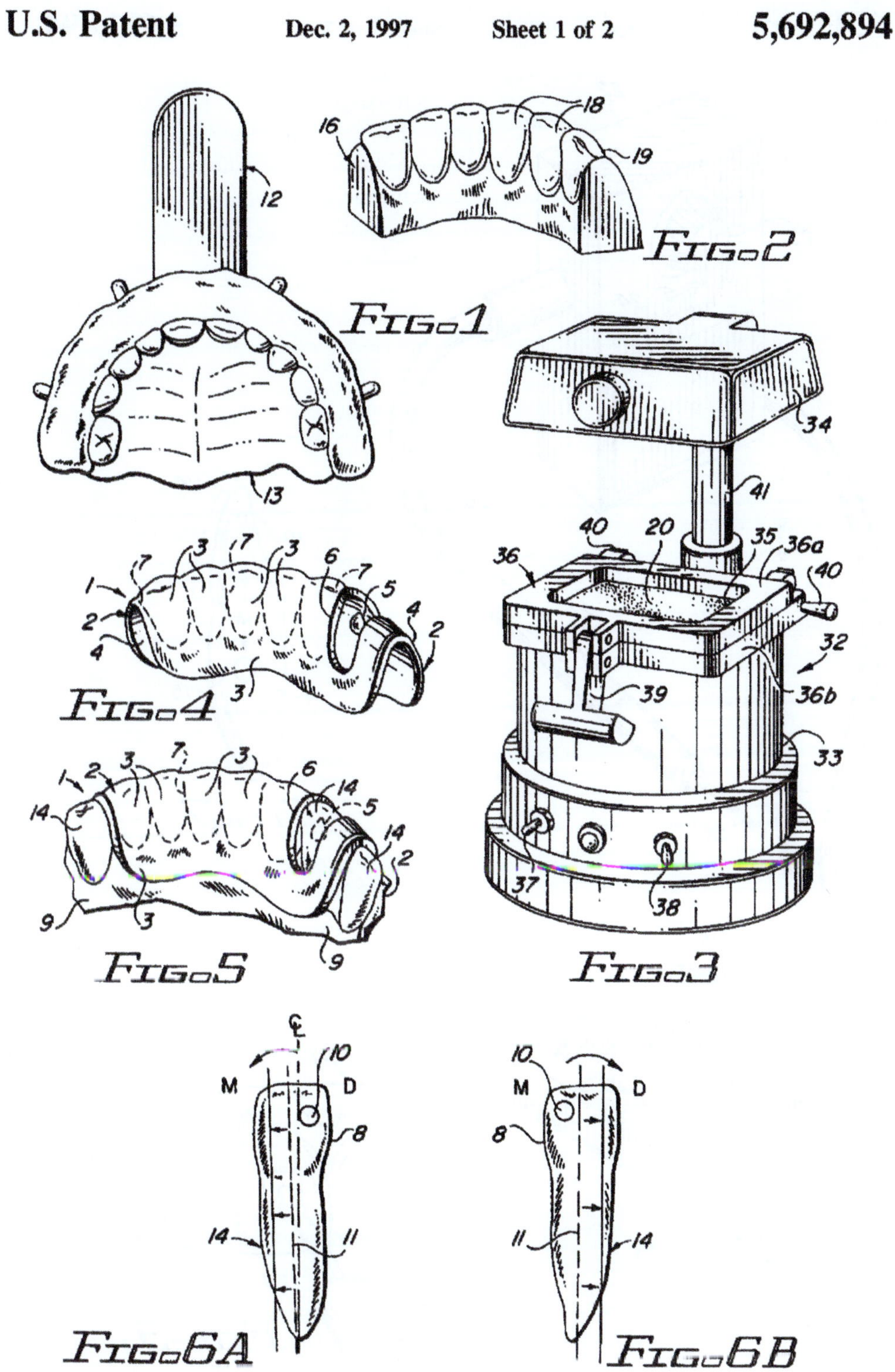

Fig. 1.3 (Cont'd)

(Continued)

U.S. Patent Dec. 2, 1997 Sheet 2 of 2 **5,692,894**

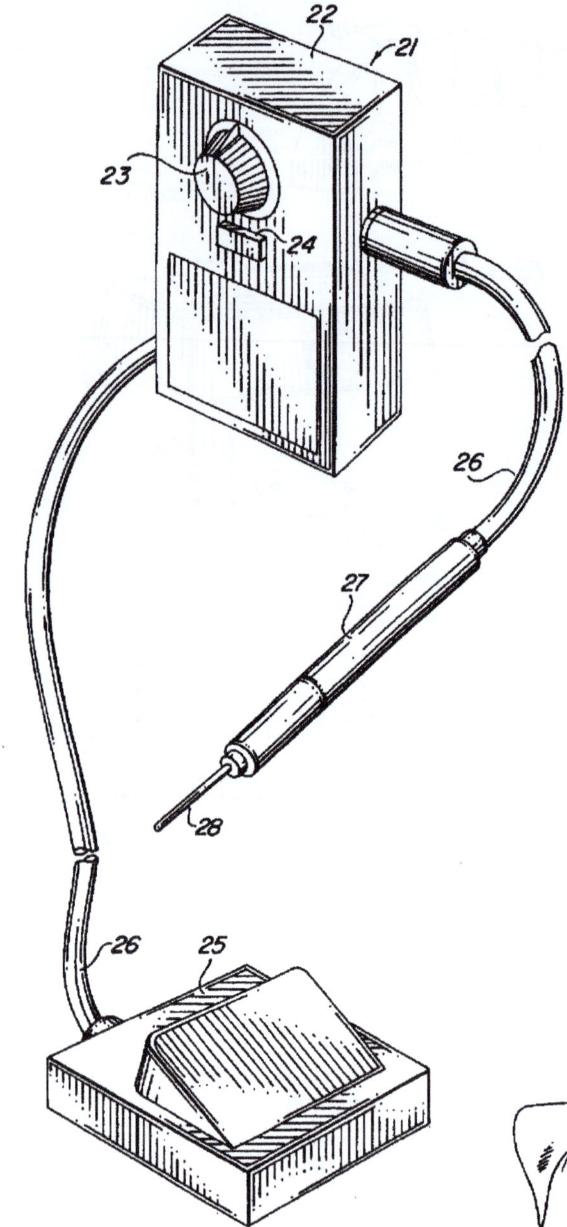

FIG. 8

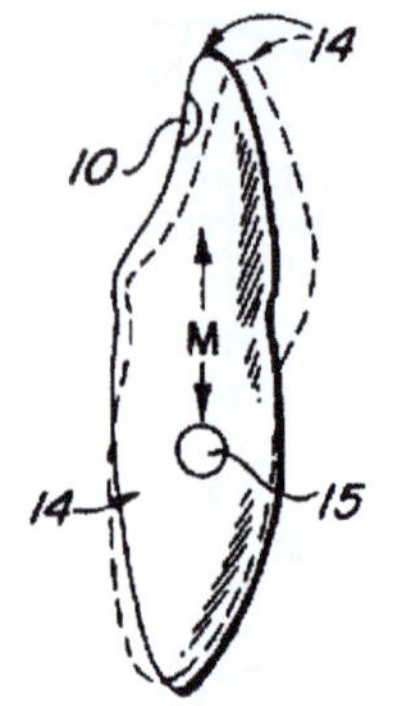

FIG. 7

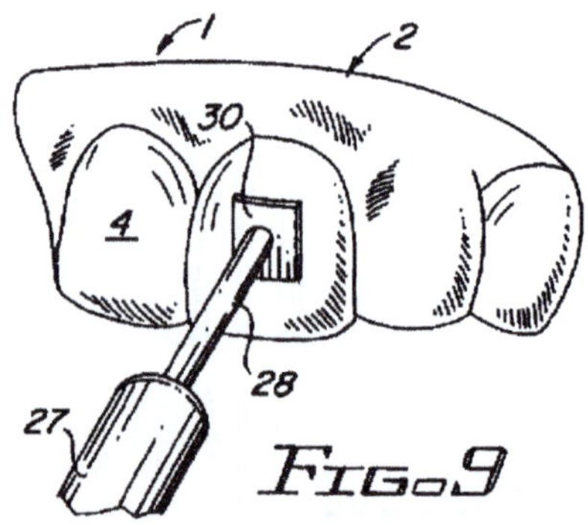

FIG. 9

Fig. 1.3 (Cont'd)

1.2 Origins of Align Technology

At the end of the 1990s a computerized aligner system was developed in the USA with promising features: namely, Invisalign, created by two Stanford students, Zia Chishti and Kelsey Wirth.

Zia Chishti was an orthodontic patient who found out that his own clear retainer might be applicable to the whole orthodontic treatment, as it might be able also to move teeth and avoid metal braces. This reasoning led to why they both started the Company, partnered with some other students in their campus, Apostolos Lerios and Brian Freyburger, who were responsible for the Computer Aid Design part of this start-up.

They then developed a software to design incremental stages of retainers to straighten teeth in a campus laboratory. In 1998, they got Food and Drug Administration (FDA) approval, and were then able to sell their product to the orthodontic community, which was resistant to this radical change, mostly owing to the lack of orthodontic experience of its founders.

In 2000, they raised $140M from venture capital companies and this allowed them to start a $31 million TV campaign that same year. In 2001, the Company went public, raising an additional $128M on NASDAQ.[6]

During this time, consumers drove more than 70% of the American Orthodontists to be trained in the system.[7] That same year, Align Technology made Invisalign available to general dental practitioners, arguing that offering it only to orthodontists would be considered unfair competition by dentists.

Fig. 1.4 Align Technology logo.

By then, Align Technology was spending most of its revenues on advertising, and losing about $18 million per year,[8] which led cofounders Wirth and Chishti to resign from Align Technology before 2003.

Fig. 1.5 Align Technology annual revenue.

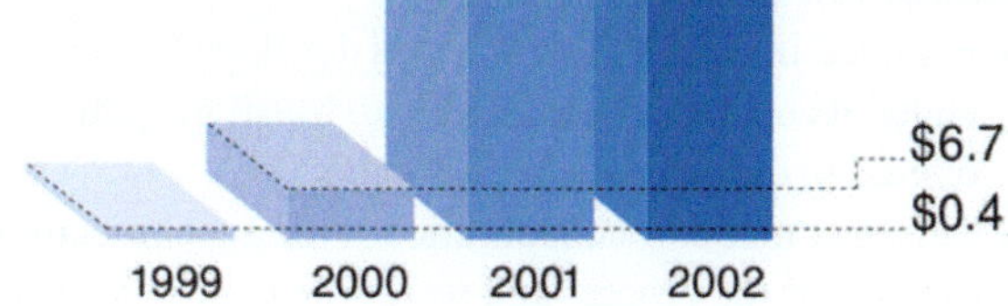

6 Feder, BJ. 'Orthodontics Via Silicon Valley; A Start-Up Uses Computer Modeling and Venture Capital to Reach Patients'. The New York Times, 18 August 2000: p. 1.

7 Bush, J. 'Stealth Braces'. YT Regional Newspapers (August 14, 2001). Retrieved January 9, 2013.

8 Lau, G. 'It has a bracing impact on patients; Align Technology' May 3, 2004.

After a cut in advertising to one-third of the original, the company grew from 80,000 patients treated in 2002 to 175,000 in 2004, while receiving awards for its stereolithography techniques, medical design and fast growth. In addition, the company finally achieved a profit for the first time in 2003.

In 2004, the FDA cleared expanded labelling for Invisalign and removed the permanent dentition requirement, making possible the launching of Invisalign TEEN and widening clinical applicability to include more complex cases and increase the age band for treatment.

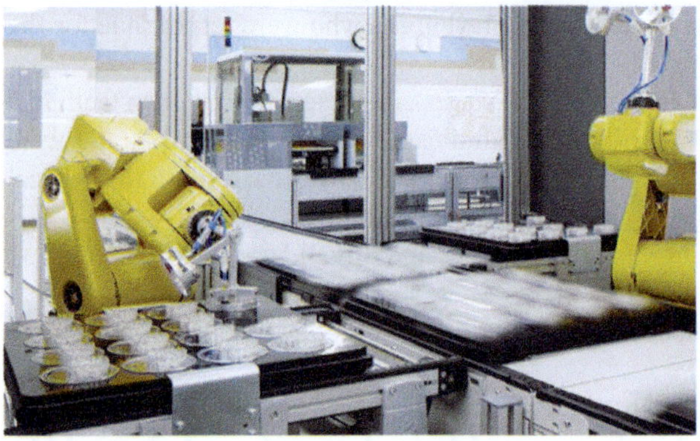

Fig. 1.6 Align Technology stereolithographic has been heavily awarded.

In 2005, the Harvard School of Dental Medicine required for the first time that its orthodontic graduate students complete Invisalign certification before they graduated.[9]

1.3 Early Clear Aligner Manufacturers

Although most patented innovations have been developed by Align Technology, other companies have been working on new functionalities since the beginning of the century.

Orthoclear

- Founded in 2005 by Zia Chishti, one of the Invisalign system founders, based in Pakistan, ended its operations in 2006 after a corporate agreement with Align Technology that followed litigations related to trademark.

ClearCorrect

- Founded in 2006 in Texas, it was developed by one of the practitioners using Orthoclear, after it ended its operations, to be able to finish his patient treatments not using the Invisalign system, offered to old Orthoclear customers.
- This was made in collaboration with a technician working with plaster models. In 2008, they digitalized the process and were able to produce larger series of aligners, which they sent to the orthodontists together with the plastic models made for every movement.
- The Company was acquired in 2008 by Straumann group, together with some other companies with previous experience in the field to build an aligner system driven by this international holding.

9 Antelman G. *International Directory of Company Histories.* St James Press. 2008; **94**: pp. 15–18.

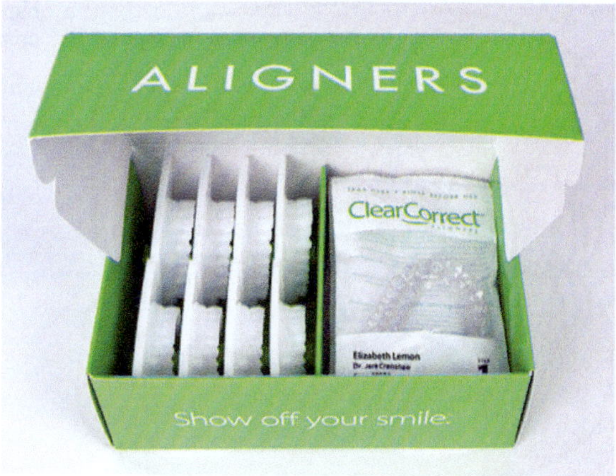

Fig. 1.7 Models and aligners by ClearCorrect.

Orthocaps

- Founded in 2006 in Germany by Khan, this system has a 'method of combining two different soft aligners for day and night time use'. These two types differ from one another in both their composition and the amount of pressure they exert. This innovation is called the TwinAligner system.

Inman aligner

- Developed by a dental technician, Donal P. Inman in 2000 in Florida, it was initially for minor alignments and finally widely used by general practitioners for veneer preparation in a simple and more affordable way than other aligner brands.

1.4 Align Technology Development

Align Technology claims an investment over $1000M, which has made them a leader in the clear aligner market over the last 20 years, with more than 900 patents currently issued at the time of writing.

This progress has been possible thanks to an increasing clinical and engineering team that has been involved with many innovations over the years, such as:

- Invisalign 1.5: this included initial SmartForces and attachments, which are attachments combined with three dimensional (3D) activations on the aligner material (by then, EX30) that help creating counterforces to achieve desired movement.
- Invisalign G3: this included passive aligners on the arch with less movement to allow class II and III elastics on patients with A-P correction needed, as well as laser cut precision cuts or hooks.
- Invisalign G4: Optimized attachments for root control movements, open bite, and pressure points on aligners on teeth with small clinical crowns that could not accommodate double attachments.

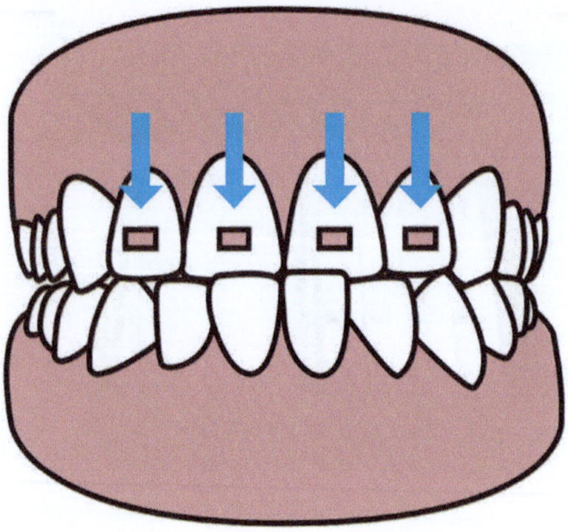

Fig. 1.8 Optimized attachments for anterior open bite.

- SmartTrack: Align Technology's proprietary material for aligners, launched for its increased fitting and elasticity.
- Invisalign G5: mostly for vertical malocclusions treatment, including specific protocols for Spee curve intrusion, passive attachments or precision ramps to help disoccluding posterior sectors.

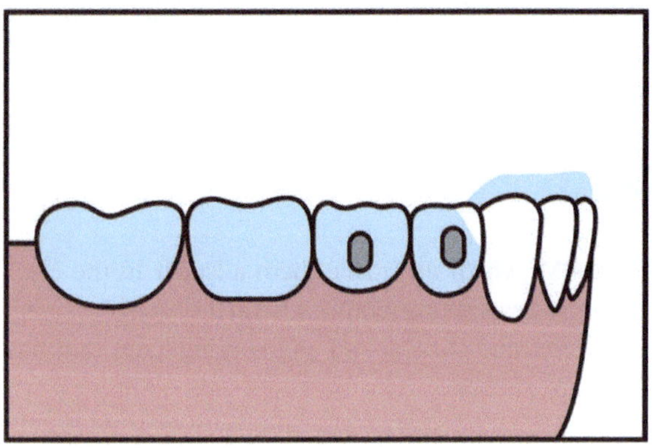

Fig. 1.9 Passive attachments for anterior intrusion.

- Invisalign G6: specific movement protocol for premolars extraction as well as exclusive attachments group designed to fulfil the best outcome in these cases.
- Invisalign G7: designed for improved finishing with functionalities such as specific lateral incisors attachments.
- One week wear: an aspect that helped to reduce the treatment length resulting from changing the aligners every 7 days instead of 14, as had previously been the case (after an internal clinical study).
- Mandibular advancement: this is one of the features that has further increased the range of cases treated, as it includes not just orthodontic treatments, but functional ones, substituting classical twin blocks or mandibular advancements for power wings.

These, together with further functionalities covered in this book can help the orthodontist to achieve the same results as with braces, and combined with auxiliary techniques such as TADs, intermaxillary elastics, buttons, surgery: any malocclusion can now be solved with aligners.

1.5 Current Situation and Future of Aligners

Since the beginning of the twentieth century there have been vast improvements in the field of orthodontics. These range from edgewise appliances to the latest straightwise ones and self-ligating braces.

If we were to search 'orthodontics' in PubMed, we would now find more than 70,000 entries, indicating that the profession is becoming more and more relevant for a global population that is demanding both health and aesthetics in their smile.

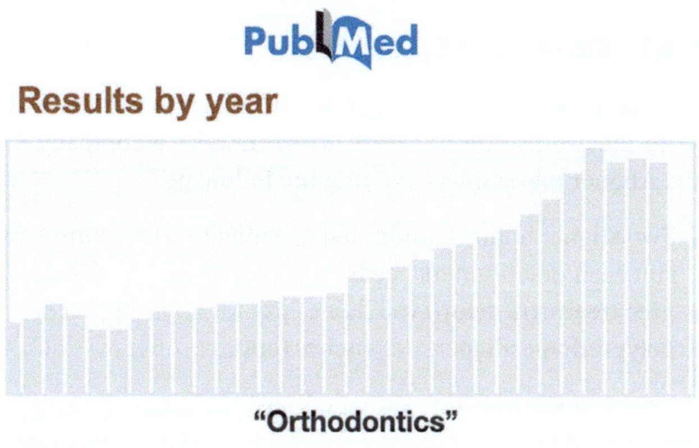

Fig. 1.10 Results in PubMed for 'orthodontics'.

As seen in the history of clear aligners, it is clear that the number of papers published on aligners is much lower than in the entire field of orthodontics, likely because of its relatively newness, with developments only coming in the last 5–10 years. The requirements for publishing a paper in a peer-reviewed journal can make it very difficult to fully appreciate their growth in the orthodontic community.

That being said, what we can see is that the popularity of aligners has been powered by Align Technology over the last 20 years, given that the majority of papers published have referred directly to the 'Invisalign' technique, and it has only been relatively recently that other brands have attempted to enter the market.

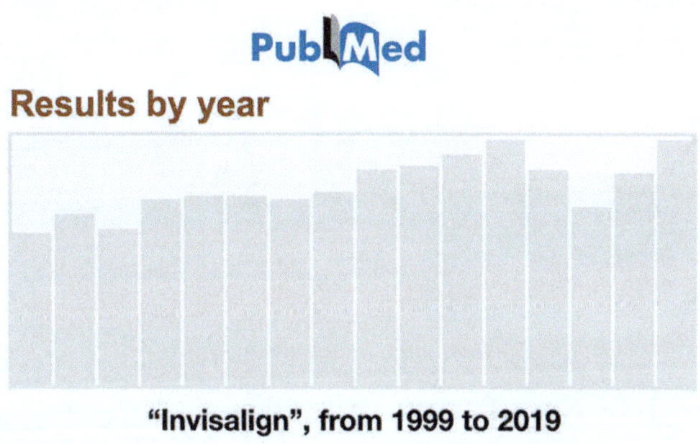

Fig. 1.11 Results in PubMed for 'Invisalign' from 1999 to 2019.

It is for this reason that the patients have been treated entirely using aligners produced by Align Technology; however, the biomechanical approach can be extended to any brand that, in the future, is able to develop a reliable product to treat any malocclusion using aligners and auxiliary techniques.

We constantly aim to analyse, study and understand what is happening within the field of orthodontics and strive to be on the edge of innovation, always one step ahead in order to provide our patients with the best solution for the situation that they face. We have focused on the most promising aligner brands available at this moment but we are aware that with technological advances everything may change very quickly.

1.6 Promising Aligner Initiatives

1.6.1 ClearCorrect by Straumann

Straumann is one of the larger dental companies in the world, and is known for dental implants. With the acquisition of ClearCorrect in 2019, a company founded in Texas in 2006, they entered the Aligner marketplace offering the following:

- Two aligner options: unlimited or individual (including just a single aligner), a flexible option to suit each practitioners needs.
- Free treatment setup (you do not pay for anything except the aligners).
- Polyurethane aligners, 0.3 inches (approx. 7.5 mm) thick, a very common material.

Unscalloped trim line extended past the gingival margin, intended to increase retention over scalloped aligners, therefore reducing the need for attachments and improving aesthetics.

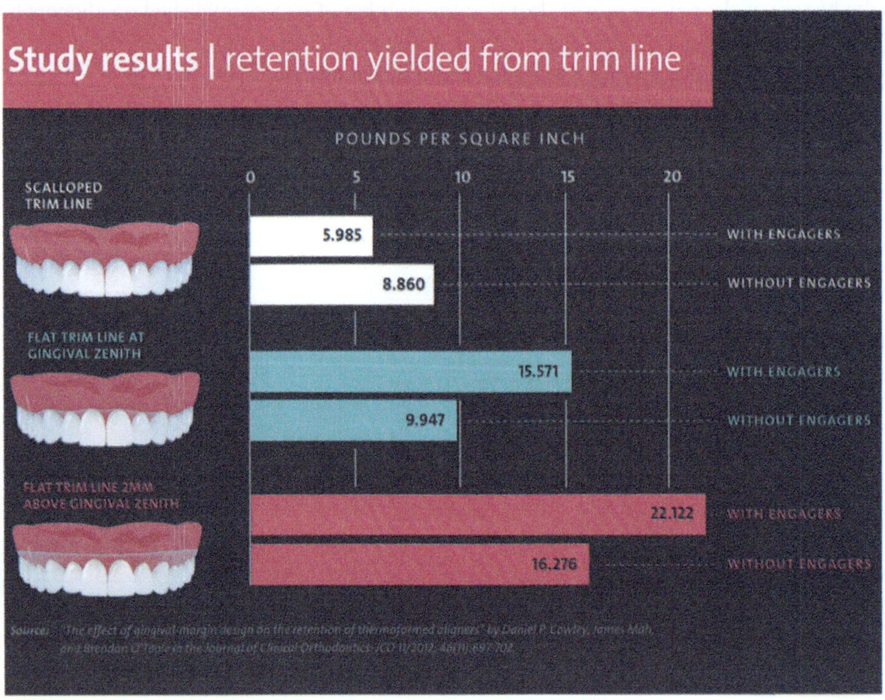

Fig. 1.12 ClearCorrect aligner retention chart. From: Cowley DP, Mah J, O'Toole B. The effect of gingival-margin design on the retention of thermoformed aligners. *J Clin Orthod* 2012; **46**(11): 697–702.

None of these aspects have been followed through a clinical study or published in a journal, so although this seems promising, we will have to wait to see how the system develops in the future.

1.6.2 SureSmile by Dentsply

Dentsply is the largest dental company in the world, with an extensive portfolio of dental products. Although initially focused on restorative dentistry they have recently incorporated dental implants and clear aligners. The acquisition of SureSmile from Orametrix in 2018 allowed them to enter the aligner market with a system displaying the following characteristics.

- The only aligner system linking cone beam computed tomography (CBCT) with cephalometric X-ray and virtual simulation of movement.
- Hybrid treatment, being able to mix braces and aligners.
- In-practice produced aligners, where the practitioner is sent the files to print three-dimensional models that are used to vacuum-form aligners with Essix plastics.

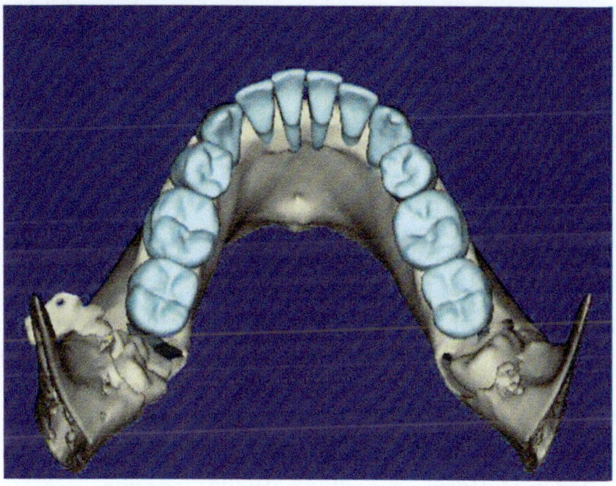

Fig. 1.13 SureSmile aligner software combined with CBCT.

1.6.3 F22 by Sweden and Martina

Sweden and Martina is a dental implant company from Italy that developed an aligner system alongside Prof. Siciliani from the University of Ferrara. The system has the following characteristics:

- Mentoring from a member of the University of Ferrara throughout the duration of the treatment.
- Chromatic stability, owing to less pigment retention from the plastic material used for the aligners, and proven through clinical study by the university.
- Optimal fitting, leaving a space smaller than 40 μm between the aligner and the teeth.
- 20% lighter force transmission than other aligner materials, according to one study by the university.
- Increased comfort, as a result of the university's trimming protocol.
- Increased retention, as a result of a design based on a paper published by Cowley[10] suggesting higher values of retention are obtained when aligners are cut regularly and straight at the level of the gingival margin zenith.

10 Cowley, DP. Effect of Gingival Margin Design on Retention of Thermoformed Orthodontic Aligners (2012). UNLV Theses, Dissertations, Professional Papers, and Capstones. 1662. https://digitalscholarship.unlv.edu/thesesdissertations/1662.

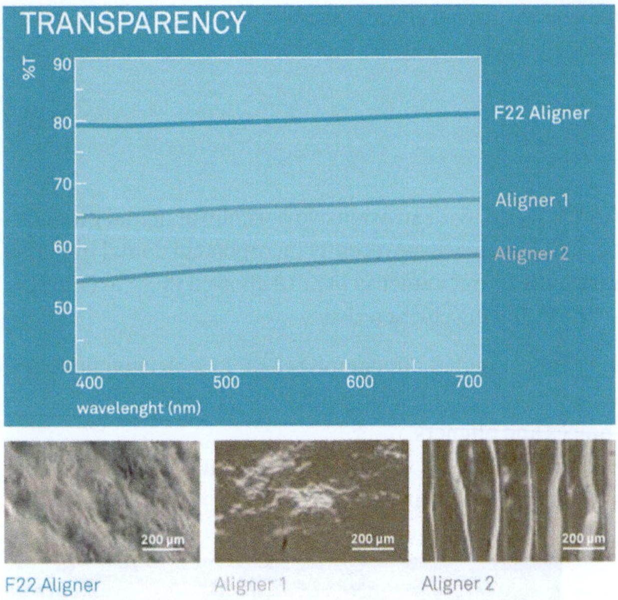

Fig. 1.14 F22 chromatic stability. From Lombardo *et al.* Optical properties of orthodontic aligners—spectrophotometry analysis of three types before and after aging. *Prog Orthod* 2015;16:41.

1.6.4 Clarity by 3M

The MBT prescription, developed by McLaughlin, Bennett and Trevisi, was successfully marketed by 3M, based in Germany, having developed many innovations in the orthodontic field and including the proprietary Incognito lingual braces system.

In 2018, they launched their Clarity aligners, with the same name they gave to their aesthetic braces system, claiming:

- Advanced analytics and software planning tools.
- Open platform accessible with any scanner.
- 3M Treatment Tracking patient App.
- Accessibility from PC and MAC.

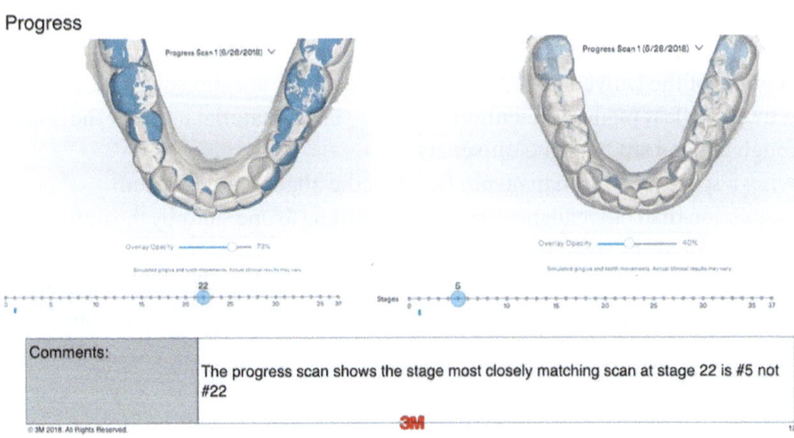

Fig. 1.15 3M superimposition for treatment evolution.

- From November 2019, the only information published in regard to this were two clinical cases published on their website, both for aligning anterior teeth, but with no A/P correction or vertical component in the treatment.

1.6.5 Spark, by Ormco

Ormco is one of the leading brackets and wires manufacturers in the world, which started offering its own aligners brand in 2019, claiming the following (data on file from the Company that we cannot access at this time):

1) TruGEN plastic aligner is clearer than the leading aligner (AKA Invisalign).
2) TruGEN plastic aligner produces higher sustained force retention in order to reach treatment goals faster than the leading aligner (AKA Invisalign).
3) Hand trimmed aligners, with scalloped edges that are meant to be more comfortable for the patient.

Apart from this, their product portfolio is similar to the one developed by Align Technology, with 3 treatment options (10, 20 or unlimited aligners), based on a 7 day wearing period of the aligners. They have as an advantage, the ability to perform single arch treatments using the unlimited aligners product, which is not available for Invisalign aligners.

In regards to their proprietary software, it has different functionalities than ClinCheck software, the most significant being the simulation of roots. None of this has been through a clinical study

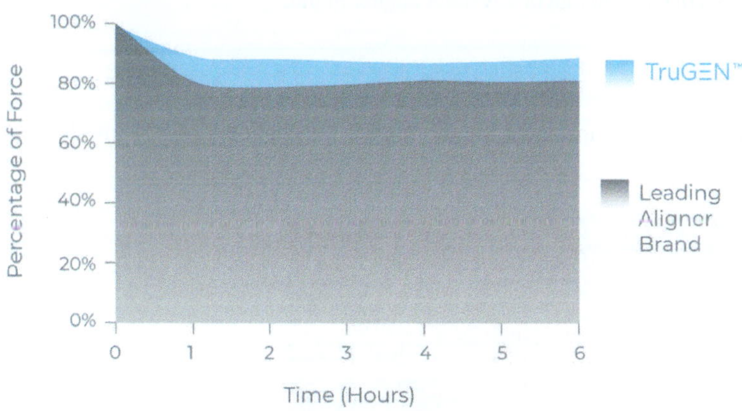

Fig. 1.16 Ormco results for their TruGEN plastic against SmartTrack (data on file).

or published in any journal so, even though these aspects are promising, we will have to wait to see how it develops in the future.

1.6.6 CA Clear Aligner by Scheu

This German aligner system enables clinicians to fully take control of aligner production, provided that there is a dental technician in the team responsible for developing models and manufacturing in-office vacuum aligners that offer several advantages:

- Integration of auxiliaries, such as expansion screws or distalizers
- Scheu biocompatible material
- Individual fabrication for each treatment step

- Three thicknesses available (0.5, 0.65 and 0.75 mm) to be changed selectively in order to exert certain forces

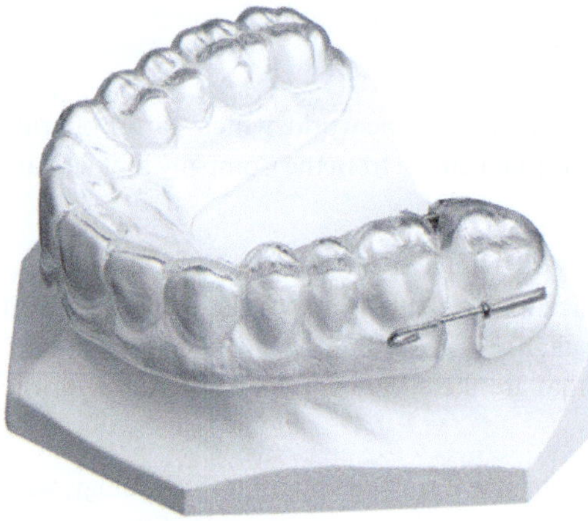

Fig. 1.17 Distalizer inserted in an in-practice aligner.

This is one of the segments that might grow in the near future when 3D printing allows direct aligner printing in the practice, thereby reducing the need for vacuum models, saving both time and money and making it cheaper to produce aligners. This will improve the affordability of the treatments for patients, as this option already provides a fit equal to that of any other aligner brand.[11]

1.6.7 Irok

This US Company is focused on the printing of digital models for aligners design, but also for retainers, indirect braces bonding.

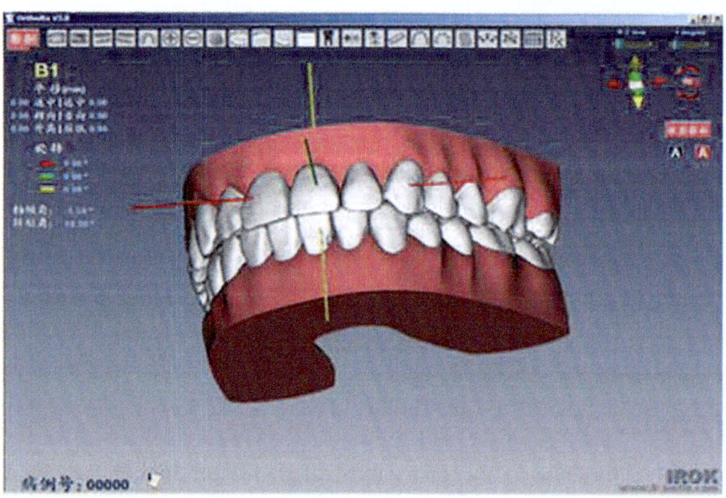

Fig. 1.18 Irok is focused on digital models that can serve different purposes.

---

11 Mantovani E *et al.* Scanning electron microscopy analysis of aligner fitting on anchorage attachments. *J Orofac Orthop*. 2019;**80**(2):79–87.

Its unique characteristic is that it provides the possibility of aligning in combination with dental implant software, based on the implant's final position, and it can be placed with a surgical 3D splint.

1.6.8 Angelalign

Founded in 2001 by Li Haumin in conjunction with Tsinghua University and Beijing Capital, Angelalign is the largest provider of transparent teeth aligners in China.

Since 2006 they have been granted 80 patents relating to processes, aligners, manufacturing and 3D technology and, for these reasons, they can offer a product with several technological advancements and functionalities through their iOrto platform:

- masterMulti, offering the opportunity to use different aligner thickness
- Mandibular advancement device, first launched globally, in 2015
- a7 extraction technology, tested over 15 years

Together with other Asian companies such as Smartee, for whom there is currently little information in Europe, Angelalign will probably become an important stakeholder in aligners development.

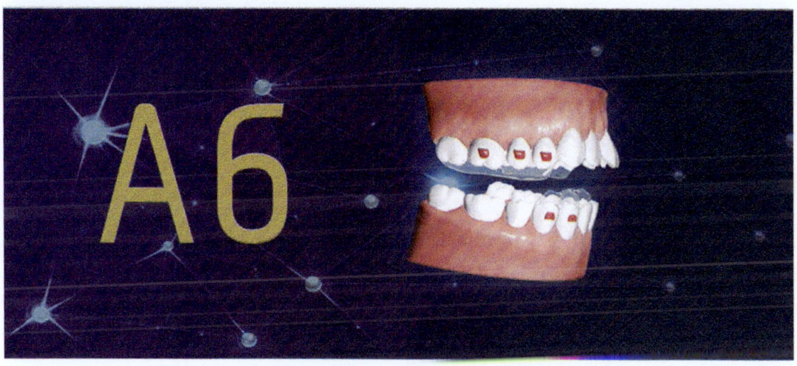

Fig. 1.19 A6 mandibular advancement launched in 2015.

1.6.9 Alineadent

This Spanish aligner Company has its origins in a dental laboratory specializing in orthodontic functional appliances, which led to the development of this aligner brand. Its characteristics are:

- Open system, compatible with any scanner brand
- Immediate validation from a dental technician
- Planning within 72 hours
- Production within 72 hours
- LineDock software for case management

Unfortunately, there is no evidence available with regard to its capability in the management of complex cases, as with some other dental companies manufacturing aligners. Their ability to improve this may rely on their approach to practitioners that may choose to use them in cases of minor tooth movements.

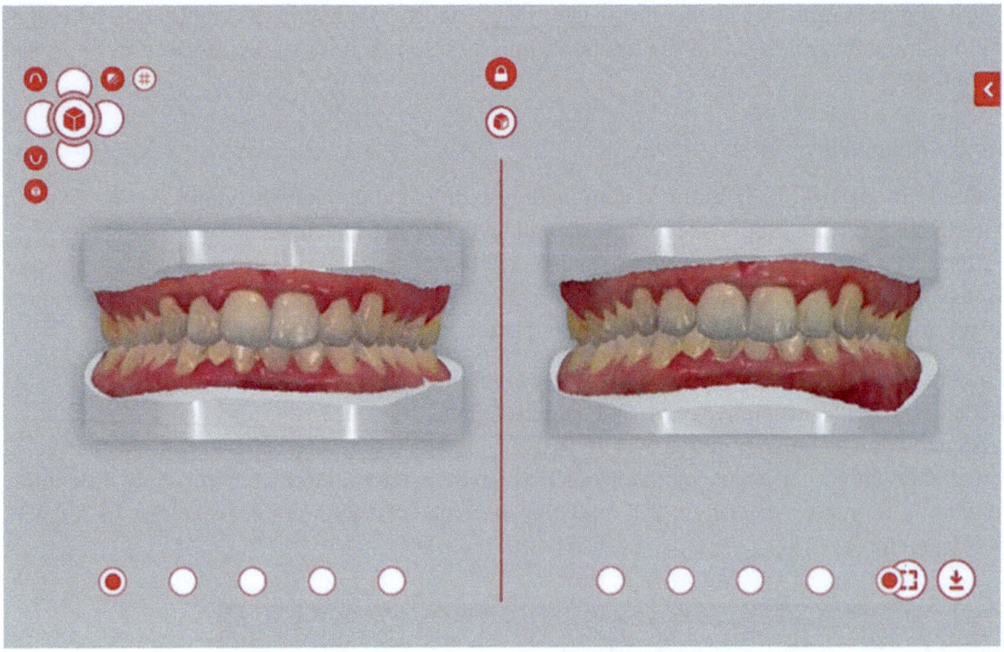

Fig. 1.20 LineDock software.

1.6.10 Remote Aligner Companies

It is important to mention direct to consumer aligners, or remote aligners initiatives, especially as Candid, one of these companies, has raised $78.4M in venture capital funds, and SmileDirectClub already has more than 300 locations in the US, UK and Australia and has treated more than 650,000 patients since its foundation in 2014.

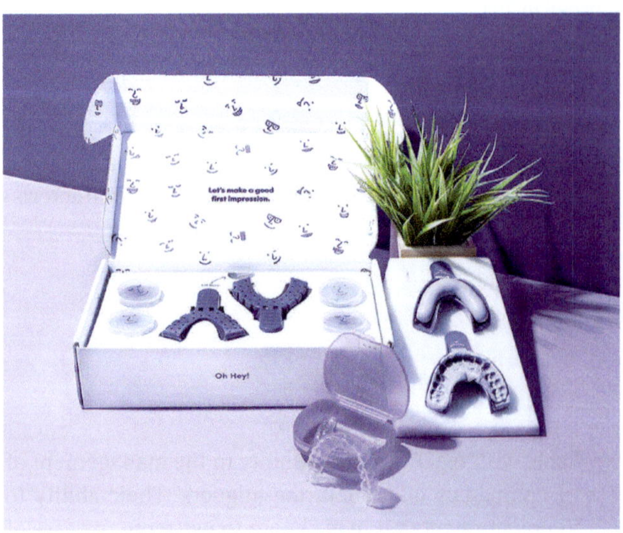

Fig. 1.21 SmileDirectClub self-polyvinyl siloxane (PVS) -impression kit.

They all are based on the following workflow:

- Scanning in a company facility similar to a store or self-taking a polyvinyl siloxane (PVS) impression at home with a kit sent from a remote aligner company, and sending it back to its headquarters
- Validating the case at the company aligners production facility
- Patients receive the aligners

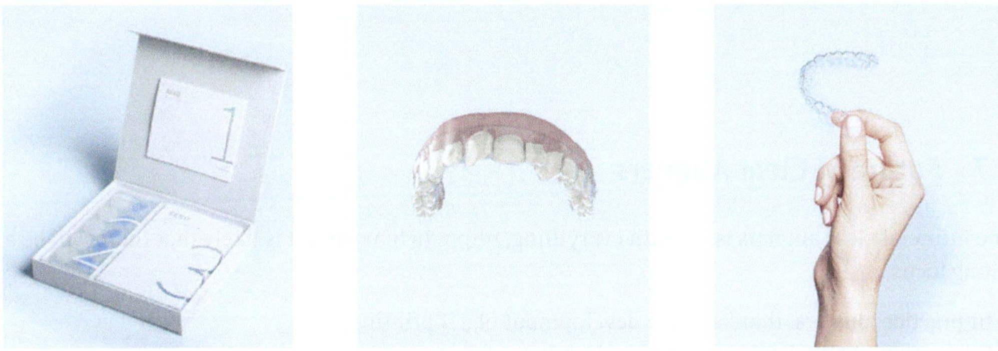

Fig. 1.22 CANDID aligners process.

In an era when people are used to a one-click-buy, particularly through their Smartphone, and when telemedicine is on the rise as a result of the growth of the internet and wearables that are part of our daily routines, this might sound 'good' for patients who want to have a cheaper treatment option, as they are usually three to four times cheaper than an average comprehensive treatment performed by an orthodontist.

There have been several blocks to the success of these companies: for, example SmileDirectClub were forced to pull out of the Spanish market after the Spanish Ministry of Health warned that their system was against Spanish Law, and the American Association of Orthodontists filed complaints with 36 state dental boards and attorney generals alleging specific statutory and regulatory violations.

These systems may lead to health problems in the future for some of their users owing to poor, improper treatment. This may lead to problems that need to be resolved in-house, resulting in a further treatment cost on top of the impact on their health.

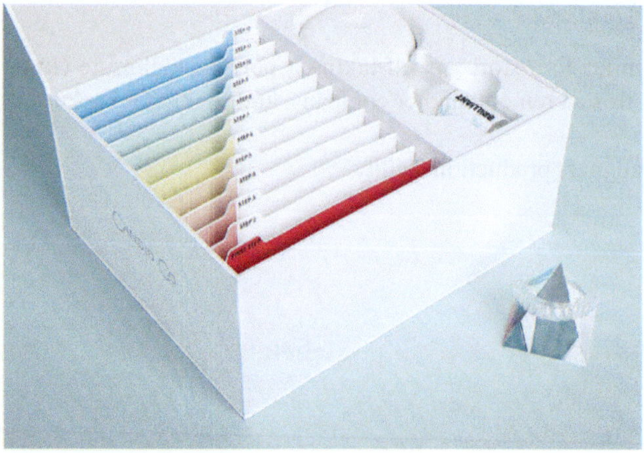

Fig. 1.23 CANDID aligners set.

1.7 Future of Clear Aligners

The future of clear aligners is, as with everything, unpredictable, but it is likely that there will be a strong focus on:

- In-practice aligners, thanks to the development of 3D printing
- Integration of CBCT with treatment planning software
- Increasing number of laboratories and aligners companies
- Price reduction

What is clear is that, thanks to this, before 2030 100% of the orthodontic treatments will be performed with aligners in every practice in the world, as it is currently in ours.

We should aim to ensure that as orthodontists we are ahead of these changes and share our views and clinical experience with the orthodontic community as a whole so we may help to improve the smiles of everyone.

2

Basic Principles with Aligners

Invisalign treatment is an orthodontic technique, not just a product. As such, orthodontic principles of force application, engagement, anchorage and biomechanics need to be applied. However, aligners move teeth differently than fixed appliances do. In order to understand this we need to have a look at how aligners work.

2.1 Forces

Aligners move teeth by exerting a push force. When the aligner is inserted over teeth, the aligner deforms over the teeth and the elasticity in the aligner material pushes the teeth into position.

Optimized attachments provide an active, flat surface that the aligner may push against to provide effective tooth movements.

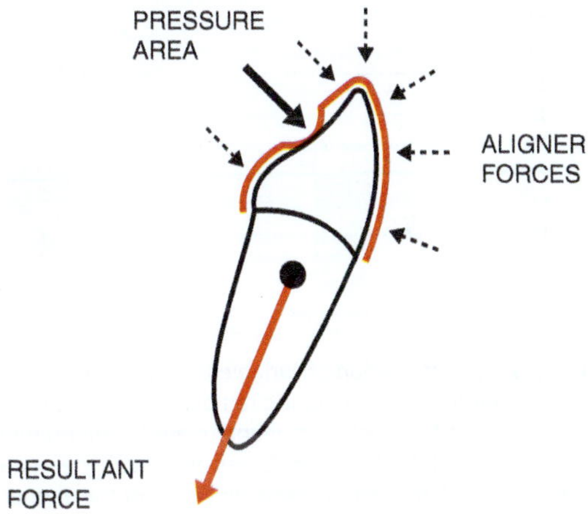

Fig. 2.1 Forces will be delivered through the combination of plastic and attachments.

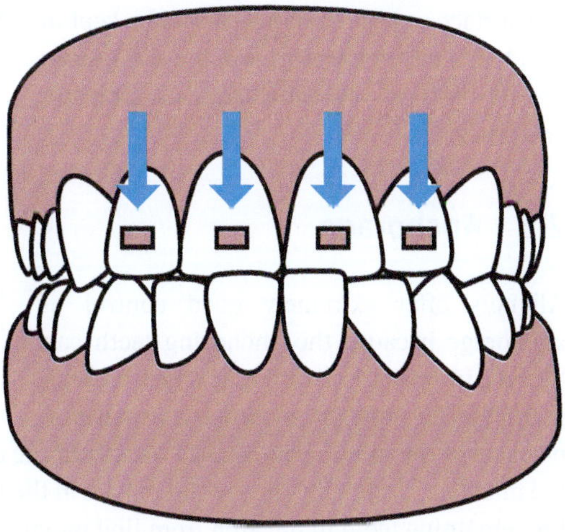

Fig. 2.2 Optimized attachments provide an active, flat surface that the aligner may push against to provide effective tooth movements.

2.2 Engagement

Aligners engage teeth by enclosing the tooth in aligner material. The more material wrapped around a tooth, the better the engagement. In teeth with a long clinical crown and larger surface area, there will be better engagement and therefore better expression of tooth movement. In contrast, in teeth with short clinical crowns and less surface area, there is less engagement and less expression of tooth movement.

Aligner Techniques in Orthodontics, First Edition. Susana Palma Moya and Javier Lozano Zafra.

Companion website: www.wiley.com/go/lozano-zafra/aligner-techniques

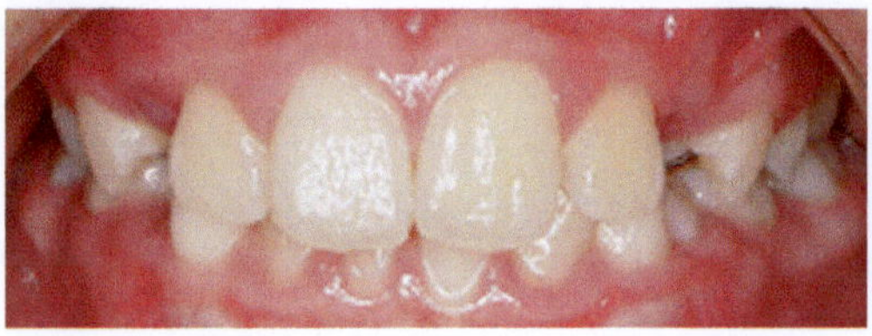

Fig. 2.3 These crowns allow enough contact from plastic to exert desired forces.

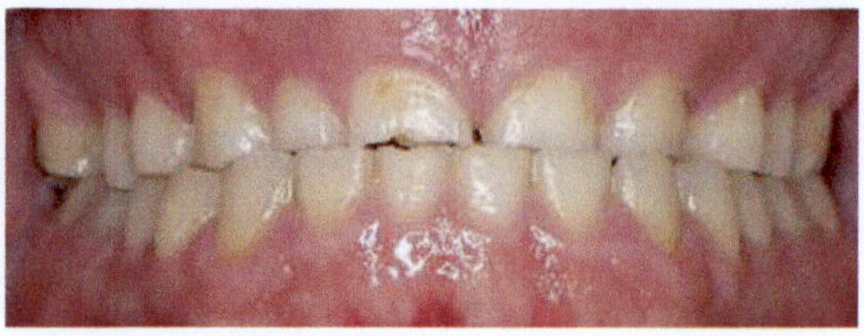

Fig. 2.4 Short clinical crowns might reduce movement predictability.

One way to increase the engagement of the aligner onto teeth with short or small clinical crowns (for example, peg-shape lateral incisors) is to place an attachment on the tooth.

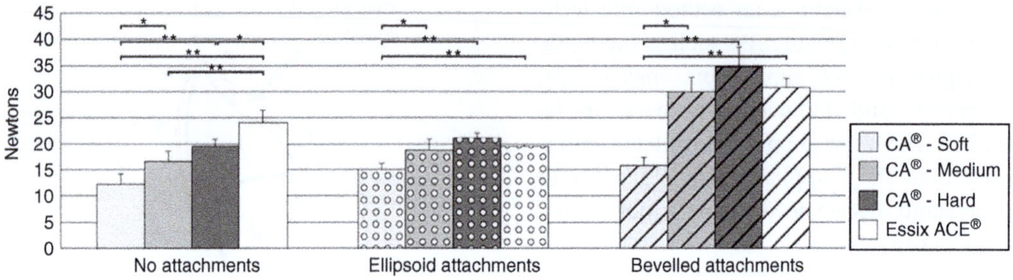

Fig. 2.5 Quantification of variable aligner material on retention. (Left) Vertical displacement forces (Newtons) of each aligner material during removal from the control cast containing no attachments. (Right) Vertical displacement forces of each aligner material during removal from the cast containing ellipsoid attachments. (Right) Vertical displacement forces of each aligner material during removal from the cast containing bevelled attachments. Each column represents one of the aligner materials tested (CA soft, medium, hard; Essix ACE).[1]

This is a different approach from that with braces, which had 'contact points' instead of a full surface contact and this should be kept in mind for a treatment plan to achieve the same results that can be achieved with brackets and wires.

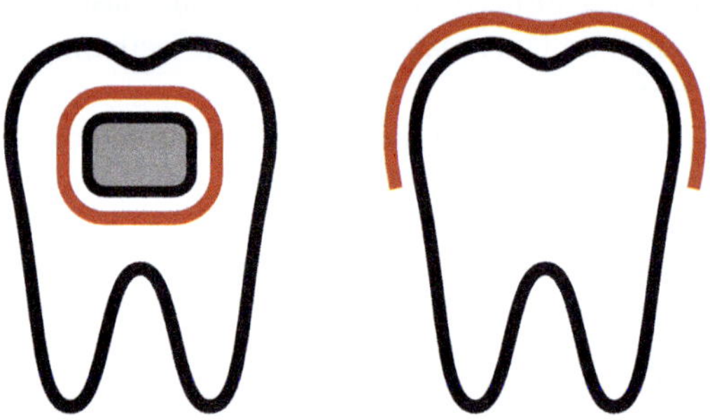

Fig. 2.6 Brackets have a strong small contact point in comparison with a soft big contact surface between aligner and teeth.

2.3 Anchorage

Aligners offer extremely good control of anchorage because the anchoring teeth can become immovable at different stages of treatment. For example, in asymmetric expansion, one side of the mouth can be used to expand the other. Alternatively, in sequential distalization of the maxillary arch, only the second molars in the initial stages of treatment can be distalized, while the remaining teeth in the arch from first molar to first molar do not move in the initial stages and act as an anchorage segment to push the second molar distally for anteroposterior correction.

1 Dasy H, Dasy A, Asatrian G, Rózsa N, Lee H-F, Kwak JH. Effects of variable attachment shapes and aligner material on aligner retention. *Angle Orthodontist* 2015;**85**(6):934–940.

Fig. 2.7 While second molars are moving, the rest of the teeth are considered as anchorage.

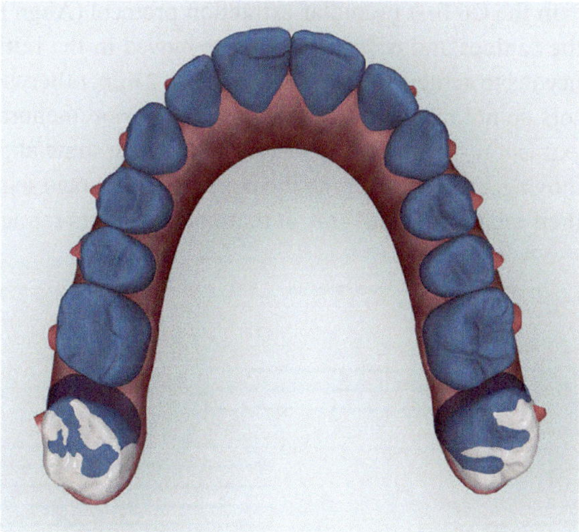

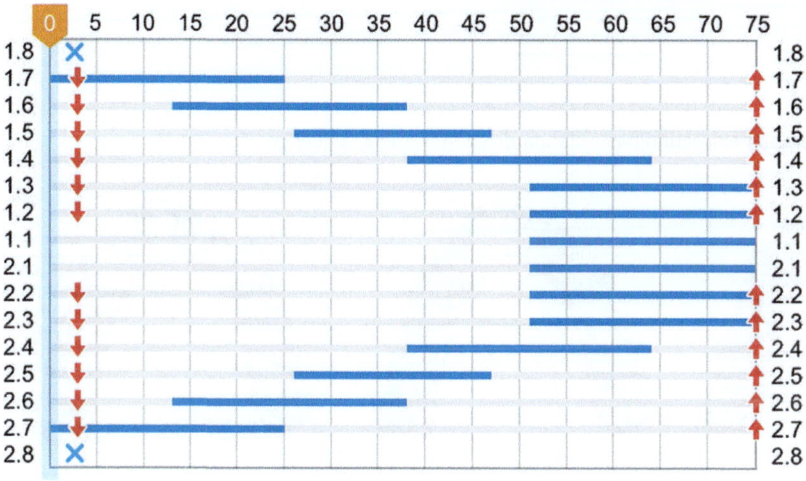

Fig. 2.8 This figure shows a horizontal 'V' movement pattern.

Fig. 2.9 The second quadrant is being expanded using the first quadrant as anchorage.

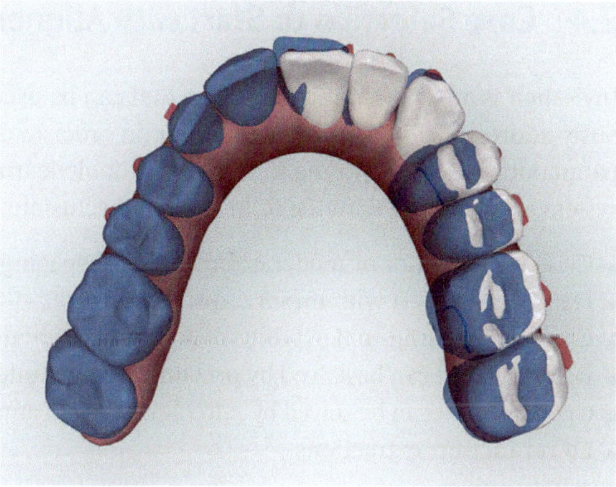

In the G6 first premolar extraction protocol (Align technology), for maximum anchorage, only the canines and posterior teeth are moved in the initial stages of treatment (if anchorage loss is needed to achieve class I, but only up to 2 mm, otherwise the G6 protocol does not apply). The incisors do not move, and they act as an anterior anchorage segment to distalize the canine into the extraction site for space closure. After using some aligners, the second premolar and molars stop moving, and they become the posterior anchorage segment. Canines will move up to one-third of their total movement and, at that point, incisors retraction will start.

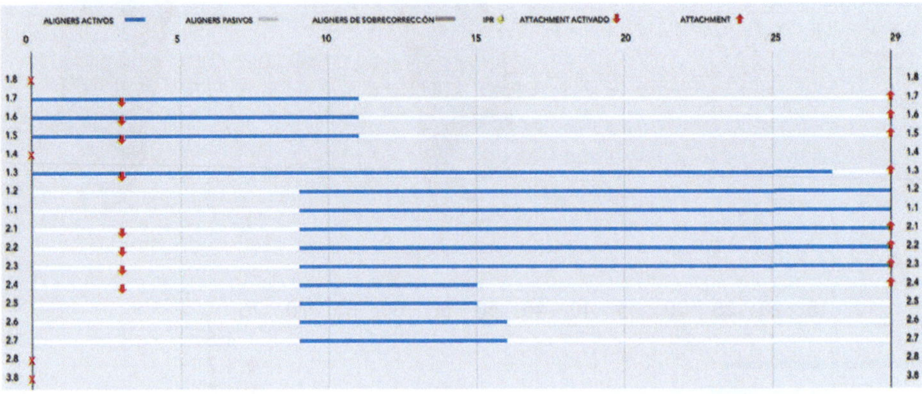

Fig. 2.10 G6 first premolar extraction has a standardized movement sequence.

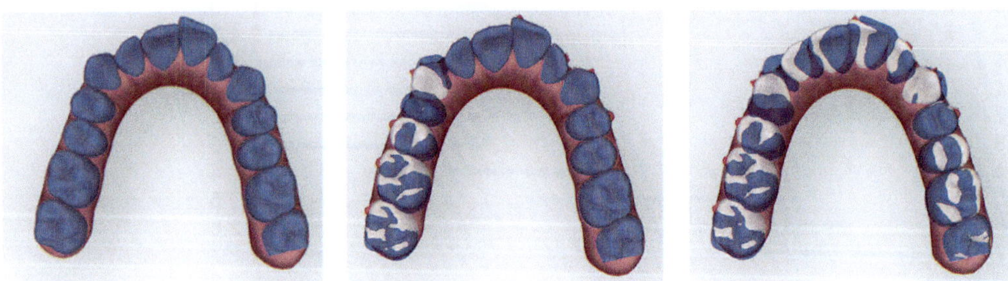

Fig. 2.11 In this G6 protocol extraction of 14 (from left to right), the posterior sector and canine move first; when the canine has achieved 1/3 of its total movement, incisors can start retruding.

2.4 Case Selection to Start with Aligners Technique

Invisalign is an orthodontic technique that can be used to treat all malocclusions that were previously addressed with brackets. However, in order to develop confidence with the technique, it is paramount in the beginning to follow a suitable learning curve to allow familiarization with the system and working with the following malocclusions is recommended:

- Class I with minor or moderate crowding or spacing
- Half-cusp Class II with minor crowding
- Class III with minimal overbite/overjet non-extraction cases
- Deep bite that can be solved by proclination and anterior intrusion (without posterior extrusion)
- Open bite that can be solved by retroclination and anterior extrusion (without posterior intrusion)
- Lower incisors extractions

However, if we are already comfortable and secure treating all types of malocclusions successfully with braces, then why should we change to aligners?

3

Why Invisalign?

We will explain why we decided to change our patients from braces to aligners and the advantages this brought to the growth of our practices and for ourselves.

3.1 Why Did We Begin Prescribing Invisalign in Our Practice?

Our reasons for prescribing Invisalign in our practice are:

- *Differentiation*: we wanted to be different from other practices that only offered brackets to their patients. Our goal was to have more contented patients in our offices, leading to more positive feedback and producing patients that would become our best ambassadors for referrals.
- *Reputation*: currently, and especially in Spain, the state-of-the-art treatment within orthodontics is Invisalign, so patients might believe that if you are not confident in Invisalign, then you might not be a good orthodontist.
- Efficiency in our practice:
  - fewer (and shorter) appointments
  - fewer emergencies
  - appointments planned ahead, so staff can use our protocols and reduce chair time
  - fewer staff members needed to attend the same number of patients
  - easier training for new staff (compared with using brackets and wires).

It was considered that all these elements would result in a more efficient workflow, and they did!

- *Aesthetics*: patients seek an aesthetic pleasing look, but not just at the end of treatment, as occurs with brackets and wires, so it is much better for them if we can offer those aesthetics during the entire treatment using an almost invisible plastic appliance.
- *Up-to-date image of practice:* it is easier if you show your treatment plan using digital tools and 3D planning using an iTero (intraoral) scanner, the outcome simulator and ClinCheck, especially compared with practitioners who are still showing their treatment plan with pictures and plaster models.
- *For the future*: this is our real motivation and the most important one for us.

Aligner Techniques in Orthodontics, First Edition. Susana Palma Moya and Javier Lozano Zafra.

Companion website: www.wiley.com/go/lozano-zafra/aligner-techniques

3.2 Our Motivation

Our prime motivation is that we strongly believe that in the not too distant future, Orthodontics will be exclusively based on aligners. Therefore, what we aim to do right now is offer our patients the treatments most practitioners will be offering in a few years' time. So, why wait if technological advances let us offer this treatment with the same goals and results as brackets and wires? We also believe this will lead us to being considered lead practitioners, further improving our practices.

The first smartphones became available just a decade ago, and it already seems as though they have been with us for a lifetime. Technology is advancing so rapidly that we will experience radical changes in society. As we undergo this rapid change, our old treatments using braces will no longer apply. Technology is creating a new set of rules that will change everything in our way of working: everything that can be digitized and customized will be. We firmly believe that soon no patients will be using braces for orthodontic treatment so, 'The sooner we transform all our patients into aligner patients, the sooner we will find the right path for our practice growth'.

4
Patient Communication Skills

The first element in our practice driving growth was word of mouth. For this, we developed a communication plan to explain that Invisalign is not just an aesthetic treatment, it is a lifestyle.

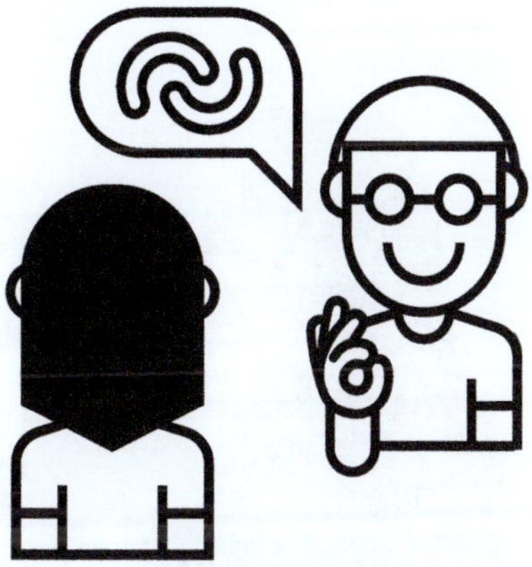

Fig. 4.1 Let's talk about aligner treatment with our patients.

4.1 Invisalign Equates to Health, Wellness and Outstanding Results

We focused on communicating to our current patients that we were using a new technique to align the teeth without braces. For this we used the following channels:

- Verbal in-office communication
- Digital and paper newsletter
- Social media

After this, we provided them with a change in mindset:

- For parents: health, wellness and guarantee of results
- For teenagers: change everything in your smile without changing your lifestyle

Fig. 4.2 The more Invisalign patients you have, the more Invisalign referrals you will have.

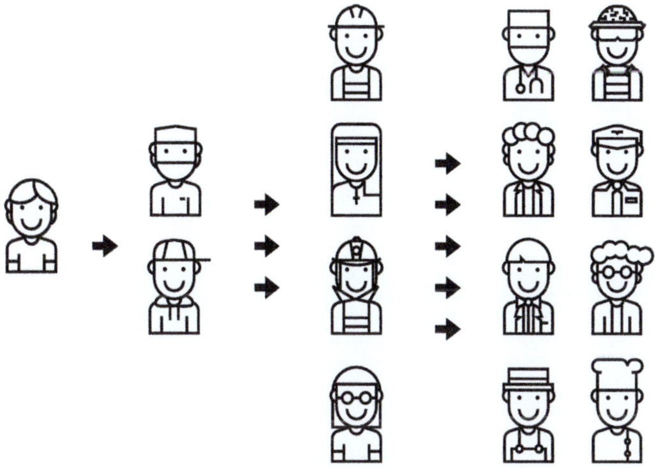

Aligner Techniques in Orthodontics, First Edition. Susana Palma Moya and Javier Lozano Zafra.

Companion website: www.wiley.com/go/lozano-zafra/aligner-techniques

4.2 Effective Patient Communication

As in-office communication is crucial and the best chance to interact with patients, we suggest having an Invisalign treatment coordinator in any office. Ideally, this would be a dental hygienist who:

- Addresses the patient's doubts about the treatment.
- Explains the whole process (the patient journey).
- Assists the patient from the moment they are given the treatment plan and quotation until they finish their treatment.

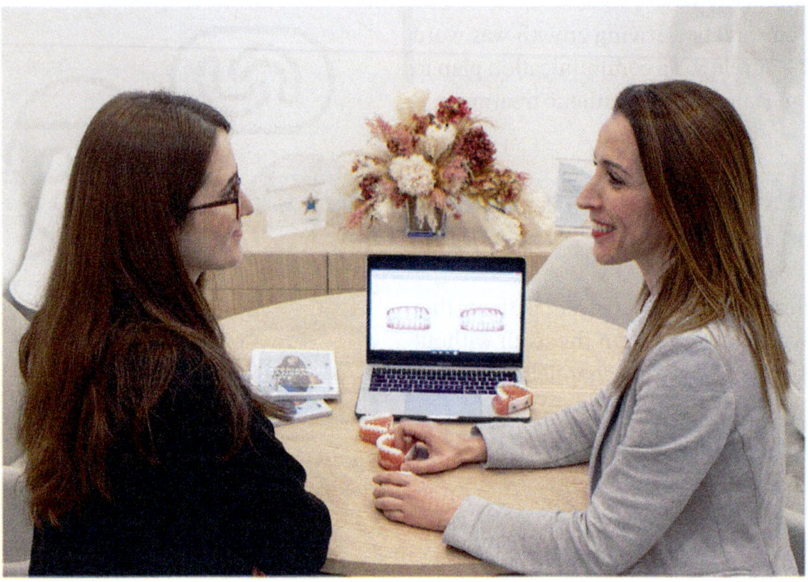

Fig. 4.3 A treatment coordinator is a key success driver for Invisalign.

5

Keys to Practice Growth

The 'four Ps' are the main growth drivers for Invisalign in our practices:

- Progress: this technique is more advanced than any other in orthodontics – it is a 100% digital and customized technique.
- Predictability: the chance of having selective anchorage during the treatment makes our movements more predictable.
- Possibility of treating every malocclusion, even in mixed dentition.
- Profitability: treat more patients with less chair time and fewer staff needed.

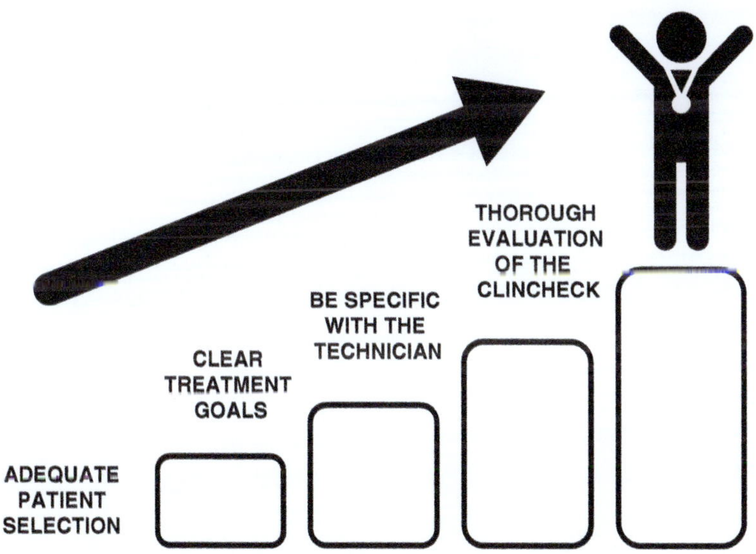

Fig. 5.1 If we plan our growth in advance, we will reach our goals.

5.1 How to Get the Best Results with Invisalign

We have come to the conclusion that the keys for success with Invisalign rely on:

- **Adequate patient selection** (motivate the patient, show them at every appointment the results he or she is obtaining due to the use of the aligners)

Aligner Techniques in Orthodontics, First Edition. Susana Palma Moya and Javier Lozano Zafra.

Companion website: www.wiley.com/go/lozano-zafra/aligner-techniques

- **Clear goals of treatment** in every plane: transversal, sagittal and vertical.
- **Being very specific with the technician** (in your instructions): communicate not only what you want to achieve but also how you want to obtain your treatment goals and the staging of movements needed for this particular malocclusion.
- **A thorough dynamic evaluation of the ClinCheck**, considering staging, differential anchorage, looking for predictable movements while avoiding those outside the predictability range of the aligners shown as black dots on the tooth movement assessment (TMA) tool.

6

Patient Selection

The Invisalign selection tool is a guide provided by Align Technology to help choose between the different treatment options that Invisalign provides, according to the patient malocclusion. This is a tool that might be used before sending the case in order to assess the predictability of the case (simple, green/moderate, blue/difficult, black) as well as the treatment option from the Align portfolio. During the learning curve, clinicians usually do this evaluation 'automatically', but we still think it is useful for beginners.

Based on Align's 'big data' it is possible to predict accurately the outcomes from every tooth movement. This is really important in order to achieve excellent results, as the practitioner will need to understand how to make movements possible using auxiliary techniques (which relies on experience), alongside aligners or attachments (which is what this tool 'analyses').

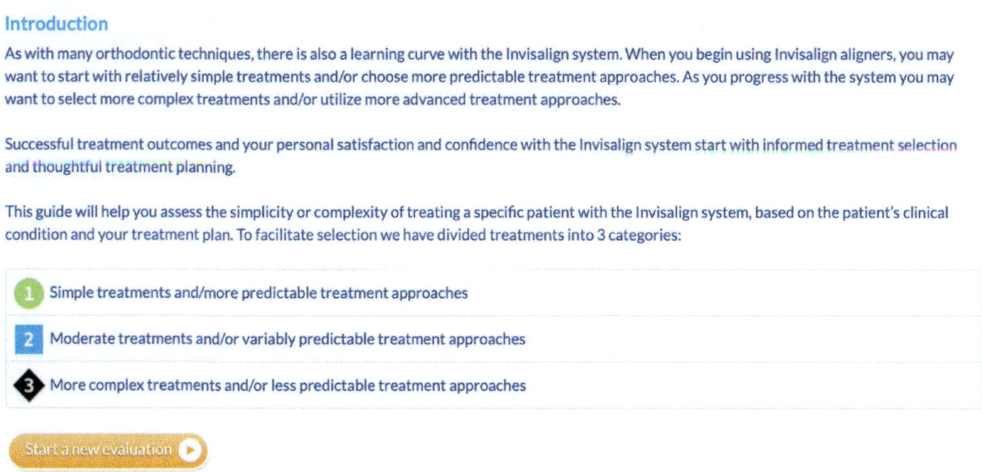

Fig. 6.1 Invisalign evaluation tool.

Aligner Techniques in Orthodontics, First Edition. Susana Palma Moya and Javier Lozano Zafra.

Companion website: www.wiley.com/go/lozano-zafra/aligner-techniques

7

Predictability of Movement

Movements are classified into three colours, according to their predictability:

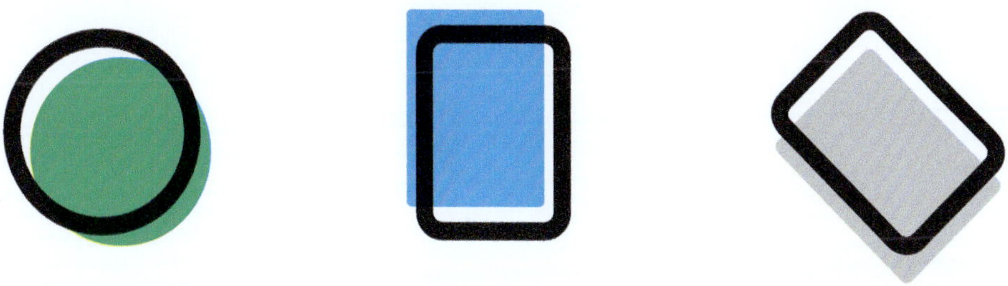

VERY PREDICTABLE MOVEMENTS

MOVEMENTS WHERE WE MAINLY MOVE THE TOOTH CROWN

1. Proclination of anterior teeth
2. Retrusion of anterior teeth
3. Tipping of the crowns
4. Expansion by changing the torque

- Anterior intrusion between 2 and 4 mm
- Incisors rotations

PREDICTABLE MOVEMENTS

- Root torque (labial or lingual)
- Midlines shift lower than 2 mm
- First molar rotations (second molars do not rotate so well)
- Distalization between 2 and 4 mm
- Asymmetric extractions

LESS PREDICTABLE MOVEMENTS

- Mesio-distal root tip
- Teeth body movement (protrusion or retraction)
- Body expansion of the arch (not expansion by changing torque)
- Posterior Intrusion
- Anterior Extrusion
- Posterior extrusion (we will always accompany this with elastics)
- Rotation of canines, premolars higher than 45°
- Mesialization (Maximum 1-2 mm and taking into consideration differential anchorage)

Fig. 7.1 All treatment predictability can be checked with the Invisalign evaluation tool before sending the case.

7.1 Treatments to Gain Familiarity with the Technique

Class I < 6 mm spacing or crowding.

- Deep bite < 4 mm
- Open bite < 2,5 mm
- Class II < 4 mm
- Class III < 2 mm (distalization of lower molars by tipping the lower molars crown to distal without moving the roots)
- Midlines shift < 3 mm

Aligner Techniques in Orthodontics, First Edition. Susana Palma Moya and Javier Lozano Zafra.

Companion website: www.wiley.com/go/lozano-zafra/aligner-techniques

8

Types of Treatments with Invisalign

Currently, although this may change in different parts of the world and in the future as a result of Align Technology commercial policies, the different options that Align provides according to the malocclusion of our patients are indicated in Fig. 8.1.

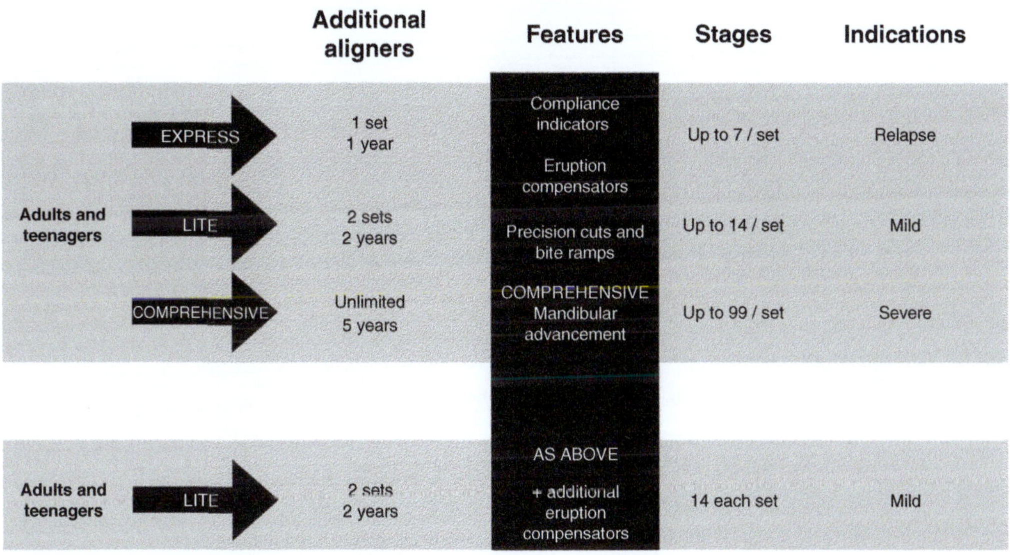

Fig. 8.1 Align Technology's 2021 portfolio.

Aligner Techniques in Orthodontics, First Edition. Susana Palma Moya and Javier Lozano Zafra.

Companion website: www.wiley.com/go/lozano-zafra/aligner-techniques

9

Pillars of the Invisalign Technique

The Invisalign system is not just a set of aligners, as other resources are needed to achieve success in each case. Based on this, we describe five pillars of the technique, which are:

- Aligners
- ClinCheck software
- Attachments and features of SmartForce
- Auxiliary techniques
- Technicians

9.1 Aligners

Aligners are made from SmartTrack material, a patented plastic formula exclusively designed for this purpose, while attachment templates are made with EX 15 and Vivera retainers with EX 40.

Characteristics of the SmartTrack technology:[1]

- Creates a soft and constant force.
- Is more elastic than other aligner materials, which results in a longer working period.
- Better adjustment of the teeth than any other alternative.
- Easier to use and provides an easier way of placing and removing the aligner.

Every aligner makes:

- 0.25 mm of lineal movement
- 2 degrees of angular movement to correct rotations
- 1 degree of torque movement (lingual–root torque or labial–root torque)

In cases where we want to slow down the amount of movement, this can be requested from the technician, which will change Align's default parameters to 50% (half of the movements indicated above).

Aligners are created to be used 22 hours per day, with changes depending on the amount of movement every 7, 10 or 14 days.

1 Bräscher AK, Zuran D, Feldmann RE Jr, Benrath J. Patient survey on Invisalign® treatment comparen the SmartTrack® material to the previous aligner material. *J Orofac Orthop.* 2016;77(6):432–438. Epub October 24, 2016.

Aligner Techniques in Orthodontics, First Edition. Susana Palma Moya and Javier Lozano Zafra.

Companion website: www.wiley.com/go/lozano-zafra/aligner-techniques

9.2 ClinCheck Software

This application, created by Align Technology, was designed specifically for practitioners. ClinCheck provides a 3D virtual representation of a treatment plan derived from the orthodontic prescription.

Each practitioner is able to send information back and forth with Align as changes are made to the treatment plan, and then aligners are manufactured in accordance with the finalized plan and sent directly to the practitioner to begin the patient's treatment.

9.3 Attachments and Features of SmartForce

These are attachments for composite structures that are bonded to the patient's teeth in order to help achieve the movements previously planned on the ClinCheck software. They can be 'conventional', with standardized shapes and sizes, or optimized, where a shape and size is determined by the software based on each patient and tooth. They are bonded throughout the treatment and will be removed at the end of it.

In 2013, Align Technology developed the SmartForce features in order to create the optimal forces to move the teeth in a predictable way. They can be placed.

- On teeth, as optimized attachments
- On the aligner, as pressure points or power ridges

Full information of these will be delivered in later sections of this book.

9.4 Auxiliary Techniques

As stated previously, clear aligner therapy needs other forms of auxiliary techniques, such as elastics, buttons, powerchains, temporary anchorage devices (TADs) and others, just as we do with fixed appliances in order to make treatments more predictable and more efficient.

We will explain some of these auxiliary techniques in the troubleshooting and auxiliary techniques section but it must always kept in mind that a great result with aligners needs a great practitioner using the five pillars: it is not just a matter of plastic and elastic, but an orthodontic treatment based on mechanics, forces and a detailed treatment plan that has to include every tool in our 'ortho' arsenal.

9.5 Technician (CAD Designer)

ClinCheck software allows practitioners to plan occlusion and tooth position but other changes, such as staging and teeth extraction still need collaboration from an Invisalign CAD designer. This makes these individuals really important to the treatment outcome and requires practitioners to adapt to the 'technician language' in order to achieve the best result from the aligner technique.

10

Conventional Attachments

Conventional attachments are passive attachments that increase the engagement of the aligner onto the tooth. They act as a handle for the aligners to move teeth. They can be placed via written request to the technician or by using the drag and drop feature on the 3D controls.

There are three types of conventional attachments:

- Ellipsoid attachments: Used for retention or anchorage when the tooth surface area is limited, for example for peg-shape lateral incisors or the lingual surface of a lingually inclined mandibular second molar.
- Rectangular attachments: These are passive attachments that can be vertical or horizontal. By default, they are placed in the middle of the tooth crown, but can be moved to any desired position to facilitate the mechanics that have been planned for the case.
    - Horizontal: can be used for root control, especially for labial root torque on the molars. These can also be used in short crowns in order to increase the retention of the aligners, which is part of the standard Align's protocols for patients that are still growing in interventions such as mandibular advancement or first protocols (similar to this, but optimized). In unilateral crossbites, horizontal rectangular attachments are used on the side without the crossbite in order to provide anchorage to correct the unilateral posterior crossbite on the contralateral side. This will be explained in Chapter 17, but they help to control the root torque so as to create an 'en masse' movement of not just the crown but of the whole tooth body.
    - Vertical: these are used for root control when the software cannot place optimized root control attachments, such as mandibular incisors in cases involving the extraction of one lower incisor.

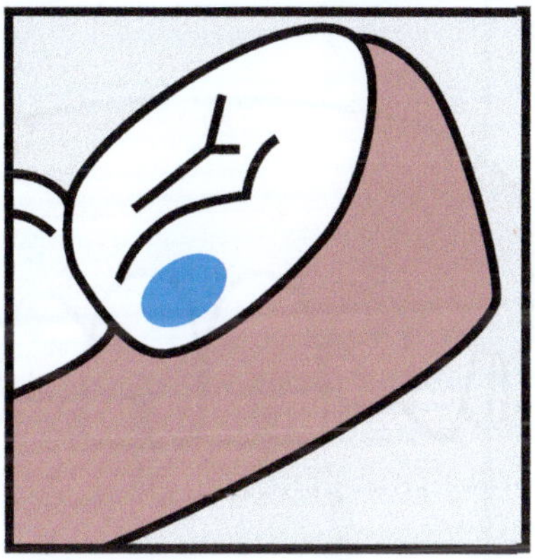

Fig. 10.1 Ellipsoid attachments.

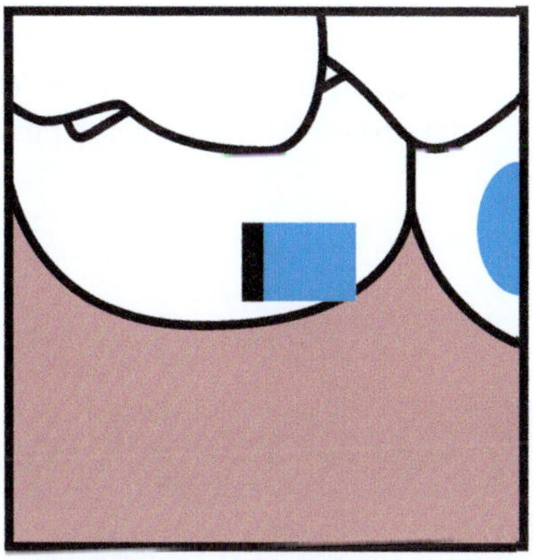

Fig. 10.2 Horizontal attachments have great clinical effects on transverse plane.

Aligner Techniques in Orthodontics, First Edition. Susana Palma Moya and Javier Lozano Zafra.

Companion website: www.wiley.com/go/lozano-zafra/aligner-techniques

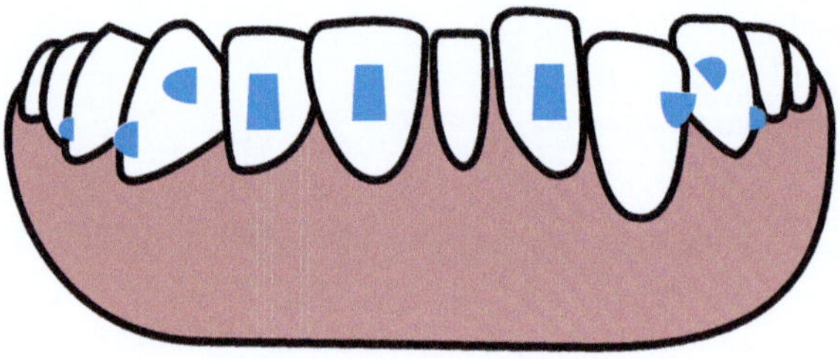

Fig. 10.3 Conventional attachments are selected whenever there are no optimized ones available.

- Bevelled attachments: both horizontal and rectangular vertical attachments can be bevelled
  - Horizontal attachments can be bevelled to the occlusal (HBO) or to gingival (HBG) to help with intrusion or extrusion movements:
    - For extrusive tooth movements on posterior molars, a horizontal attachment bevelled to gingival can be used
    - For intrusion, use the horizontal attachment bevelled on the occlusal on the teeth adjacent to the one that has to be intruded

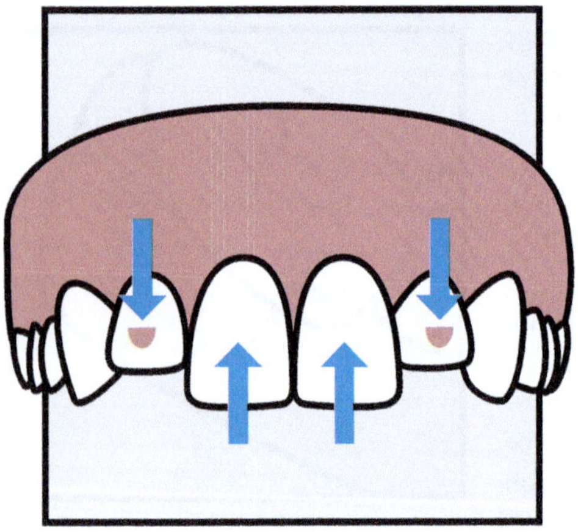

Fig. 10.4 Extrusion attachments are placed on teeth adjacent to the ones to be intruded, so as to create a counter-movement that will lead to a force couple. This is a great example of how biomechanics are applied on aligners.

  - Vertical attachments can be bevelled to mesial (VBM) or to distal (VBD): for rotation movements when the software has not placed optimized rotation attachments, for example when correcting first molar rotation. The bevelled surface is the active one, as the bevel provides a flat surface for the aligner to push against to achieve the desired tooth movement.

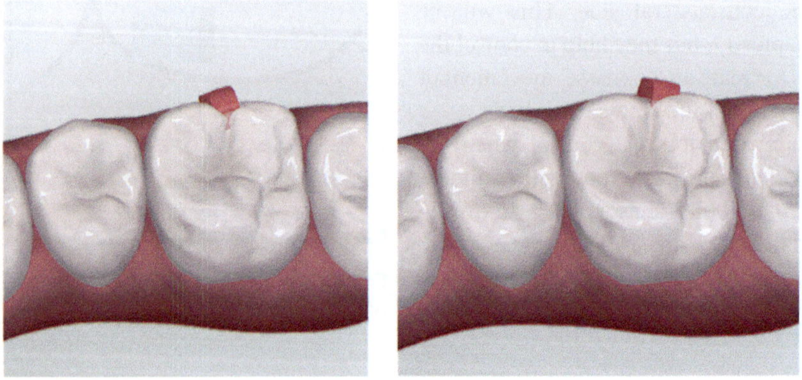

Fig. 10.5 Vertical attachments bevelled to mesial (left) and distal (right).

- Conventional and optimized attachments might have similar functions:
  - Double root control attachment: AT conventional rectangular vertical
  - Optimized rotation attachment: AT conventional rectangular vertical bevelled to mesial VBM or distal VBD
  - Optimized extrusion attachment: AT conventional horizontal bevelled to gingival HBG

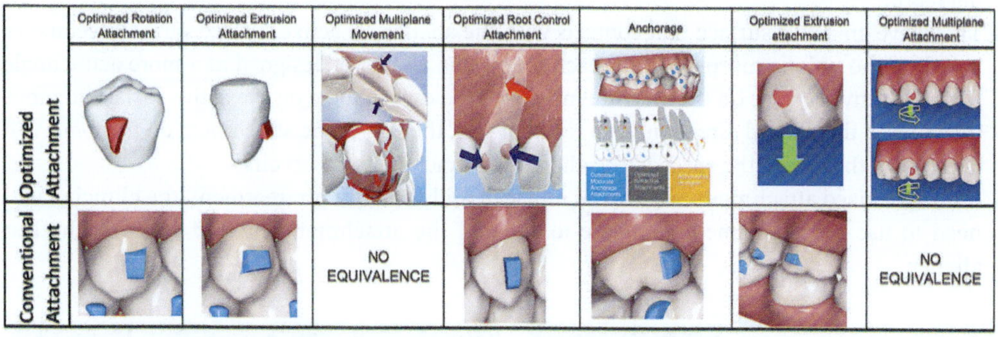

Fig. 10.6 Conventional attachments might be placed to achieve similar movements to the optimized ones.

10.1 Features of SmartForce

10.1.1 Optimized Attachments

These area attachments with different characteristics from the conventional ones. They are:

- Designed to provide optimal force to achieve a more predictable movement
- Tailor-made for each tooth's width, long axis and contour
- Positioned precisely to deliver the forces while simultaneously eliminating interferences

All these characteristics are defined by the ClinCheck software and do not permit changes by the practitioner, a feature that may change in the future.

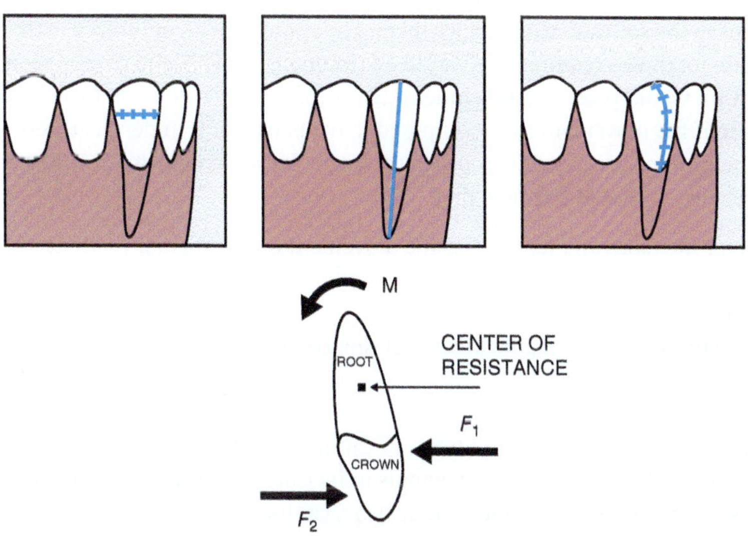

Fig. 10.7 Research and development investment has led to a very powerful biomechanical system.

Optimized attachments provide SmartForces applied to the teeth. They provide the amount of force necessary to create the ideal movement of the tooth. In addition:

- They are automatically placed by the software when it detects certain thresholds of tooth movement. They are designed to control the point of application of the force, the direction of the force and the amount of force applied. Every optimized attachment is customized to each individual tooth.
- They have an active surface that contacts with the aligner. Its active surface varies in geometry based on the unique morphology of each tooth. The aligner is designed at a more acute angle than the active surface on the attachment in order to exert a force on the active surface to move the tooth in the desired direction. As a result of this, the size of the attachment on the tooth will differ from the size of the space in the aligner for attachment (reservoirs).
- If an optimized attachment needs to be replaced midway through treatment, the clinician will need to use the attachment template to re-bond the attachment, instead of using the last aligner.

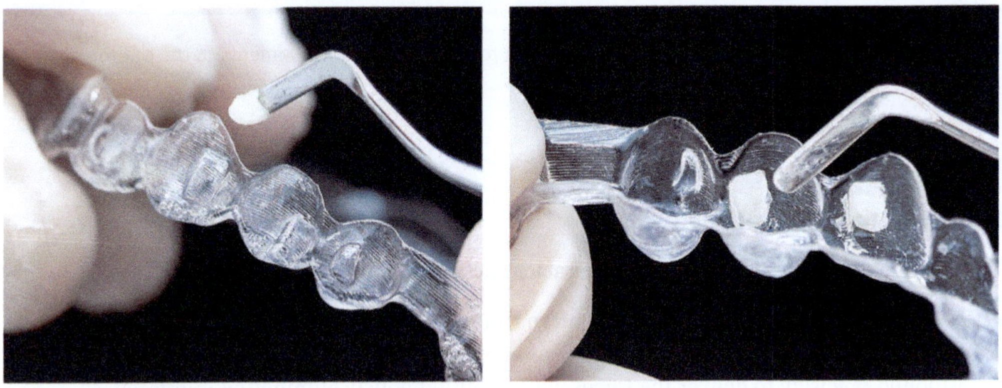

Fig. 10.8 Conventional dental composite is the material chosen for attachments.

In the past, the practitioner could not ask the technician to place an optimized attachment, but could ask for the movement so the software would place them. For example, if an optimized extrusion attachment on a certain tooth was required, we would ask for more than 0.5 mm of extrusion in that tooth and the software would place the attachment. However, it is now possible to ask for optimized attachments even if the movement is not supposed to happen (or it is under the threshold), which could prove helpful for certain situations (lower premolar anchorage to level lower Spee curve by incisor intrusion). It should be noted that:

- They are individualized for the tooth and for the specific movement that particular tooth needs
- Their position, shape or size cannot be changed
- They cannot be placed lingually
- They are not compatible with other lingual attachments or SmartForces

Currently available optimized attachments include:

- Optimized rotation attachment (for rotation movements in canines and premolars)
- Optimized extrusion attachment (for extrusion movements in incisors, canines and premolars)
- Optimized root control attachment (for root control in incisors, canines and premolars)
- Optimized attachment for upper lateral incisors

  - Multiplane attachment (for lateral incisors with rotation and vertical movement)
  - Optimized support attachment (to support lateral incisors when there is an intrusion movement on adjacent canine or central incisors); deep bite correction.
- Optimized attachments on molars:
  - Multiplane attachment (for molars with rotation + vertical movement)
  - Extrusion optimized attachments (for extrusion movements on molars)
- Optimized support attachments: to provide support for predictable dental arch expansion in mixed dentition.

Optimized Rotation Attachment

These are placed for rotation of canines and premolars greater than 5 degrees:

- Placed when more than 5 degrees of rotation is needed.
- The predictable rotation is between 30 and 45 degrees.
- If one needs to be replaced for a conventional one, it will be a vertical rectangular attachment bevelled to mesial or distal.

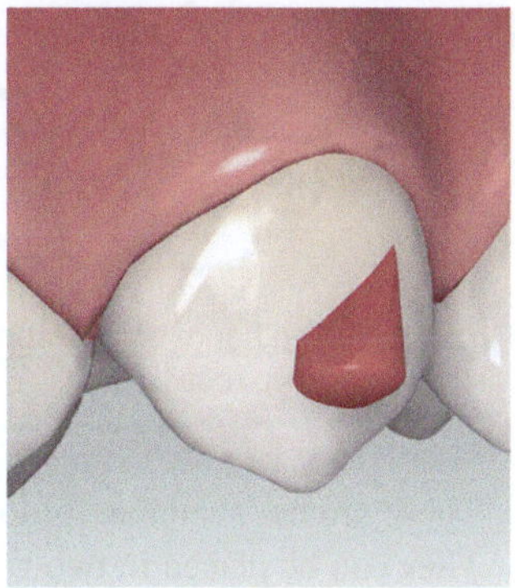

Fig. 10.9 Placement on canines and premolars.

Optimized Extrusion Attachment

Designed for extrusion of incisors, canines and premolars, these attachments are bonded in the middle of the crown:

- They are placed when the extrusion is more than 0.5 mm and have a wedge shape
- When they are placed on lower premolars, they are used as an anchorage for the anterior intrusion of the incisors and they have a different shape
- They can also be activated to provide an extrusion force on the premolars during the anterior intrusion
- When extrusion of the four upper incisors is greater than 0.5 mm the four teeth will act as a single unit

We will look at these attachments in more detail later, but note that they are mandatory when an anterior open bite is part of the patient's malocclusion, otherwise the aligner will not be able to apply a clean extrusion vector.

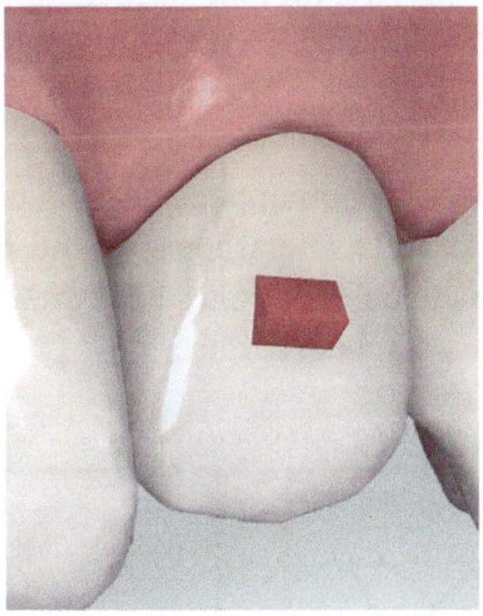

Fig. 10.10 Placement on incisor.

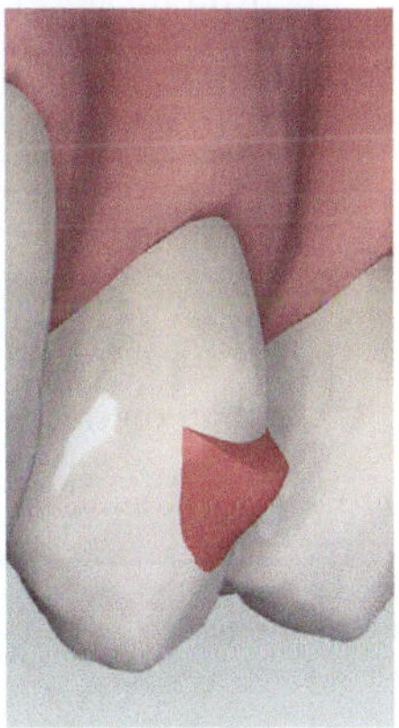

Fig. 10.11 Placement on premolar.

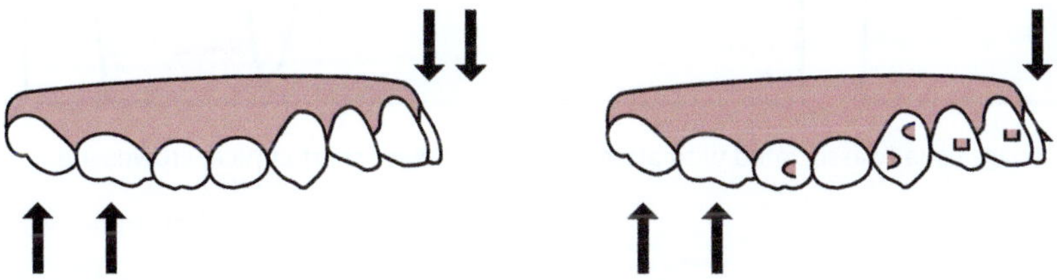

Fig. 10.12 The right side shows how anterior extrusion attachments help to create a counterforce to posterior intrusion, achieving predictable movements.

Optimized Root Control Attachments

These are are designed for upper central upper incisors and lower canines, where they will control root movement, for tipping management and 'en masse' translation:

- They have two active surfaces and are placed when there is a translation of the tooth centre of resistance greater than 0.75 mm

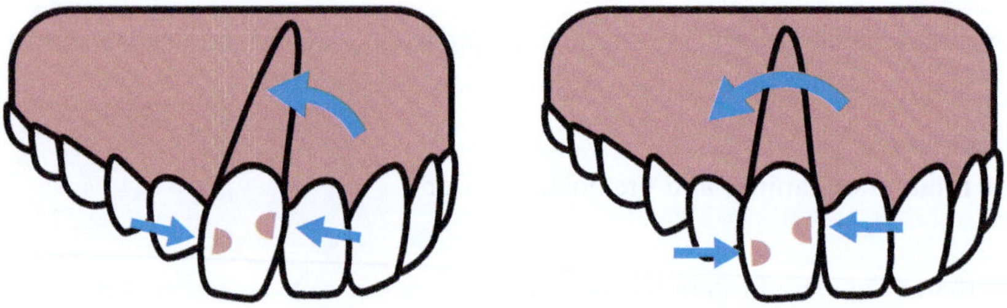

Fig. 10.13 The figure on the right shows how optimized root control attachments create a couple of forces to improve root tipping.

- These are not available for lower incisors
- They can be placed in two ways:
  - In opposite orientations on both central incisors (like a mirror image): they are used to close a diastema (mesial root tipping of 11 and 21 to close the diastema)
  - Parallel to each other on both central incisors (they are placed in the same directions in both central incisors). In this case they are used to move the upper midline in one direction
- They are automatically placed by the software:
  - When the centre of the root on upper and lower canines and premolars moves more than 0.5 mm
  - When the centre of the root on upper central incisors moves more than 0.75 mm
  - They can also be placed in lateral incisors and premolars, but because of the short crown, instead of a 'double attachment' it is sometimes shown as a half-moon and a pressure point applied on the aligner's lingual surface

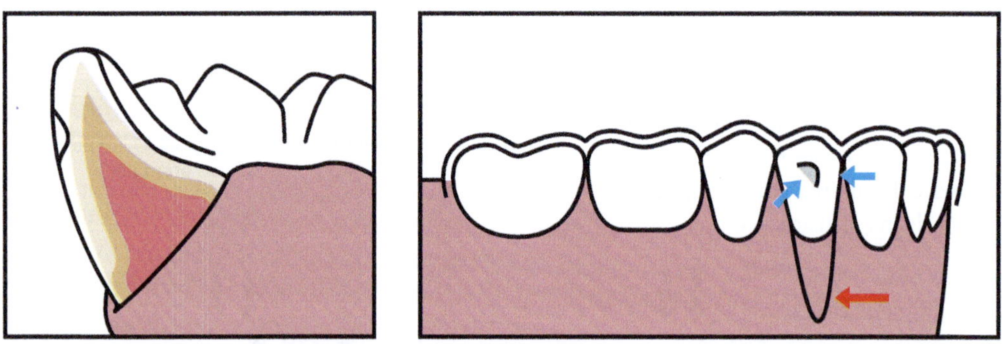

Fig. 10.14 Pressure points are usually associated with attachments whenever short clinical crowns are detected.

Optimized Attachments for Lateral Incisors

Multiplane Attachment

- Placed when the lateral incisors need intrusion or extrusion while simultaneously requiring rotation, torque or tipping movements
- They have an active surface on the attachment and a lingual pressure point

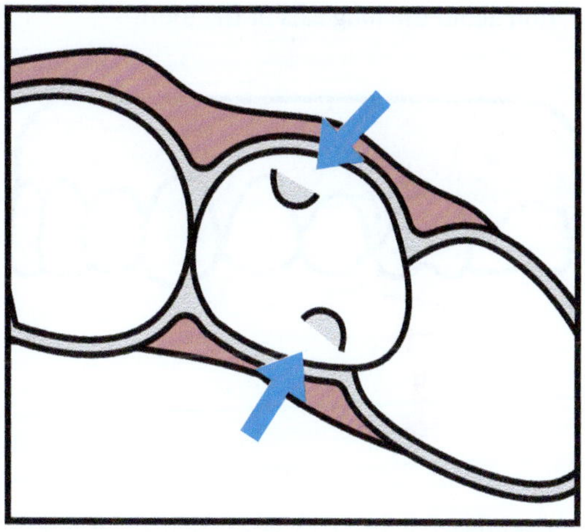

Fig. 10.15 Combination of attachments and lingual pressure points help creating an excellent force system.

Optimized Support Attachment

- Placed on lateral incisors when 1 mm or more of intrusion is planned on adjacent canine or central incisors, similar to the example given for posterior intrusion, but with characteristics adapted to lateral teeth clinical crowns
- The aim of these attachments is to prevent tracking problems on the lateral incisors during the vertical correction of the central incisors and the canines

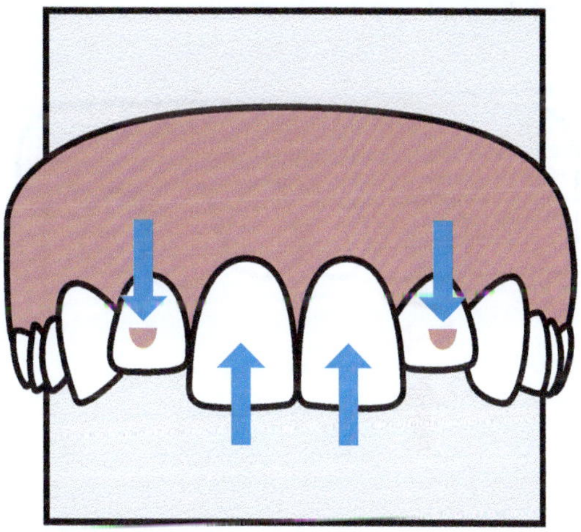

Fig. 10.16 Sometimes attachments are designed for support instead of movement.

Optimized Attachments for Molars

These are automatically placed by the software for anchorage purpose and to assist the molars to move in different planes of space.

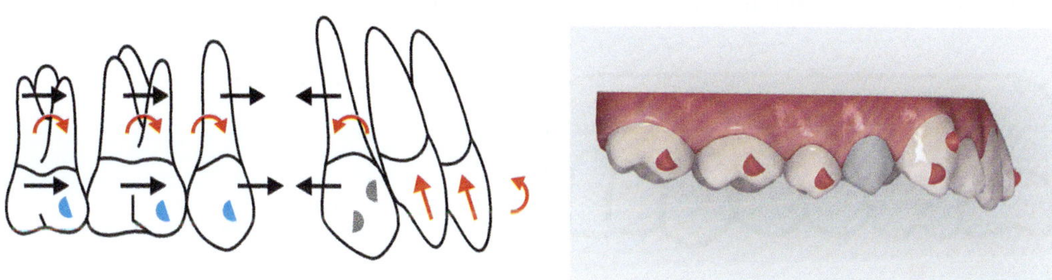

Fig. 10.17 Attachments for molars are relatively new and provide improved root movement.

Multiplane Attachments for Molars

- Optimized multiplane attachments are designed for molars that require rotation correction and a vertical correction of intrusion or extrusion at the same time.
- For extrusion + rotation, equal to or more than 0.5mm extrusion and 5 degrees of rotation about the long axis of the tooth.
- For extrusion/intrusion, between 0.5 mm intrusion/extrusion and more than 5 degrees of rotation about the long axis of the tooth.

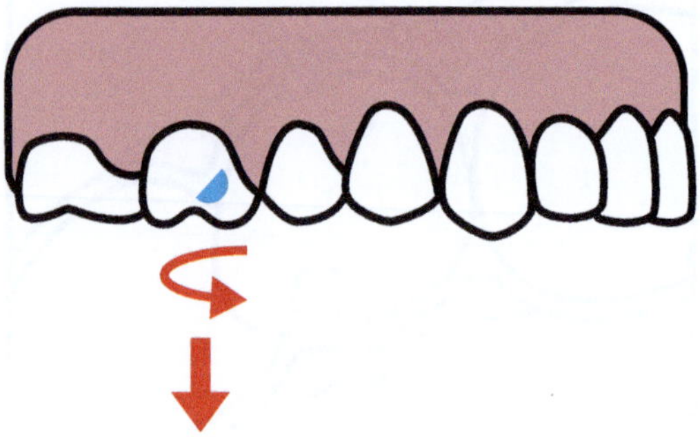

Fig. 10.18 Mesiobuccal rotation combined with extrusion.

- For intrusion, equal to or less than 0.5mm intrusion and 5 degrees of rotation about the long axis of the tooth.

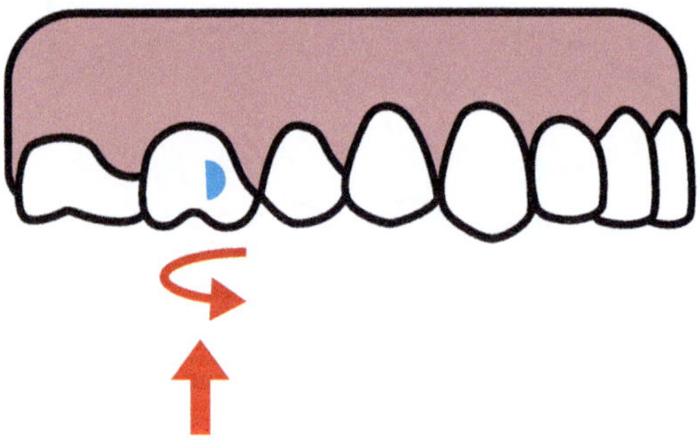

Fig. 10.19 Mesiobuccal rotation combined with intrusion.

Optimized Extrusion Attachments for Molars

These help with the extrusion of the molars, for extrusion + rotation, more than 0.5mm extrusion and less than 5 degrees of rotation about the long axis of the tooth.

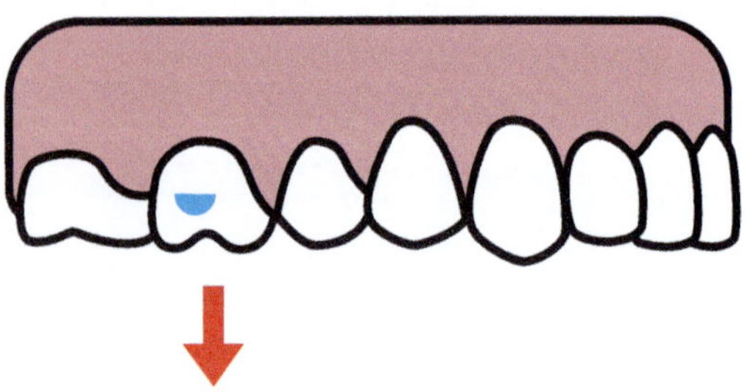

Fig. 10.20 Molar extrusion.

10.2 Optimized Support Attachments

These provide support for predictable dental arch expansion.

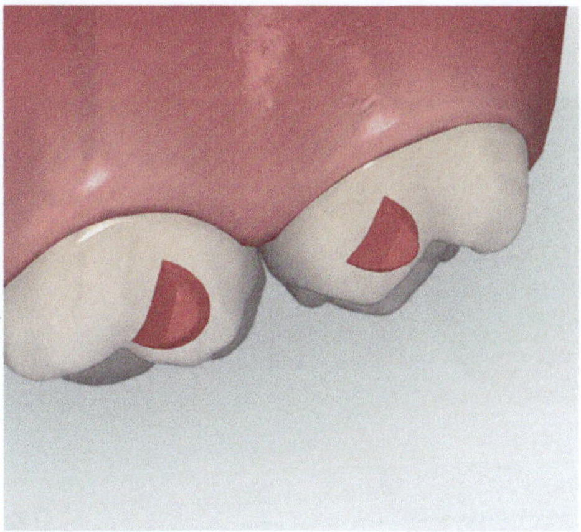

Fig. 10.21 Optimized support attachments are commonly used in first treatments.

10.2.1 SmartForces

There are other types of SmartForce attachments, such as those placed on the aligners (not on the teeth, as attachments) to help achieve the desired movement, which have been developed after more than a decade of research and development from Align Technology.

Power Ridges

They might be placed alone, and are not compatible with attachments, usually stablishing a force couple, for example, for incisors torque:

- Buccal
  - Available on upper and lower incisors
  - They produce lingual root torque (LRT)
  - Threshold for placement is 3 degrees LRT
  - 1 degree/aligner

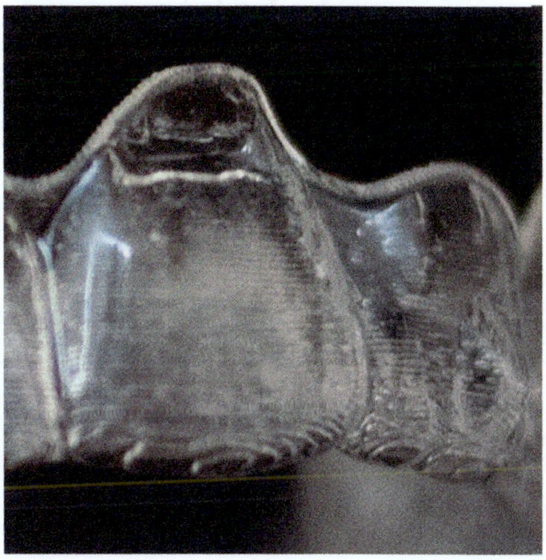

Fig. 10.22 Power ridges are plastic bends exerting 'push' forces.

- Buccal + lingual
  - Available on upper incisors
  - They produce LRT + incisor retraction
  - Threshold for placement is 3 degrees LRT + anterior retraction
  - 1 degree/aligner +0.25mm retraction

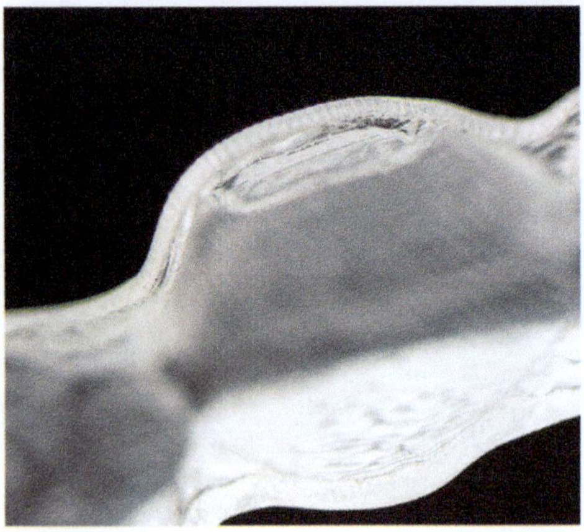

Fig. 10.23 Activation exerts forces translated to crown or root.

Pressure Points

As previously stated, they can be placed in combination with attachments, for example, to promote teeth rotation or intrusion.

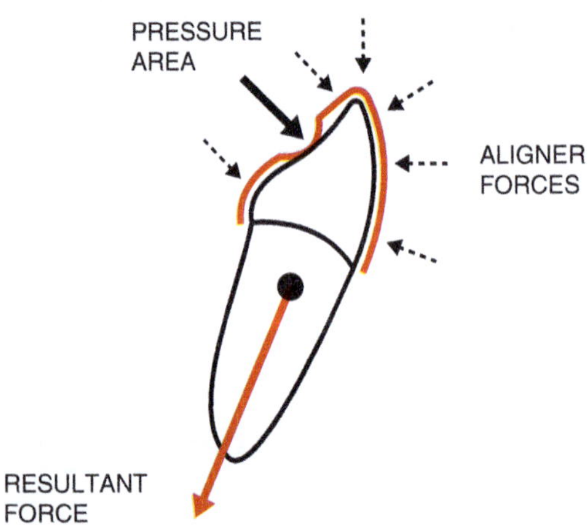

Fig. 10.24 Effect of pressure point on the tooth.

Precision Ramps

These are usually dynamic, changing on every aligner, adapting to tooth movement, and constitute a differential aspect to braces, which can only change when the practitioner has the patient in office.

This is especially useful for precision bite ramps which, in contrast to fixed turbo bites help create only the required tooth disocclusion, being more comfortable for the patient's TMJ and, as they 'disappear' whenever the patient removes the aligner to eat, improve their quality of life.

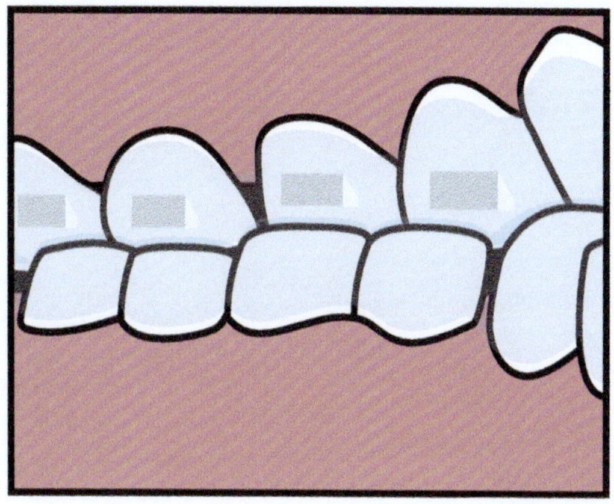

Fig. 10.25 Precision Ramps are much comfortable for the patient than conventional bite ramps.

Precision Wings

This is the latest innovation from Align Technology on SmartForces applied to the aligners, developed for Mandibular Advancement Features. They help the patient by advancing the mandible on a preset basis, which is now the gold standard whenever mandibular hypoplasia is found on young, growing patients.

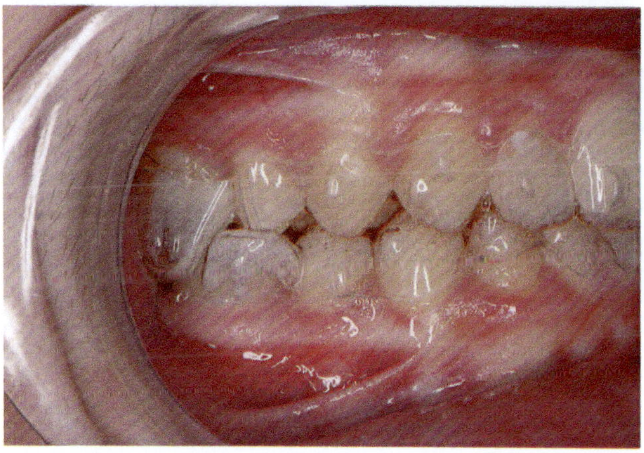

Fig. 10.26 Clinical view of Precision Wings in a growing patient.

11

Clinical Preferences

The software and the technician (CAD designer) will work on the ClinCheck based on your clinical preferences. They can be modified when desired or for a specific patient. However, it is important to dedicate time to specify what the expectations are for each treatment as this will help save time and produce more accurate results in the years to come.

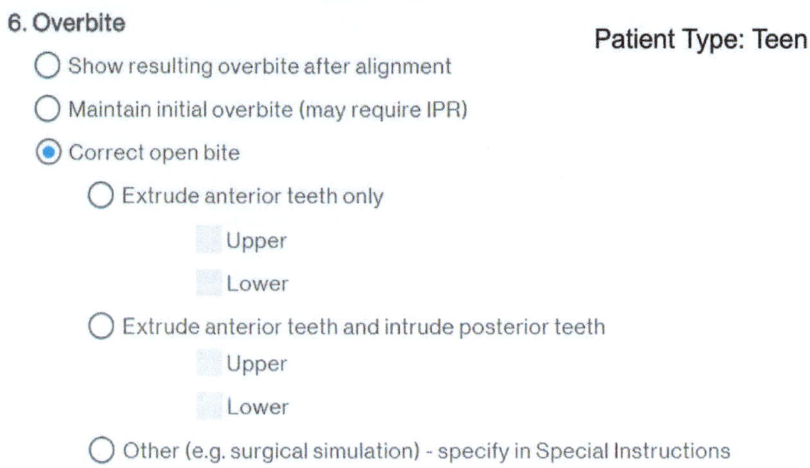

Fig. 11.1 Dedicate time to setting up clinical preferences.

Treatment software will act automatically based on 'Clinical Preferences' to create ClinCheck Treatment Plans. However, every time the clinician submits a new patient they can, if needed, modify the clinical preferences exclusively for this patient.

Aligner Techniques in Orthodontics, First Edition. Susana Palma Moya and Javier Lozano Zafra.

Companion website: www.wiley.com/go/lozano-zafra/aligner-techniques

12

Bonding Attachments and Interproximal Reduction

12.1 Bonding Attachments Protocol

The following Align Technology recommendations are suggested for a bonding attachments protocol, as summarized below and in Fig. 12.1.

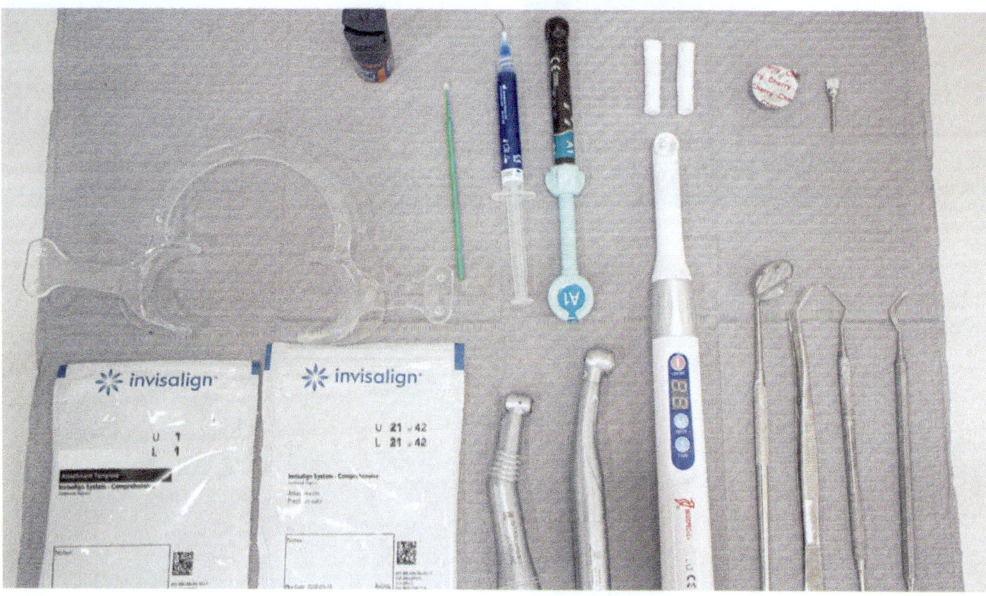

Fig. 12.1 Have materials and equipment ready before any appointment.

- Check the adjustment of the attachment template
- Isolate with Nola dry field cheek retractor and prepare teeth: apply etching for 30 s, wash the surface carefully and then dry until the surface of the teeth becomes completely white.

Aligner Techniques in Orthodontics, First Edition. Susana Palma Moya and Javier Lozano Zafra.

Companion website: www.wiley.com/go/lozano-zafra/aligner-techniques

- Use the bond on the surface of the teeth and cure it following manufacturer's instructions.
- Apply the composite roughly in the attachment template. Clinicians must use one of the composites recommended by Align Technology to prevent erosion of the attachment or debonding. SmartForces are only guaranteed with certain composites, as attachments might change their shape or surface easily if made with different brands from those tested (refer to the Invisalign Doctor Site to check suggested composite brands).
- Place the template in the mouth and apply pressure while curing the attachments.
- Remove template and remove excess composite with a bur.
- Test first aligner fit. The active bevel of the attachment must be in contact with the aligner.

Repeat the same process in the other arch.

Show the patient how to insert and remove the first aligner.

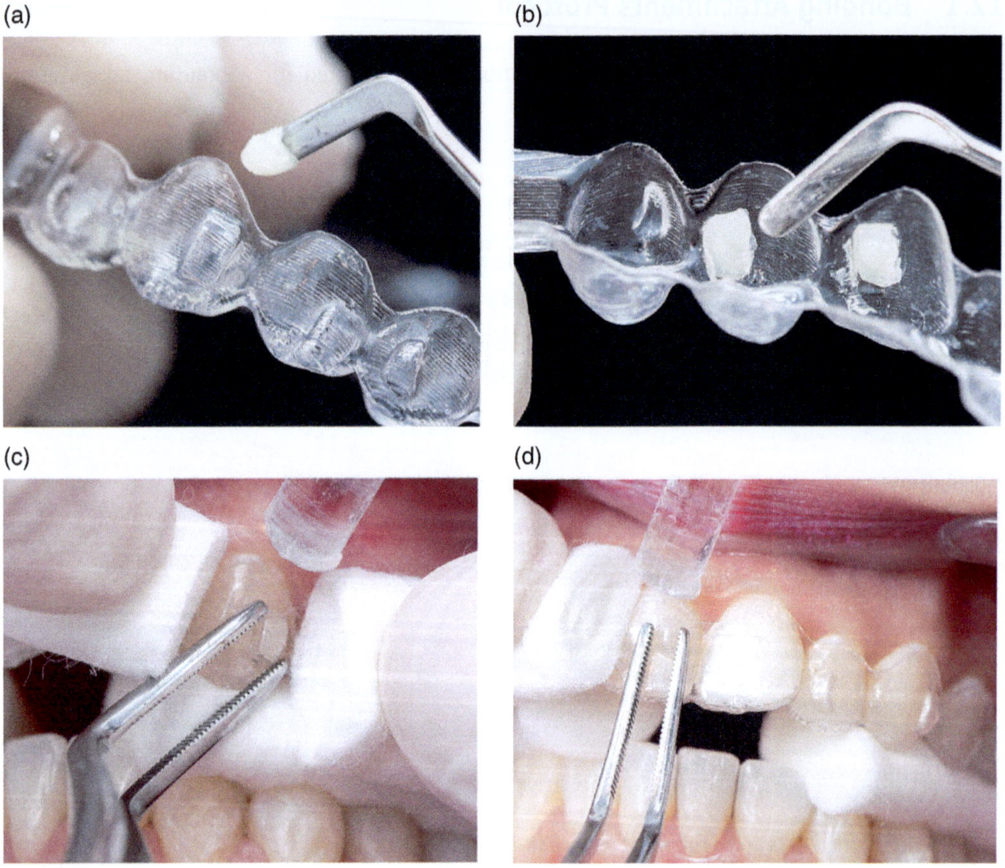

Fig. 12.2 (a) Place composite on template and (b) ensure there is no composite excess. (c) Bonding is best performed by two operators and (d) start from distal to mesial to avoid unexpected light-curing.

Following Align Technology's instructions on composites is strongly advised, as they have been previously tested, and results optimized, which cannot be ensured when using other brands.[1]

1 Barreda GJ, Dzierewianko EA, Muñoz KA, Piccoli GI. Surface wear of resin composites used for Invisalign® attachments. *Acta Odontol Latinoam* 2017;**30**(2):90–95.

12.2 Interproximal Reduction Procedure

Interproximal reduction (IPR) is the term usually applied to the Invisalign technique for stripping. This is a clinical procedure characterized by the interproximal enamel reduction of the teeth.

When applied to orthodontics, the space created is used for tooth alignment in cases of crowding[2] and the camouflage of class II/III malocclusions with an overjet excess/lack,[3] as well as improving dental aesthetics by teeth recontouring.[4]

It is important to develop a good technique as enamel irregularities/scratches, resulting from an inadequate technique could increase the susceptibility of these teeth to the accumulation of plaque. That said, it should be stressed that both clinical teams from Craig and Sheridan[5] and Sheridan and Ledoux[6] concluded that posterior teeth whose interproximal enamel was stripped were not more susceptible to decay or periodontal disease, so it can be considered a safe and convenient procedure.

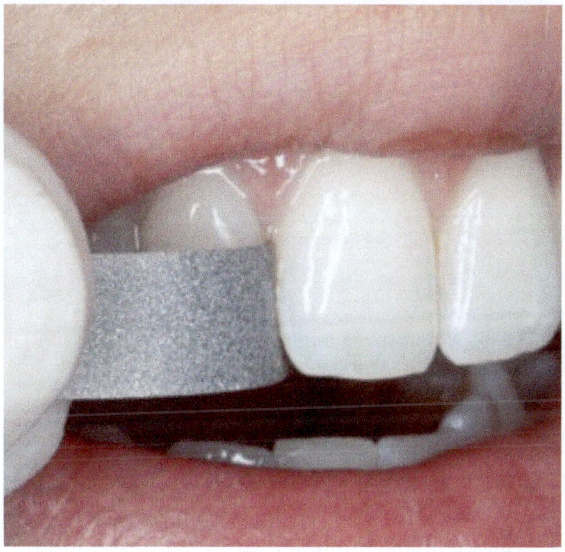

Fig. 12.3 A metal interproximal reduction strip is the most common type used.

Any IPR should be performed upon the practitioner's criteria, usually using any of the most common techniques:

- Manual diamond strip
  - Particularly effective for <0.2 mm IPR, mostly on anterior teeth
  - Start with the thinnest strip
  - Patient's gums should be protected with any retraction technique

---

2 Betteridge MA. The effects of interdental stripping on the labial segments. *Br J Orthod*. 1981;**8**:193–197.

3 Vanarsdall RL, Jr. Periodontal-orthodontic relationships. In: Graber TM, Vanarsdall RL JR, eds. *Orthodontics: Current Principles and Techniques*. 2000: pp. 801–838.

4 Zachrisson BU. Zachrisson on excellence finishing. Part I. *J Clin Orthod* 1986;**20**:460–482.

5 Craig G, Sheridan JJ. Susceptibility to caries and periodontal disease after posterior air-rotor stripping. *J Clin Orthod*. 1990;**24**:84–85.

6 Sheridan JJ, Ledoux PM. Air rotor stripping and proximal sealants: an SEM evaluation. *J Clin Orthod*. 1989;**23**:790–794.

- Slow speed diamond disk
  - First break tight contacts using diamond strips
  - To isolate, use interproximal wedges to loosen contacts
  - Patient's soft tissues can be protected using a dental mirror
- High speed bur
  - Suggested for 0.5 mm IPR
  - To isolate, use interproximal wedges to loosen contacts
  - Be careful around cervical regions to avoid ledges
  - Use water spray to reduce clogging and overheating

(a) (b)

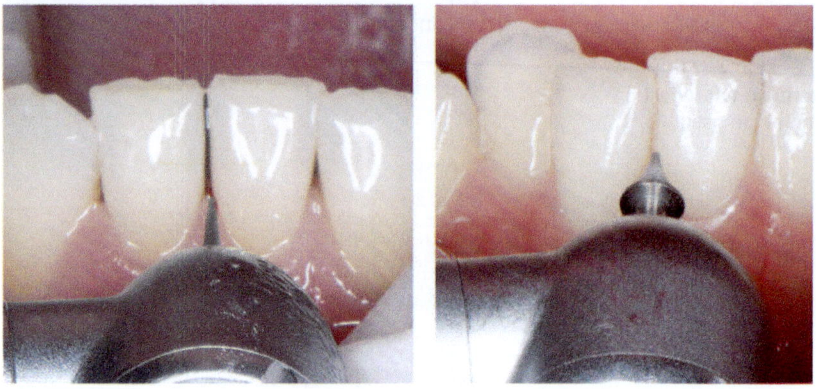

Fig. 12.4 A high-speed bur interproximal reduction (IPR) is suggested for 0. 5mm IPR, using both interproximal bur (a) and (b) edge rounding.

- Oscillating technique
  - Single/double-sided disks used in conjunction with oscillating hand pieces for enamel reduction
  - Start with the thinnest disk
  - Use water spray

Suggested IPR Protocol

Anterior IPR:

- <0.4 mm: oscillating technique
- >0.4 mm: diamond disk + oscillating technique

Posterior IPR:

- <0.4 mm: oscillating technique
- >0.4 mm: diamond bur + oscillating technique

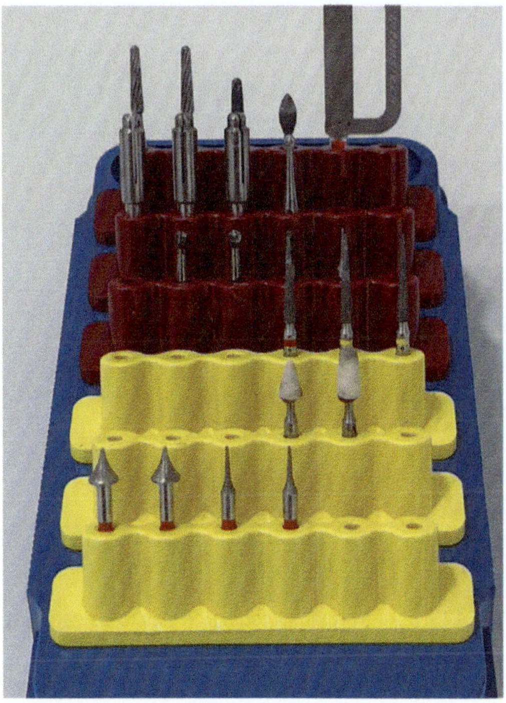

Fig. 12.5 Interproximal reduction and attachments removal bur set is ideal for an Invisalign practice.

Suggested IPR Procedure

- Check space between teeth to decide if IPR is required
- Check that the clinical situation is equal to the ClinCheck
- If the space is less than 0.4 mm, protect soft tissue with wet jet. Use 0.15 mm metal strip (both sides) to break the contact point. After breaking the contact point with this strip, use the oscillating technique from thinner to thickest until the desired measurement is achieved.
- If the IPR is more than 0.4 mm, rotatory instruments are necessary:
  - Use drill with a high-speed bur for posterior teeth
  - Contra-angle with diamond disk for anterior teeth, while always protecting the soft tissue
- Measure with gauges. Do not use pressure to insert the gauge. After 3 minutes, check it again as the resilience of the periodontal tissue can tend to close this space again.
- Polish and verify: polish with a polishing strip, apply fluoride varnish to prevent sensibility and note down in the patient file the amount of IPR done.

  In our clinical template we register:

- IPR, at what stage of treatment this has to be done and between which teeth
- When we have to begin using elastics
- If we need to use any extra auxiliary techniques and at what stages
- If any attachment appears or disappears during the treatment
- Note potential problem teeth (the chief complaint of the patient and the black movement of the ClinCheck)
- The number of aligner we are on, and the next appointment with us

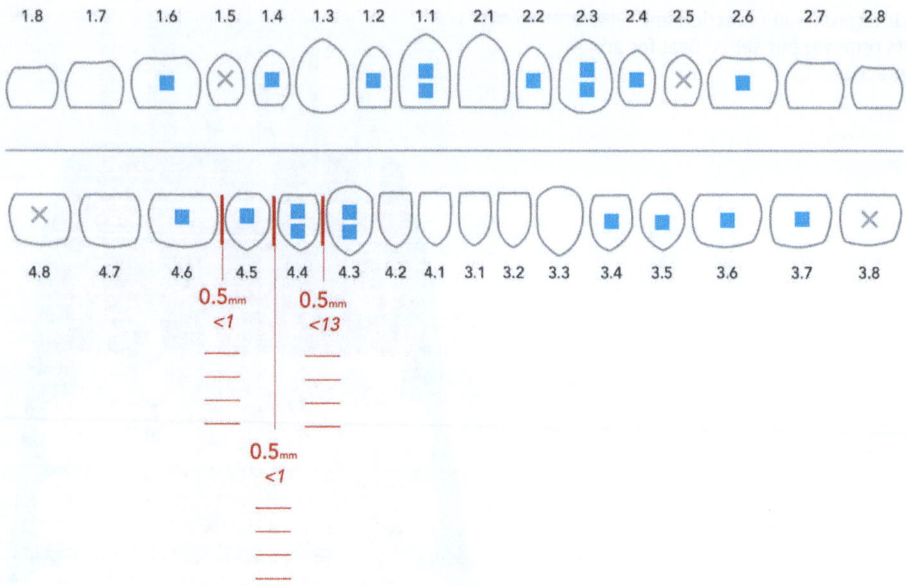

Fig. 12.6 Interproximal reduction has to be carefully planned and performed.

13

Digital Workflow

With any orthodontic technique, as with clear aligners, records routinely include study casts, intraoral and extraoral photographs, and panoramic and lateral cephalometric radiographs.

Additional diagnostic records may include a 3D cone beam computed tomography (CBCT) scan, periapical radiographs and any other diagnostic records necessary to begin the case.

One of the main advantages with clear aligners is that the whole procedure can be performed digitally, tracking every single movement and it is possible to 'time lapse' it.

13.1 Records

13.1.1 Photographs

Extraoral

Extraoral pictures should be taken with the following parameters on your camera:

- Manual mode
- F5.6
- 1/125
- ISO 100
- Flash ¼ (ring flash is strongly advised)

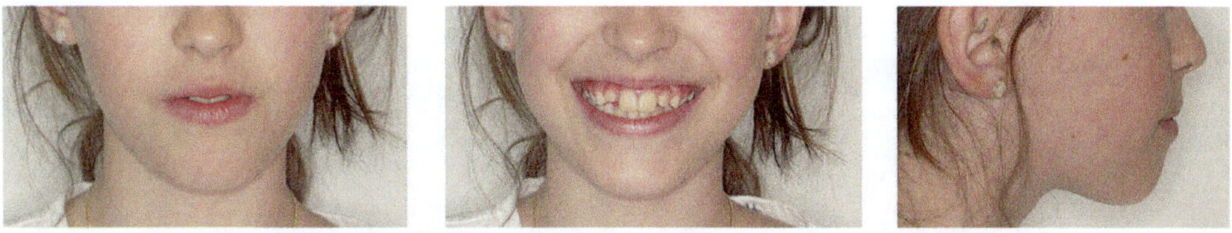

Fig. 13.1 Frontal, smile and lateral photographs.

A plain white background is recommended to avoid distortion on the images.

Intraoral

Lateral pictures must be exactly at 90 degrees: if lateral photos with any other angulation are sent, it will not be possible to check if the technician has set the occlusion for the real patient situation.

Aligner Techniques in Orthodontics, First Edition. Susana Palma Moya and Javier Lozano Zafra.

Companion website: www.wiley.com/go/lozano-zafra/aligner-techniques

For this, note that 'teeth' will be set up by the system with the pictures, so a poor quality picture might lead to a 'false' initial occlusion and, if this was not identified from the very beginning, it would lead to a 'false' or inappropriate treatment plan.

(a) (b)

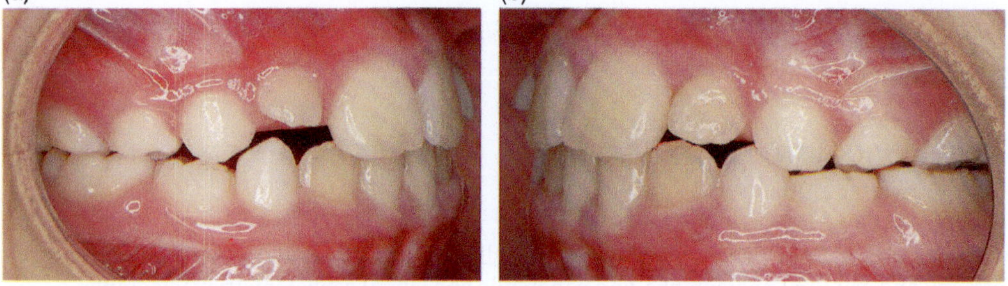

Fig. 13.2 90 degree pictures are mandatory both in right (a) and left (b) intraoral views.

It is important to send an overjet photograph. In the intraoral frontal view, it is also possible to check the upper and lower midlines.

(a) (b)

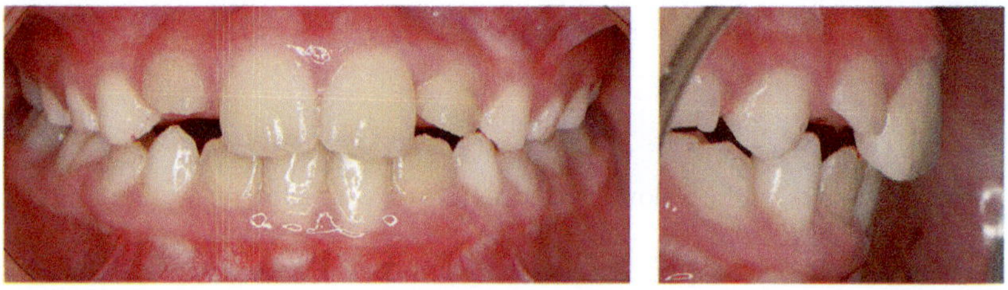

Fig. 13.3 Intraoral frontal (a) and overjet (b) pictures will help create a good treatment plan.

Occlusal photographs must be sent with articulating paper marks to assist the technician in setting up the initial occlusion.

(a) (b)

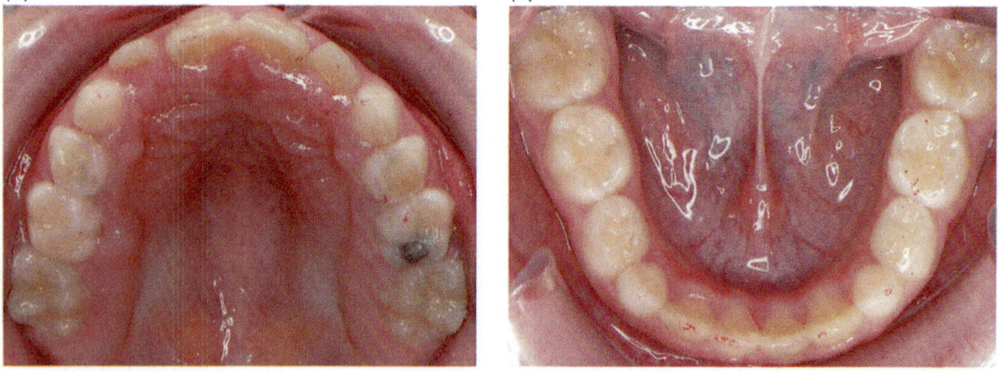

Fig. 13.4 Blue or red ink on both upper (a) and lower (b) occlusal pictures will help in setting up initial occlusion.

13.1.2 Impressions: PVS vs Scan

PVS Impressions

Flexitime or Aquasil Ultra are the materials recommended for PVS impressions. It is important also not to use latex gloves to mix the PVS material, as they might interfere with its properties, and to follow the manufacturers' instructions in regards to the working time of the product.

Choose the size of the tray carefully: in case of doubt, choose a bigger one and check that the third molars are included in the tray.

The impression has to be made in two stages: first the heavy material and second the light material.

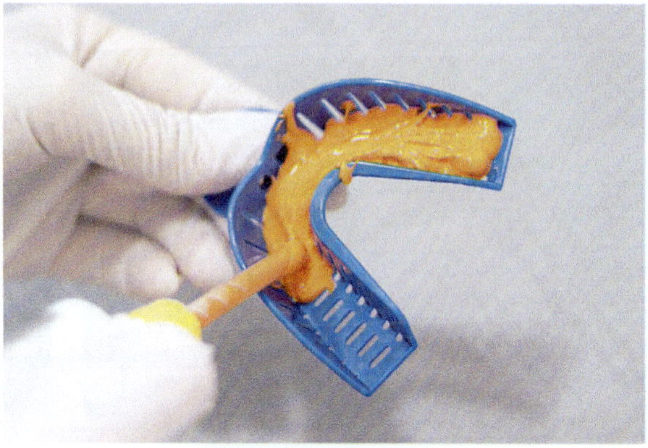

Fig. 13.5 Polyvinyl siloxane (PVS) material placement.

Procedure:

- Mix the PVS material with vinyl gloves (do not use latex)
- Place a small amount of PVS material in the tray's posterior zone
- Insert the tray and press slightly in the molar zone, use a smooth movement

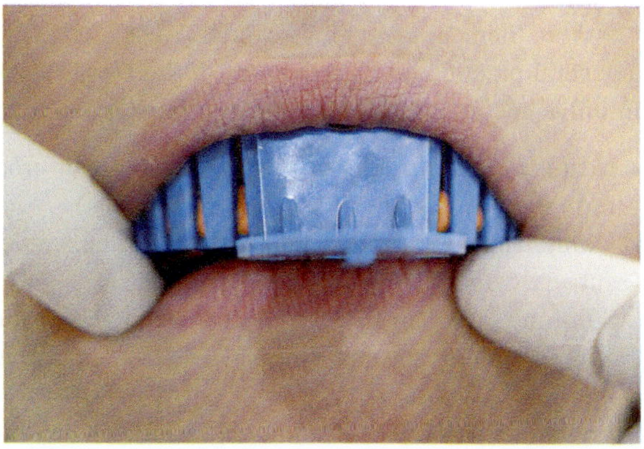

Fig. 13.6 Inserting tray with polyvinyl siloxane (PVS) material into the patient's mouth.

- Remove the tray immediately and exert pressure on the PVS material to open space for the light PVS silicon.

- Fill the tray with light silicon.
- Insert the tray into the mouth, it must be inserted from back to front in the upper arch and from front to back in the lower arch. Do it slowly to allow air to escape.
- Maintain the tray with no movement until the setting time is over.

A perfect impression is one in which the heavy PVS cannot or can only just be seen, and where we can visualize all the teeth, including the distal part of the second molars; 1–2 mm of gum should also be observed.

As a result of Align's efforts and investment in research and development, digital detailing is now available to us, which is something that is not available with impressions for lingual appliances, for example, but nevertheless it is still essential to take a really good impression in order to achieve a great digital model.

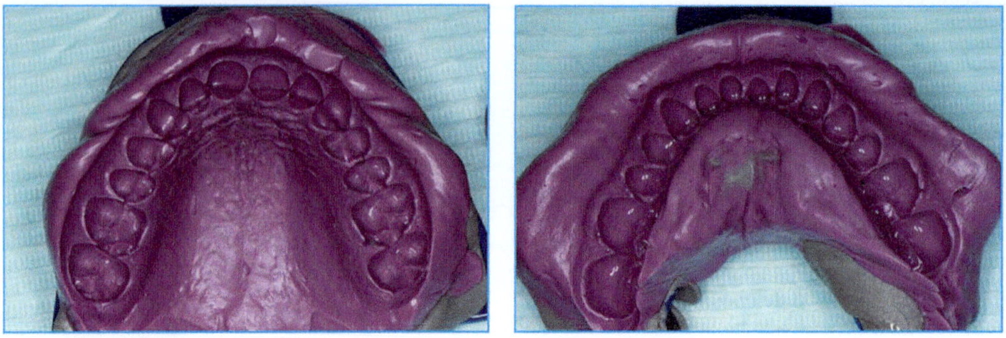

Fig. 13.7 Upper (left) and lower (right) impressions. Source: Images from Align Technology database.

Shipping boxes on the IDS Webstore, which will be delivered free of charge to the practice will need to be ordered to send PVS impressions. The impressions and patient prescription are placed in these boxes and sent to Invisalign, and instructions for this are provided inside the boxes.

iTero Scan

The iTero Element 2 Intraoral Scanner is designed to fit in practice even better than before. Whether a general practitioner or orthodontist, the iTero Element is designed to deliver speed, reliability, intuitive operations and outstanding visualization capabilities that include:

- Next-generation processor giving reduced scan processing and a faster start-up time (can perform a full arch scan in as little as 60 seconds)
- Uninterrupted scanning: long-lasting, rechargeable battery for easy mobility from surgery to surgery without plugging in or rebooting
- Stunning colour imaging: enhanced colour offers a more thorough look at the patient's oral health
- High-definition visuals: slim, 21.5-inch monitor with 16:9 widescreen viewing format and improved resolution for highly detailed images
- Ergonomic wand placement: designed with a centre-mounted wand cradle for easy ergonomics during scanning
- Smarter scanning: improved wand touchpad is as intuitive as gesturing on a smartphone: the touchpad can be used to switch between scanning segments or rotate the model on screen

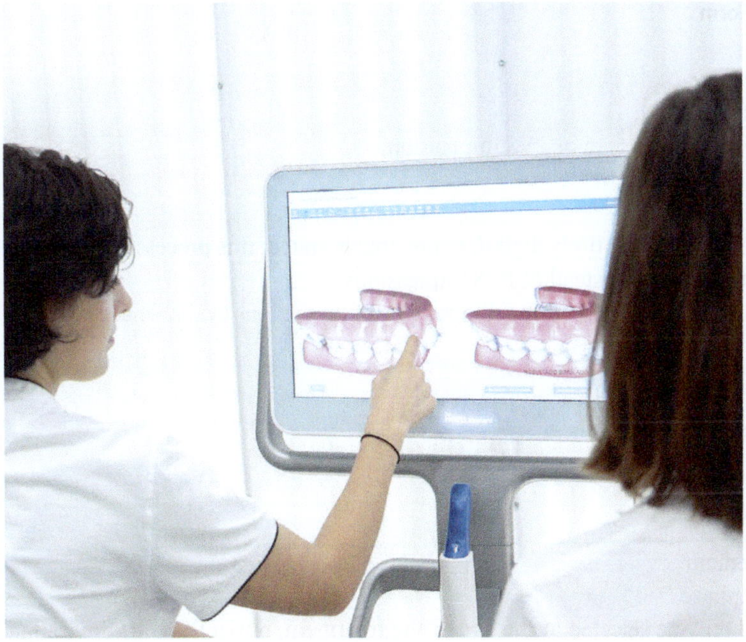

Fig. 13.8 iTero scanner has several advantages, such as the Outcome Simulator.

X-rays

It is recommended that, as a minimum, both panoramic and lateral radiographs are submitted.

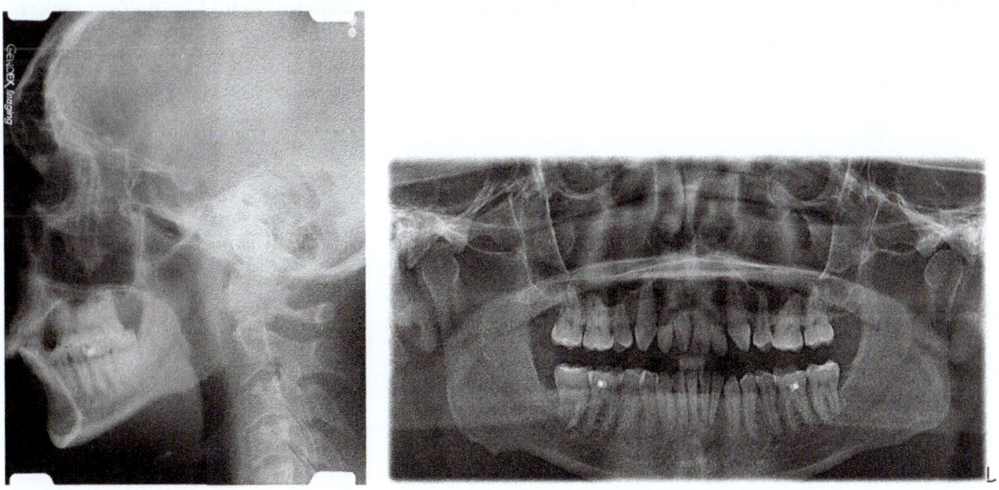

Fig. 13.9 Lateral and panoramic X-rays.

13.2 Creating a New Patient Record

To create a new patient record, the facial and intraoral photographs and the X-rays need to be uploaded. This, together with the patient data: name, surname, date of birth will create a unique profile on the Invisalign Practitioner Site.

Submitting a Prescription Form

- Create a patient
- Take patient's records
- Complete prescription form
- Package records: photos and iTero scan or PVS impression

Prescription Form

From this moment on, the process is entirely digital, as previously stated, this process can be 100% fully digital if a iTero scanner is used instead of PVS impressions.

After adding a new patient, select between the different treatments plans available according to the patient profile, choosing between:

- Adult (20 years or older)
- Teenager (13 to 19 years)
- Growing (6 to 12 years)

Next, select a product type:

- Aligners, for active treatment
- Retainers, for retention phase
- 'Vivera retainers' would only be selected at the end of the treatment, but at the start 'Invisalign Clear Aligners' will always be selected, which provides us with the following treatment options:
- Comprehensive, for a complex malocclusion
- 'Lite', for a simple treatment
- Express, for a relapse or really simple treatment

Finally, the prescription form needs to be filled in step by step depending on the malocclusion of the patient. How to fill in the prescription form is explained for every space plane at the beginning of each chapter.

14

ClinCheck Software

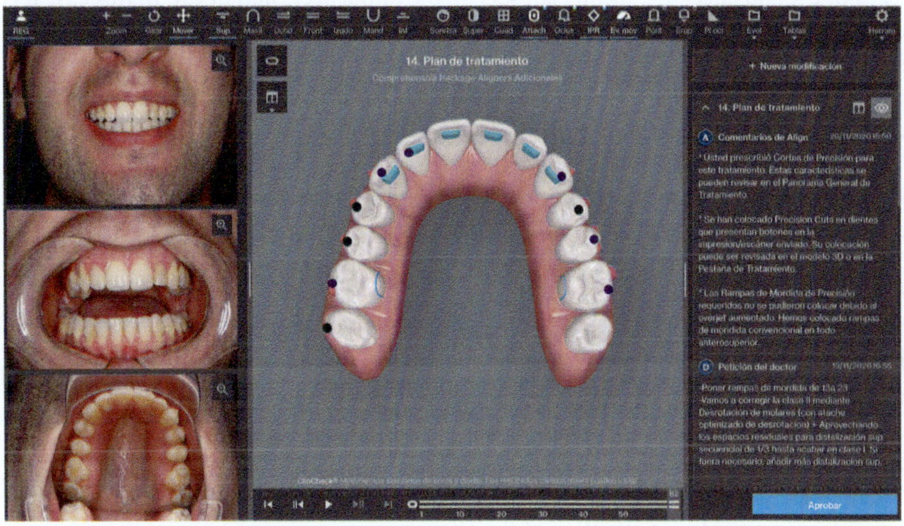

Fig. 14.1 ClinCheck software on-screen.

After the clinician sends the patient's records, diagnoses the malocclusion, formulates a treatment plan and fills in the prescription form, this is communicated to the technician.

Using this data, the software generates a simulation of the tooth movements into the final occlusion that will have to be reviewed by the practitioner to ensure the best orthodontic goals and sequences.

14.1 The Perfect ClinCheck Review in 10 Steps

1. Check initial occlusion
2. Review comments tab
3. Review the final position
4. Check the number of stages in treatment
5. Dynamic evaluation of the ClinCheck
   i. Simultaneous movements
   ii. Sequential movements
   iii. Reciprocal movements

Aligner Techniques in Orthodontics, First Edition. Susana Palma Moya and Javier Lozano Zafra.

Companion website: www.wiley.com/go/lozano-zafra/aligner-techniques

6. Check the superimposition tool
7. Review the Tooth Movement Assessment (TMA)
8. Review attachments
9. Review IPR
10. Review precision cuts

14.1.1 Check Initial Occlusion

Review the initial occlusion with the photographs sent to make sure the occlusion is set correctly. Note that you can send the bite registration if taking impressions, although it is not mandatory.

- If there is a discrepancy between centric occlusion (CR) and centric relation (CR), we must send every record in CR and check the technician sets up the initial occlusion in CR. In this case it is suggested that occlusal photographs be taken with articulating paper marks to assist the technician in setting up the initial occlusion.
- If the initial position in the ChinCheck is not the same as the initial position for the patient, ask the technician to set up the occlusion to the point of initial contact; sometimes new photographs may be required.
- Check the initial occlusion from all points of view: anterior view, right and left buccal views and the anterior overjet view. Check also if there is canting of the occlusal plane, as the initial position of the malocclusion must be set up with the same canting (for this purpose, the smiling photograph and the intraoral frontal are mandatory).
- Review the initial occlusion for incisors with gingival recession at the beginning (ask the technician not to procline and do the IPR in earlier stages to avoid round-tripping). In addition, check that the technician does not cover the enamel–cement line or maximum contour of the tooth with the gum recession.
- Look for implants in the initial occlusion, and check that those teeth do not move in the ClinCheck. In these cases, also ask the technician to cut the gingival margin 3 mm towards the occlusal in order to prevent over-retention of the aligner.

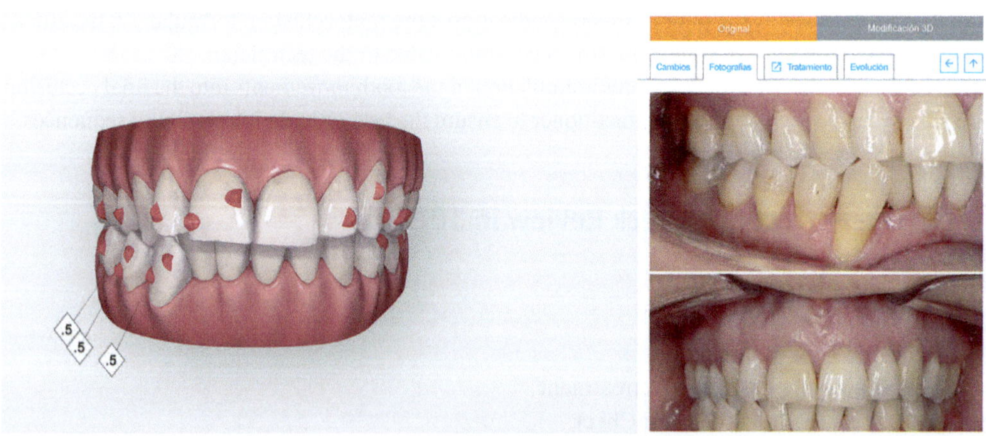

Fig. 14.2 Compare ClinCheck with pictures on the same plane before you start planning the case.

14.1.2 Review Comments Tab

This is the tab where the technician communicates with the practitioner. This tab may include:

- Problems with the impressions or the scan: for example if, due to soft tissue, the most distal teeth have not been included in the appliance. In this case, the clinician will have to decide whether to take new impressions/scan or surgically remove the soft tissue to enable a better registration of the distal teeth.

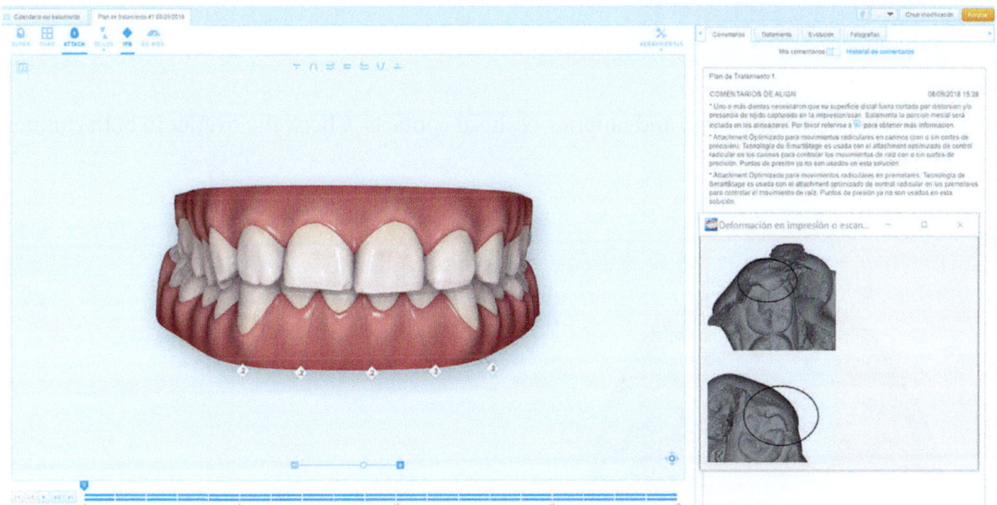

Fig. 14.3 Distortions of the impression might affect aligner coverage, so it is important to pay attention to technician comments about this.

- A request for further instructions in order to solve the malocclusion. For example, if the clinician asked to correct the class II, but did not indicate how (e.g. by upper distalization, lower mesialization, mandibular advancement or posterior IPR) the technician might ask for further instructions to achieve the final goal. It is therefore really important to provide these, as practitioner's treatment plan is the key to a positive treatment outcome.
- Comments on attachment and precision cuts placement.

14.1.3 Review the Final Position

The final occlusion setup should be checked to see if the occlusion meets the treatment goals. The panoramic X-ray should also be checked at this time to ensure that all pretreatment root inclinations have been corrected in the final occlusion.

Views that have to be evaluated:

- Anterior view: check midlines, crown tipping of the incisors, aesthetic alignment, overbite, arch form and buccal corridors

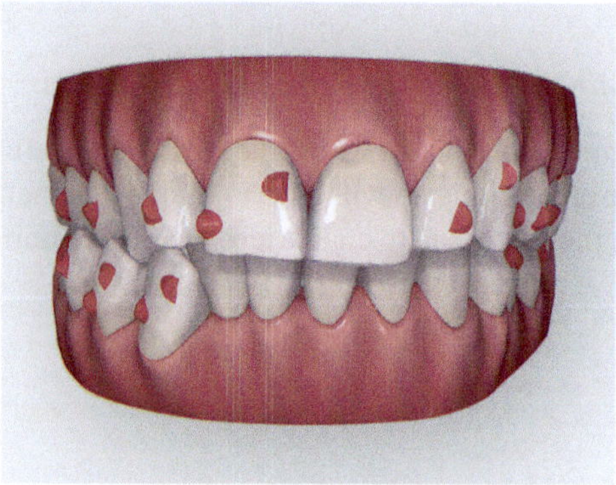

Fig. 14.4 Anterior view.

- Overjet view: anterior overjet and anterior occlusal contacts. Check the overjet in both canines is the same

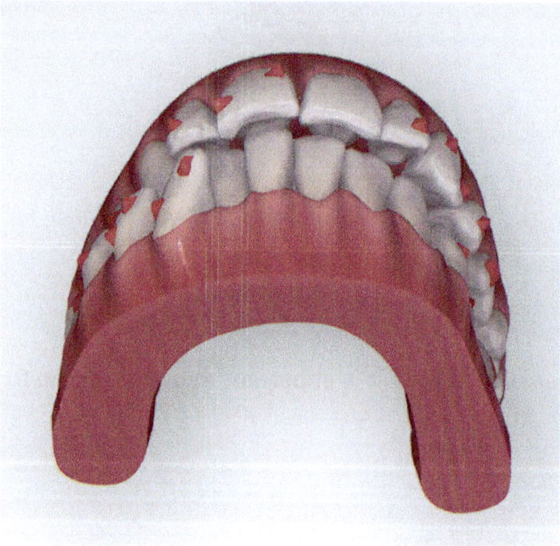

Fig. 14.5 Overjet view.

- Buccal right and left view: review the incisor torque, the interincisal angle, canine and molar relationships right and left, buccal interdigitation

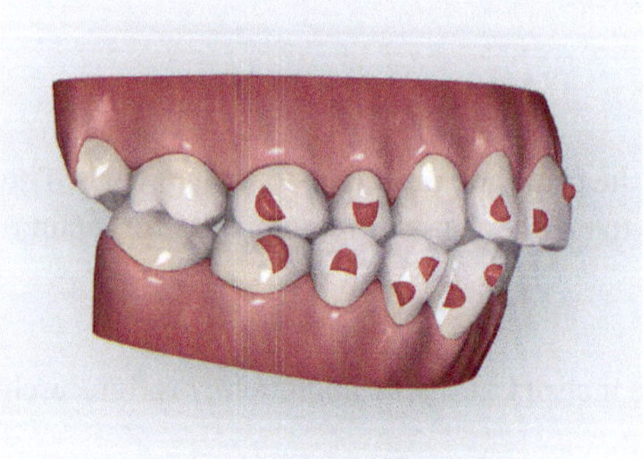

Fig. 14.6 Buccal right view.

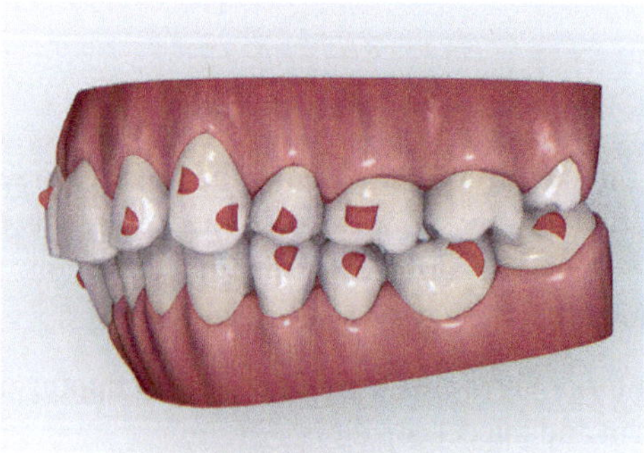

Fig. 14.7 Buccal left view.

- Occlusal views (maxillary and mandibular): symmetry of the arches, arch form, alignment, marginal ridges and central fossae

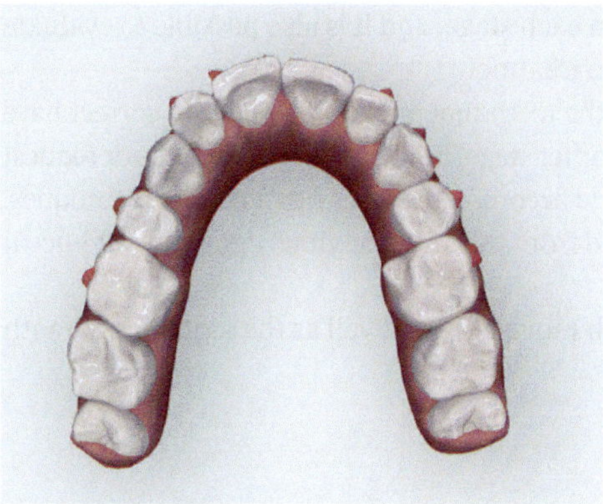

Fig. 14.8 Occlusal view: maxillary.

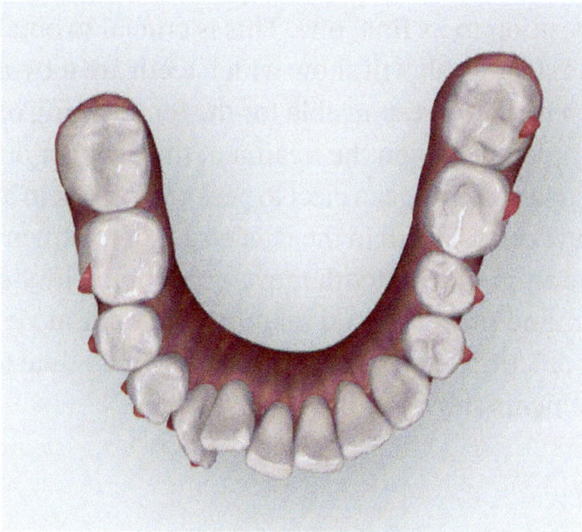

Fig. 14.9 Occlusal view: mandibular.

- Posterior view: cup-to-fossa relationships, buccolingual torque of posterior teeth

Fig. 14.10 *Posterior view.*

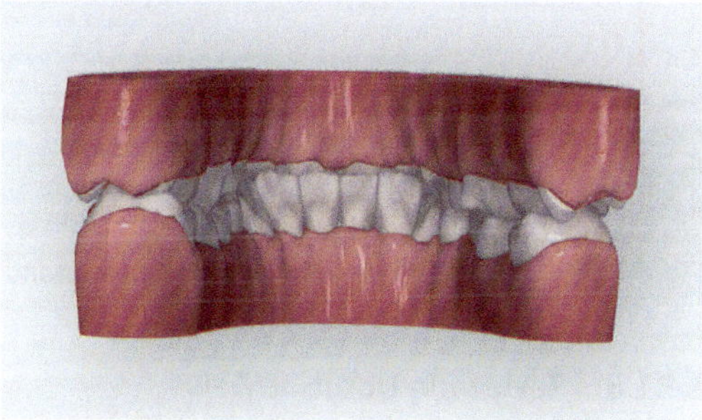

14.1.4 Check the Number of Stages in Treatment

The number of stages of active and passive treatment is indicated on a bar at the bottom of the screen (Fig. 14.11). Colours define characteristics of the aligners:

- Active aligners are represented in blue
- Passive aligners are light blue
- Overcorrection aligners are brown

If the correction of the malocclusion depends on the use of elastics, we must ensure that there are enough aligners to achieve the correction of the malocclusion (this topic will be covered in Chapter 20).

If the correction of the malocclusion depends on mandibular advancement (MA), we must ensure that we have at least 25–30 stages of the advancement phase so the malocclusion can be resolved.

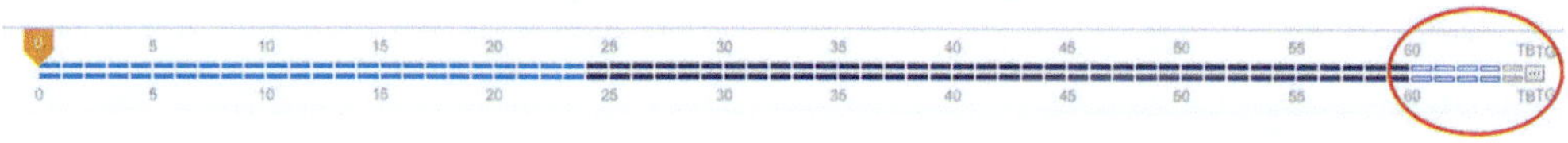

Fig. 14.11 Mandibular advancement.

14.1.5 Dynamic Evaluation of the ClinCheck

This phase is essential: hit the play button and check each tooth movement carefully from the initial position to its final one. This is crucial to obtaining a predictable treatment result.

The staging tab will show which teeth are moving in each stage, and it is also possible to evaluate which teeth are responsible for the lengthening of the treatment.

In order to shorten the treatment time further once the teeth that are taking longer to correct have been addressed, we can elect to perform the IPR in an earlier stage, limit certain movements or request to move certain teeth in the later stages of treatment, and accompany these with auxiliary techniques.

The animation of tooth movement should be viewed from the anterior view, right and left buccal views, and maxillary and mandibular occlusal views.

As practitioners, we must assess the individual tooth movements as well as the sequence of tooth movements shown in the staging tab.

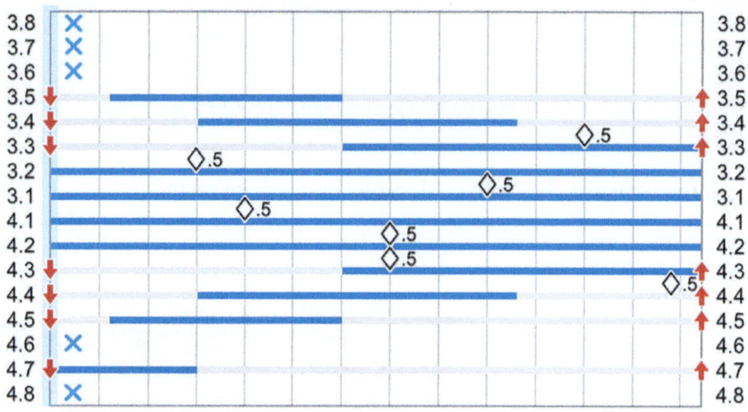

Fig. 14.12 Treatment overview helps us understand general structure of the treatment plan.

14.1.6 Reviewing Occlusal Views

When starting to review occlusal views:

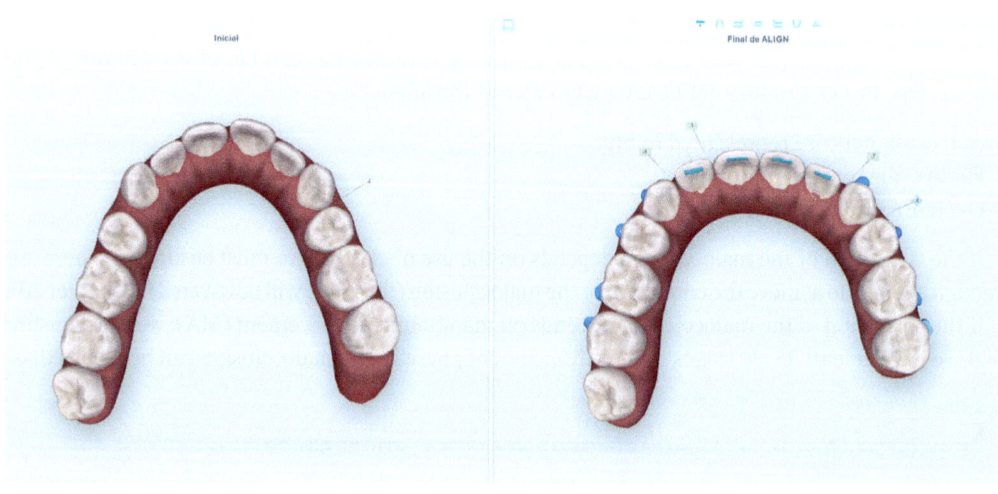

Fig. 14.13 Reviewing occlusal views.

- Decide whether a symmetric or an asymmetric expansion is going to be performed.
- Proclination: establish anteroposterior limit of the proclination depending on the periodontal tissue and the initial position of the incisors.
- Do not move teeth which have no space to be moved. Take special care with lateral incisors and second premolars in lingual positions: first, create enough mesio-distal space, then move them to their ideal position. Teeth require space to move, if there is not enough space, then teeth will collide with adjacent teeth and tooth movement may not be fully expressed. Delay the movement of a lingually displaced tooth until after space has been provided.
- *Anchorage attachments*, consider what attachment is needed to solve the malocclusion. For example, to level the curve of Spee, anchorage attachments distal to the incisors are needed in order to intrude them.
- Differential anchorage: analysis of the force vectors.

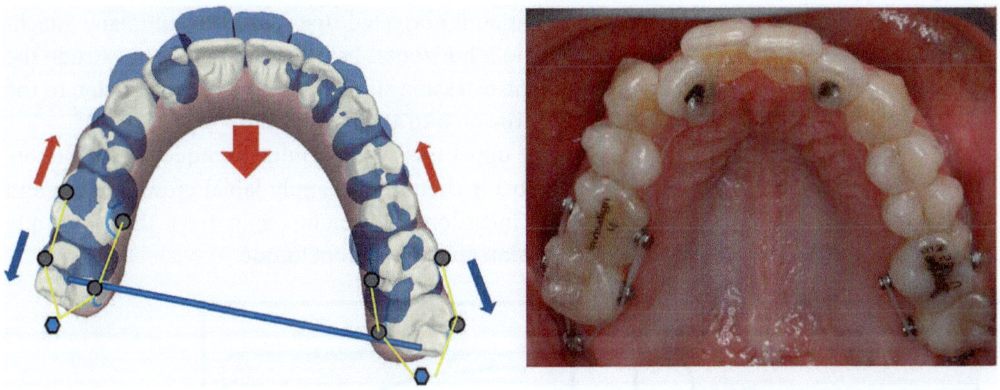

Fig. 14.14 Analysis of the force vectors: in simultaneous distalization, if all teeth are moving simultaneously to distal, additional anchorage can be planned, for example temporary anchorage devices in the tuberosity.

Simultaneous Movements

These are movements that the ClinCheck software plans simultaneously with potential issue for misfitting, as they are part of previously proven protocols that allow the overlapping of several movements at the same time:

- Expansion + incisor retraction: can ask for expansion and reduction of the arch length simultaneously (in this way, both movements can be enhanced)
- Expansion + correction of rotated teeth (canines, premolars and molars)
- Movement of incisors in class II (intrusion, retrusion and lingual root torque)

Sequential Movements

These are movements that should not be done at the same time or they will create tracking problems. A thorough examination of the staging of movements in the ClinCheck must be made, while being alert to the fact that some of these movements may create problems of maladjustment in the aligner during the treatment.

- 'En masse' expansion and proclination: If the expansion is not produced by changing torque but by body expansion, the proclination and the expansion must not be done at the same time. First expand and then protrude.

- Expansion vs distalization: It is difficult to execute tooth movements in two planes of space simultaneously, for example, in a clinical situation where there is a posterior crossbite, it becomes more difficult to correct the crossbite in the event that distalization is also required. In this case, the crossbite could be corrected in the initial stages in order to move teeth to the sponge bone using criss-cross elastics and expansion before starting distalization.
- Asymmetric expansion: if there is differential torque in both sides of the arch, the side with normal torque should not be moved until the contralateral side is corrected. In this way, the side with normal torque is used as an anchorage and flaring of the posterior molars prevented (with a labial tipping of the crown in the final occlusion).
- Class II subdivision: use the side in class I as an anchorage to correct the side in class II; once you have a bilateral class I, continue moving both sides simultaneously.
- Rotation and extrusion of upper lateral incisor: even though the multiplane attachment is designed to provide a vertical correction in the lateral incisors at the same time that the rotation is corrected, it is recommended that the rotation is corrected first with the multiplane attachment and after that change the attachment to a horizontal bevelled to gingival to extrude the incisor. Whenever possible, aim to perform the extrusion simultaneously to the retrusion of the upper incisor in order to turn an absolute extrusion into a relative one.
- Deep bite correction with negative torque of upper incisors: the lingual torque of the incisors needs be corrected before attempting to intrude them. First, apply labial crown torque and then ask the technician to perform the intrusion movements to correct the deep bite using pressure areas and finally ask for retrusion and lingual root torque.

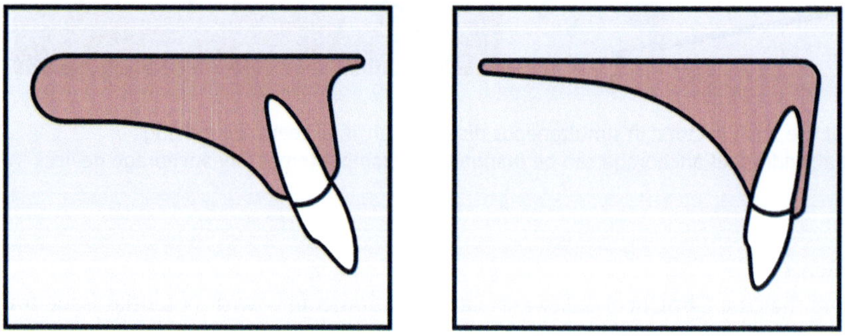

Fig. 14.15 Anterior positive torque (left) allows pure intrusion to resolve a deep bite, while a negative one (right) forces us to correct it before intrusion.

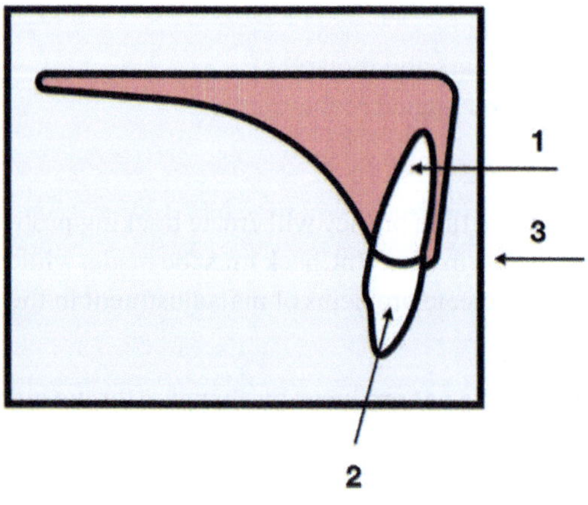

Fig. 14.16 The sequence will always be based on three steps: (1) procline incisors/retrocline root, (2) intrude and (3) retrude.

Rotation + Tipping Movement on Incisors In this clinical situation, the tooth position should be corrected during the anteroposterior movement, asking the technician for round tripping movement of the incisors.

Movements of the same tooth in different planes of space might be difficult with the aligners if they are not sequenced. As an example, for a 1.1 rotated mesial-in and with distal tipping of the crown ask the technician:

- First: to rotate 1.1 mesial-out simultaneously to proclination
- Second: for IPR to make space for the retraction movement in between lateral and central incisor
- Third: for intrusion + retrusion, applying a 10 degree mesial-tipping of the crown + distal-in rotation

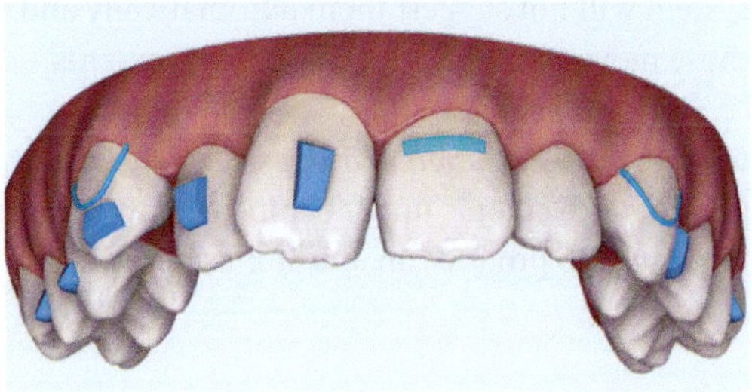

Fig. 14.17 Staging is mandatory to help in achieving desired final position.

One needs to be especially careful with uneven intrusion of maxillary central incisors during the treatment and review the ClinCheck stage by stage to verify tooth positions in the interim stages. To maintain level incisal edges throughout treatment it is important to request that both maxillary central incisors have to be moved together and that even incisal edges be maintained through the various stages of tooth movement.

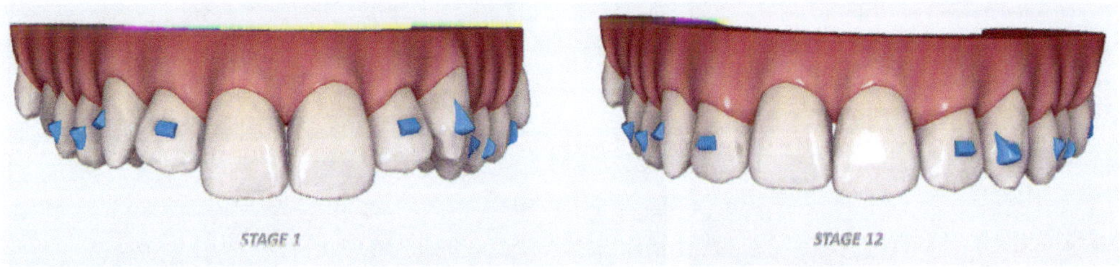

Fig. 14.18 Checking every stage on anterior sector will prevent from unaesthetic situations.

Rotation + Tipping Movement on Canines As with the incisors, these two movements done in a simultaneous way can end in maladjustment of the aligner and fitting problem in the canines. In order to make both movement predictable we must sequence the movements:

- First: rotate distal-out simultaneously to expansion labial crown torque of the canine
- Second: IPR between lateral incisor and canine of 0.3 mm to make space for the mesial-in rotation
- Third: rotate mesial-in simultaneously to 10 degrees tipping root to mesial and tipping crown to distal

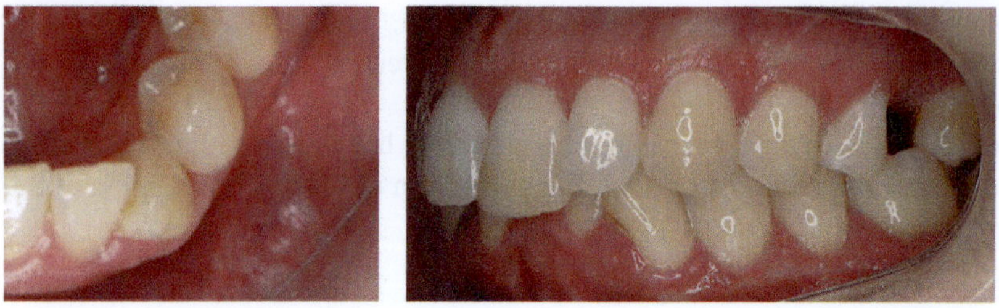

Fig. 14.19 Round tooth rotations (canines and premolars) require perfectly staged movements.

Reciprocal Movements

These are movements that can be carried out simultaneously in order to increase effectiveness. The system will not suggest them automatically and will rely on the clinicians' preferences. We refer to these movements as antagonistic movements.

Upper Canine Extrusion and Upper Lateral Intrusion It is common to find a number of cases that present with ectopic upper canines that have erupted high in the gum and extruded lateral incisors that erupt to produce an anterior crossbite.

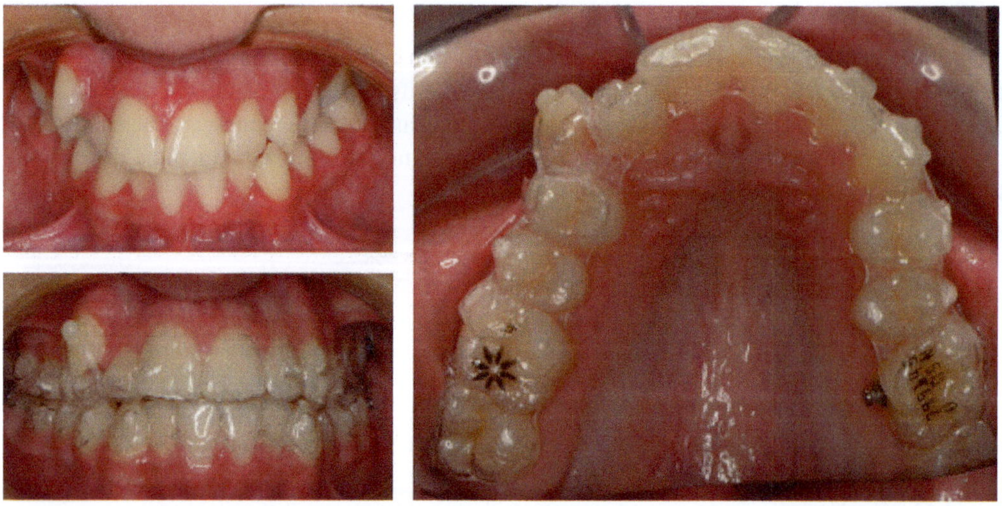

Fig. 14.20 Ask the technician to perform the extrusion of the canine simultaneously to the intrusion of the lateral. Provided that the space has already opened up to allow for these movements, this will help to make both vertical movements more predictable.

***Molar Compression Simultaneously with Incisor* Protrusion** This is very useful to correct anterior crossbites. This is also known as the 'pearl necklace' effect: if a pearl necklace is placed on a table and the posterior zone compressed, the anterior zone will move forward. This is exactly what happens with the incisors when the premolars and molars are compressed using the aligners.

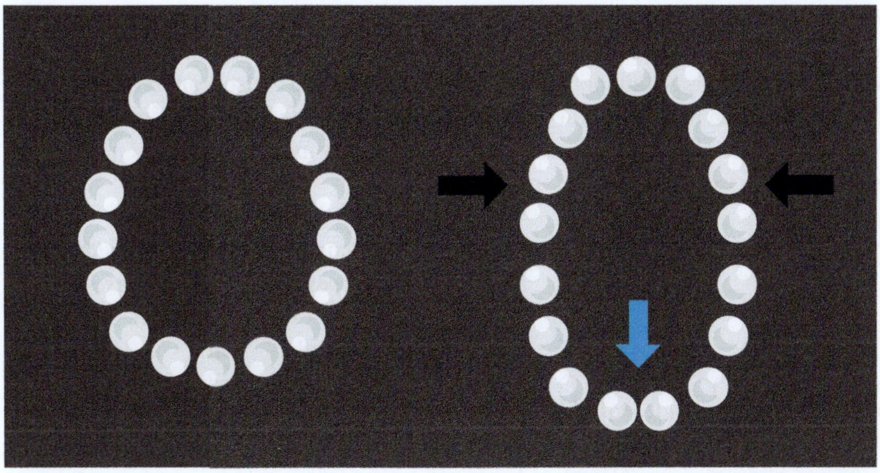

Fig. 14.21 The pearl necklace effect explains how to use these mechanics in order to shorten the length of treatment.

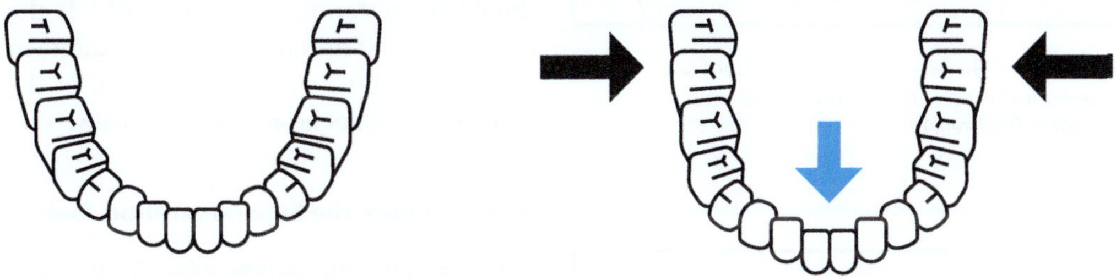

Fig. 14.22 Simultaneous expansion for reduction in arch length (incisor retrusion).

These movements together are highly predictable and are favourable to correct an open bite.

In the same way as before, if the premolars and molars are expanded (opening the pearl necklace in the posterior zone), the incisors will automatically naturally move backwards into a more retruded position. If the technician is asked to perform those movements at the same time, the expansion will be much more effective.

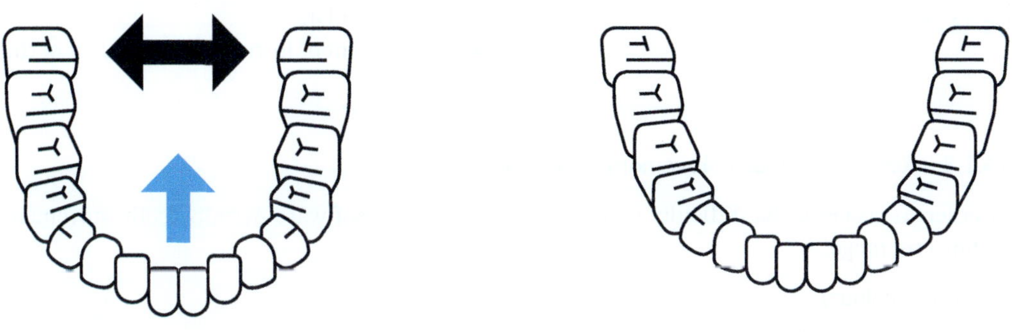

Fig. 14.23 Expansion leads to arch depth loss and anterior retraction.

Simultaneous Molar Mesialization with IPR and Incisor Retraction Mesialization of the molars and premolars is a less predictable movement with aligners than distalization. For this reason, in order to make it more effective, the loss of anchorage that happens when the incisors are retruded needs to be used. By performing both movements at the same time it is possible to achieve a more effective posterior mesialization especially, if previously to this simultaneous movement, extra anchorage is achieved by relating the incisors root to the cortical bone.

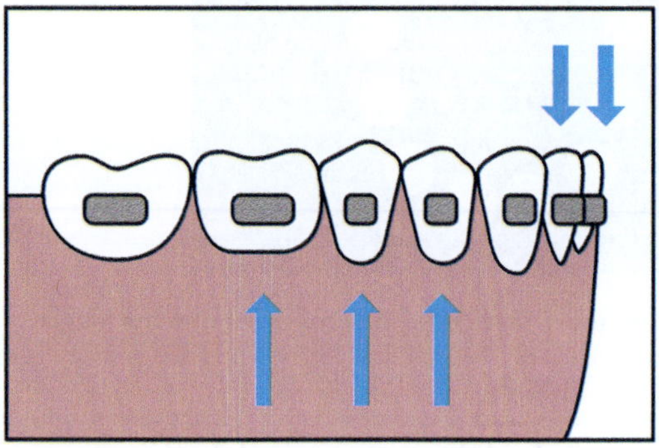

Fig. 14.24 Whenever possible, simultaneous anterior intrusion and posterior extrusion enhances final result.

Centre Upper and Lower Midlines Simultaneously with Anteroposterior Movements During proclination or during incisors retraction midline correction with a transversal movement will not be predictable.

Simultaneous Extrusion of the Premolars with Intrusion of the Incisors (in Growing Patients with a Hypodivergent Skeletal Pattern) In order to level the curve of Spee, these movements should be performed simultaneously. If the ClinCheck first intrudes the incisor and then extrudes the premolars, the extrusion of the premolars will not be achieved clinically.

14.1.7 Check the Superimposition Tool

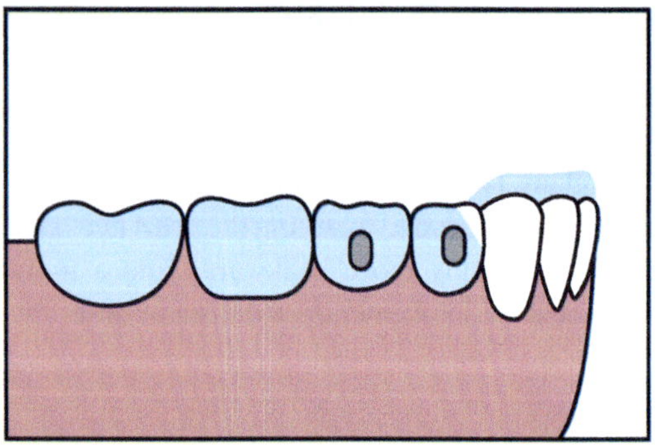

Fig. 14.25 Superimposition tool.

With the superimposition tool, the pretreatment situation can be compared with the post-treatment position of each tooth. In this way it is possible to check:

- The total amount of proclination or retraction of upper and lower incisors
- The amount of expansion
- The round tripping of each tooth during the treatment
- The amount of distalization or mesialization of the molars
- The amount of intrusion or extrusion of the incisors

14.1.8 Review the Tooth Movement Assessment

In order to visualize the difficulty of tooth movements, the software permits tooth movement within a set range:

- Easy (no colour)
- Moderate (blue dot)
- Advanced (black dot: which means the practitioner should plan to use auxiliary techniques in order to improve the predictability of the movement)

When clicking on the TMA tool these colours will show us the range of difficulty for intrusion, extrusion, rotation and root movements.

If some teeth fall into the advanced category, the clinician can choose between reducing those movements, adding attachments to make them more predictable or the use of auxiliary techniques.

Practitioners should focus on designing tooth movements in the ClinCheck that fall within the easy to moderate TMA range to make the treatment more predictable.

For this, practitioner should redesign the ClinCheck plan towards easier tooth movements. For example, the extrusion of the maxillary second molar and intrusion of the mandibular second molar are advanced tooth movements with aligners; if the maxillary second molar extrudes but the mandibular second molar fails to intrude, this will result in a prematurity in the posterior occlusion, resulting in a buccal open bite. The way to make an easier and more predictable treatment plan would be by modifying the plan to extrude the maxillary second molar and intrude the mandibular second molar to a lesser degree thereby moving them into the easy movement range and increasing predictability.

The practitioner can also make difficult tooth movements more predictable by using auxiliary techniques such as buttons and elastics, segmental fixed appliances, class II or class III elastics, TADs, etc. For example, in the case of a second upper molar that has erupted buccally, a resin stop can be used on the occlusal surface of the aligner to disocclude the teeth and an elastic used to correct the scissor bite.

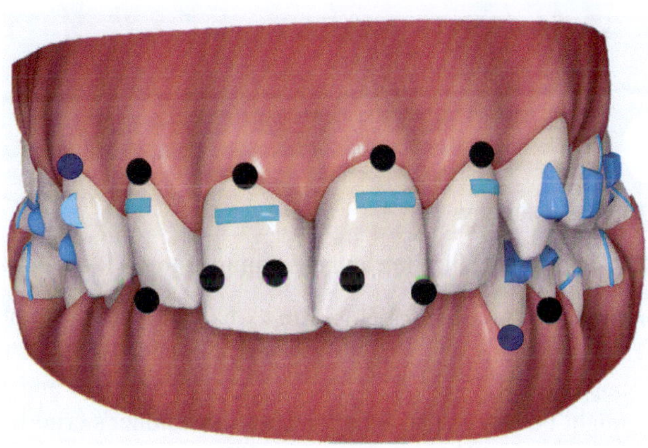

Fig. 14.26 Black dots indicate complex movements.

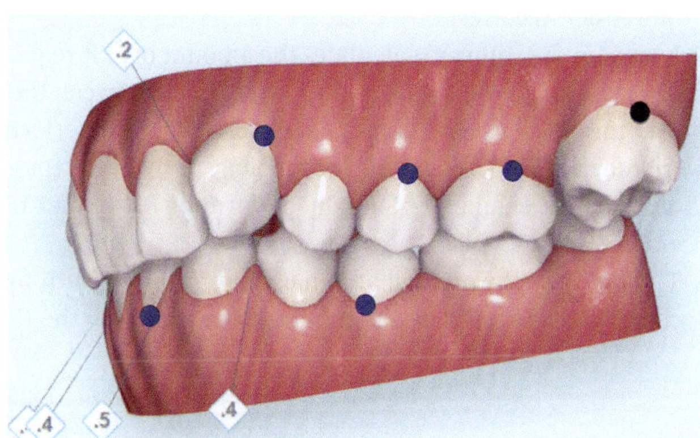

Fig. 14.27 Blue dots indicate moderate movements.

14.1.9 Review Attachments

The software will automatically place the required attachments when performing movements of intrusion, rotation and crown tipping. Tooth movements on the molars and mandibular incisors need to be evaluated to check whether any attachments are necessary.

Situations where the software will not place the attachment automatically are:

- Horizontal attachments bevelled to gingival or occlusal on premolars and molars in cases with severe expansion, in order to maintain the labial root torque and prevent the labial tipping of the molar crowns after the expansion
- The use of rectangular attachments in cases with short crowns to increase the retention of the aligners in anteroposterior movements
- Attachments for anchorage, like the ones required in deep bite cases on the premolars

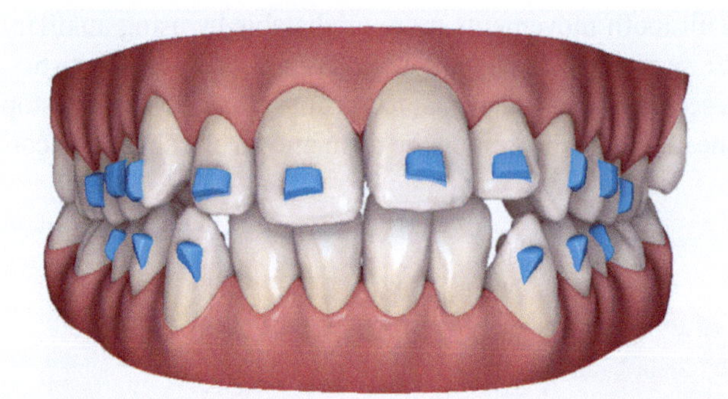

Fig. 14.28 Attachments.

14.1.10 Review IPR

The amount, the location and the timing of the IPR needs to be carefully reviewed.

- Amount: In young patients, aim to make the treatment plan without or with minimal IPR. For older patients with black triangles, especially those with periodontal problems, in order to approximate the roots at the end of the treatment and reduce the black triangles, more IPR might be prescribed, depending on practitioner's criteria. Open bites with maxillomandibular protrusion will benefit from more IPR; conversely, deep bite cases will benefit from less IPR, by allowing more proclination of the incisors, generating a relative intrusion and making the deep bite easier to correct.
- Location: the software calculates the amount of IPR required to solve the crowding or tooth size discrepancy. The IPR required will be divided between the contact areas. For example, if there is 0.4 mm IPR between 3.2 and 3.3, the clinician can perform IPR of 0.2 mm on each tooth or distribute the IPR based on the morphology of the teeth (more IPR on the morphology of the teeth with thicker enamel) potentially performing 0.4 mm of IPR on the canine and none on the lateral incisor.
- Timing: the software will automatically align the teeth first to allow the clinician to access the contact areas for IPR and then retract the teeth into the IPR space.

If there is excessive round tripping, or if the periodontal tissue does not allow proclination of the incisors, the technician can be requested to:

- Plan the IPR at an earlier stage.
- Restage tooth movement and perform posterior IPR to avoid round tripping.
- By doing so the space created by the posterior IPR can be used to move each tooth distally one by one to avoid incisor proclination.

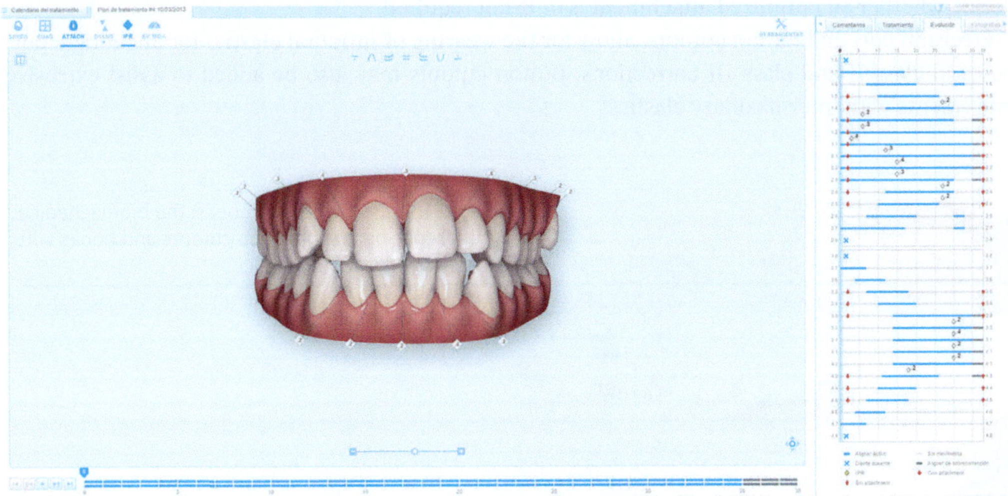

Fig. 14.29 White boxes indicating interproximal reduction turn yellow at the stage in which this has to be performed.

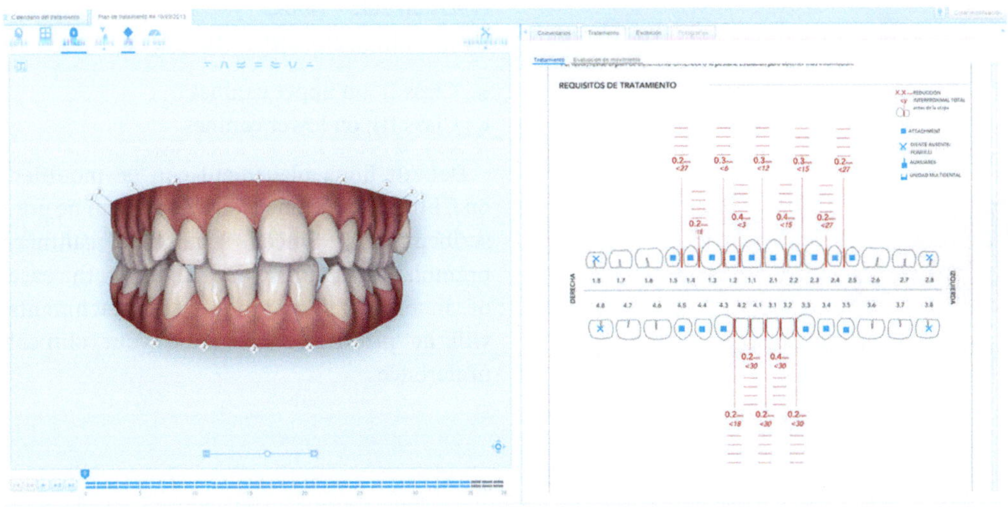

Fig. 14.30 Treatment overview also addresses interproximal reduction needs.

14.1.11 Review Precision Cuts

Prescribing precision cuts on the initial prescription form is not recommend in order to allow the software to position attachments more adequately for the movement of the teeth (note that optimized attachments are incompatible with precision cuts, so the system might not place one even if it is needed for the tooth movement).

In the second evaluation of the ClinCheck, precision cuts can be added by dragging and dropping either a precision-cut hook or button cutout. This is important because it is then possible to decide whether an optimized attachment is or is not required.

Precision cuts and button cutouts, allow for the wearing of intraoral elastics for anchorage purposes in class II and class III corrections. Button cutouts may also be added to assist extrusive movements with intermaxillary elastics.

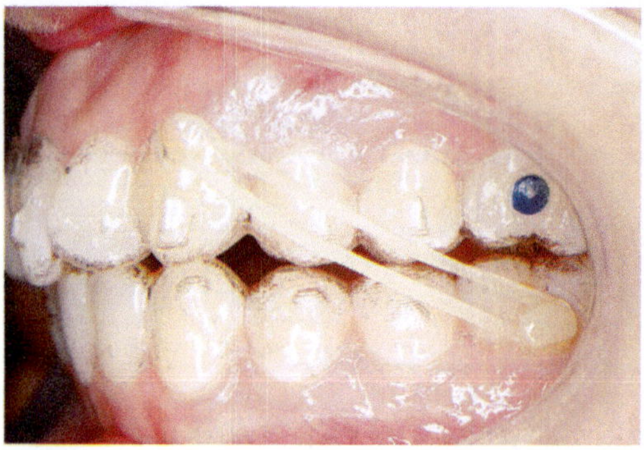

Fig. 14.31 Buttons and hooks: the biomechanical difference between button cutouts and hooks will be covered later.

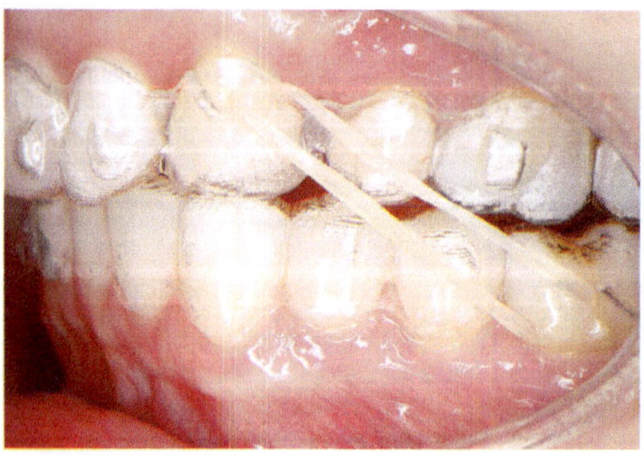

Fig. 14.32 Hooks on both upper and lower arch will affect anterior torque.

Precision Cuts – Hooks

By default, hooks will be placed:

- Class II: on upper canines
- Class III: on lower canines

Default hook placement can be modified on Clinical Preference #14. Hooks can be prescribed on the buccal surfaces of canines, premolars and molars. By default, in the case of incompatibility, optimized attachments will be prioritized based on your clinical preference.

Precision Cuts – Button Cutouts

By default, button cutouts will be placed:

- Class II: on lower first molars
- Class III: on upper first molars

Default button cutouts placement can be modified on Clinical Preference #14. Button Cutouts can be prescribed on the buccal and palatal/lingual surfaces of canines, premolars, and molars. By default, in the case of incompatibility, optimized attachments will be prioritized based on clinical preference.

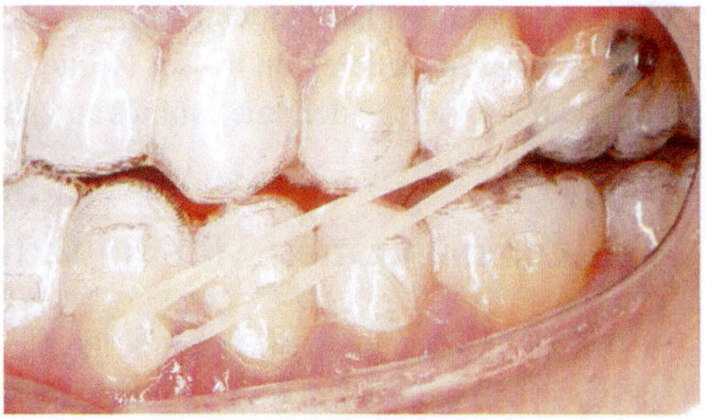

Fig. 14.33 Button cutouts will allow composite or metal buttons to be bonded onto the tooth.

Compatibility of Precision Cuts and Optimized Attachments

- Root control optimized attachments can be modified to accommodate precision cuts on the canine, enabling the use of elastics
- Precision cuts can coexist with optimized attachments for rotation, extrusion, and now optimized root control, deep bite, retraction and anchorage attachments, provided that there is sufficient room
- In cases where a precision cut and an optimized attachment cannot be placed because of insufficient space, clinical preference can resolve the conflict
- Whenever there are two different orders, the default will be placing optimized attachments instead of precision cuts

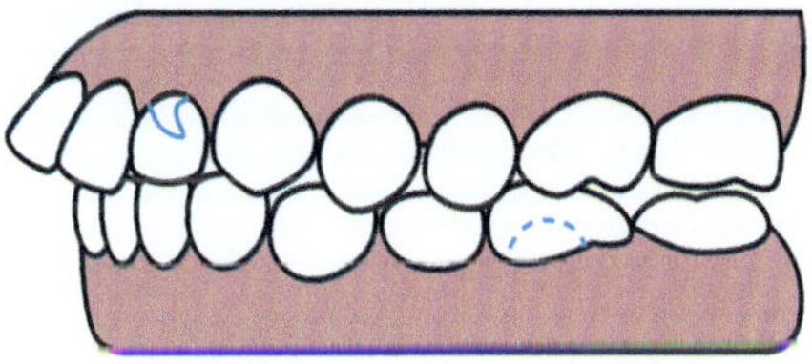

Fig. 14.34 Upper hook will affect upper anterior torque.

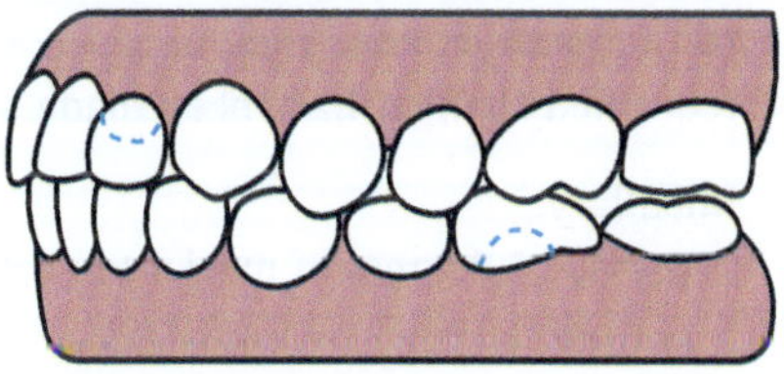

Fig. 14.35 Upper cutout for bonded button will have less effect on anterior torque when elastics are used.

Within the patient prescription form, a direct link to the drag-and-drop precision cuts interface makes it easier to set up a treatment.

Upper Canine Hooks and Lower Buccal Cutouts for Class II, div 1

Upper Buccal Cutouts and Lower Canine Hooks for Class II, div 2

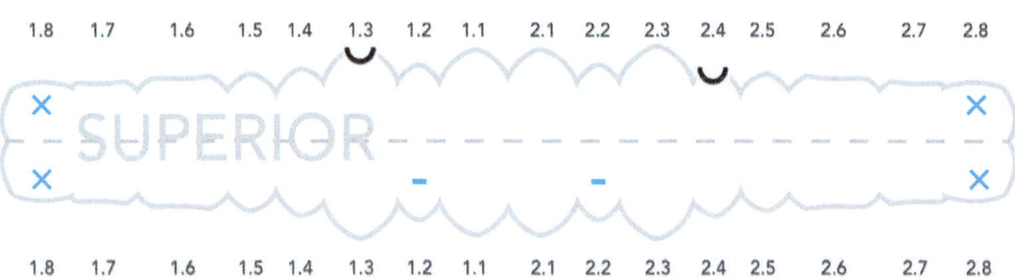

Fig. 14.36 Treatment overview also refers to hooks or button cutouts.

Cases are discussed later in which practitioners might change this default placement of precision cuts/hooks, depending on incisor torque (which is affected more by hooks than by buttons). Buttons can also help to derotate canines and molars as needed.

14.2 Communication with the Technician

- Be specific in instructions: for example, if you want to level the incisal edges between 1.1 and 2.1, specify which incisor you want to intrude or extrude or if you want to move both teeth during the correction (e.g. extrude 1.1 until the edges of both incisors are levelled):
  - When possible state the amount of tooth movement desired in a numerical quantity: e.g. 'overcorrect the extrusion of 1.1, 0.2 mm at the end of the treatment'
  - Specify the direction of the tooth movement: e.g. rotate 0.3 mm distal in the 2.3
- Identify the view: ensure that the technician is looking at the same view when trying to make the modifications. For example, in anterior view please centre lower midline with upper midline. Use IPR 3 to 3 during the correction. The clinician can also take a screenshot to allow the technician to see the same view.
- State the problem and give a solution. For example, in order to have anchorage during the asymmetric expansion, do not move the second quadrant until the posterior crossbite on the right side has been corrected.
- Use reference points: e.g. using the torque of 2.3 as a reference, give labial torque to the 1.3 until equal torque in both upper canines is achieved.
- Make a numerical checklist of all the changes required. This will help the technician keep track of the modifications they need to do and will also help the clinician to verify whether all the requested changes have been made. For example:

  Maxillary:
  - provide 5 degrees of mesial-out rotation to 1.6
  - extrude 1.1. by 0.5 mm to level incisal edge with 2.1

  Mandibular:
  - procline lower incisors until labial surface is perpendicular to the bone
  - overcorrect by 0.5 mm the mesial-out rotation of 4.2

Whenever it appears that the technician has not followed instructions, review them: practitioners might not be 100% clear in their instructions or theses instructions may be ambiguous.

15

Treatment Monitoring and Appointments Protocol

This chapter provides the 10 steps you and your team should check in every appointment to properly track the treatment progress.

15.1 Tracking Treatment Progress

1. Check Patient Compliance

- Ask them if they have worn the aligners for the number of hours required
- If compliance is not good enough, try to reach an agreement with your patient, for example if they do not want to use the aligners 22 hours a day, instead of changing the aligners every 7 days, plan a 10- to 14-day intervals protocol

2. Oral Health

If the teeth are dirty or the gums swollen, hygiene instruction should be reinforced and perhaps an appointment with the periodontist should be scheduled before continuing with the treatment.

3. Tooth Tracking

- Check the patient with the *last aligner in the mouth*: if there is a maladjustment on any tooth, this will need to be addressed before continuing treatment
- Check the *adjustment of the attachment on the reservoirs of the aligner*: the active part of the attachment must be in contact with the aligner, colour the attachment, if necessary, in order to check
- *Review the teeth position and their position on the ClinCheck:* compare the current stage in the ClinCheck with the intraoral position of the teeth, always using anatomic references

For example, in a class II correction, check that the intermaxillary position of the canines corresponds with the stage the patient is at the ClinCheck using an anatomic reference in the lower arch, or in severe rotation of a premolar or canine, check that in the ClinCheck the correction observed corresponds with the intraoral one.

4. Interproximal Contacts

- Remove the tartar and use dental floss to look for tight contact areas, especially in crowded teeth

Aligner Techniques in Orthodontics, First Edition. Susana Palma Moya and Javier Lozano Zafra.

Companion website: www.wiley.com/go/lozano-zafra/aligner-techniques

- If there are tight contacts, loosen them with a diamond metal strip, even if no interproximal reduction has been requested

  Other situations in which we should loosen the contact point, even if the software does not require any IPR are:

- Between the incisors before starting the absolute intrusion movement
- Between the premolars and molars in severe expansion
- In rotated canines

5. Check the Actions Required for the Actual Stage

- Perform all the planned IPR for the current stage and for the aligners that are going to be given to the patient.
- Check if any new attachments appear or any existing ones disappear in the aligners that we give to the patient.
- Check if the patient needs to wear elastics during the current stage and if so, bond buttons for the elastics.

6. Check the Next Aligner in the Patient's Mouth

- Check fitting of the new aligner. Ask the patient to place and remove the aligner by themselves, to ensure they are doing so correctly.
- Pay special attention to the problem teeth, which must be noted down on the clinical template. A problem tooth or the teeth marked by the software with a black dot because of difficult movement are major concerns in the patient.
- If there is a fitting problem with this tooth, auxiliary techniques might be required at this stage.

7. Fill the Pontics

- If the patient has any missing tooth, these gaps can be filled using orthodontic wax or flowable composite.
- There are few tips to do this, depending on your clinical preferences.

8. Note the Dates

Record the dates that each aligner should be changed on the aligners' envelope.

9. Take Pictures to Monitor Evolution

10. Show the Patient their Evolution

The patient should be shown their evolution and the result they can expect from each aligner. Explain the use of elastics if necessary.

15.2 Appointments Protocol for Invisalign Patient

1) Aligner #1 without attachments (3 weeks): give welcome kit and instructions to the patient
2) Aligner #2 bonding attachments (use attachment template), with extractions if required
3) Aligner #3 begin IPR (as requested on clinical preferences)

4) Aligner #4: begin regular appointments protocol, as indicated below (we suggest that you make a checklist with all these steps so that staff can follow a protocol when helping out with the patient's appointment)

15.3 Protocol on Each Appointment

1) Check the fit of the last aligner in the patient's mouth
2) Try in the new aligner (check adjustment), ask the patient to do it themselves in order to check the insertion and removal of the aligner
3) Check dental alignment (first in the ClinCheck and then in the mouth)
4) Check attachments (mark with a pencil in the case of any doubt), check there are no empty spaces in the incisal edge of the teeth and check there are no missing attachments
5) If there are pontics, fill them with wax
6) Check the problem tooth
7) Check the expected tooth movements for the new set of aligners the patient will receive using the ClinCheck (soften the contact points in intrusion and rotation of round teeth)
8) Remove tartar and soften contact points in crowding (check with dental floss without wax) and prepare for IPR if planned
9) Check in the ClinCheck if any attachments appear or disappear
10) Note the dates when aligners should be changed on the boxes
11) Take photographs if considered necessary

16

Troubleshooting and Retention

A great orthodontic treatment with the Invisalign technique starts with a great ClinCheck plan, which is why it is important to have a deep fundamental knowledge of the system and its pillars of success.

That said, during any treatment there will be changes from the original planning, as with brackets in the past, where we used auxiliary techniques, rebonded brackets, used coil springs, auxiliary root torque devices. We should therefore expect to face similar challenges with aligners: these issues can be resolved either by asking for additional aligners or by following our troubleshooting tips and finishing strategies.

16.1 Auxiliary Techniques

Auxiliary techniques will be required when there is a fitting problem, which might be caused by a bad treatment plan, patient biology or poor patient compliance:

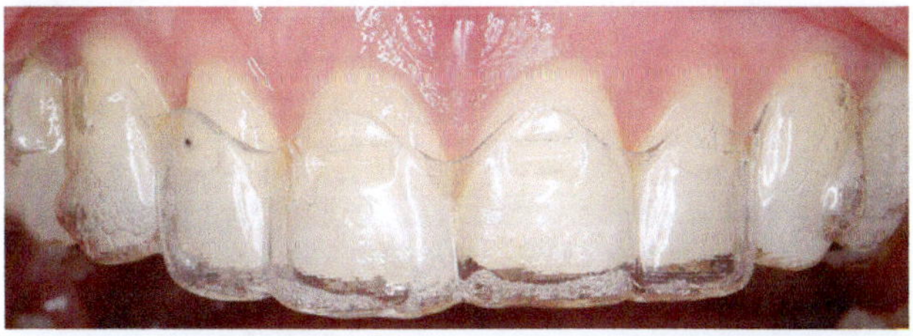

Fig. 16.1 An example of poor fitting.

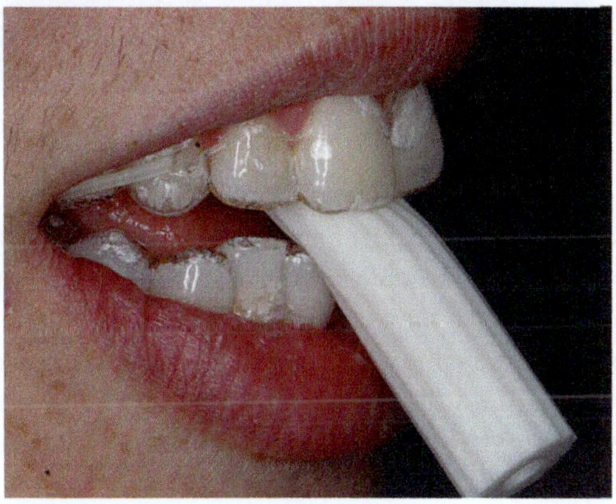

Fig. 16.2 Fitting can improve with 'fitters' chewing.

Aligner Techniques in Orthodontics, First Edition. Susana Palma Moya and Javier Lozano Zafra.

Companion website: www.wiley.com/go/lozano-zafra/aligner-techniques

- If it is less than 1 mm: this means there are blue or black movements or patient compliance is low, and so the patient should be asked to wear the aligners for a longer period (10–14 days)
- If it is between 1 and 2 mm: use detailing plier (anterior rotations and in/out movements) or auxiliary techniques (posterior rotations, extrusion, root tipping)
- More than 2 mm: scan again

In order to achieve a successful orthodontic treatment, we need to know how to troubleshoot and solve the complications as they arise. Complications commonly encountered with aligners are described below.

16.1.1 Tooth Does Not Follow Rotation Movement

When there is a gap between the aligner and the incisal edges of the teeth or a space around the attachments upon insertion. There is a discrepancy between the tooth position in the aligner and intraorally; the tooth is more rotated in the mouth than in the ClinCheck.

This might occur when there has not been enough compliance and the patient has changed the aligner before the full movement has been completed. One possible solution is to revert to previous aligners and attempt to recover the movement. Try the aligner that best fits and continue the treatment from that aligner.

Another possible cause of a discrepancy between the tooth position and the aligner is that in the software this tooth has started to move before enough space has been created or the clinician did not perform a sufficient amount of the prescribed IPR. To correct the rotation of an incisor, use detailing pliers.

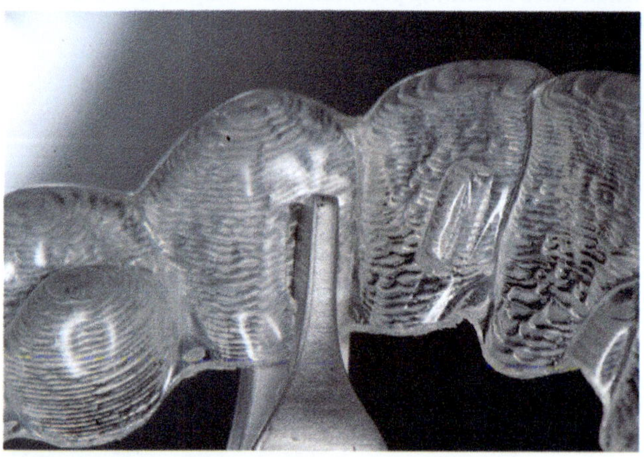

Fig. 16.3 Detailing pliers are helpful for case finishing.

At this point we should stress the importance of asking the technician to make sure there are open contacts mesial and distal to any rotated or lingually positioned tooth. Be especially careful with rotated second premolars rotated and lingual lateral incisors, as the default staging in the software is to move teeth simultaneously, which is not predictable. To increase predictability, we suggest restaging the rotated tooth movement to create space first before moving it into alignment.

In canines that have rotation and tipping problems at the beginning of the treatment, if the software tries to solve the problem of the rotation and root tipping simultaneously, a discrepancy between the canine position and the aligner will appear. To solve this problem, buttons linked with a Powerchain can be used, performing IPR mesial and distal to the canine and maintaining the same aligner until the position of the attachment inside the reservoir of the aligner is corrected.

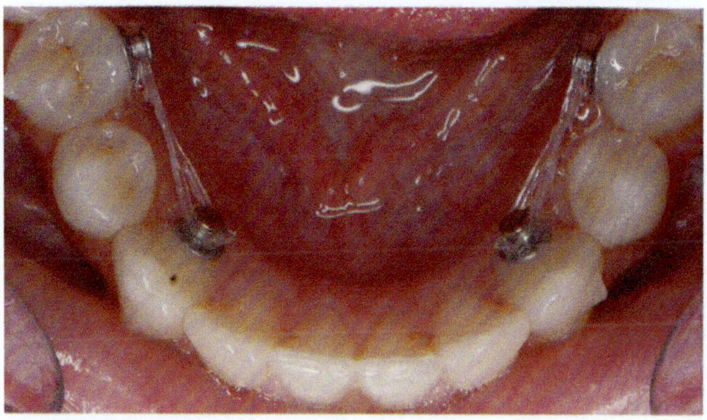

Fig. 16.4 Auxiliary technique to recapture a rotated lower canine with button and power chain.

16.1.2 Tooth Does Not Follow Vertical Movement

A common cause of intrusion is lack of space. If teeth collide into each other, even if they receive the required force to move, they cannot reach their final position and they become intruded.

In order to prevent the intrusion of the teeth, check the contact points with dental floss at every appointment and if they are found to be tight, perform slight IPR to ensure the teeth have space to move.

Extrusion issues may also be encountered during the treatment which may be resolved easily using the tips provided here.

Auxiliary Technique to Extrude a Lateral Incisor

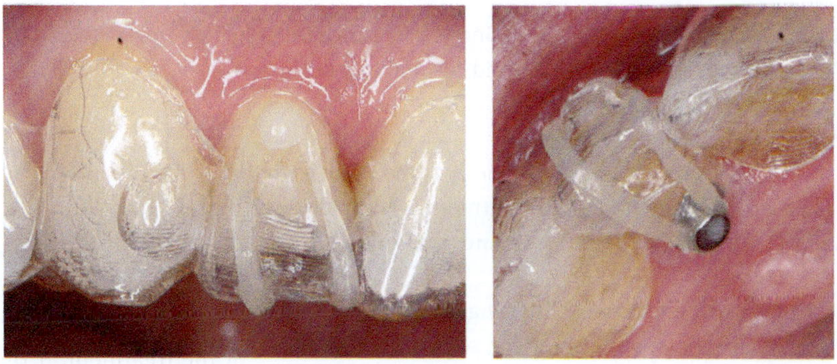

Fig. 16.5 Buccal (left) and palatal (right) view of a lateral incisor extruded with buttons and elastics.

There is a common auxiliary technique to extrude a lateral incisor that has become intruded during the treatment.

- The aligner has to be trimmed on the buccal and lingual sides to allow the tooth to extrude
- It is important to ensure that there is enough clearance between the button and the edge of the aligner: 4.5 ounces, 3/16' elastics can be used to extrude the tooth, placed from the buccal to the lingual button

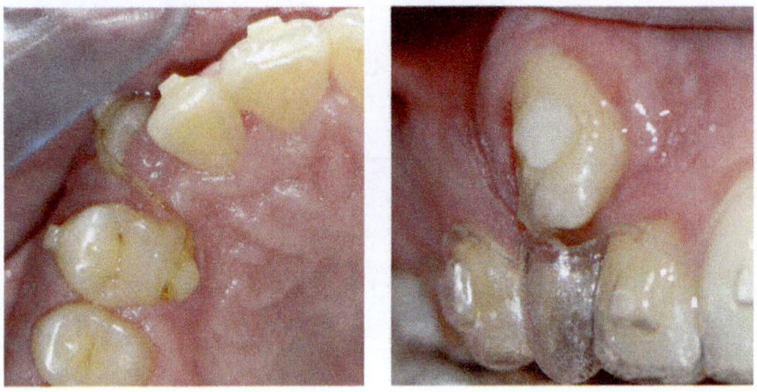

Fig. 16.6 Ectopic canines not covered by the aligner.

When there is an ectopic canine, this must be virtually eliminated to avoid tracking problems and the ectopic canine will need to be guided to its final position using extrusion elastics once space has been opened for it. In these cases, the prescription from the practitioner will be used to request that the technician places a large pontic that overlaps the lateral incisor in order to provide space for the ectopic canine.

- After opening space for the canine, extrusive elastics may be used to extrude canines into the virtual pontic
- Buttons can be used on both the buccal and lingual surfaces of the canine to extrude them
- The pontic must be trimmed to avoid interference with eruption of the tooth
- Once the canine has erupted, a new scan is taken to include the newly positioned canine and additional aligners are requested

16.1.3 Managing Root Tipping

This is another important aspect in extraction cases and is performed during these treatments or in cases of agenesis in order to properly close spaces and re-establish occlusion.

Uprighting a Molar Root

The patient shown in Fig. 16.7 presented with severely tipped molars in the right and left mandibular quadrants after previous orthodontic treatment. Molar uprighting was built into the aligner assisted by TAD mesial to the molars and sectional wire from the molars to the microscrew.

The patient shown in Fig. 16.8 had a mesial tipping of the second premolar root. A power arm was used to upright the root of the second premolar, with a power chain from the power arm to a button on the second molar.

Fig. 16.7 Uprighting a premolar root.

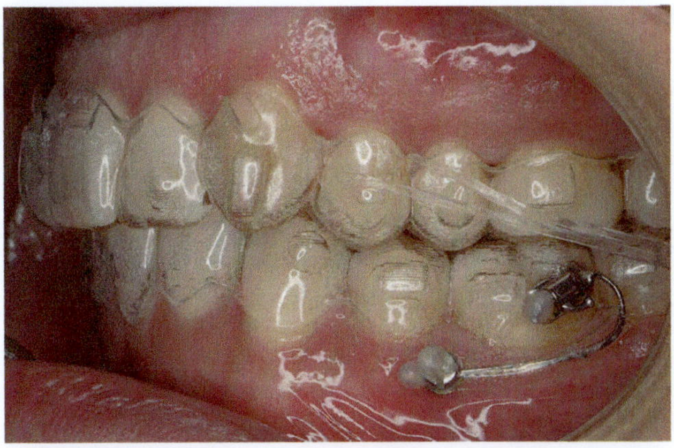

Fig. 16.8 This patient had a distal tipping of the second premolar root. A Power Arm was used to upright the root, with a coil spring to another Power Arm bonded to the canine.

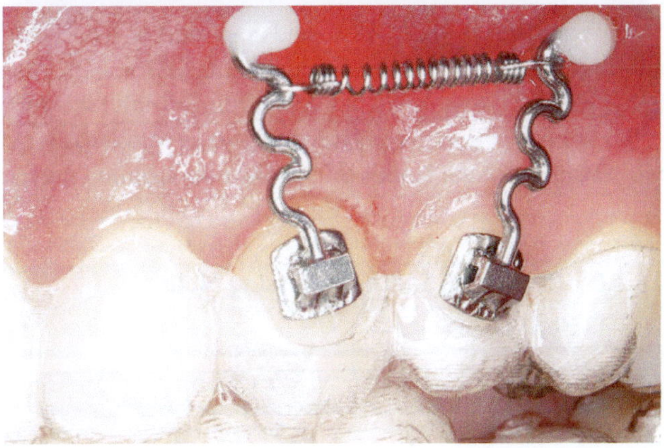

16.1.4 Managing Posterior Mesialization

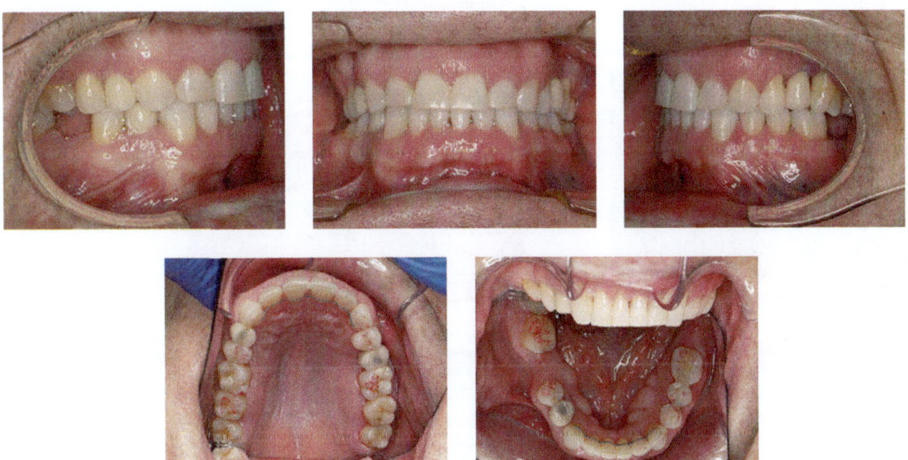

Fig. 16.9 In this case, the goal was to mesialize 47 and 48 in order to close 46 space.

Evolution of Mesialization

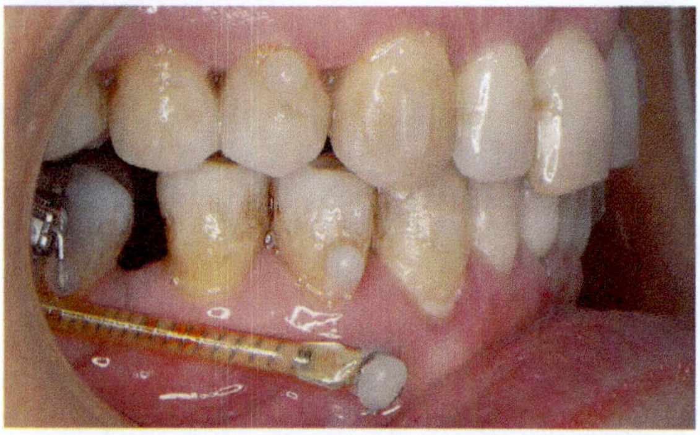

Fig. 16.10 Patient with missing 46.

The patient shown in Fig. 16.10 had a missing 46. The treatment goal was to mesialize the second and third molars in order to avoid placing an implant. Aligner wear was accompanied by a sectional wire on the molars and a coil spring from the second molar to a microscrew.

It is important that the coil traction goes as parallel as possible to the TAD in order to prevent the mesial tipping of the molars during the mesialization movement.

16.1.5 Reopening Space for Missing Molars

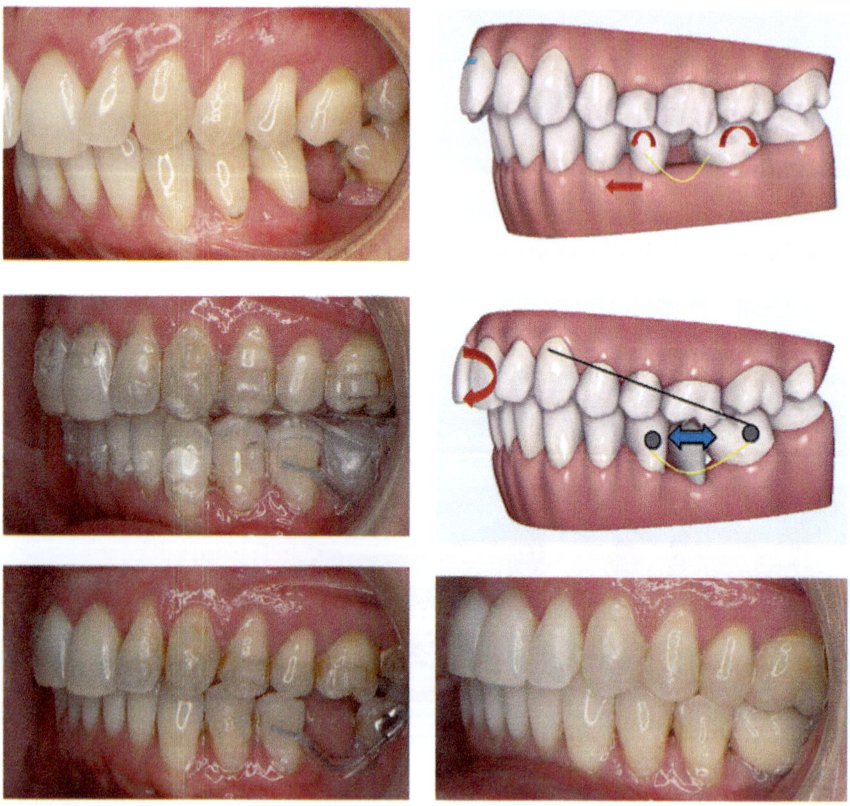

Fig. 16.11 The patient had missing 36 and 46.

The patient shown in Fig. 16.11 had a missing 36 and 46, so it was decided to open space for both missing molars in order to assist the correction of the dental class II, using the space opened to mesialize the lower arch. As the third lower molars were present, they were used as anchorage to avoid the distal tipping of the molars, and the Locatelli anchor was placed in the second molar and the second premolar.

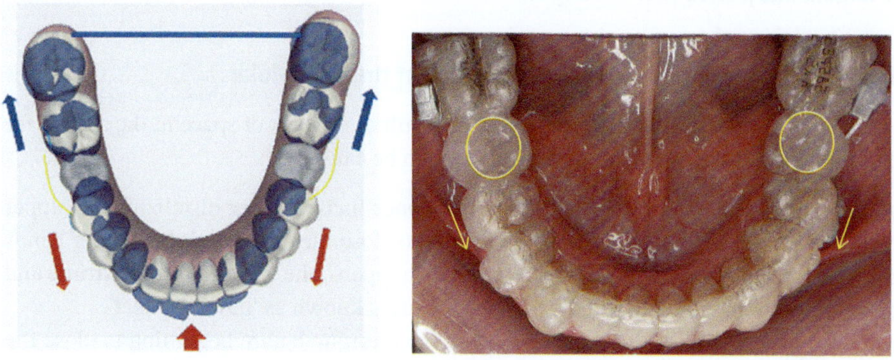

Fig. 16.12 A Locatelli helps to open space.

The second lower molar will not tip distally thanks to the third lower molar and the second premolar will move mesially at the same time as the expansion of the lower arch.

16.1.6 Achieving More than 4 mm of Anterior Intrusion

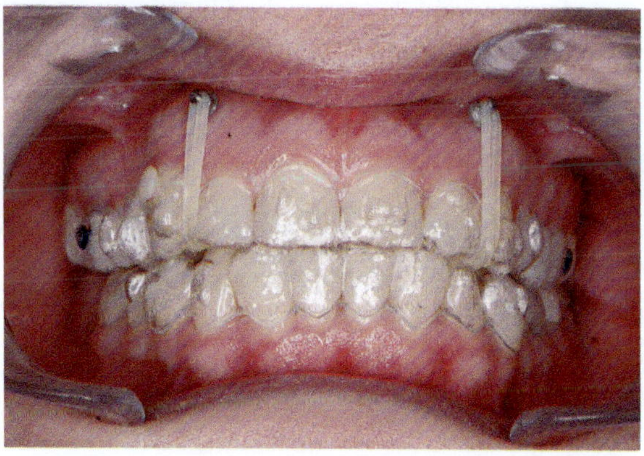

Fig. 16.13 Temporary anchorage devices help intruding teeth in severe deep bite cases.

Whenever the intrusion of the incisor is more than 4 mm, TADs need to be used to assist and these can be placed between the root of lateral and upper canines. This positioning of the TADs allows intrusion of the incisors by placing two TADs instead of four. In these cases, the clinician can bond aesthetic buttons on the cervical margin of the four upper incisors and use light elastics (2 ounces) to intrude the incisors. Note that:

- The elastic must be worn for 12 hours under the four incisors, as shown in Fig. 16.13, and another 12 hours of wear only under the central incisors, in order to prevent the lateral incisors intruding more than the central incisors.
- The patient should be informed about the possible need for a gingivectomy during the intrusion movement. Control X-rays of the incisor's roots should be taken every 6 months to prevent resorptions.

- The aligner should be trimmed only on the labial side to accommodate the aesthetic buttons. Precision cuts may also be planned on the ClinCheck.

Where a clinician prefers to use TADs between lateral and canines, four TADs will need to be used, two in the labial side and the other two lingual with an elastic used from the labial micro-screw to the lingual one passed over the aligner.

16.1.7 Managing Intrusion of the Mesiobuccal Cusp of the First Molar

The mesial tipping of the first molar crown occurs as a result of the lack of space in the aligner for arch length reduction. This lack of space in the aligner can be caused by:

- Loss of anchorage: when attempting to retrude the upper incisors after distalizing the upper molars or in extraction cases, the arch length reduces to close the space and the aligner bends because of a lack of space anteroposteriorly. When this happens, the upper incisors extrude and the mesial cusp of the maxillary first molar intrudes. This is known as 'bowing effect'
  - To prevent the bowing effect, build in adequate incisor torque before beginning to close the extraction space or before incisor retraction and while also strengthening the posterior anchorage during incisor retraction
  - The use of adequate staging techniques for space closure in premolar extraction cases is also recommended
- Insufficient IPR during space closure or incisor retraction: to prevent this situation ensure that the prescribed IPR is carried out at the correct stage of treatment

To solve the tipping of the first molar, once it has occurred, cut the upper aligner distal to the second upper premolar and make a button cutout in the lower molar and place an intermaxillary elastic from the upper first molar to the lower first molar (1/8'–3/16', 4.5 ounce elastics).

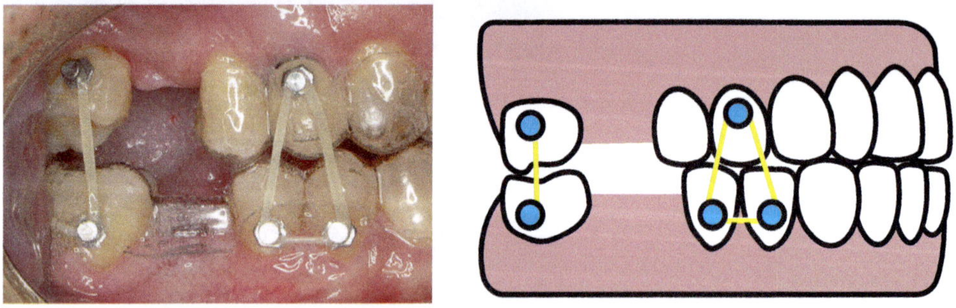

Fig. 16.14 Posterior extrusion is achieved here with auxiliary buttons and elastics.

16.1.8 Managing Premolar Rotation Greater than 45 Degrees

In order to maintain a shorter length of treatment, ask the technician to correct the rotations of these premolars in the later stages of treatment, as in doing it will be possible to considerably reduce the number of active aligners.

- Requesting the correction in this manner will mean that the software will not use these premolars as guide teeth and will therefore not slow down the movement of the other teeth
- To address the premolar rotations, buttons and lingual Powerchains will need to be placed at the point in the ClinCheck where the premolars start to move: place the buttons and power chain lingually to assist the rotations and make their correction predictable

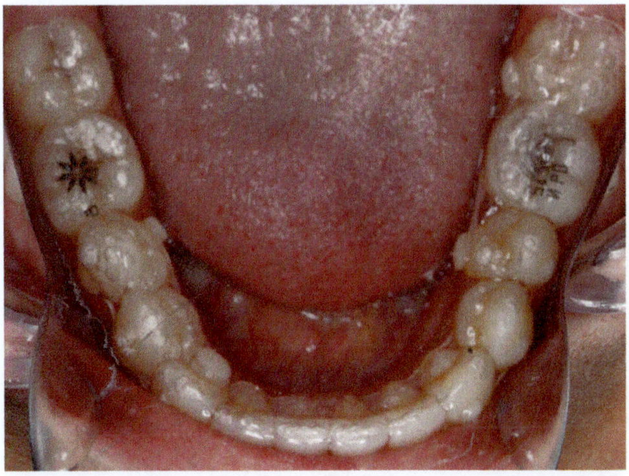

Fig. 16.15 Auxiliary buttons and elastics help derotating teeth.

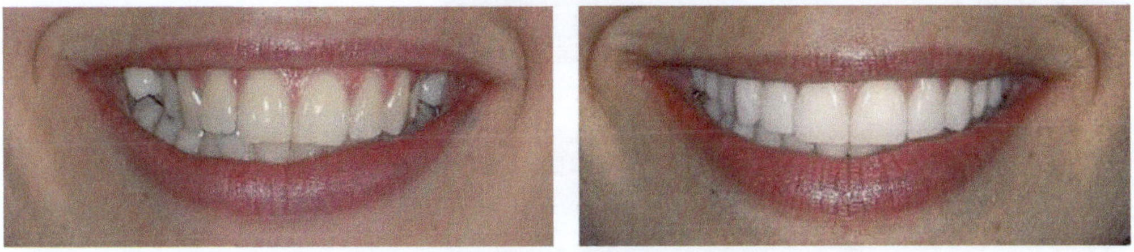

Fig. 16.16 Change in smile after expansion of upper arch and offset and rotation of 15 and 25 using aligners, buttons and lingual Powerchains.

16.1.9 Solving a Posterior Open Bite

A posterior open bite during treatment can happen for various reasons:

- Bowing effect resulting from lack of space in the aligner during the arch length reduction.
- Premature contact in the anterior zone, which might happen after an expansion that did not take into consideration a possible lack of overjet and the secondary effect of retraction of the incisors during expansion movements or because of lingual torque of the upper incisors during the anterior retraction. If premature contacts happen on the anterior zone, a posterior open bite will appear.

To prevent this, the practitioner needs to create positive overjet when attempting a substantial arch expansion and provide enough labial torque on the upper incisors before closing the anterior space through retraction.

To solve a posterior open bite:

- If the posterior open bite is light, i.e. gap equal to or less than 1 mm, section the aligners distal to the canines to allow the posterior teeth to erupt into occlusion. These sectioned aligners should be worn for several weeks
- If the posterior gap is more than 1 mm, section the aligners distal to the canines, bond buttons on the posterior teeth, and attach settling elastics
- If there is a residual curve of Spee in the lower arch, make button cutouts in the maxillary aligner and section only the lower aligner distal to the canines. The extrusion of the lower teeth will correct the remaining curve of Spee
- An alternative solution when ordering additional aligners is to ask the technician to give extra labial torque to the upper incisors, perform IPR 3 to 3 in the lower arch and retrude and intrude the lower

incisors. In this way, a positive overjet can be achieved and afterwards the technician can make a virtual jump (simulation jump) to adjust the occlusion, providing a posterior open bite closure
- Do not ask the technician to close the posterior open bite by extrusion of the posterior molars and premolars, as the extrusion movement is a difficult movement with aligners

16.1.10 Correcting Canine Rotation as well as Anteroposterior Discrepancy

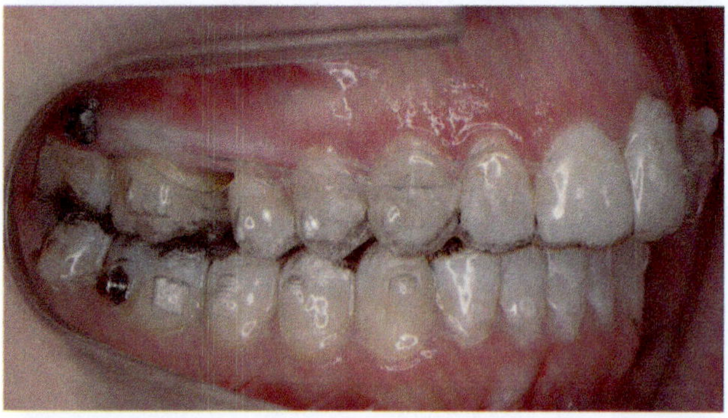

Fig. 16.17 Mesial-in rotation of the canine.

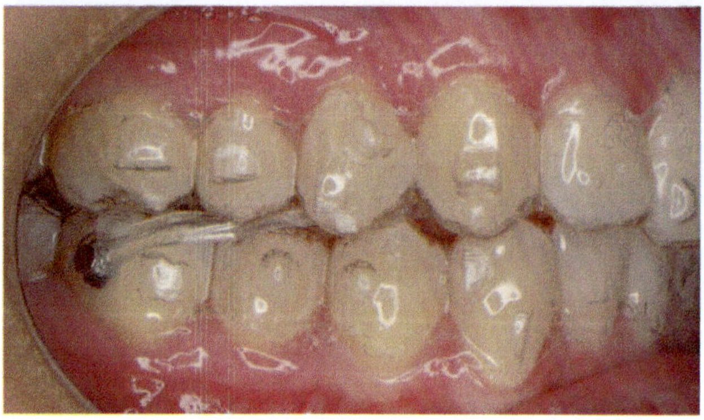

Fig. 16.18 Mesial-out rotation of the canine.

- If in the initial position of the upper canine, it is rotated mesial-in, place the precision cut on the labial side.
- If in the initial position of the upper canine, it is rotated mesial-out, bond a button on the lingual surface of the upper canine and place the elastic on the lingual surface in order to provide a mesial-in rotation at the same time as correcting the class II malocclusion.

16.2 Finishing Techniques

Finishing bends made with the detail pliers may be used in the last aligners. The practitioners should consider whether overcorrection aligners are going to be needed when reaching the last three aligners of the treatment.

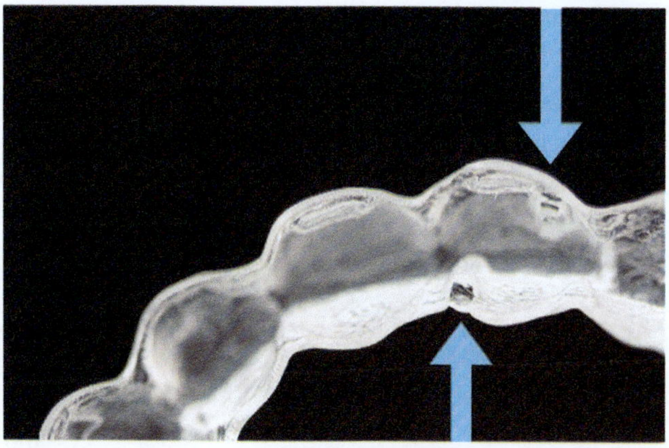

Fig. 16.19 Finishing bends.

16.2.1 Overcorrection

Overcorrection refers to overcorrection of the individual tooth position in the final occlusion in the ClinCheck by using either the 3D controls or by written request to the technician in the three last aligners of the treatment.

To overcorrect the rotation of round teeth such as lower canines, there is the option to dispense these last three aligners to the patient or not, depending on the patient's final tooth position.

16.2.2 Overtreatment

Overtreatment refers to setting up a final occlusion in the ClinCheck that is beyond the desired clinical outcome as we should expect that all the movements requested will not be fully expressed on the aligners.

- Overtreat vertical discrepancies deep bite and open bites:
  - In deep bite cases, overtreat the anterior intrusion to a final 0 mm of overbite and overtreat the extrusion of the posterior teeth to create strong contact points at the end of the treatment (red posterior contact points).
  - In open bite cases, request an overtreatment of the anterior extrusion to + 2 mm of overbite.
- Overtreat transversal expansions: ask the technician to expand by applying labial root torque simultaneously to the posterior teeth until the lingual cusp of the upper molars contact with the buccal cusps of the mandibular posterior teeth. This is especially important in growing patients with class III malocclusion.
- Overtreat root tipping in extraction cases: ask the technician to overtreat root inclinations adjacent to the extraction site, leaving the roots in the ClinCheck with a final tip toward the extraction site.
- Overtreat the lingual root torque of the upper incisors: In class II malocclusion, extraction and deep bite cases with retroclined upper incisors at the beginning. As these cases are going to use class II elastics that will torque the upper incisors lingually during the treatment, so the final inclination of the upper incisors might be different from the final one we visualize on the ClinCheck.

Virtual C-chain

Do not apply virtual C-chain, if:

- There are no open diastemas to be closed.
- There is not enough overjet (if we try to close an upper diastema with C-chain and there is not enough overjet, we will generate premature anterior contacts and a posterior open bite).

16.3 Retention

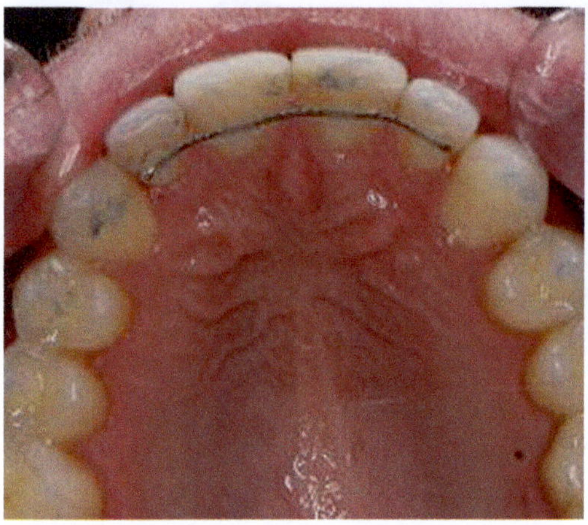

Fig. 16.20 Fixed retention from lateral to lateral.

Retention is the phase of orthodontic treatment that maintains the teeth in their orthodontically corrected positions following the cessation of active orthodontic tooth movement. This approach is supported by histological studies which have shown that the supracrestal periodontal fibres remain stretched and displaced for more than 7 months after the cessation of orthodontic tooth movement, suggesting that the retention period should generally be at least 7 months. The paradigm today is that retention is for life.

Advantages of fixed retention are:

- More effective than removable one
- Minimum patient cooperation
- It is great for debonding and retaining in the same appointment

Disadvantages of fixed retention are:

- The technique is sensitive to place
- It is difficult for patients to maintain, as it can impact oral hygiene
- They must return to the clinic when the retainer breaks or debonds
- If the wire is broken it may become active, producing unwanted movements
- Usually limited to anterior teeth

Fig. 16.21 Vivera retainers are manufactured by Align Technology.

Advantages of removable retention are:

- Aesthetic and effective
- Vivera are good for debonding and retaining in the same appointment (they can be ordered via the IDS based on the last stage or by taking a new scan)
- Fit properly
- More hygienic than fixed retainer

Disadvantages of removable retention are:

- More patient compliance is needed
- Laboratory cost
- Patients might lose them
- Retainer aesthetics are reduced over time

17

Arch Length Discrepancies

Arch length discrepancies result in crowding or spacing of the teeth. As most cases of dental crowding show a higher prevalence for the anterior region, clinicians need to have efficient methods of relieving dental crowding, such as arch expansion, proclination of the anterior teeth, sequential distalization, tooth extraction or interproximal enamel reduction. The method used will be determined by the amount of crowding, facial profile, and patients' age.

This chapter will cover crowding management by interproximal reduction (IPR), mainly on the anterior segment. This is a safe clinical procedure involving the reduction, anatomical recontouring and protection of interproximal enamel surfaces of permanent teeth. For patients with mild or moderate crowding (4–8 mm): this is a really good alternative to dental extraction.

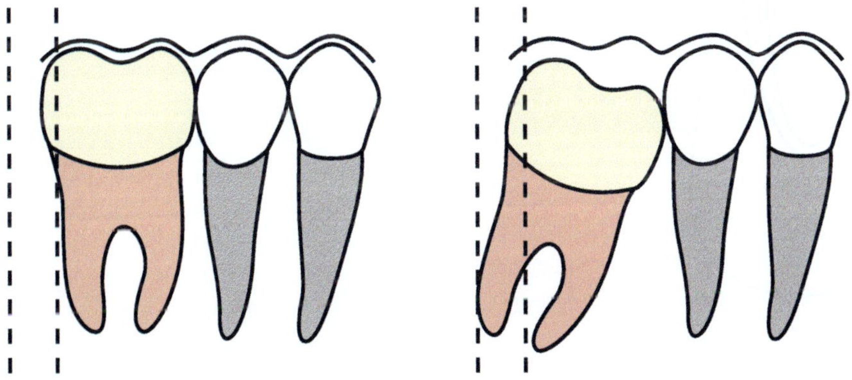

Fig. 17.1 Interproximal reduction has to be performed carefully in order to avoid tooth intrusion caused by insufficient space inside the aligner.

Aligner Techniques in Orthodontics, First Edition. Susana Palma Moya and Javier Lozano Zafra.

Companion website: www.wiley.com/go/lozano-zafra/aligner-techniques

Apart from crowding there are some other indications for IPR on adults, such as Bolton Index discrepancy, changes in tooth shape and dental aesthetics (e.g. macrodontia), normalization of gingival contour and elimination of black gingival triangles.

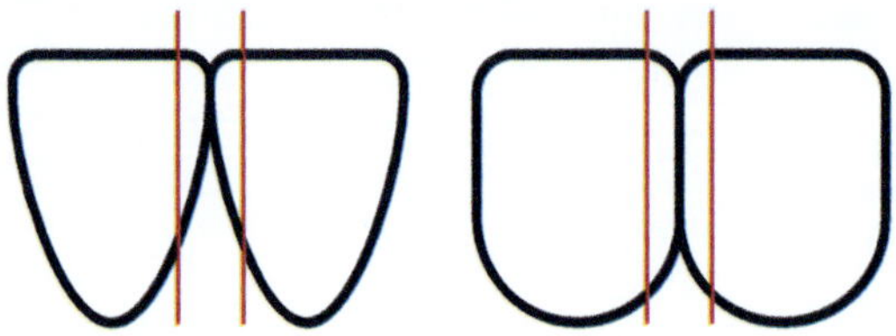

Fig. 17.2 Interproximal reduction might improve the shape and size of teeth, reducing unaesthetic black triangles.

There is also another clinical point to this as, after creating proper interdental contacts, the risk of loss of alveolar bone or root cement is decreased.

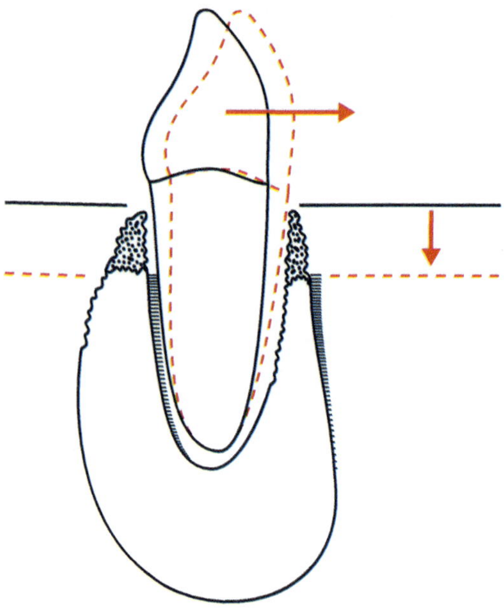

Fig. 17.3 Interproximal reduction in cases of crowding might improve contact points thereby reducing alveolar bone or root cement, so it has clear indications for periodontal patients.

Tooth spacing, which might be related to tooth shape or size, also needs to be considered. In some cases we might perform IPR on the opposite arch to compensate the Bolton discrepancy or go for restorative treatment alternatives such as ceramic or composite veneers to re-establish the ideal size of teeth.

Spacing can also be related to any clinical conditions other than tooth size, which will need a specific clinical approach to obtain the best clinical and aesthetic results with the aligners technique.

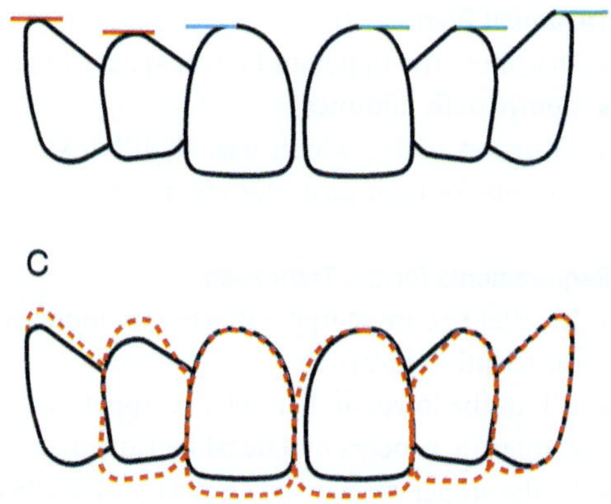

Fig. 17.4 Spacing cases are usually related to abnormal tooth size, which leads to a need for aesthetic planning, which will be covered in Chapter 25.

Key to this, as we will see in the clinical cases review, is adding extra palatal root torque (PRT) to teeth in which we are closing space, so crown retraction is accompanied by a root movement, creating an 'en masse' retrusion to close the space.

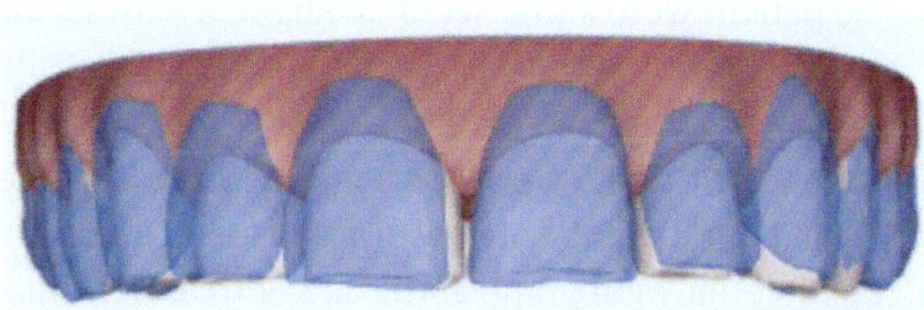

Fig. 17.5 Palatal root torque is seen on the ClinCheck Pro as blue areas on the superimposition areas in which the roots were previously placed.

17.1 Spacing

17.1.1 Spacing, Case 1

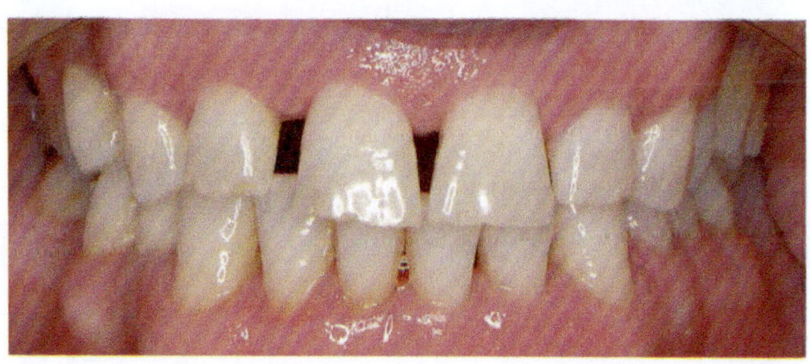

Fig. 17.6 Skeletal class I with spacing.

Diagnosis

A 45-year-old, symmetric, normodivergent patient presented with dental class I with missing 14/25/37 and 46 and an implant in 44. The patient had upper and lower diastemas, which were bigger in the upper arch, with abrasion on the incisal edges of upper incisors. A Bolton discrepancy with microdontia of lateral upper incisors was also found. First right upper molar was slightly extruded because of a missing 46.

Treatment Plan
- Distribute the upper and lower spaces to place implants for the missing teeth
- Centre both midlines
- Intrusion of 16, which was slightly extruded, leaving final space of 0.5 mm distal to lateral incisors for their posterior reconstruction

Requirements for the Technician
- In order to correct upper diastemas, increase the overjet (requested on special instructions in the prescription form)
- IPR in the lower arch and leave upper diastemas distal to lateral upper incisors for the posterior composite veneers on lateral incisors to correct Bolton discrepancy
- In the upper arch a strong posterior anchorage is needed to create a movement of retrusion, intrusion and lingual root torque of upper incisors
- Third molars not to be moved in order to have posterior anchorage to retrude upper and lower incisors

Treatment Summary
- Treatment was completed in 20 months
- The patient wore a first set of 34 aligners with 10-day change intervals and one set of additional aligners. Upper and lower diastemas were successfully closed
- Class I occlusion was maintained
- 16 was intruded and levelled with the occlusal plane
- The patient did not use intermaxillary elastics during treatment.
- A panoramic radiograph at the end of treatment shows root parallelism and the implants placed for the missing teeth
- The patient is still waiting to have the crown for 14 and the implant for 46 placed as well as the distal reconstruction in 12 and 22

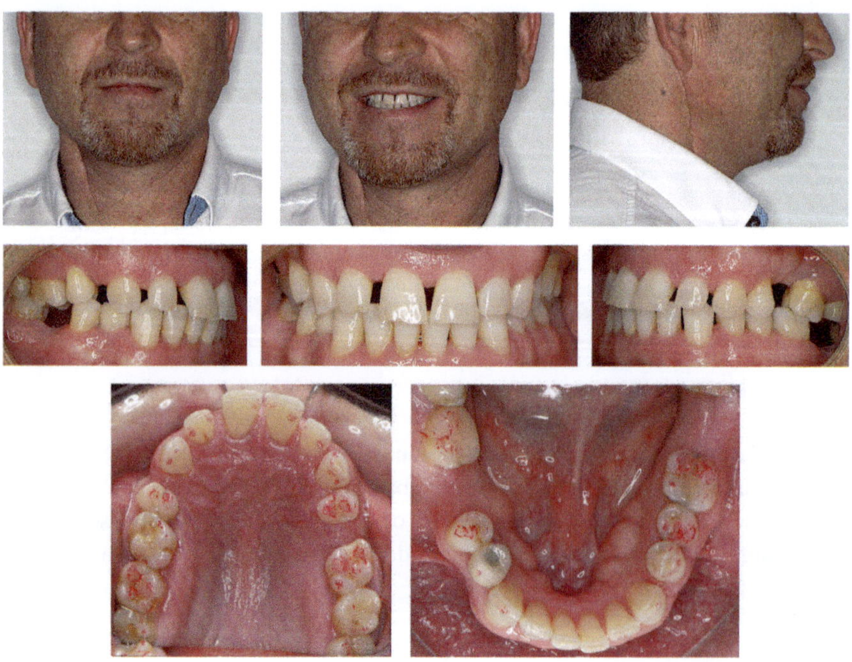

Fig. 17.7 Pretreatment views.

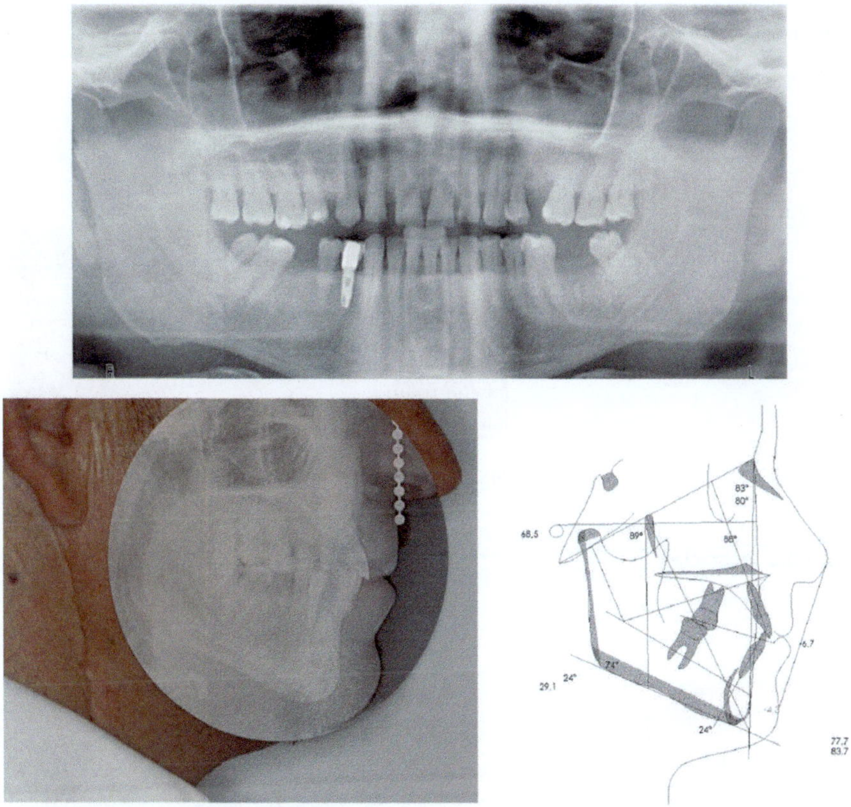

Fig. 17.8 Pretreatment panoramic X- ray, teleradiograph and cephalometry.

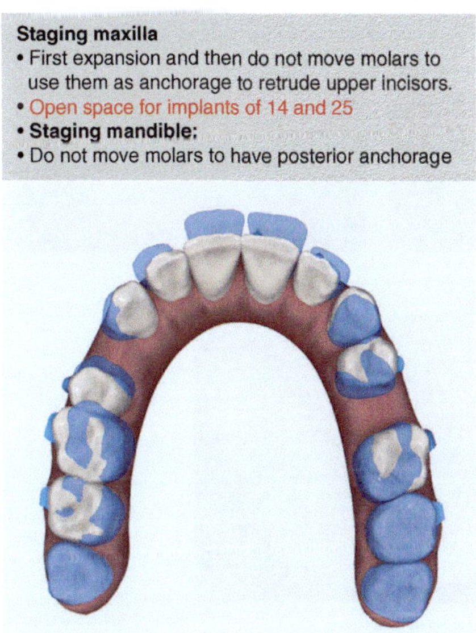

Fig. 17.9 Upper CC superimposition and instructions to CAD designer.

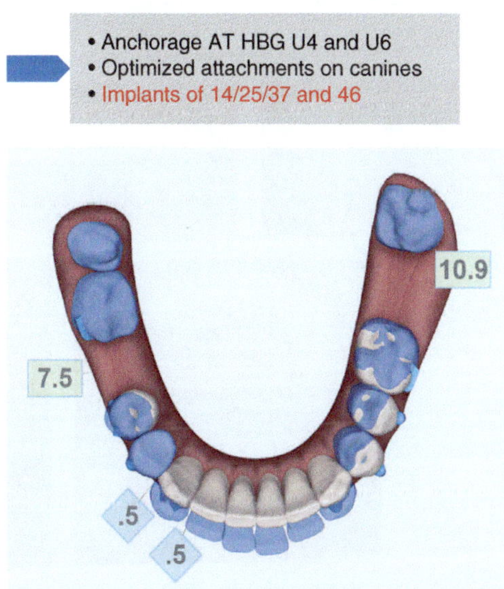

Fig. 17.10 Lower CC superimposition and instructions to CAD designer.

IPR in lower arch to create overjet to close upper diastemas

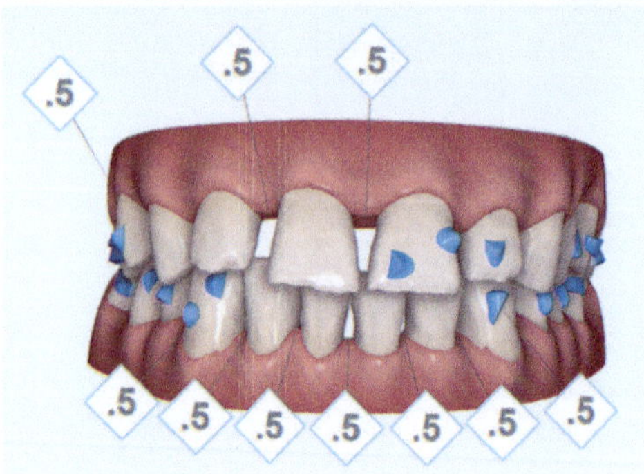

Fig. 17.11 Front CC view.

- Many anchorage attachments in posterior zone.
- IPR + TRL at the same time to lower incisors (final position of lower incisors –1 degree)

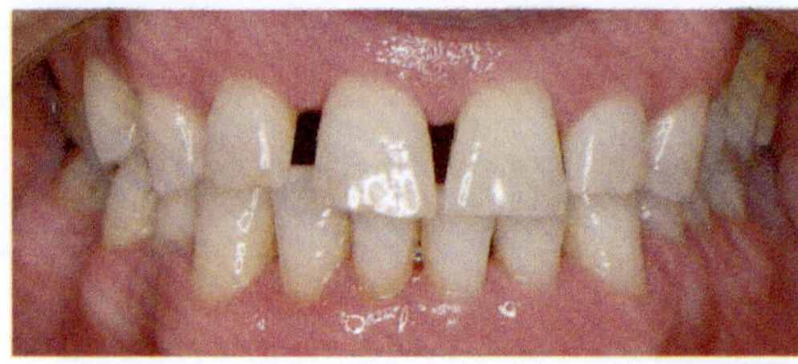

Fig. 17.12 Front intraoral picture.

Communication with the Technician

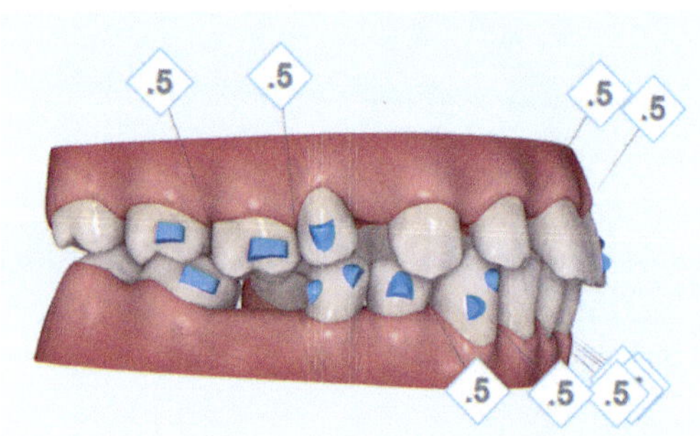

Fig. 17.13 Right ClinCheck view, initial situation.

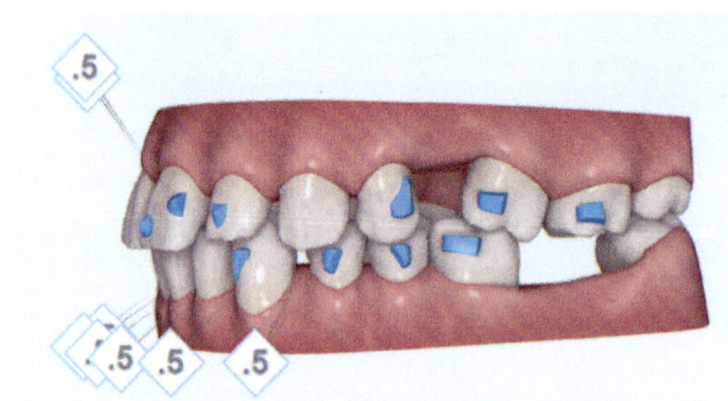

Fig. 17.14 Left ClinCheck view, initial situation.

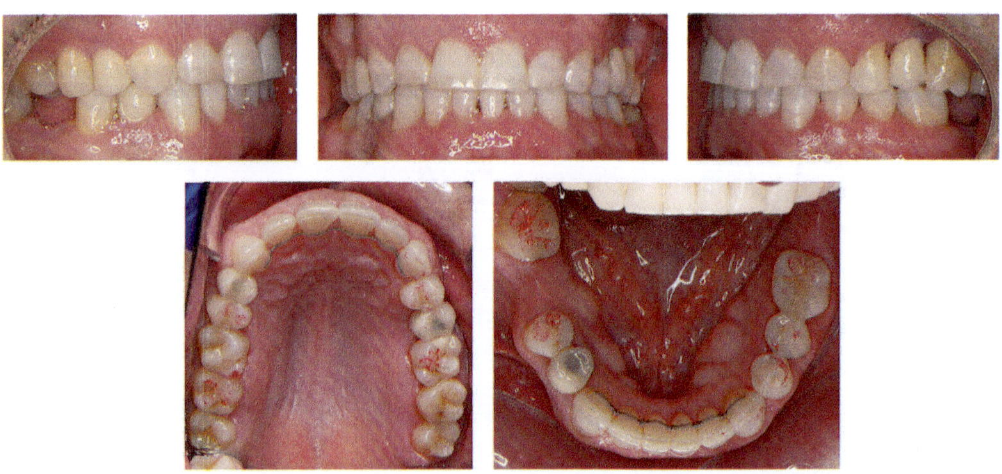

Fig. 17.15 Post-treatment views.

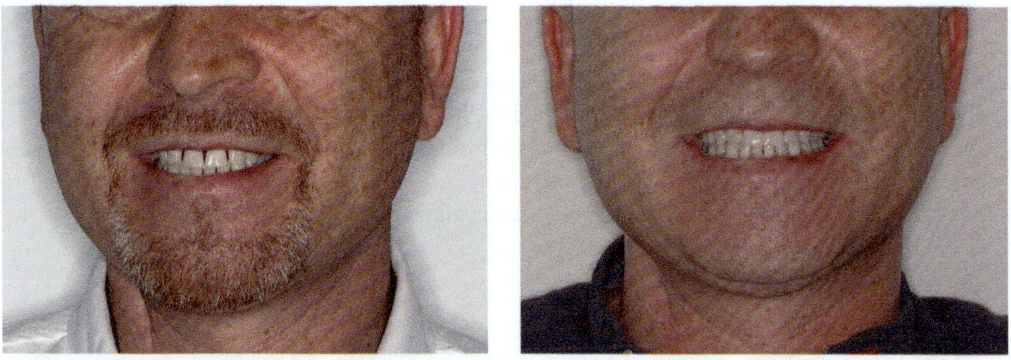

Fig. 17.16 Pretreatment and final smile.

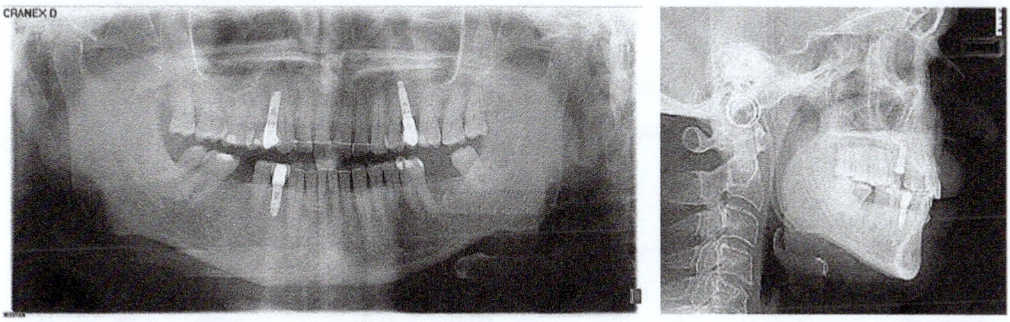

Fig. 17.17 Post-treatment panoramic and lateral X-rays.

17.1.2 Spacing with Frenulectomy

Fig. 17.18 Skeletal class I with spacing.

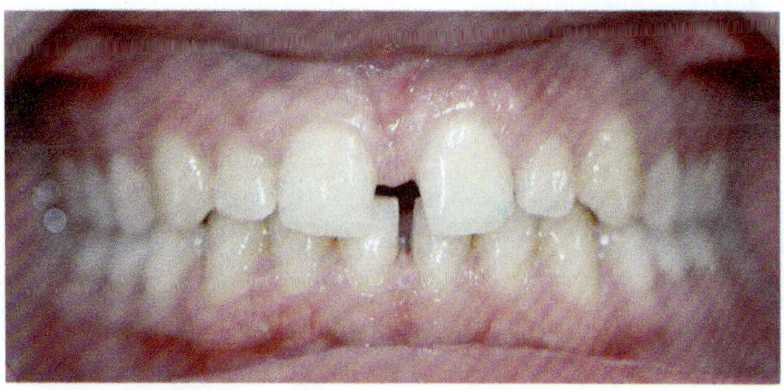

Diagnosis

A 20-year-old, symmetric patient who presented with a dental class I and a gummy smile. The patient had a large upper diastema. Short clinical crowns on upper incisors were also found.

Treatment Plan

- Closing spaces and maintaining anterior torque by adding extra lingual root torque
- Perform a frenulectomy at the initial stage so as to increase clinical crown size; however patient refused and postponed it to the end of treatment, together with a frenulectomy to prevent space relapse

ClinCheck 1: Requirements for the Technician

- Close spacing by crown retrusion, both in upper and lower
- Intrude both upper and lower incisors to solve deep bite and gummy smile by applying deep bite sequence with optimized extrusion or bevelled to gingival attachments on distal tooth
- Upper laterals extrude at the same moment as central incisors are intruding, producing a countermovement and levelling gingival architecture
- In order to correct upper spacing, 10 degrees extra palatal root torque added to upper incisors, as well as the lower ones, with ClinCheck PRO

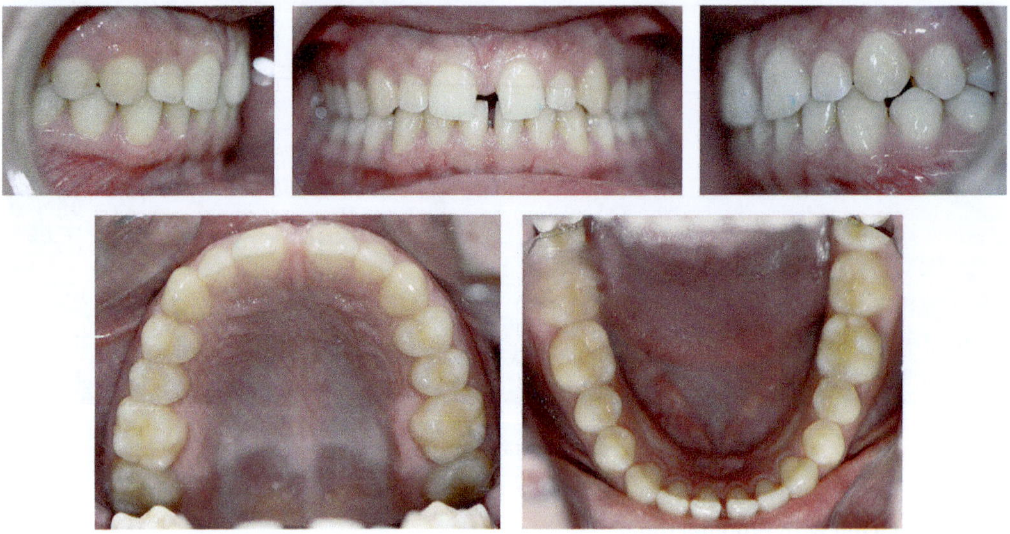

Fig. 17.19 Intraoral views left, front, right, upper, lower.

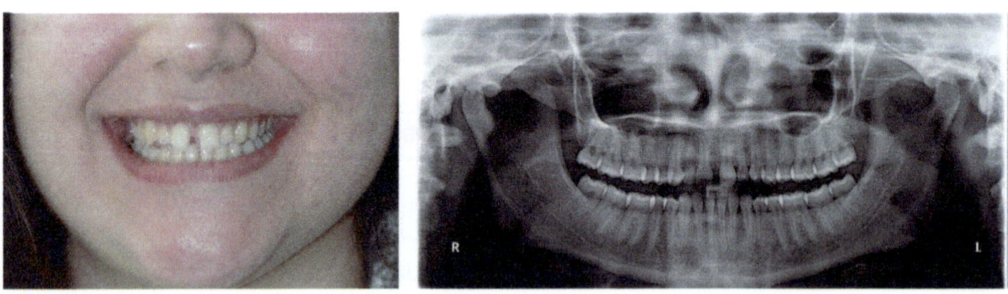

Fig. 17.20 Smile and pretreatment panoramic X-ray.

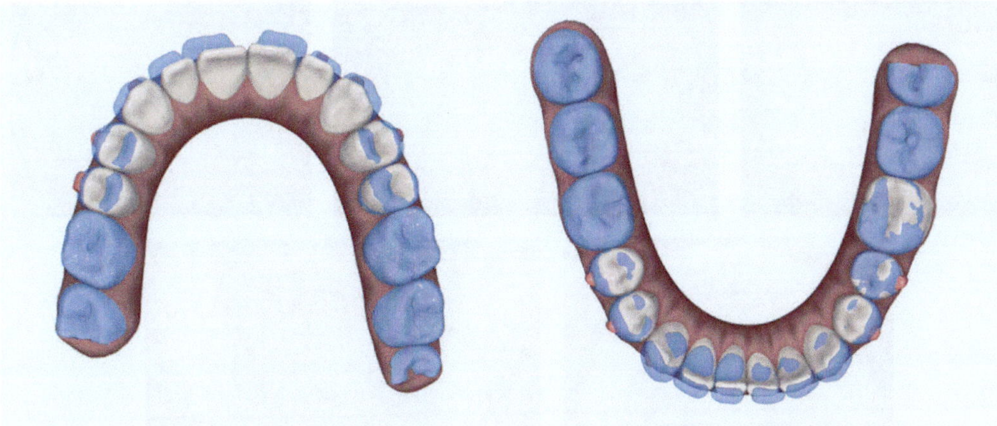

Fig. 17.21 Pretreatment ClinChecks.

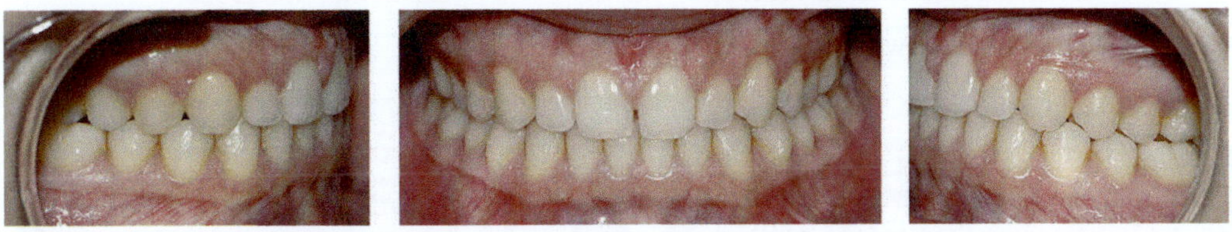

Fig. 17.22 Refinement: intraoral views, left, front, and right.

ClinCheck 2: Requirements for the Technician

- Hypercorrect diastema space closure
- Add buccal horizontal attachments 12–22 to ensure space closure
- Add palatal horizontal attachments 11–21 to create additional retention
- Patient decided to stop lower treatment and retention was bonded, so no more aligners were made for this

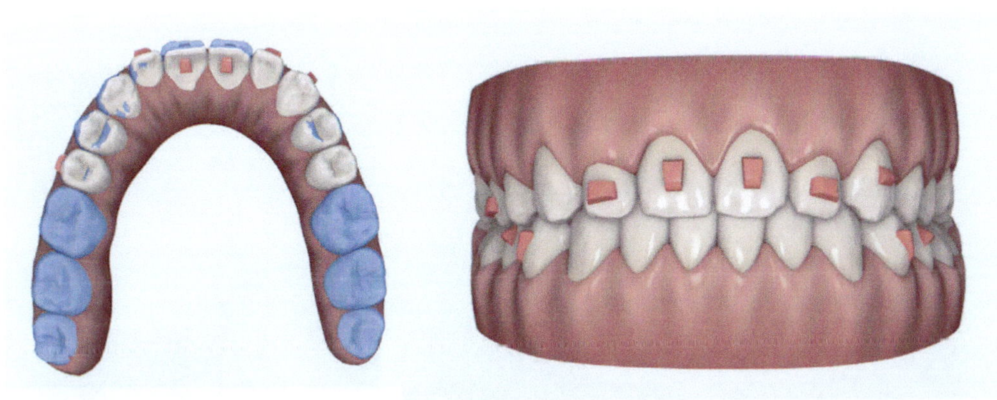

Fig. 17.23 Refinement ClinChecks.

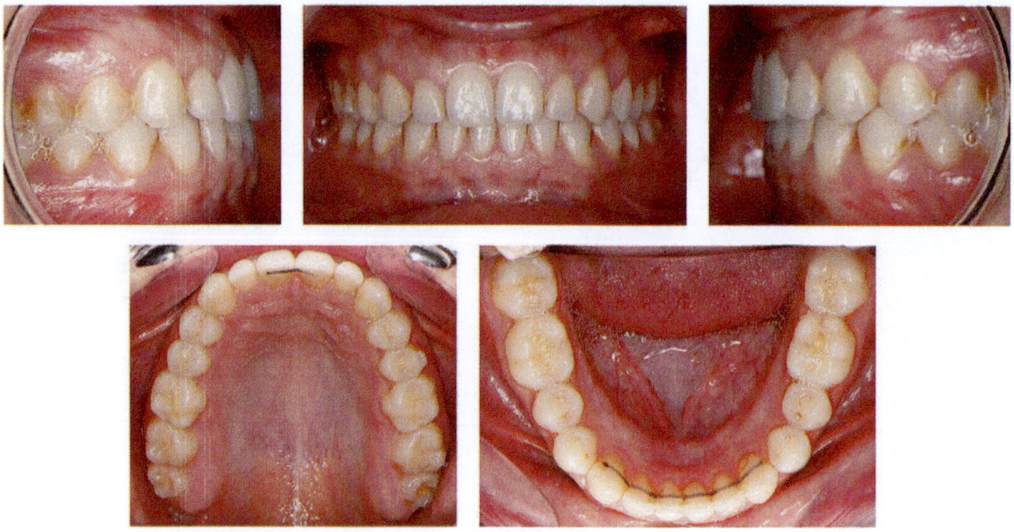

Fig. 17.24 Final intraoral views left, front, right, upper, lower.

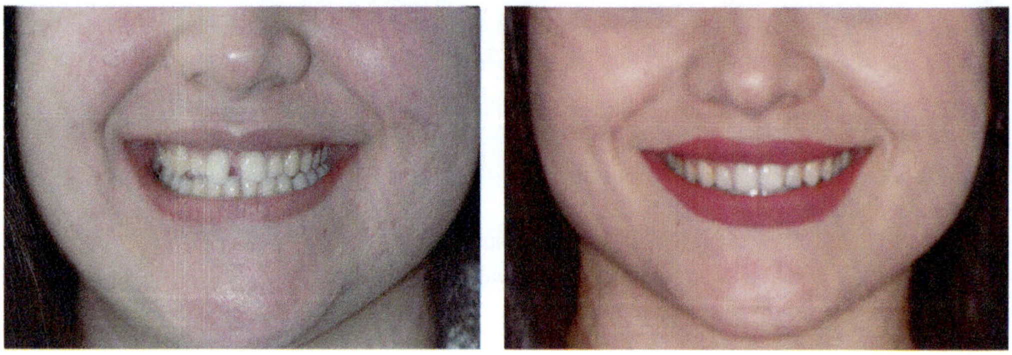

Fig. 17.25 Before and after smile.

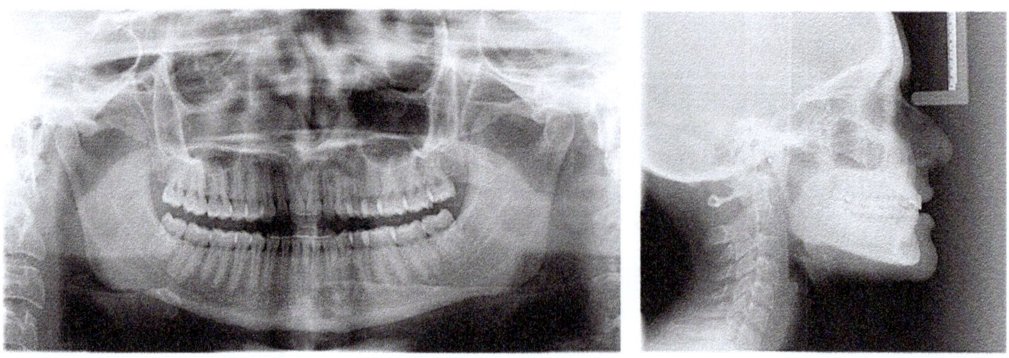

Fig. 17.26 Final panoramic and lateral X-rays.

17.2 Crowding

17.2.1 Crowding, Case 1

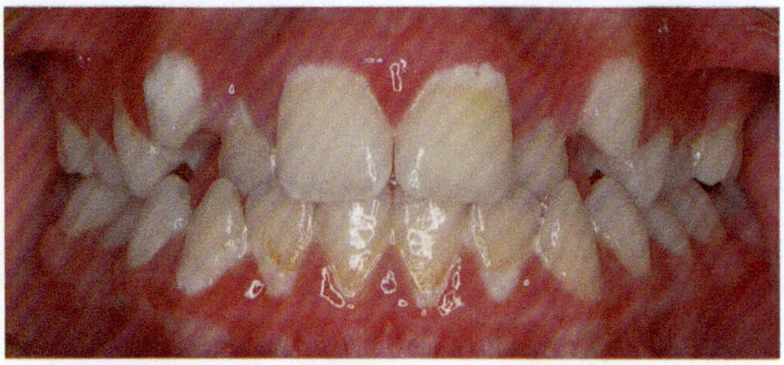

Fig. 17.27 Skeletal class III with upper maxillary compression and anterior crossbite of 12 and 22.

Diagnosis

A 12-year-old patient with hyperdivergent skeletal class III presented with upper compression with no space for 13 and 23. The extraoral view showed a symmetric patient with slight labial incompetence and right-side deviation of upper midline. He had an ectopic eruption of 13 and 23 with anterior crossbite of 12 and 22.

Treatment Plan

- Before sending the case the patient was provided with oral hygiene techniques
- The treatment plan included the virtual elimination of upper canines as well as pontics for 13 and 23
- The use of intermaxillary elastics to extrude canines
- Once space is made, extrusion of 13 and 23 at the same time as the intrusion of the upper lateral incisors
- In order to achieve a final buccal occlusion in class I, class III elastics were scheduled during the treatment

Requirements for the Technician

- Place AT HBG bevelled attachment to gingival in 12 and 22 to provide labial root torque to the upper lateral incisors during the protrusion
- In order to create positive overjet and avoid premature contacts in the anterior zone at the end of the treatment, anterior IPR 3 to 3 and retrusion of lower incisors is required
- AT vertical bevelled to distal in 25 to shorten the treatment (rotation of 25); do not use the 25 as a guide tooth and correct the rotation at high speed in the last eight stages (with that objective labial buttons on 25 and 26 and Powerchain were used to correct the rotation of 25
- AT horizontal bevelled to gingival in molars, to control posterior torque during the expansion

Treatment Summary

- Treatment was completed in 19 months.
- The patient wore 21 aligners to make expansion and open space for the ectopic upper canines
- After 21 aligners, the patient was scanned again so that the aligners would cover 13 and 23, and additional aligners were asked for
- Patient was required to use class III elastic from the upper first molars and lower canines at night during the refinement

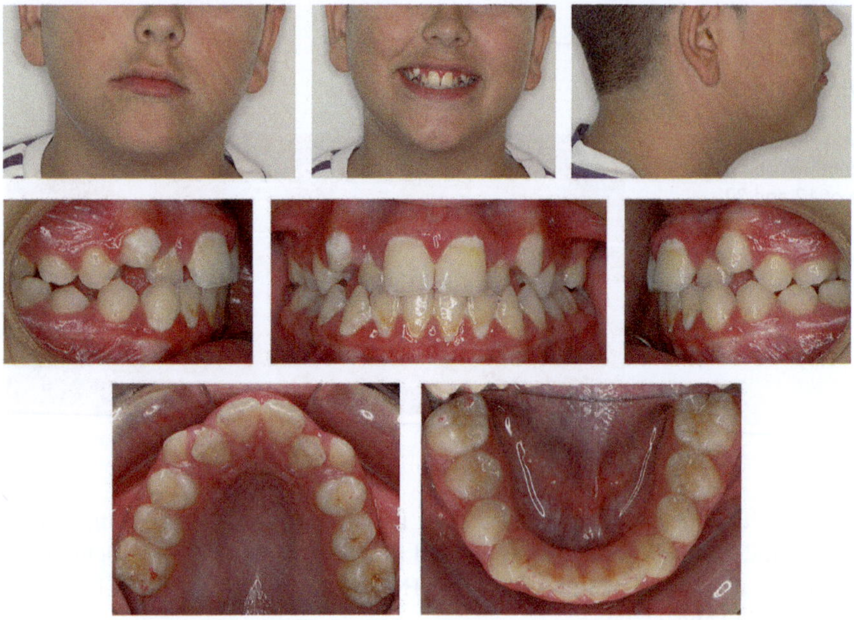

Fig. 17.28 Pretreatment views.

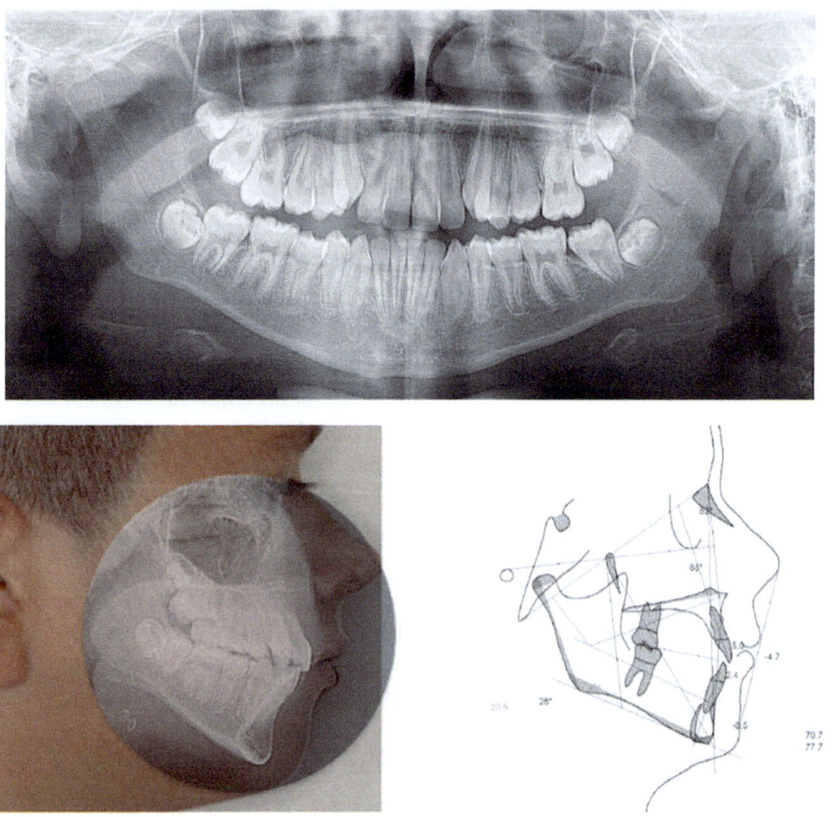

Fig. 17.29 Pretreatment panoramic X-ray, teleradiograph and cephalometry.

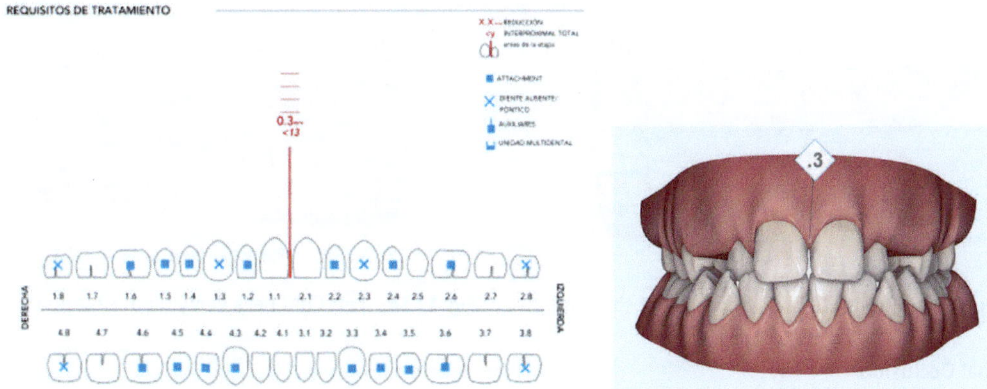

Fig. 17.30 Planned IPR on midline can be seen in several areas of the ClinCheck software.

Instructions to the Technician

Maxillary:

- Expansion + mesial-out rotation of 1.6/2.6
- Upper lateral protrusion + labial root torque during protrusion
- Bevelled attachments HBG in 1.2 and 2.2 for torque control during proclination

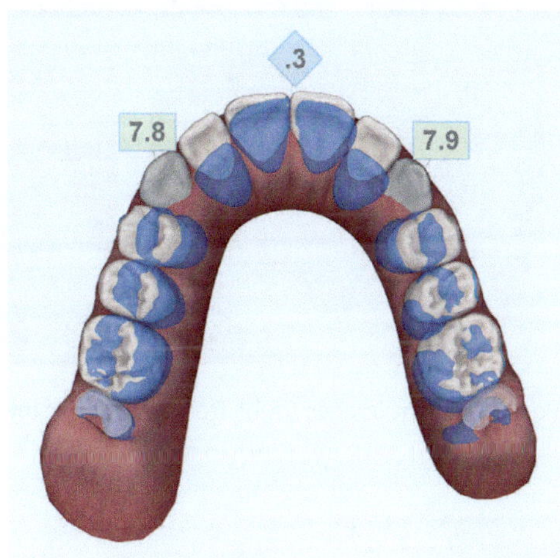

Fig. 17.31 Upper CC superimposition and instructions to CAD designer.

Mandible:

- Expansion + TRL lingual root torque of lower incisors + IPR
- Rotation of 3.3 and 4.3 during expansion (hinged rotation). Virtual removal of 1.3 and 2.3. Pontic for 1.3 and 2.3

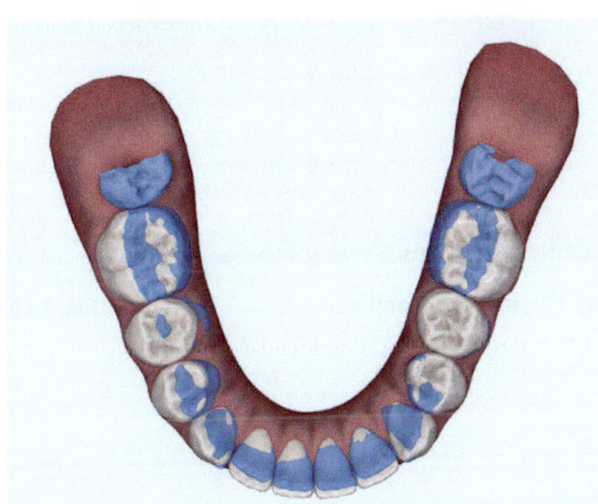

Fig. 17.32 Lower CC superimposition and instructions to CAD designer.

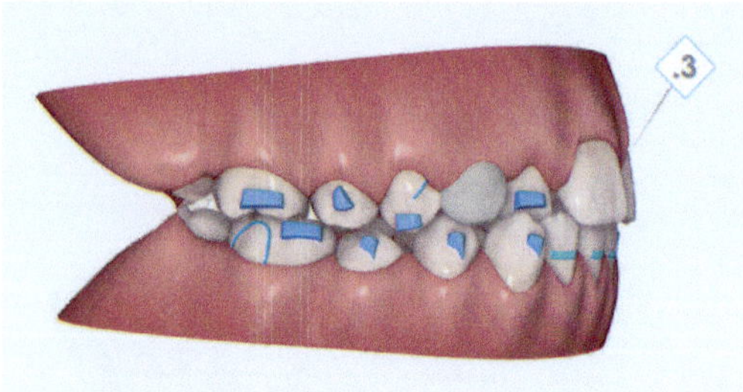

Fig. 17.33 Right ClinCheck view, initial situation.

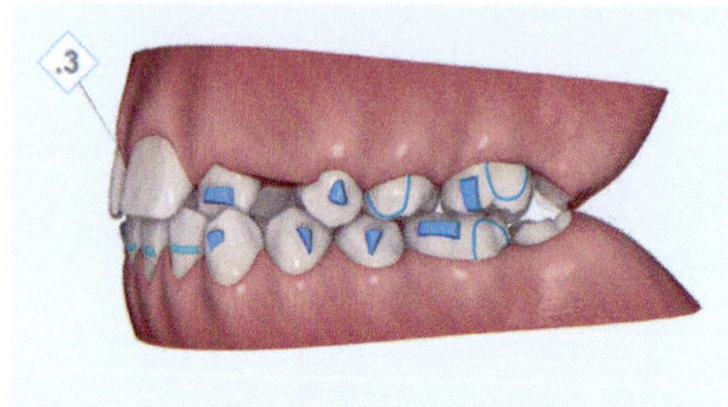

Fig. 17.34 Left ClinCheck view, initial situation.

Final Occlusion

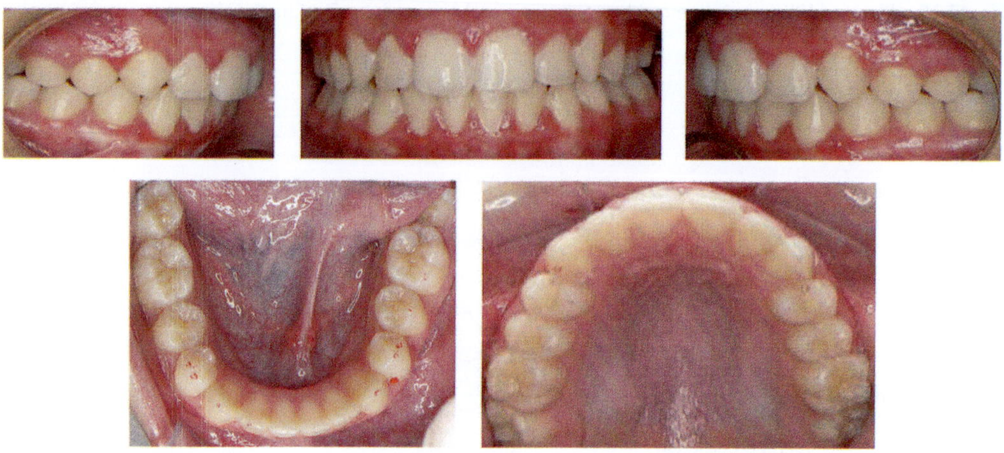

Fig. 17.35 Post-treatment images (right, front, left, upper, lower).

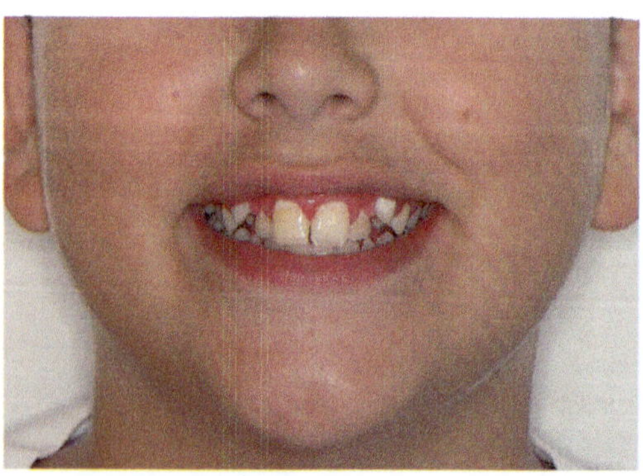

Fig. 17.36 Pretreatment smile.

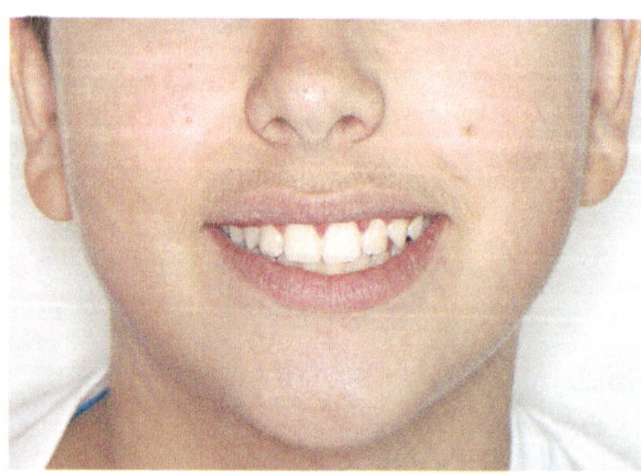

Fig. 17.37 Final smile.

17.2.2 Crowding, Case 2

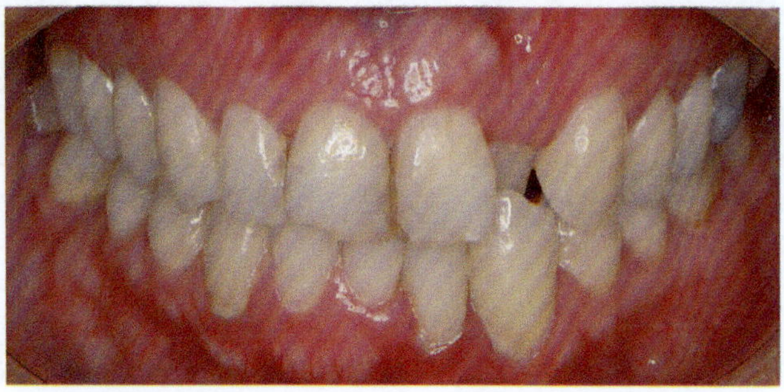

Fig. 17.38 Upper crowding and anterior crossbite 'Lite' treatment in a class III normodivergent patient.

Diagnosis

A 46-year-old patient with normodivergent skeletal class III, presented with anterior crowding and anterior crossbite of 22; she had a missing lower incisor and missing 46. She had a prognathic profile with open nasolabial angle and gummy posterior smile.

Treatment Plan

- Maintain the buccal class I relationship and not move molars in the first treatment phase.
- Procline upper incisor and provide labial crown torque to 13 and 23 to open space for 22.
- Correct anterior crossbite of the lateral upper incisors and the lower crowding.
- Second right lower molar was not planned to be upright with the Lite treatment.

Requirements for the Technician

- Asked not to move the molars to allow enough anchorage to correct the anterior crossbite of the upper left lateral incisor.
- A horizontal attachment bevelled to gingival placed on 22 to provide labial root toque to the lateral incisor during the proclination.
- In the lower arch, molars not to be moved to use them for anchorage and apply IPR and lower incisor retraction to increase the final overjet.

Treatment Summary

- Total treatment time was 14 months.
- The patient used the 14 first aligners with 2-week interval change protocol.
- After the first phase the anterior crossbite of the lateral incisor had been corrected.
- During the second set of 14 aligners the technician was required to expand the upper arch, in this case using the anterior incisors as anterior anchorage to reduce the gum posterior exposure.
- Anterior crossbite was completely corrected.
- A good anterior guide was achieved and the smile improved considerably after the expansion and the reduction of the gummy posterior exposition.

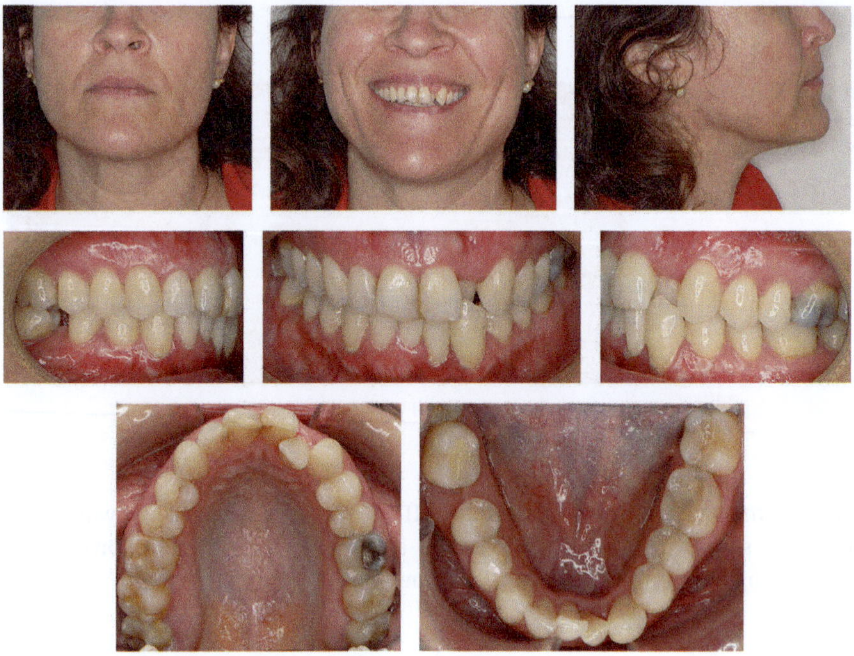

Fig. 17.39 Pretreatment extraoral and intraoral (right, front, left, upper, lower) views.

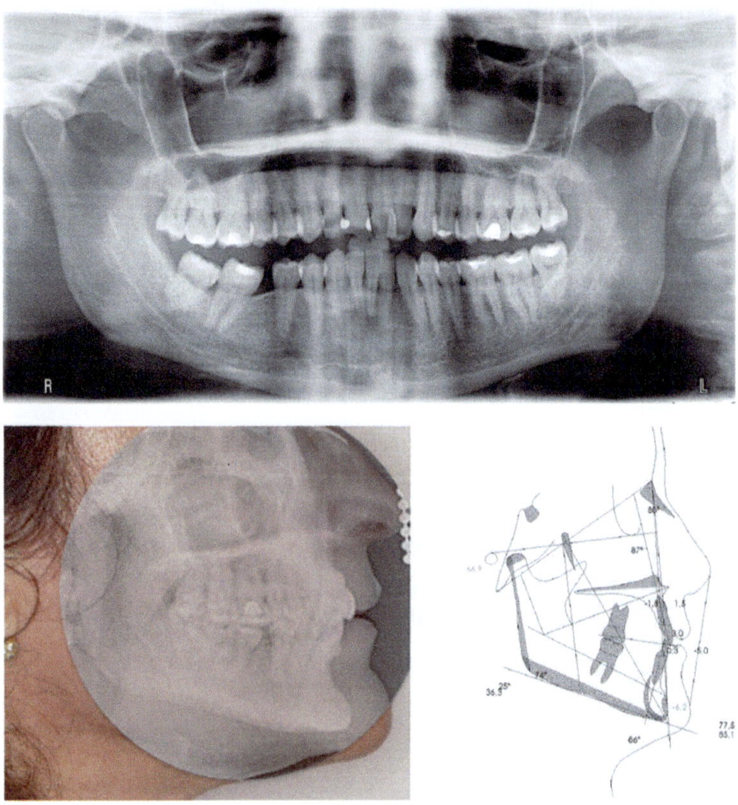

Fig. 17.40 Pretreatment panoramic X-ray, teleradiograph and cephalometry.

- Do not move molars to have anchorage
- Round tripping of upper incisors to open space for 22
- Reciprocal movement of 23 extrusion + 22 intrusion

- **AT HBG 4 mm 22** (ask the technician to move first the root of lateral incisor to labial and then the crown)
- **AT U4 and U6** anchorage attachments **HBG 3 mm**

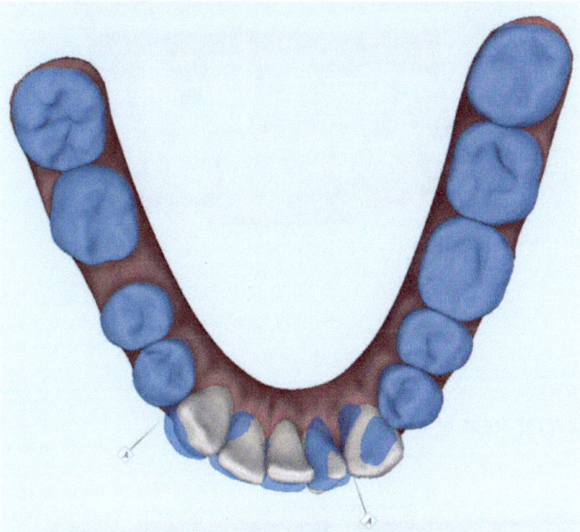

Fig. 17.41 Upper CC superimposition and instructions to CAD designer.

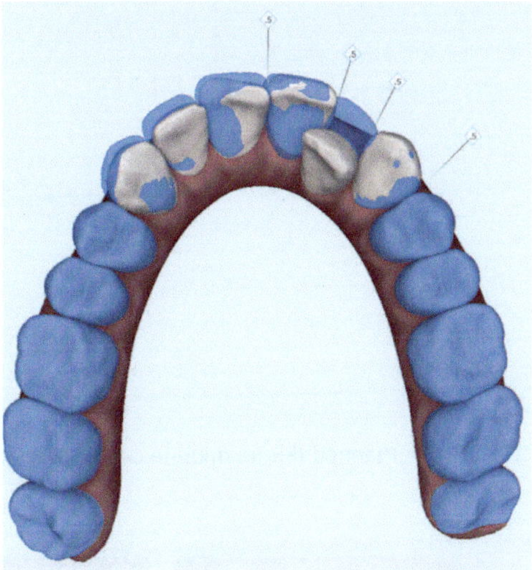

Fig. 17.42 Lower CC superimposition and instructions to CAD designer.

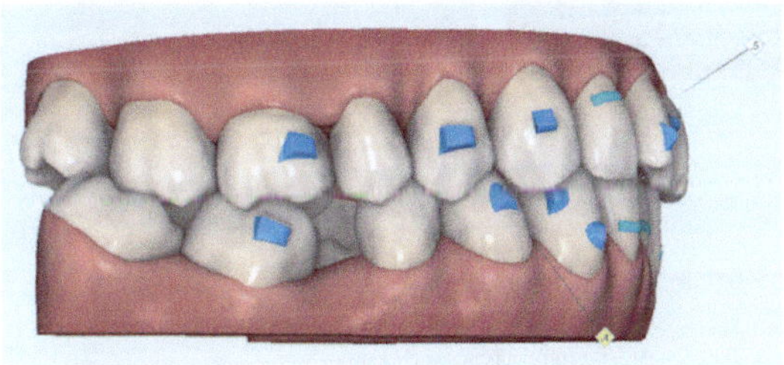

Fig. 17.43 Right ClinCheck view, initial situation.

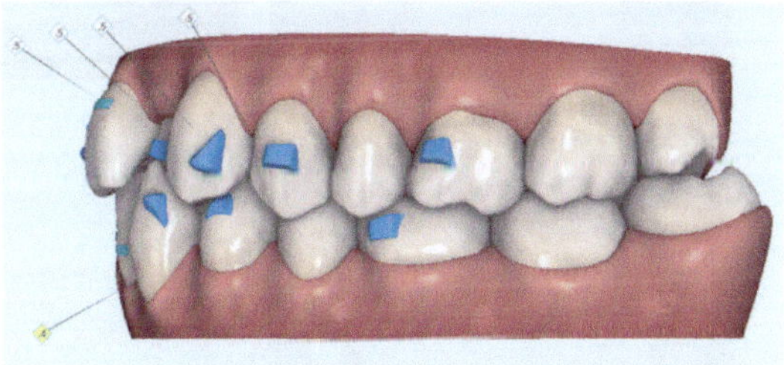

Fig. 17.44 Left ClinCheck view, initial situation.

- Correct crowding by proclination + IPR
- Centre upper midline in the middle of 3.1 (only has three incisors)

- AT HBG 4 mm in 2.2
- Round tripping 2.1 and TCV labial torque 2.3 to open space for 2.2

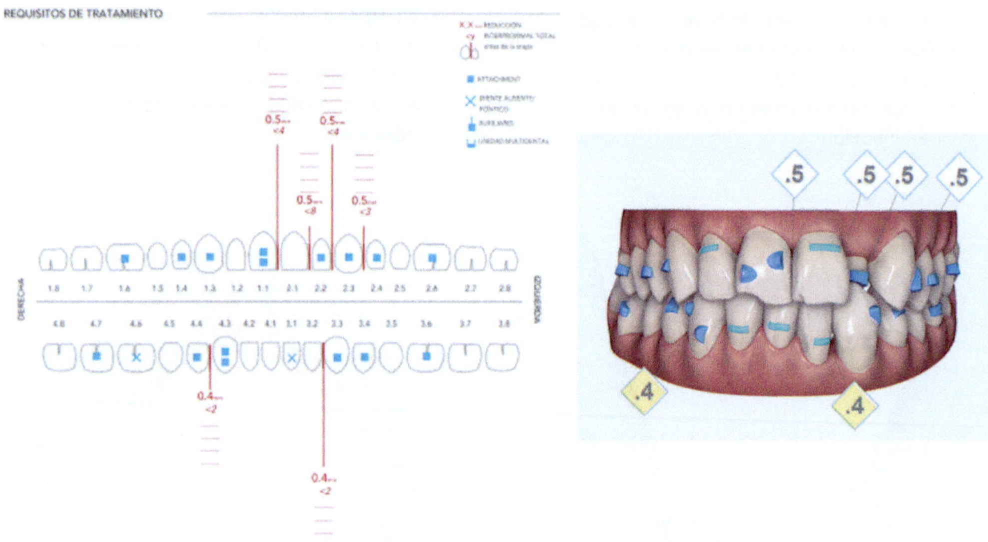

Fig. 17.45 Planned IPR on midline can be seen in several areas of the ClinCheck software.

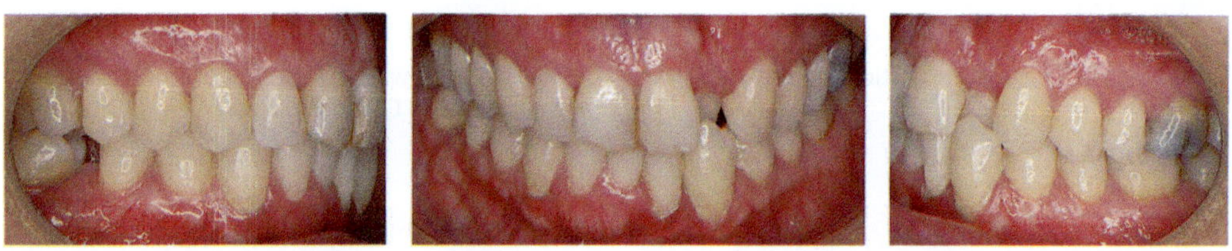

Fig. 17.46 Initial intraoral views.

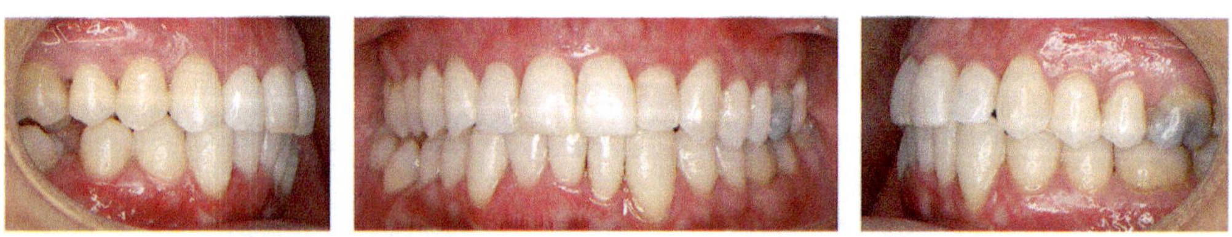

Fig. 17.47 Final intraoral views.

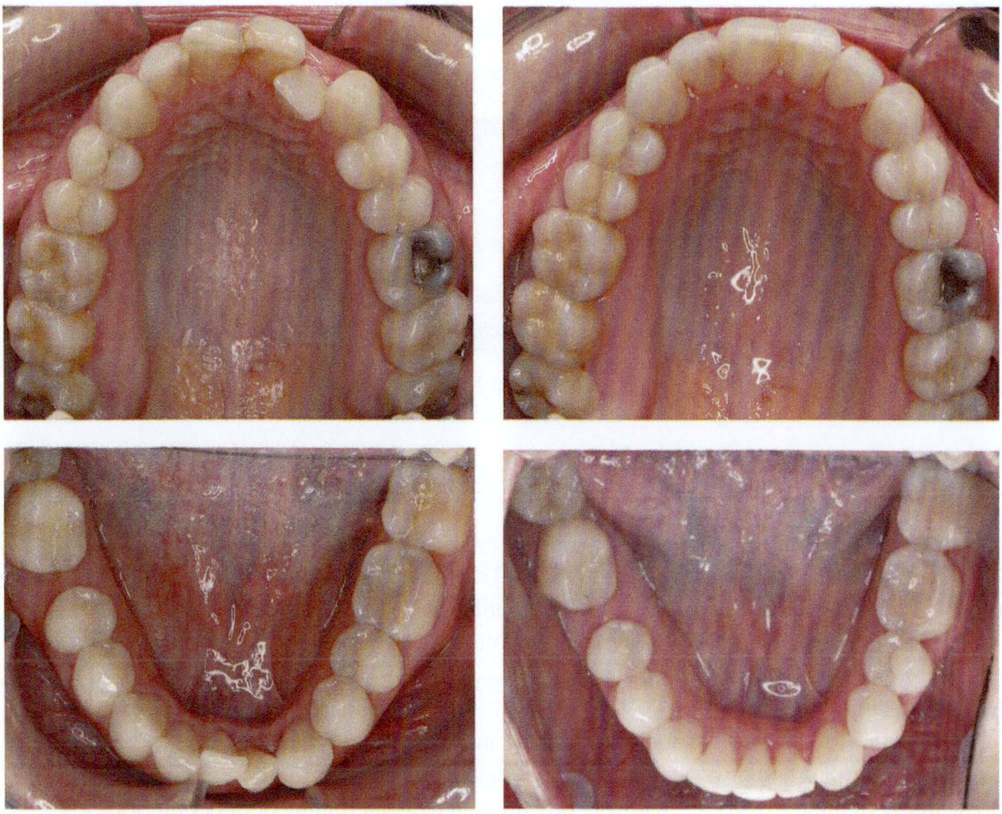

Fig. 17.48 Initial and final occlusal (upper and lower).

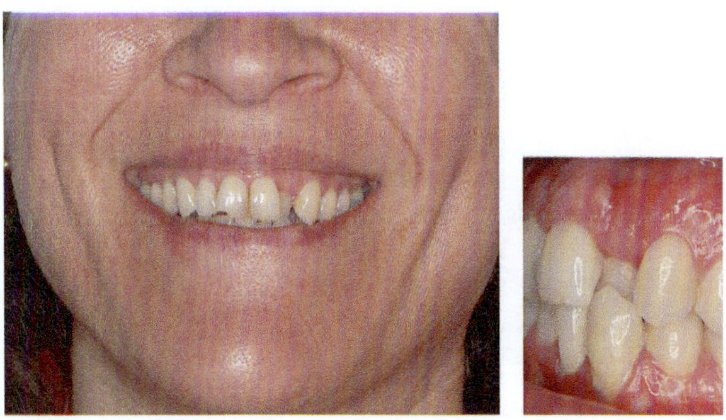

Fig. 17.49 Pretreatment smile and overjet.

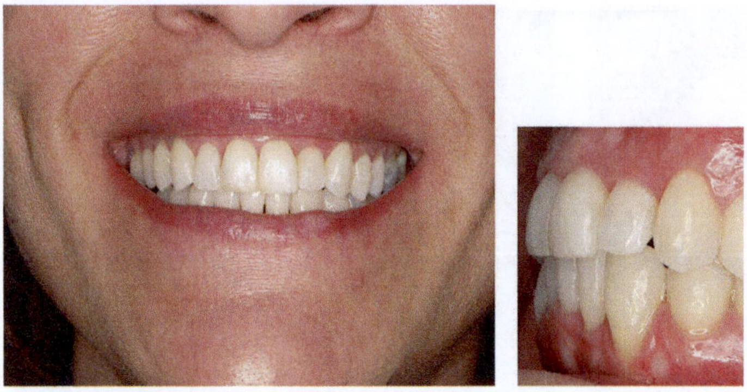

Fig. 17.50 Final smile and overjet.

17.2.3 Crowding, Case 3

Diagnosis

A 43-year-old patient with hyperdivergent skeletal class III, presented with anterior crowding and anterior crossbite of 22. They had a prognathic profile with open nasolabial angle, a left-side deviation of the upper midline and periodontal recession in 33.

Treatment Plan

- Open a space for 22 by expansion, proclination and IPR
- Correct anterior crossbite of the lateral upper incisors and correct the lower crowding
- The upper midline to be centred during proclination to avoid tipping of upper incisors

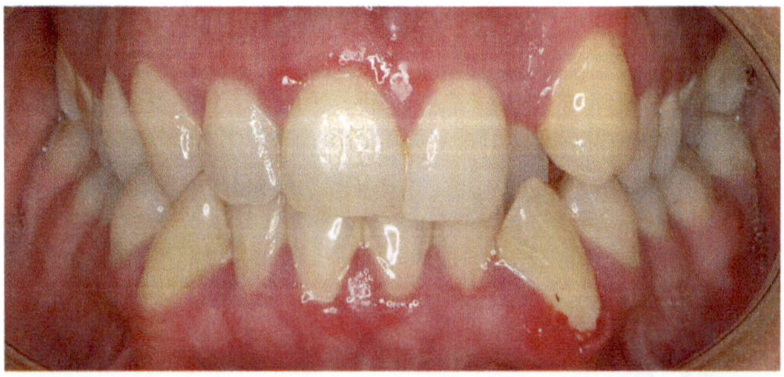

Fig. 17.51 Upper and lower crowding with anterior crossbite of 22.

Requirements for the Technician

- Asked not to move the molars in order to have enough anchorage to correct the anterior crossbite of the upper left lateral incisor
- A horizontal attachment bevelled to gingival to be placed on 22 to provide labial root torque to the lateral incisor during the proclination
- To correct the rotation of lower canines, do not rotate the canines mesial-in until there is a space of 0.2 mm provided between lateral and canines

Treatment Summary

- Total treatment time was 18 months
- The patient used 47 aligners with a 7-day change interval protocol
- After the first set of aligners the anterior crossbite of the lateral incisor was corrected
- During the second set of aligners in refinement the patient used intermaxillary elastics to settle the occlusion
- Anterior crossbite was totally corrected
- A good anterior guide was achieved and the smile improved considerably after the expansion, improving the periodontal final situation in 33 and 43

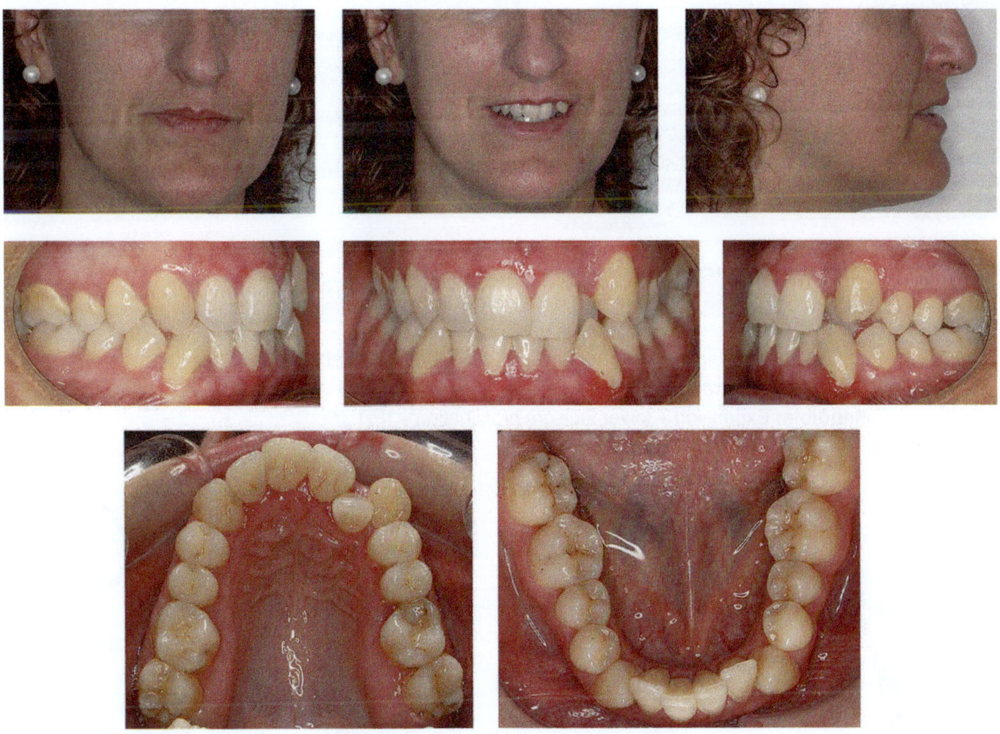

Fig. 17.52 Pretreatment: extraoral and intraoral (right, front, left, upper, lower) views.

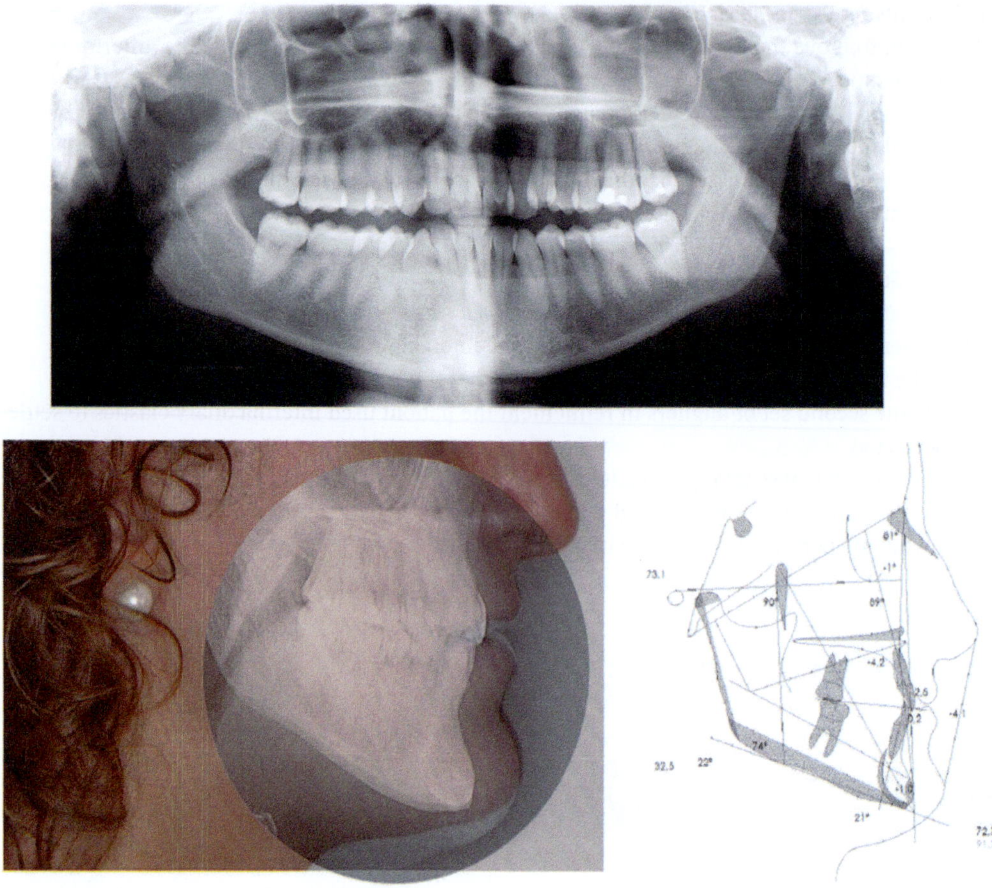

Fig. 17.53 Initial panoramic X-ray, teleradiograph and cephalometry.

Maxilla: symmetric expansion + upper incisors protrusion at the same time that we centre upper midline to the right side
Mandible: Expansion + lower incisors proclination + IPR

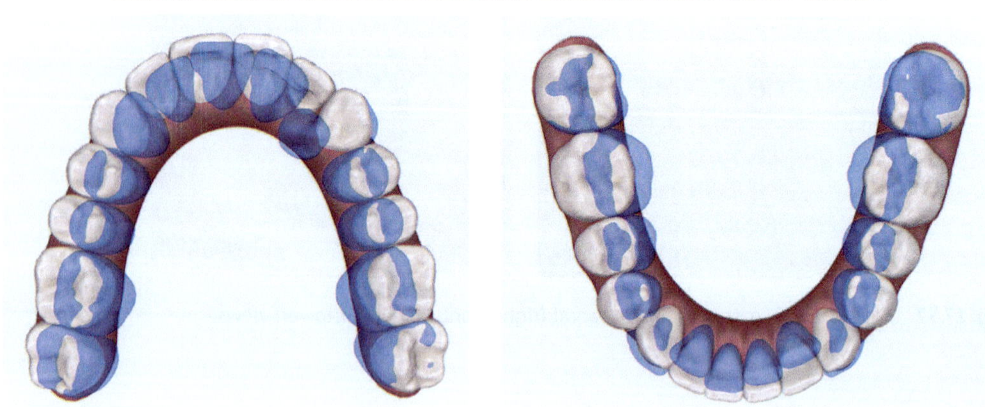

Fig. 17.54 Upper and lower CC superimposition and instructions to CAD designer.

- Symmetrical expansion of upper and lower arches (AT horizontal HBG 3 mm to control posterior torque during expansion)
- Upper incisors proclination at the same time that we centre upper midline to the right
- AT HBG 3 mm in 22 to provide labial root torque to the lateral incisors during protrusion

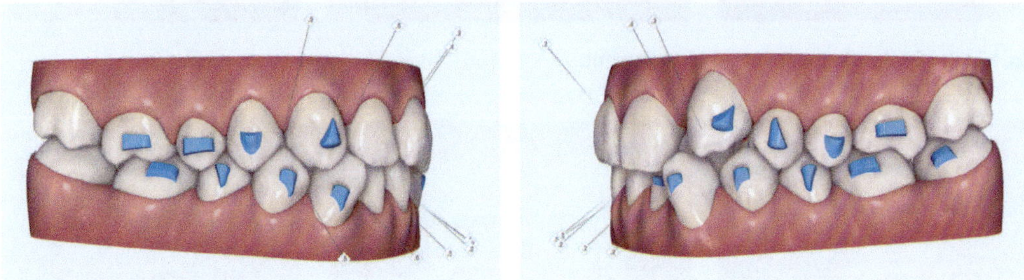

Fig. 17.55 Right and left ClinCheck view, initial situation and instructions to CAD designer.

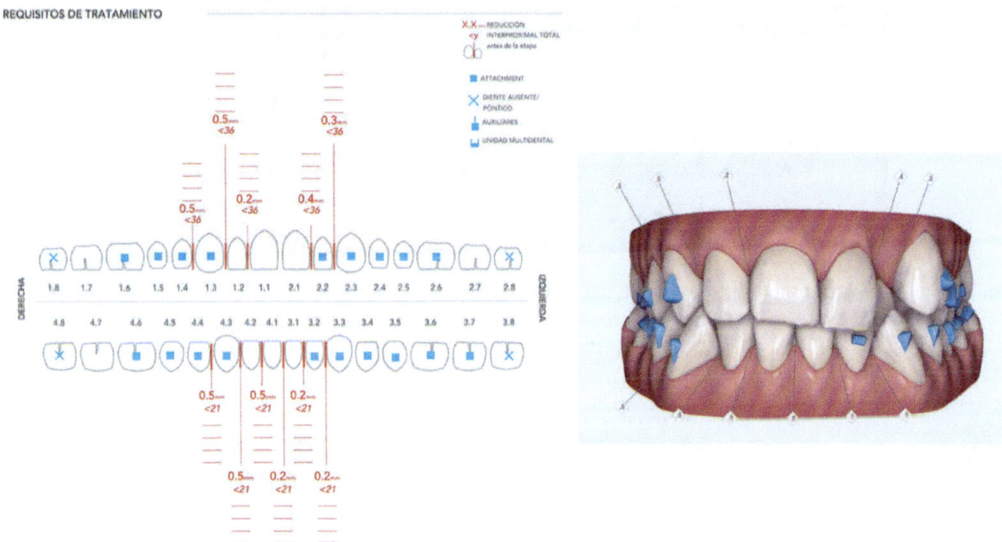

Fig. 17.56 Interproximal reduction after improving contact surface between incisors.

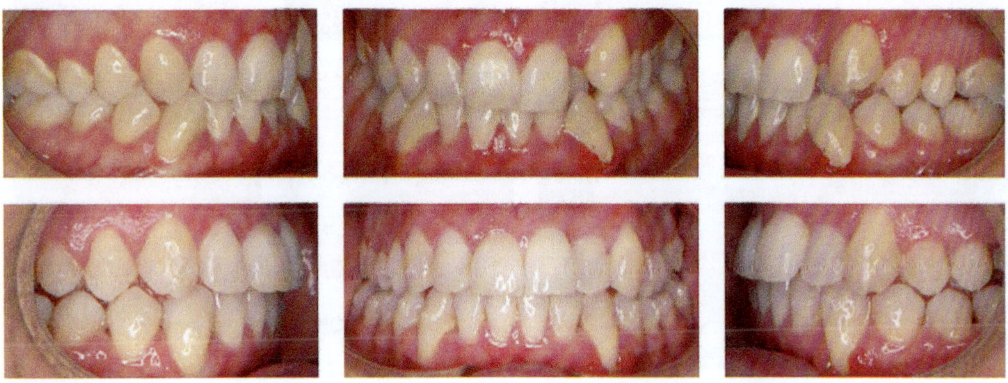

Fig. 17.57 Evolution in month 13 of treatment.

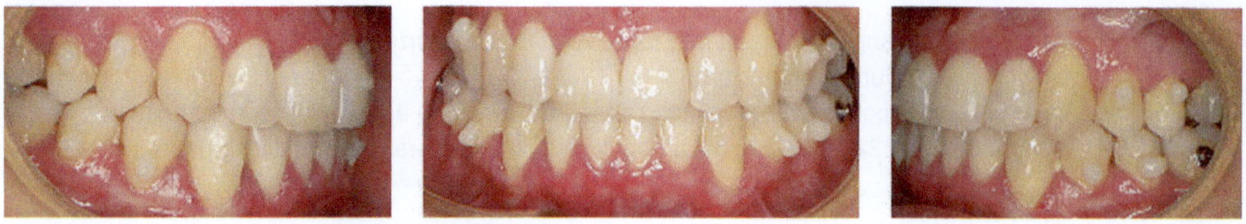

Fig. 17.58 Evolution in month 17 of treatment.

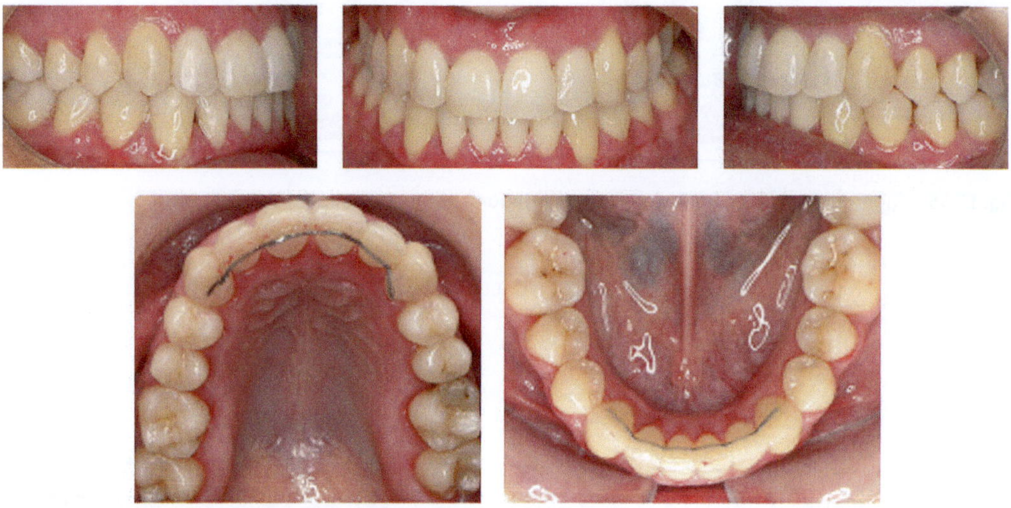

Fig. 17.59 Final intraoral (right, front, left, upper, lower) views.

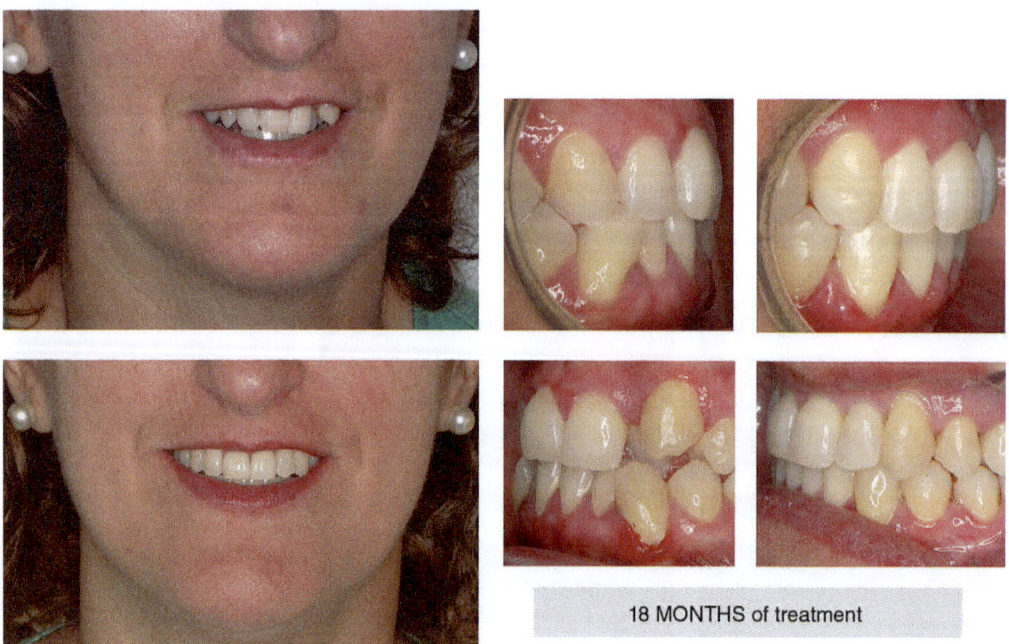

Fig. 17.60 Initial and final smile and overjet.

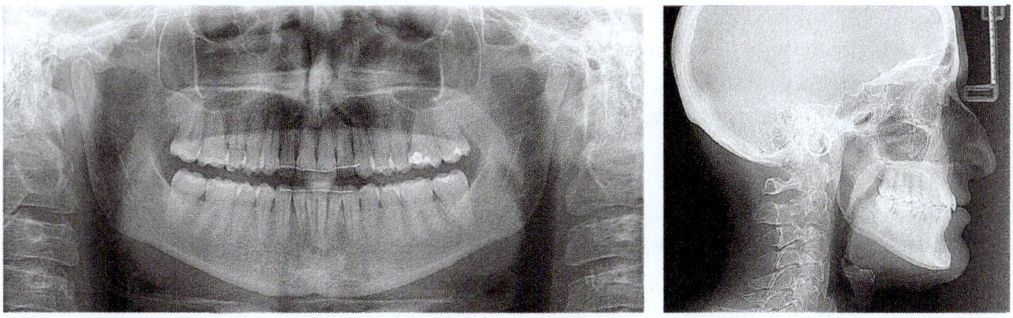

Fig. 17.61 Final panoramic and lateral X-rays.

Tips for Upper Crowding with Anterior Crossbite of Lateral Incisors

- Open space using the different space achievers depending on the malocclusion diagnosis:
  - expansion
  - proclination
  - distalization
  - mesial-out rotation of the first molars
  - labial torque to canines
- Design a symmetric parabolic arch form
- AT HBG bevelled attachment to gingival of 4 mm on lateral incisors

Tips for Lower Crowding

- In lower crowding cases, lower canines always need an attachment, if the technician does not place an optimized attachment, use the 3D control to place a vertical conventional attachment.
- Soften the contact points
- Correct canine rotation at the same time as expansion (hinge rotation)
- Be specific about how much proclination is needed
- IPR as soon as the surface allows it
- Rotation and tipping problem in canines: first correct rotation in favour of solving crowding and then correct the root tipping.

17.2.4 Crowding, Case 4

Fig. 17.62 Skeletal class I with crowding.

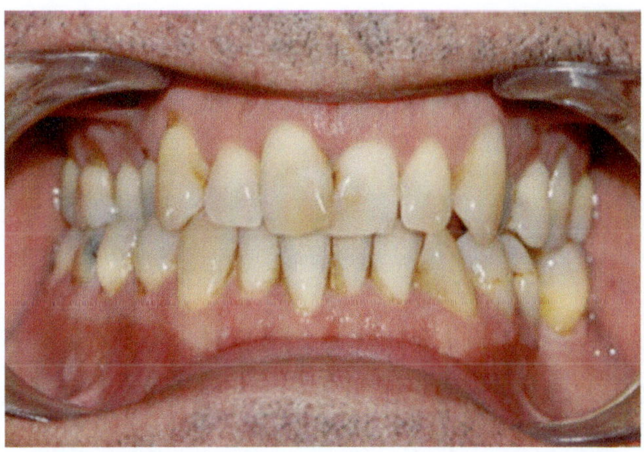

Diagnosis

A 49-year-old patient, with a symmetrical skeletal pattern, presented as dental class I with proper display and posterior compression. The patient presented upper and lower crowding, with thin gingival biotope and 36 missing. The patient had a posterior crossbite on premolars.

Treatment Plan

- Align the anterior sector using posterior as anchorage
- Initial scan did not register 37, having a lack of anchorage that was solved on the next set of aligners
- Crossbite protocol was applied without needing criss-cross elastics

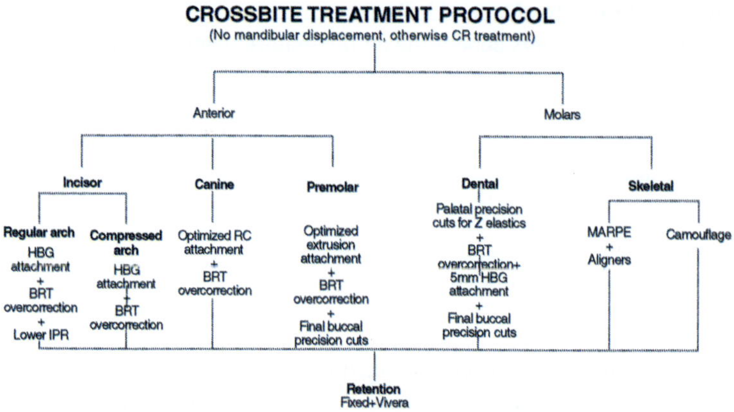

Fig. 17.63 Protocol excludes criss-cross elastics to solve premolar crossbite.

ClinCheck 1: Requirements for the Technician

- In order to prevent recessions add 10 degrees extra palatal root torque to premolars, simultaneous to crown positive buccal torque
- Plan lower IPR to avoid excessive arch development or incisors protrusion

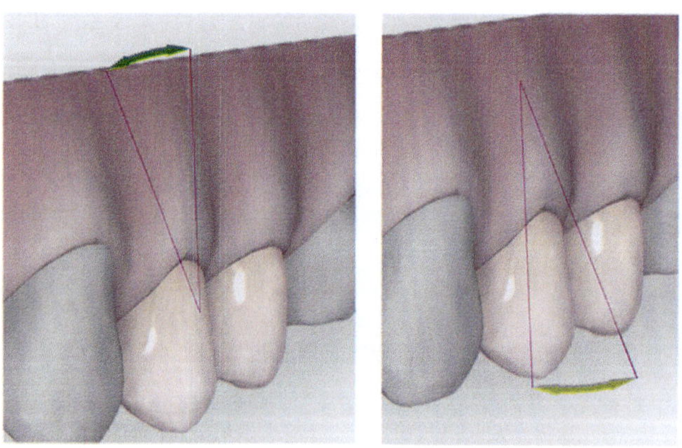

Fig. 17.64 Extra palatal root torque premolars, selecting multiple teeth with ClinCheck PRO, followed by extra crown buccal torque to solve crossbite.

- Gingival margin of 21 aligned having 11 as a reference, owing to the fact that the patient refused final incisal edge composite restoration
- Extrusion attachments on first quadrant, rotation attachments on second quadrant
- 43 staging to prevent recession: distal out, mesial protruded

Treatment Summary

- Treatment was completed in 14 months with a Lite treatment.
- Teeth were aligned and final gingival situation was stable
- Class I occlusion was maintained
- Patient did not use criss-cross elastics to solve posterior crossbite because he had molars in a proper transverse relationship, which helped as anchorage.

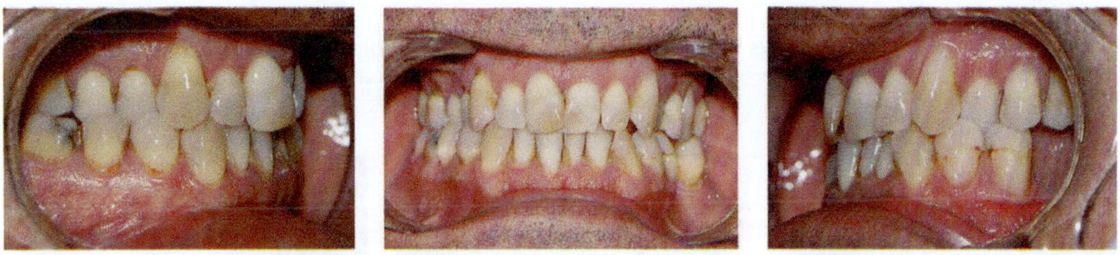

Fig. 17.65 Pretreatment intraoral views (left, front, right).

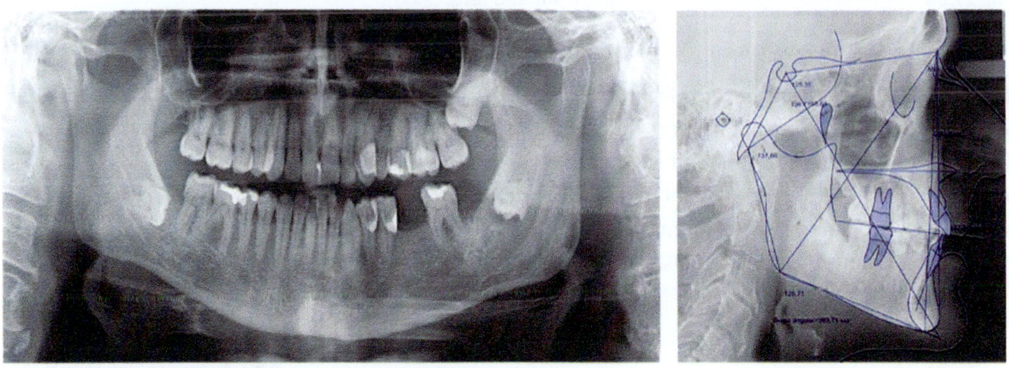

Fig. 17.66 Initial panoramic and lateral X-rays.

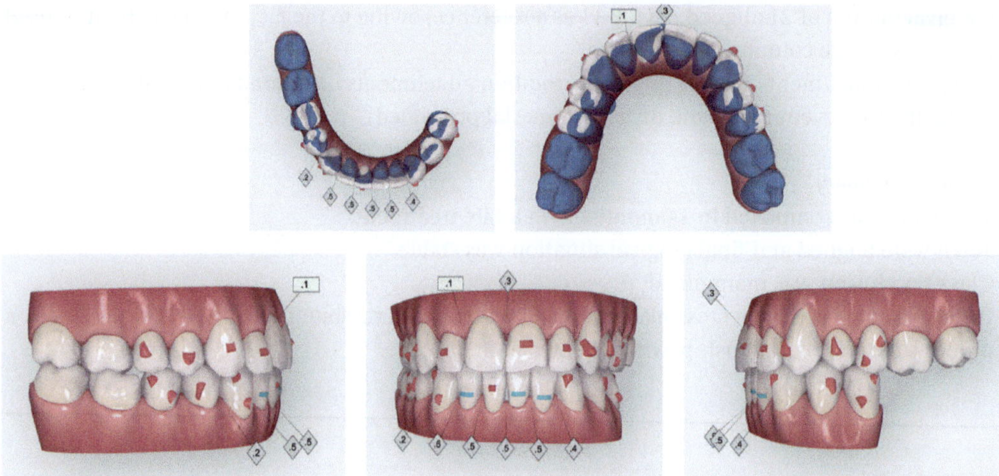

Fig. 17.67 Pretreatment ClinChecks with interproximal reduction to avoid expansion and black triangles.

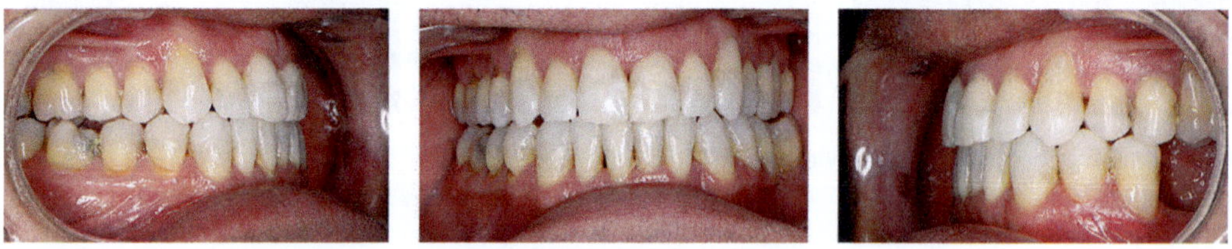

Fig. 17.68 Refinement: intraoral views (right, front and left).

ClinCheck 2: Communication with Technician

- Optimized extrusion attachments on premolars to close posterior open bite
- Space closure on lower anterior sector to close spacing
- Rotate lower premolars to distal to improve occlusion with upper ones
- On upper arch plan IPR between central incisors to avoid black triangle and use optimized extrusion attachment to level 21 incisal edge to 11 by extrusion

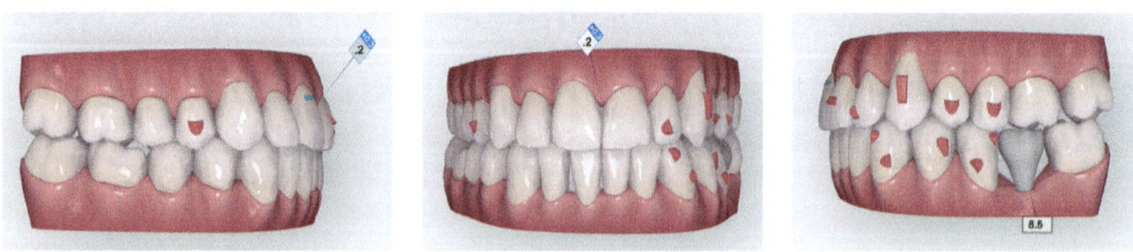

Fig. 17.69 Refinement ClinCheck: right, front and left (in this set, 37 is included to increase anchorage).

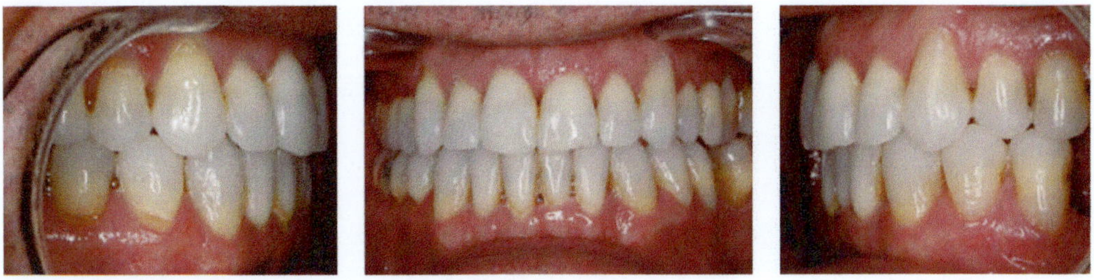

Fig. 17.70 Final intraoral views (left, front, right).

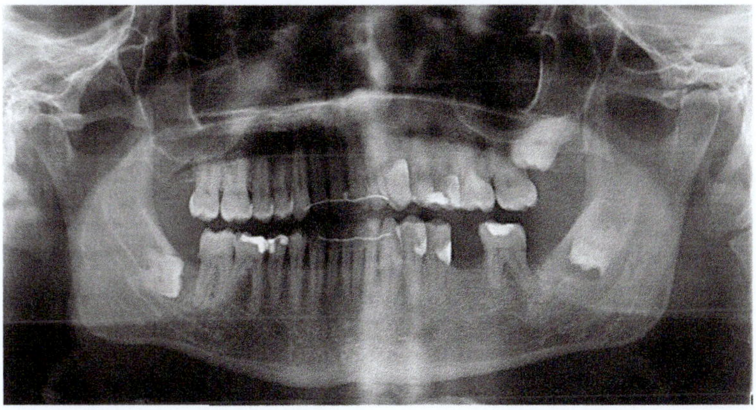

Fig. 17.71 Final panoramic-X-ray.

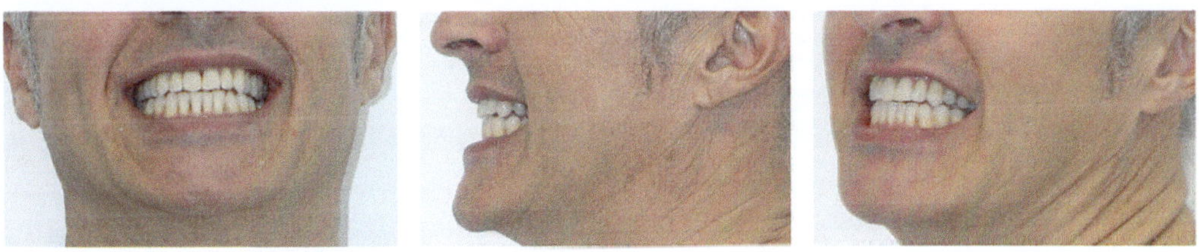

Fig. 17.72 Final extraoral views.

18

Growing Patients

After first permanent molars and incisors erupt, clinicians face a mixed dentition period in which they have to determine whether there is need for orthopaedic/orthodontic treatment or not, mostly related to skeletal rather than dental correction. Based on this, phase I treatment is usually done early in this period.

To create a treatment plan practitioners must understand the growth and development patterns, as jaw growth affects orthodontic treatment. For this, we have to focus on our knowledge of mixed dentition and growth in order to determine whether early treatment has a benefit to patients.

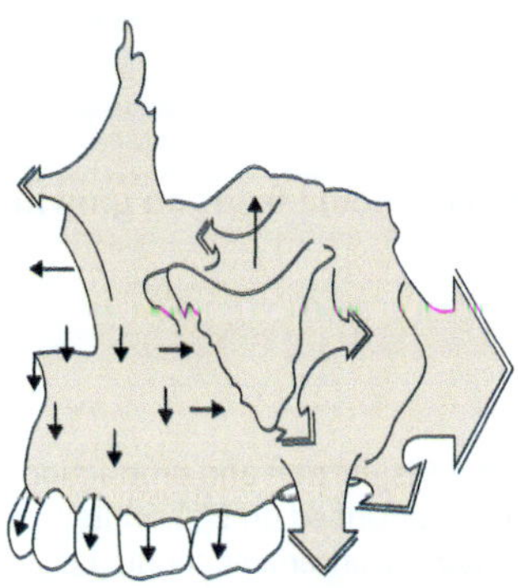

Fig. 18.1 Skeletal growth pattern has to be carefully evaluated in growing patients.

Clinicians must therefore diagnose and intercept certain developing problems with early treatment, while in other cases treatment should wait until permanent teeth have fully erupted, depending on clinical and social aspects related to the patient.

Aligner Techniques in Orthodontics, First Edition. Susana Palma Moya and Javier Lozano Zafra.

Companion website: www.wiley.com/go/lozano-zafra/aligner-techniques

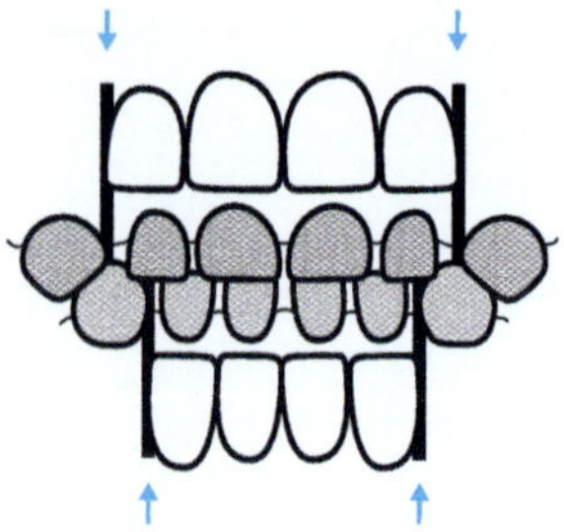

Fig. 18.2 Upper temporary spacing is 3 mm, on average, while tooth discrepancy between these and permanent ones is 7.6 mm, therefore giving a tendency to crowding.

To summarize, when crowding is severe intercanine distance has to be accelerated (6–8 years old in boys, 6–9 years old in girls) to prevent permanent severe crowding and increase arch development. Achieving arches with widths of 35–39 mm leads to prevention of extraction, and hence to better dentoskeletal and muscular adaptation.[1]

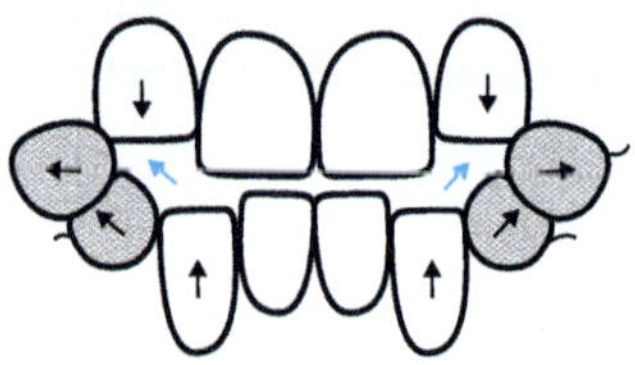

Fig. 18.3 Severe crowding on temporary teeth leads to future extractions or more complex treatments, suggesting that it must be addressed at an early stage.

In deciding whether early treatment is convenient or not, the clinician should focus on growth peaks, following the clinical considerations established by Bacetti *et al.*[2]

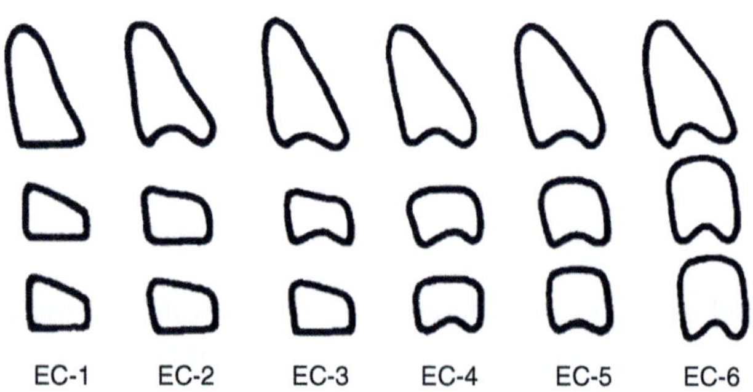

Fig. 18.4 Disjunction and protraction should be performed on EC1, while mandibular advancement should be planned on EC3/4.

1 Howe RP, McNamara Jr JA, O'Connor KA. An examination of dental crowding and its relationship to tooth size and arch dimension. *Am J Orthod*. 1983;83:363–373.

2 Baccetti T, Franchi L, McNamara Jr JA. The Cervical Vertebral Maturation (CVM) method for the assessment of optimal treatment timing in dentofacial orthopedics. *Semin Orthod*. 2005;11:119–129.

Disjunction cannot be performed exclusively with aligners, so mixed treatment with functional devices has to be considered, as we will learn later in this chapter. This is mandatory for class III patients, in which anterior crossbite also has to be resolved.

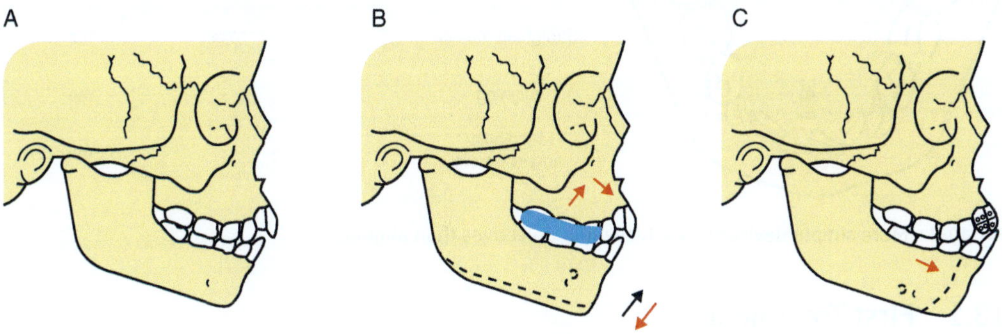

Fig. 18.5 Anterior crossbite management should be addressed early.

The same applies to class II patients if overjet is higher than 6 mm, regardless of whether it has a skeletal or exclusively dental component, as it reduces the risk of trauma on anterior incisors. Thanks to aligner improvements this can be achieved solely with Precision Wings, avoiding uncomfortable old functional devices such as Klammt or Twin Block.

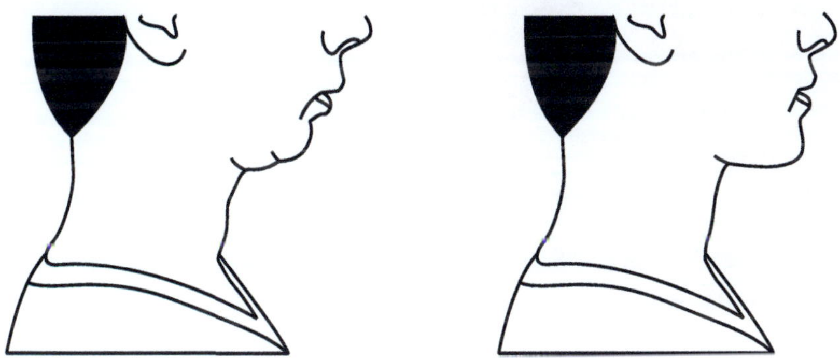

Fig. 18.6 Skeletal class II can be achieved before than usual if overjet is >6 mm.

The advantages of aligners technique in these patients are as follows:

- Single device use instead of different classic orthodontic treatments (functional, braces, wires, etc.), which leads to comfort and easy use and comprehension
- Enhanced dental hygiene
- Digital control of growth with ClinCheck models and iTero scans
- Easy to replace devices if they are lost or broken
- Compatible with sports or any other activities

For this, we strongly suggest treating growing patients with aligners, which will lead to happier patients and improved treatment outcomes.

It is also important for the orthodontist to understand that simpler devices such as Schwartz expansion devices offer simple solutions to basic problems, but good aligner management leads to good outcomes with wider objectives in the first treatment phase.

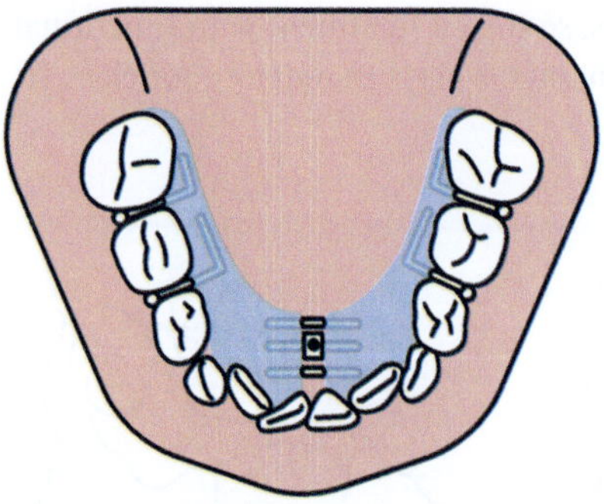

	Schwartz appliance	Lip bumper	Aligners
Lower dental expansion	Yes	Yes	Yes
Straighten molars	-	Yes	Yes
Aligning	-	-	Yes
Mandibular advancement	-	-	Yes

Fig. 18.7 More simple devices can achieve less objectives than aligners.

18.1 First Treatment

18.1.1 Upper Maxillary Compression

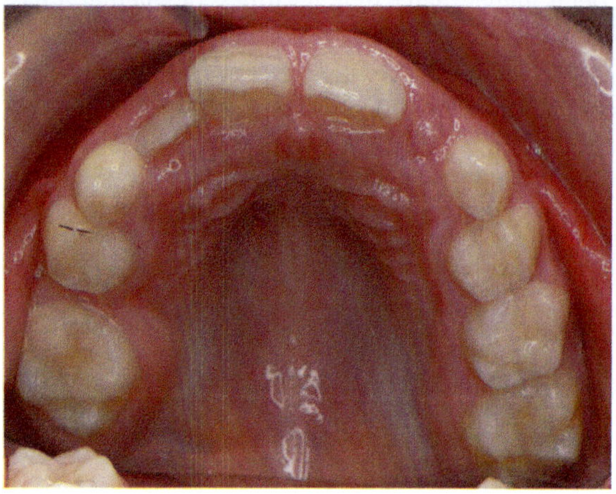

Fig. 18.8 Upper compression with posterior and anterior crowding.

Diagnosis

An 8-year-old patient with normodivergent skeletal class I presented with missing 55 and mesial ectopic eruption of 16. They had maxillary compression, deep bite and upper and lower crowding.

Treatment Plan

- Transversal expansion by Hyrax (Hygienic Rapid Expander) for basal expansion and distalization of 16 to open space for 15
- After 8 months with the Hyrax, the patient did not receive any more treatment until the complete eruption of 11 and 21; by that time the patient was 10 years old
- The case was sent to receive Invisalign First treatment and correct the upper and lower crowding and the posterior deep bite that generated after the upper incisors' eruption

Requirements for the Technician

- In the maxilla, dentoalveolar expansion was requested to open space for 13 and 23 and to provide space for aligning the upper incisors

- Further distalization for 16 was requested until eruption of 15
- In the mandible, crowding was requested to be solved by expansion and lower proclination
- To solve the deep bite, we asked for intrusion of the lower incisors
- No IPR was requested for the case

Treatment Summary

- Patient wore a Hyrax for 8 months and currently has been using the aligners for 1 year on a 7-day intervals protocol, after the eruption of 33 and 43 in the middle of the first set of aligners
- Additional aligners were requested to cover the upper and lower canines once they had erupted

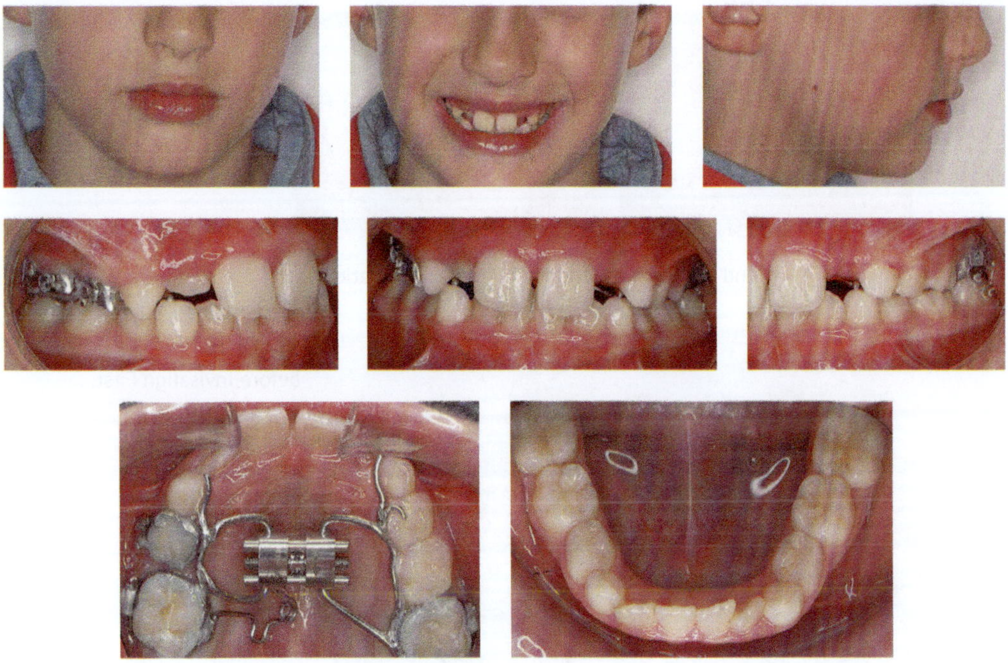

Fig. 18.9 Views with the Hyrax before Invisalign First.

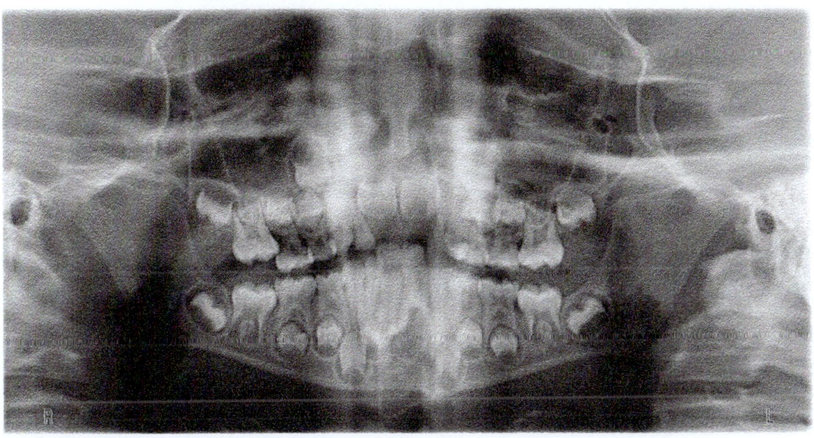

Fig. 18.10 Panoramic X-ray before Hyrax.

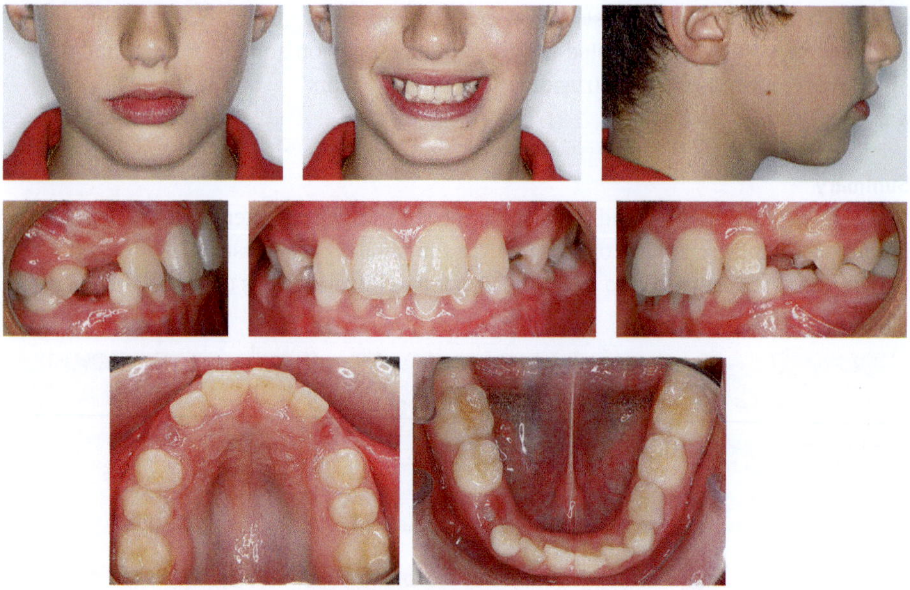

Fig. 18.11 After the Hyrax and before Invisalign First (10-year-old patient).

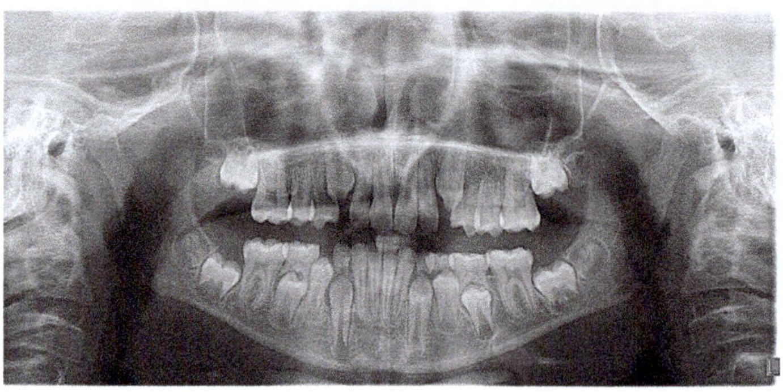

Fig. 18.12 Panoramic X-ray before Invisalign First.

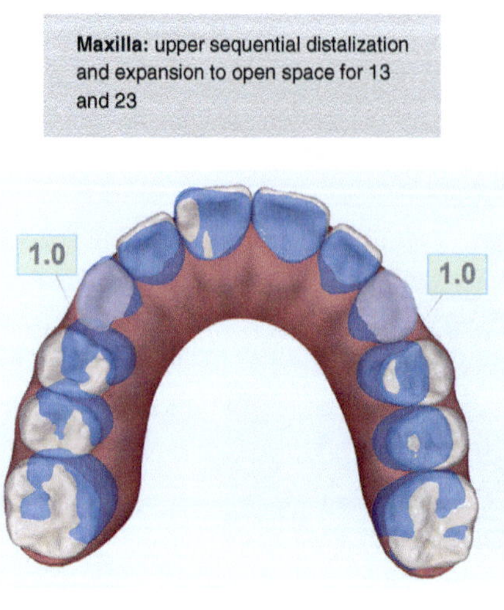

Fig. 18.13 Upper CC superimposition and instructions to CAD designer.

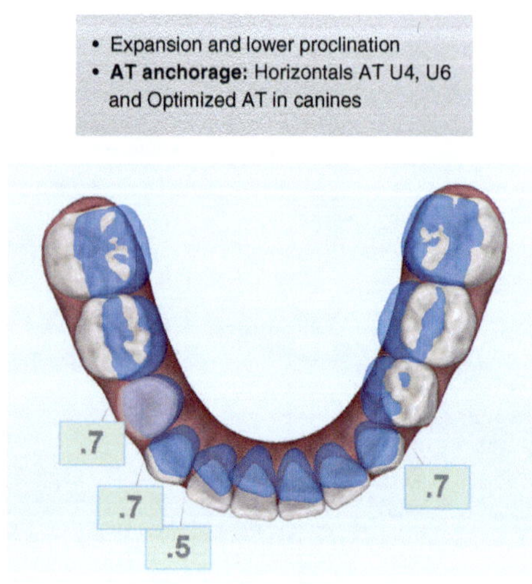

Fig. 18.14 Lower CC superimposition and instructions to CAD designer.

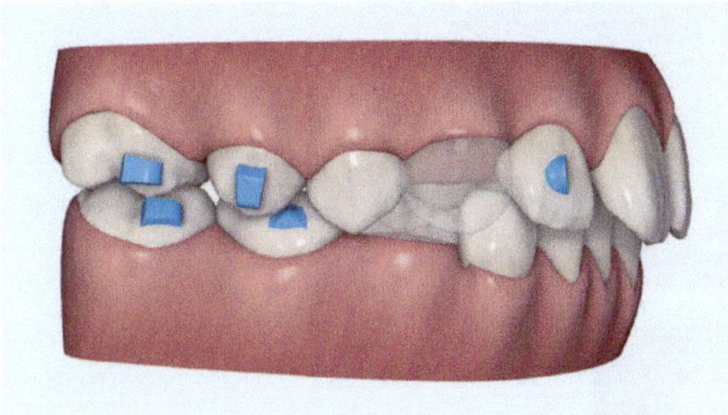

Fig. 18.15 Right ClinCheck view, initial situation.

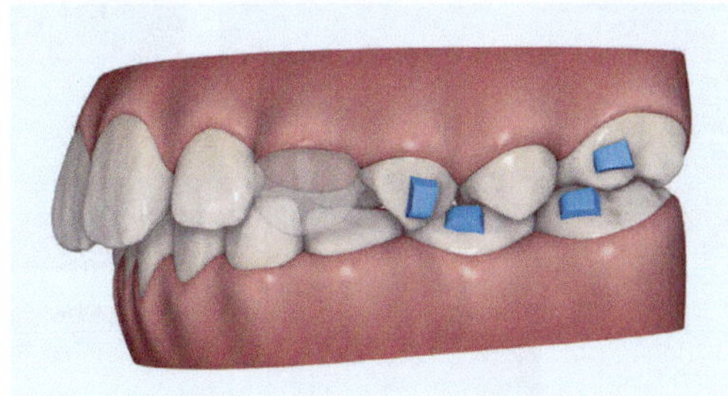

Fig. 18.16 Left ClinCheck view, initial situation.

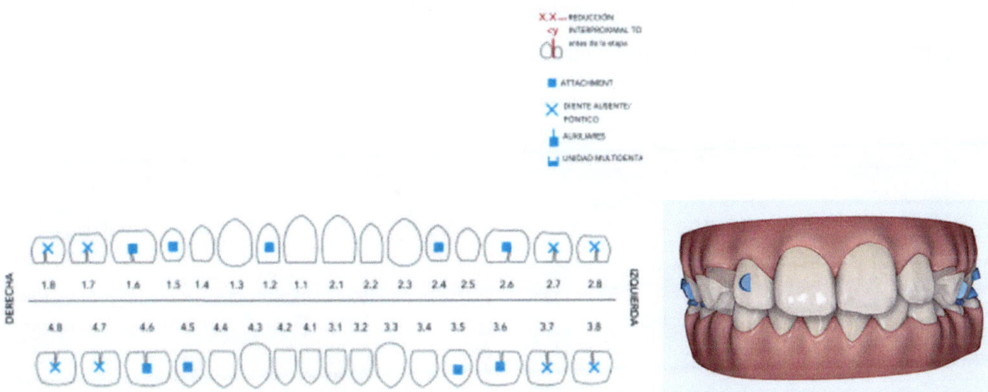

Fig. 18.17 Attachments can be seen in several areas of the ClinCheck software.

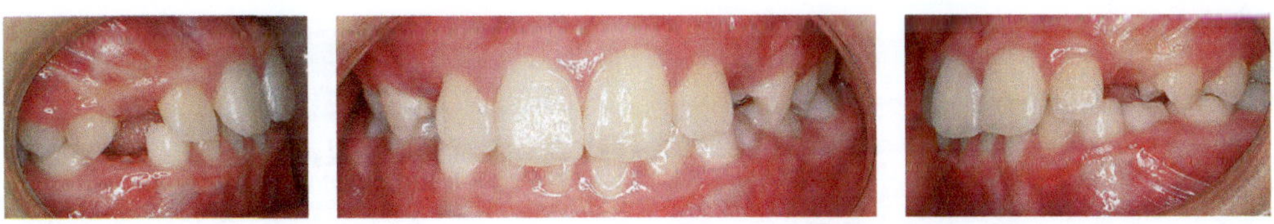

Fig. 18.18 Pretreatment intraoral views (left, front, right) before Invisalign First.

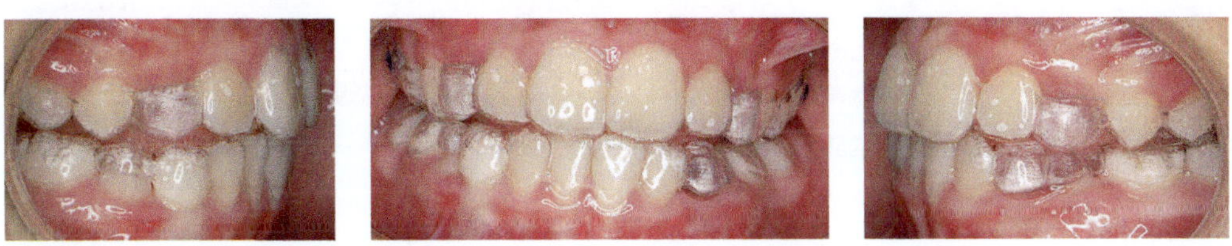

Fig. 18.19 Intraoral views (left, front, right) with first aligner.

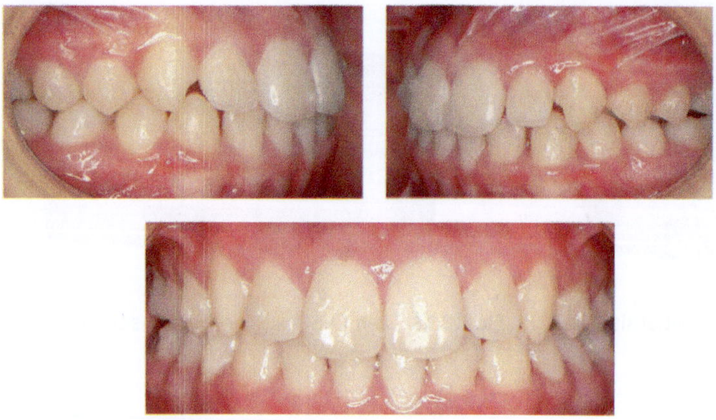

Fig. 18.20 Actual situation in additional aligners.

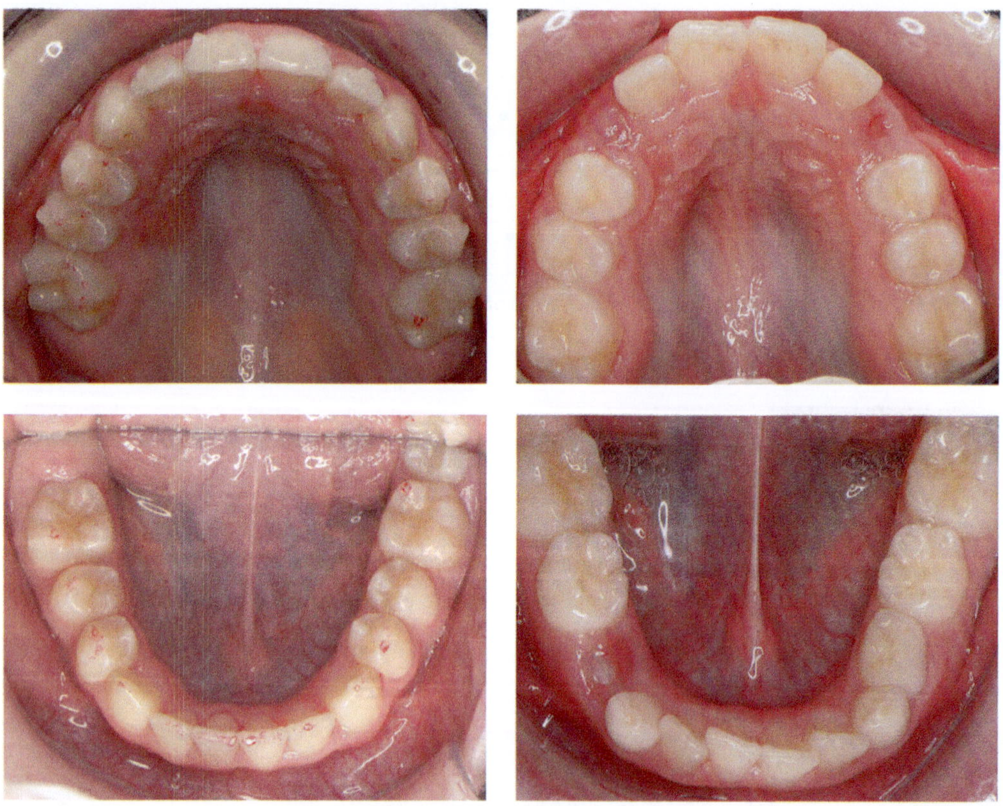

Fig. 18.21 Initial and final occlusal (upper and lower).

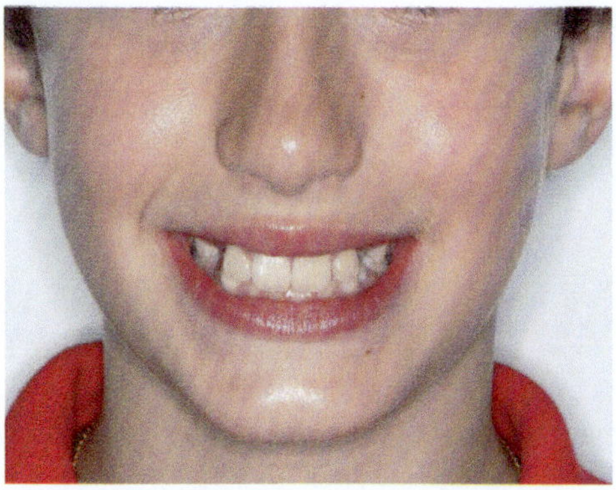
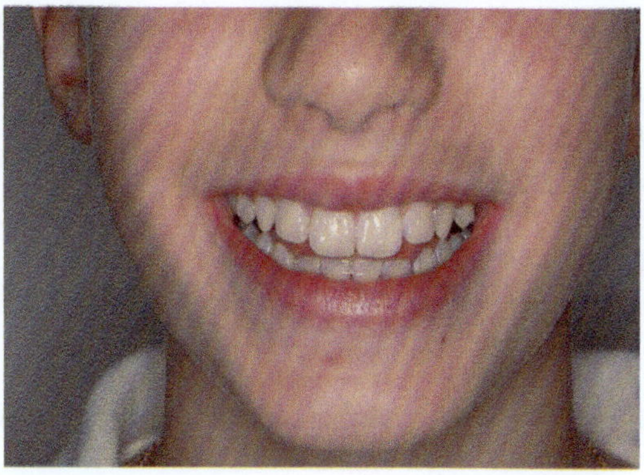

Fig. 18.22 Initial and final smile.

18.1.2 First Severe Crowding Treatment

Fig. 18.23 Severe crowding impeding proper lateral incisor eruption both in upper and lower jaw.

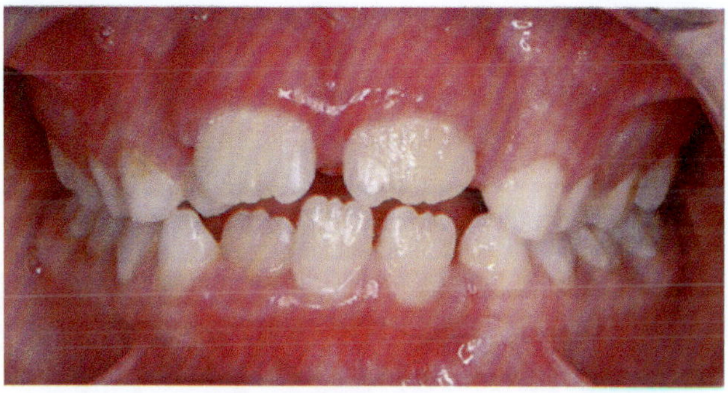

Diagnosis

A 7-year-old boy with a hypodivergent skeletal class presented with severe crowding, left tipping of lower incisors, blocking 32 eruption, facial competence and gummy smile.

Treatment Plan

- Open space for lower laterals, centring lower midline by lower incisor straightening
- Open space for upper laterals
- Achieve left molar class I
- Improve overjet
- Centre midlines
- Solve anterior crossbite, as upper lateral incisors erupted during treatment on a palatal position

ClinCheck1: Requirements for the Technician

- Request opening space for laterals centring midline simultaneously to this
- Distalize sequentially second quadrant, and planned without using class II elastics, in order to gain overjet by upper incisor protrusion

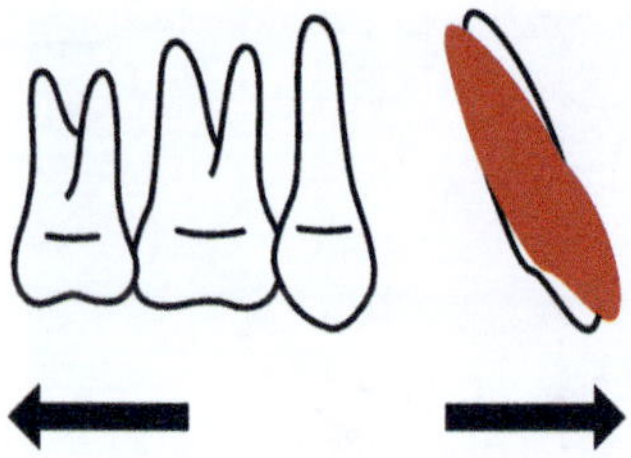

Fig. 18.24 Taking advantage of aligner biomechanics by distalizing the second quadrant, which led to anterior protrusion and mesialization.

- Expansion was requested in both upper and lower jaw, to correct posterior compressed torques and create bigger arches

Treatment Summary

- Treatment time was 18 months for the first phase
- Second phase will come with eruption of permanent teeth
- Left molar class I relationship was achieved
- Midlines were centred and direction of permanent tooth eruption improved
- Better eruption guide for 33 owing to lower incisor straightening
- Better position for 24, 25 after distalization of 26
- Improvement of smile
- Space gain for teeth alignment
- Transversal arch development

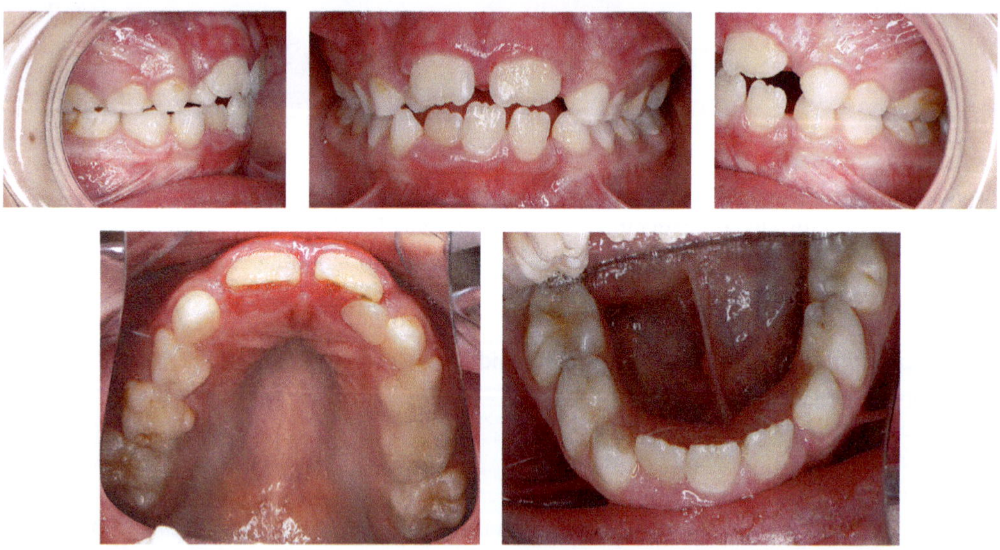

Fig. 18.25 Pretreatment intraoral views (right, front, left, upper, lower).

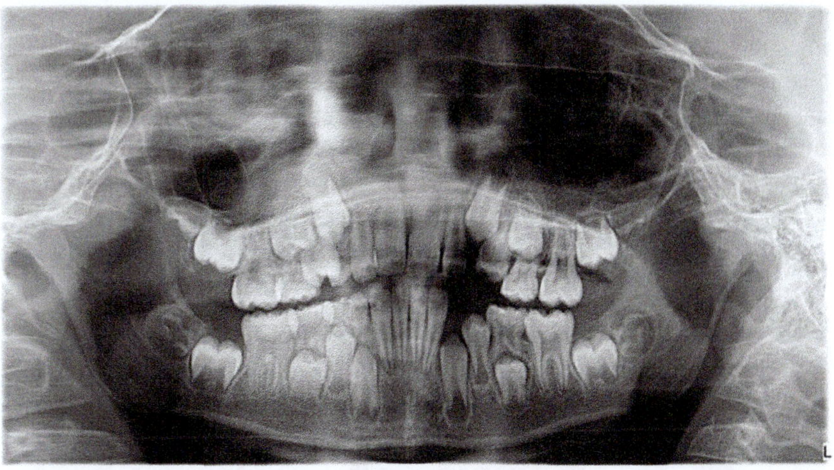

Fig. 18.26 Pretreatment panoramic X-ray showing current dentition status and lack of space for lateral incisors as well as second quadrant teeth.

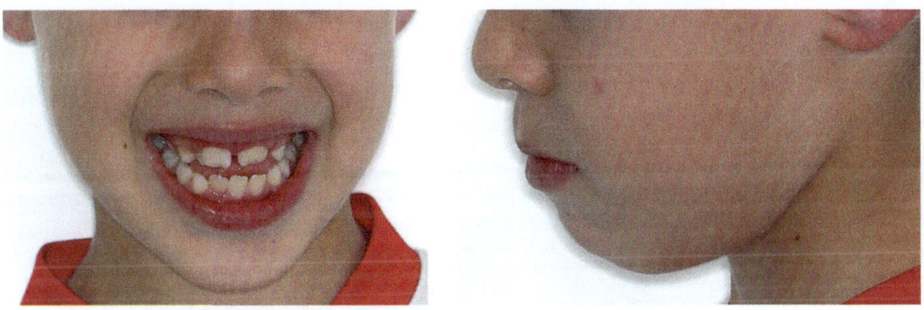

Fig. 18.27 Initial extraoral views.

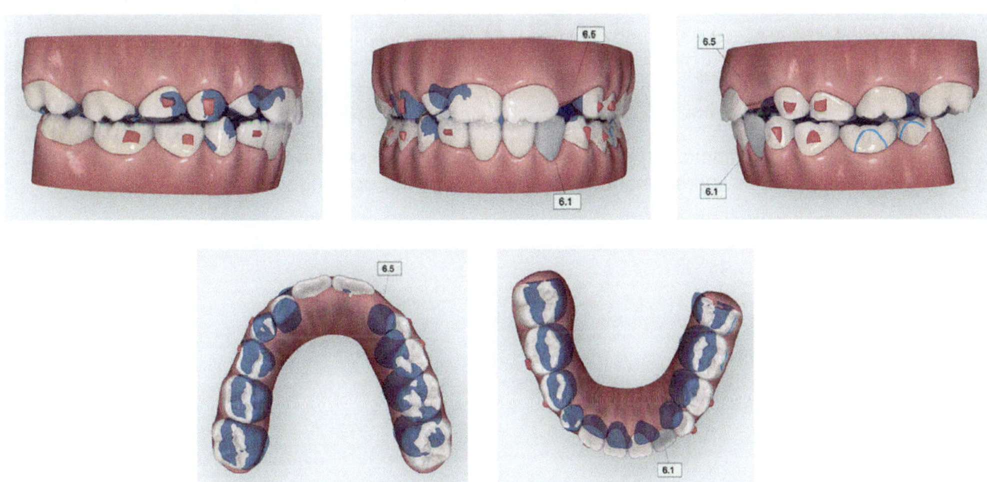

Fig. 18.28 Pretreatment ClinChecks (right, front, left, upper, lower).

ClinCheck2: Communication with the Technician

Seven aligners later, at the follow-up visit, we detected that the lower lateral incisor was erupting lingually, so the patient was rescanned to include its incisal edge on the aligner, so the crown could be moved to its ideal position.

The goals remained the same, therefore providing a big advantage in comparison with any other device that might have been used for the same goal, as adaptation of the new set of aligners is easy, there are no additional changes and we get a brand new set of aligners adapted to the situation.

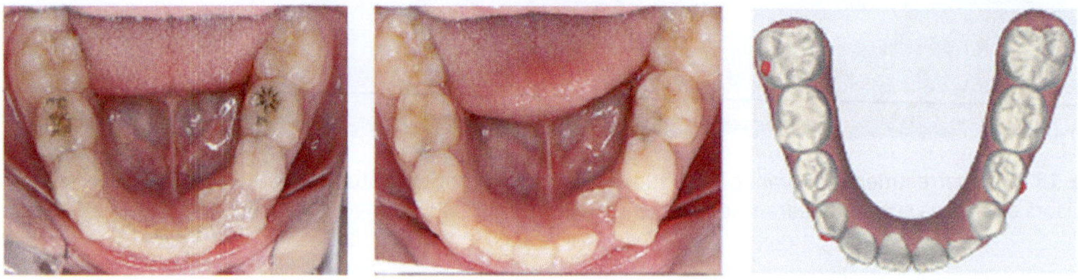

Fig. 18.29 Refinement: (left) 32 has erupted and does not fit in the aligner; (centre) 53 has increased mobility; (right) the patient is rescanned and additional aligners ordered.

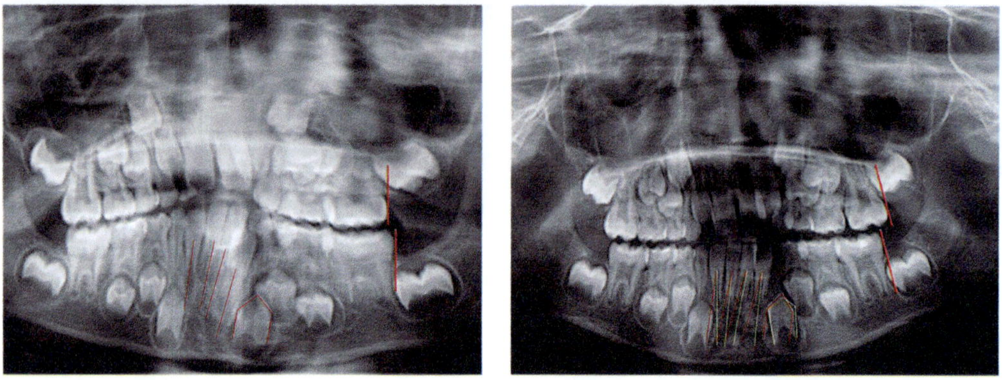

Fig. 18.30 Refinement: panoramic X-rays show the evolution of the sagittal molar relationship on second and third quadrant, as well as improvement in lower incisor tipping, opening space for 33.

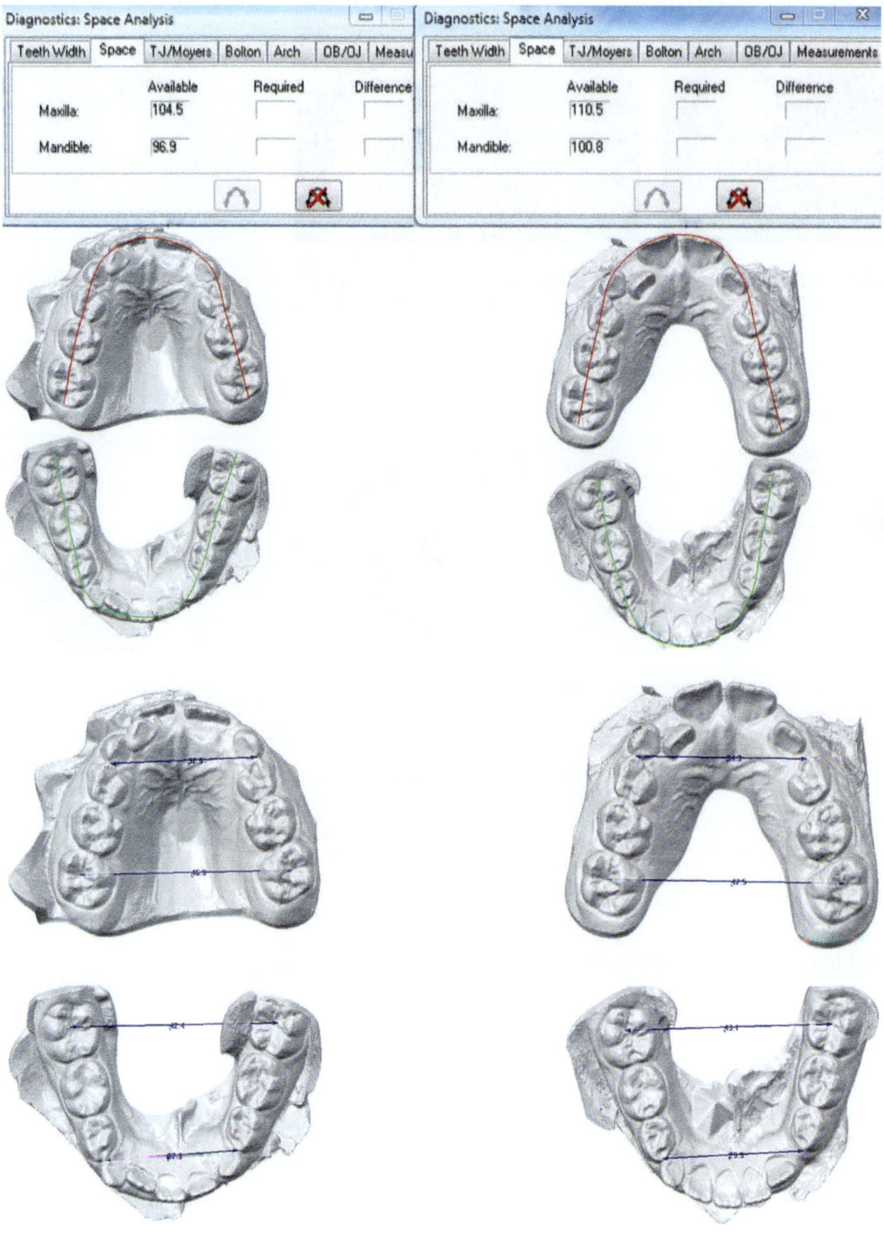

Fig. 18.31 Refinement development: Both available arch space and transverse development were achieved by distalization, proclination and expansion.

ClinCheck3: Communication with the Technician

It was discovered later that upper laterals had erupted on a crossbite, which made rescanning the patient essential to the ordering of additional aligners. The treatment plan should stay the same, except for the movement of these two teeth. The technician was asked for:

- Extrusion attachment
- Extra buccal root torque to help creating an 'en masse' movement that will take the apex of these two teeth to their ideal position

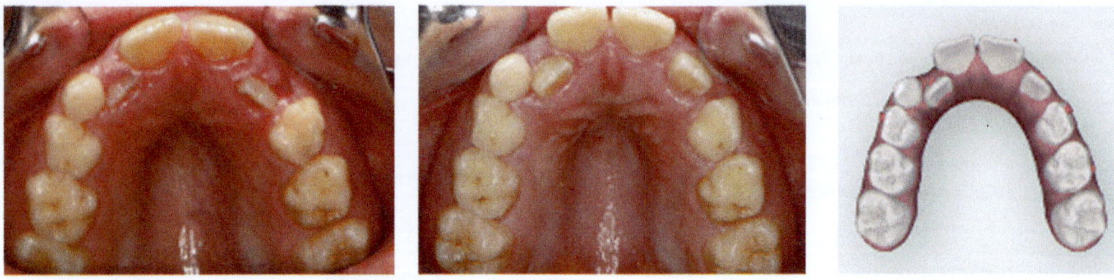

Fig. 18.32 Refinement: 12, 22 have erupted but their clinical crowns are not yet exposed (left), so patient is rescanned when clinical crowns are bigger (centre); planning an additional ClinCheck (right).

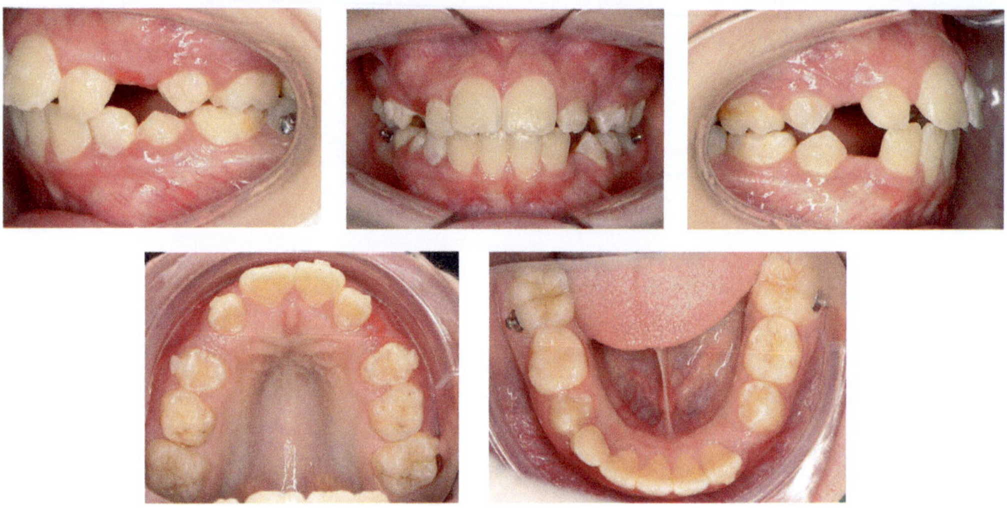

Fig. 18.33 Final Intraoral views (right, front, left, upper, lower) showing a space gain.

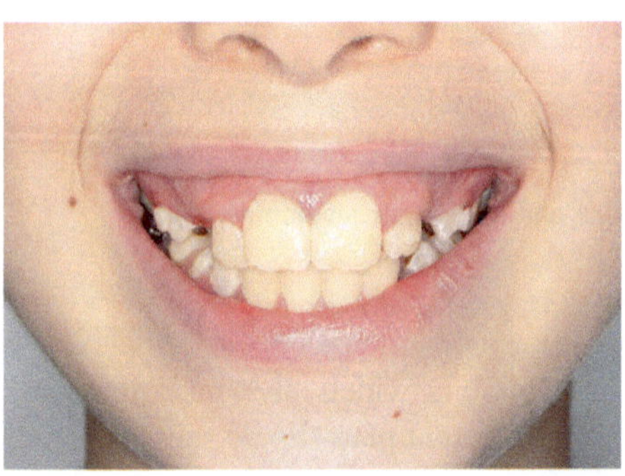

Fig. 18.34 Final and final smile views show an improvement in arch development.

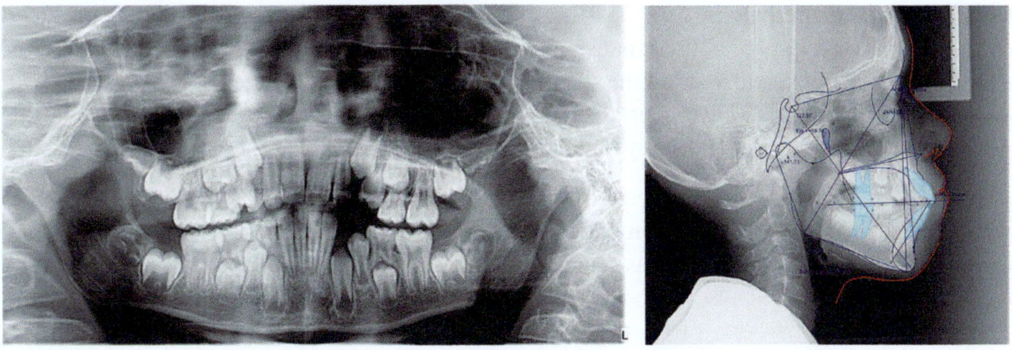

Fig. 18.35 Lateral X-ray shows incisor proclination as a result of the mechanics applied, while the panoramic X-ray shows a great improvement in space for permanent dentition.

18.2 Teenage Patients

18.2.1 Class II Corrected with Lite Treatment

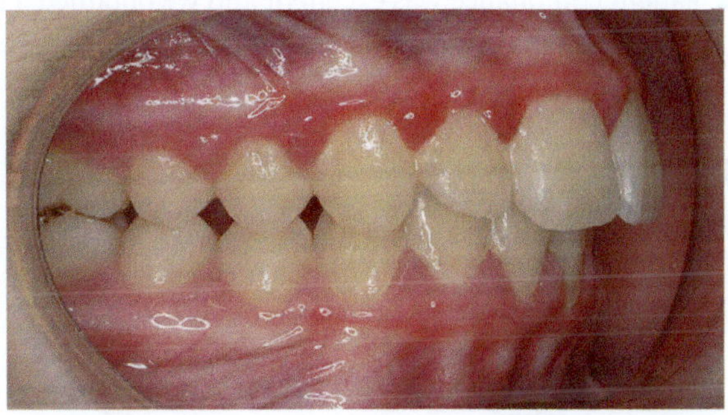

Fig. 18.36 Class II growing patient, Lite treatment.

Diagnosis

An 8-year-old patient with basal compression and macrodontia with severe crowding was treated with Hyrax and lower D-gainer in a 12-months first phase to open space for missing lower canines and for upper incisors.

- The patient came back at 15 years old, after having all his permanent dentition. At that time he presented an incomplete class II on both sides, narrow arches, 16 and 26 rotated and deep bite with minor lower crowding.
- As he was a growing patient with narrow arches and rotated upper molars, we decided to correct the class II case with a Lite treatment instead of the normal teen treatment.

Treatment Plan

- To correct the malocclusion by expansion and simultaneous upper incisors retraction
- In the lower arch, we needed to upright the lower incisors to create the overjet necessary to correct the class II malocclusion relationship

Requirements for the Technician

- Expand and use the space of the expansion to move distally the teeth on the upper arch
- In the lower arch, expand and use the space of the expansion to mesialize the lower teeth
- No upper distalization or lower mesialization was requested, only use of the space gained by the expansion to move the teeth distally in the upper arch and mesially in the lower arch

The goal was that the technician could coordinate the arches in a final class I relationship, simulating the use of class II elastics, even when precision cut or virtual jump could not be requested for this case as it had been a Lite case (note: precision cuts can now be requested in Lite treatment cases).

Treatment Summary

- Total treatment time was 16 months
- As we knew that more than 14 aligners would be necessary to correct the class II with elastics, we asked the patient to wear every aligner on 3-week change intervals during the first phase so that the elastic could have time to act and direct the lower arch into a class I
- After the first set of aligners, we asked for additional aligners that were changed on a 2-week interval protocol as the class I canine has already been achieved during the first phase
- Full-time wearing of the elastic was essential for a successful outcome
- Patient compliance was excellent and we obtained a bilateral class I with both midlines centred, corrected the deep bite through lower incisor intrusion and the smile improved considerably owing to the expansion of the arches

First-phase Records at 8 Years Old

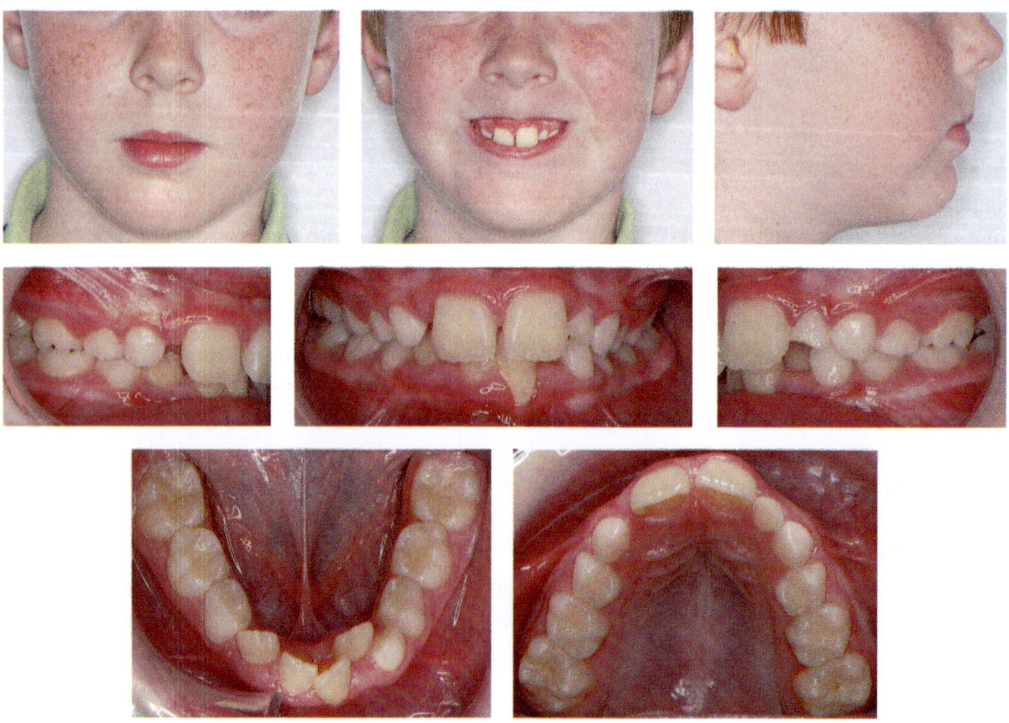

Fig. 18.37 Pretreatment views before phase 1 with Hyrax and D-gainer.

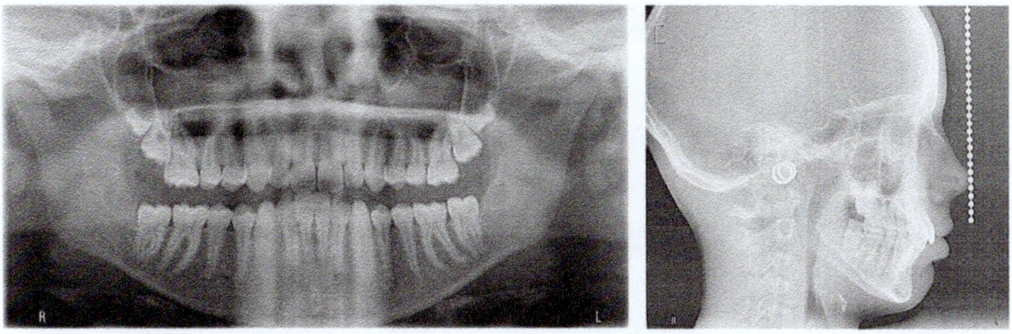

Fig. 18.38 Lateral and panoramic X-rays before phase 1 with Hyrax and D-gainer.

Second Phase Records at 15 Years Old

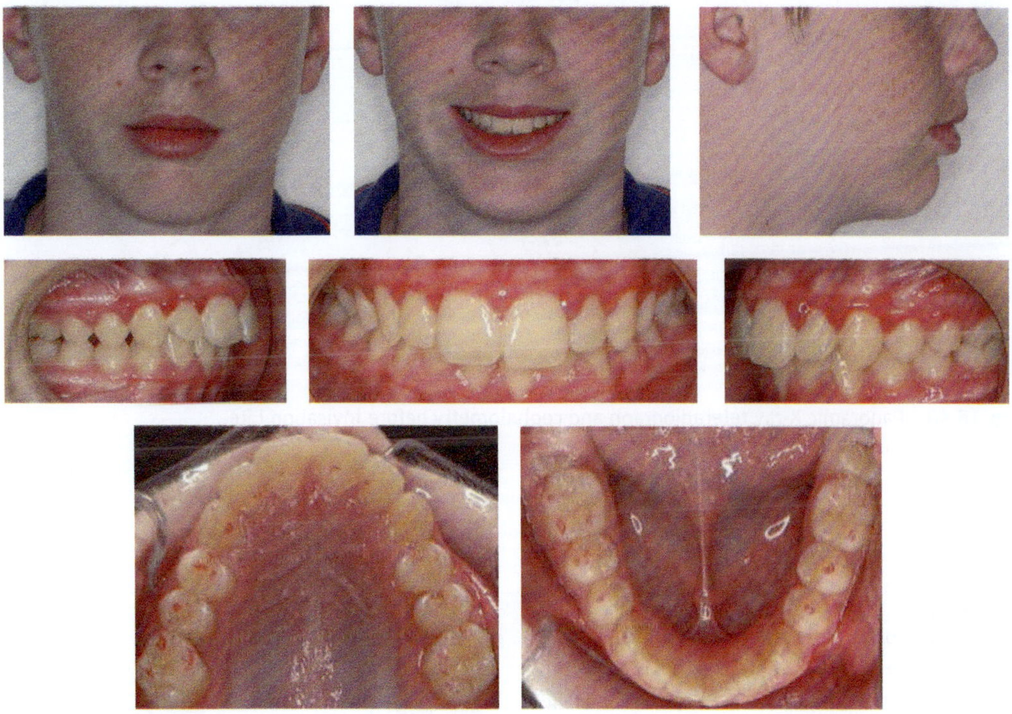

Fig. 18.39 Extraoral and intraoral (right, front, left, upper, lower) views before Invisalign Lite.

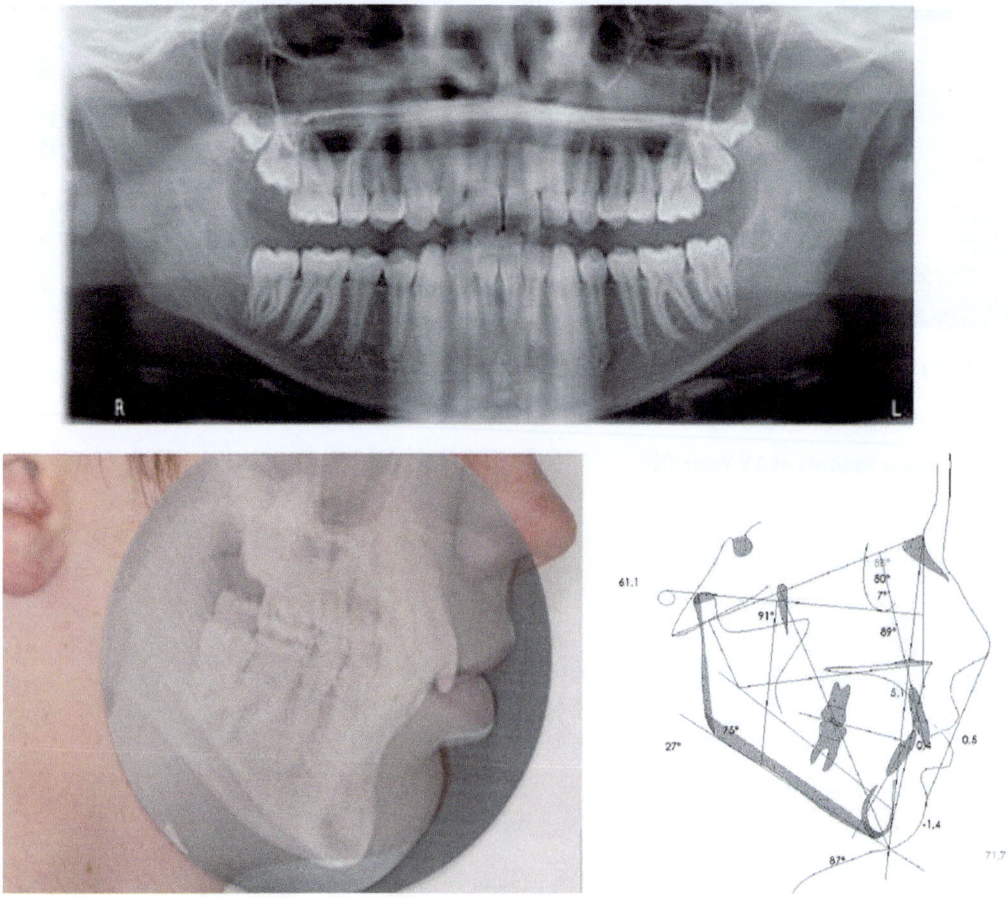

Fig. 18.40 Panoramic X-ray, teleradiograph and cephalometry before Invisalign Lite.

Maxillary:
- Expansion + mesial-out rotation of 1.6 and 2.6 + reduction of arch length simultaneously to expansion
- Ask the technician to use the space gained by expansion to move distally upper teeth. Do not ask for distalization

Fig. 18.41 Upper CC superimposition and instructions to CAD designer.

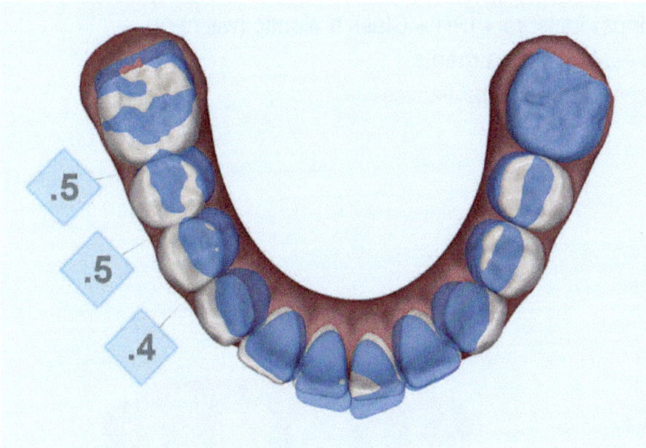

Mandible:

- Expansion and use of the space gained for mesialization of lower teeth
- Simultaneous reduction of arch length
- Overjet is needed to correct class II with elastics
- Expansion + posterior mesialization simultaneously to lower incisors retraction (this will increase predictability of mesialization)
- **Anchorage attachment:** Horizontal U4 and U6 and optimized attachment in canines

Fig. 18.42 Lower CC superimposition and instructions to CAD designer.

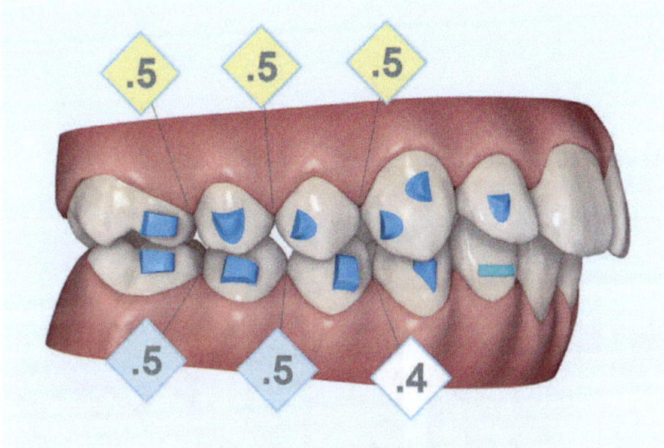

- Coordinate arches
- Level the curve of Spee to allow mandibular growth

Fig. 18.43 Right ClinCheck view, initial situation.

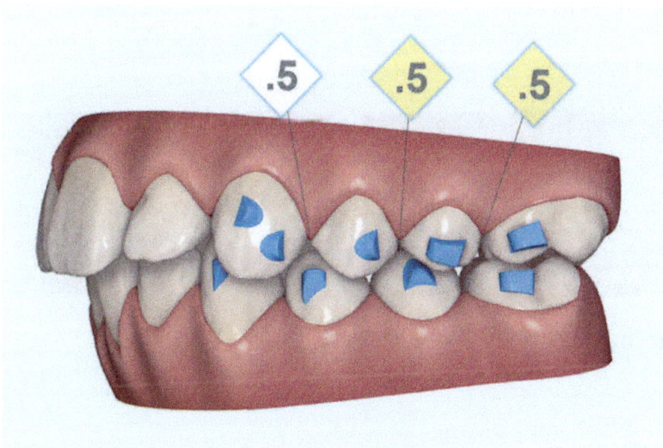

- Coordinate arches to allow class II elastics to work

IPR to engage posterior occlusion in class I

Fig. 18.44 Left ClinCheck view, initial situation.

- Expansion + lingual root torque of upper incisors + IPR + Class II elastic (will need to make the precision cut by ourselves, in Lite treatments)
- Change aligner every 21 days (need more time with elastics)

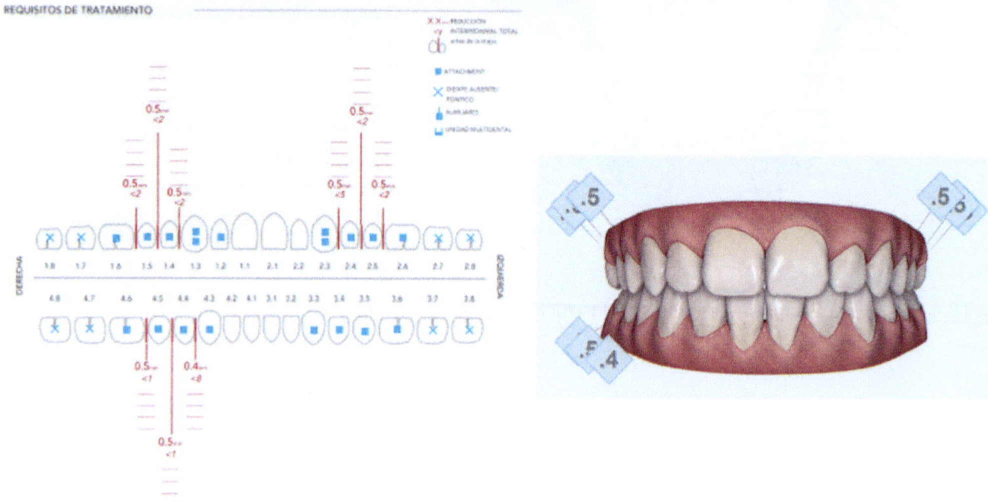

Fig. 18.45 Attachments and IPR can be seen in several areas of the ClinCheck software.

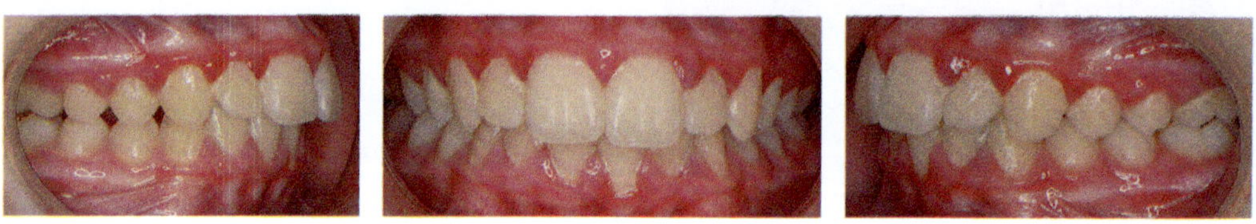

Fig. 18.46 Intraoral views (right, front, left, upper, lower).

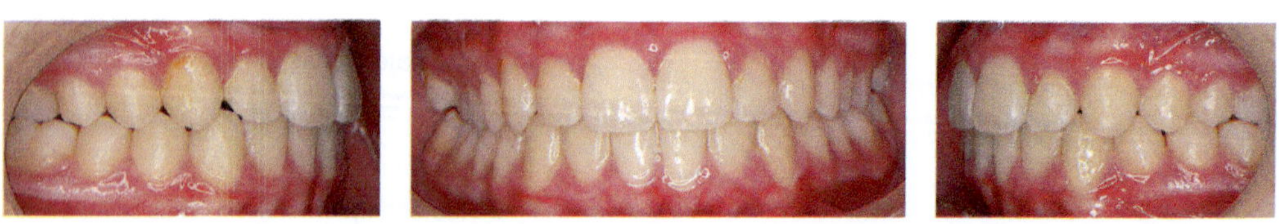

Fig. 18.47 Intraoral views (right, front, left, upper, lower).

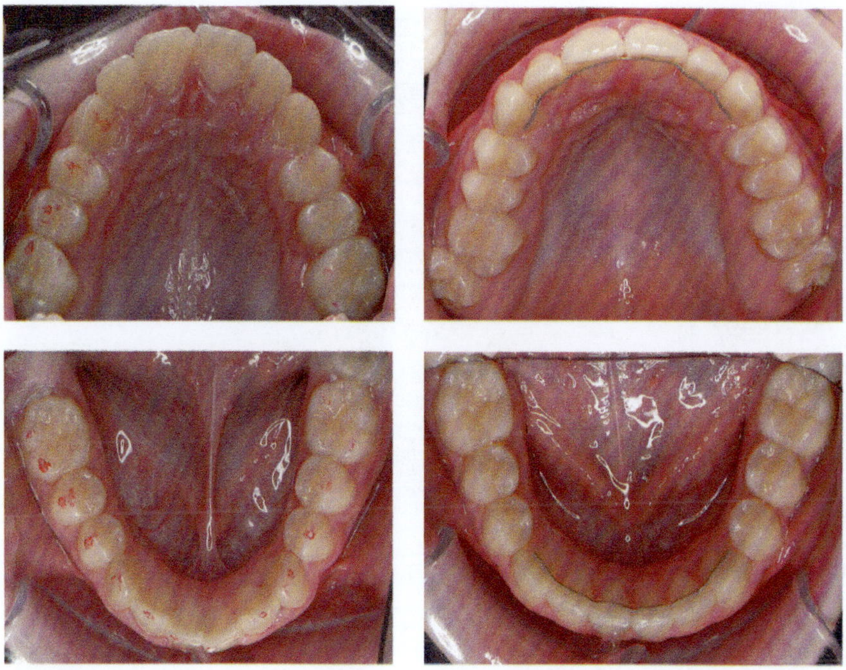

Fig. 18.48 Initial and final occlusal views (upper and lower).

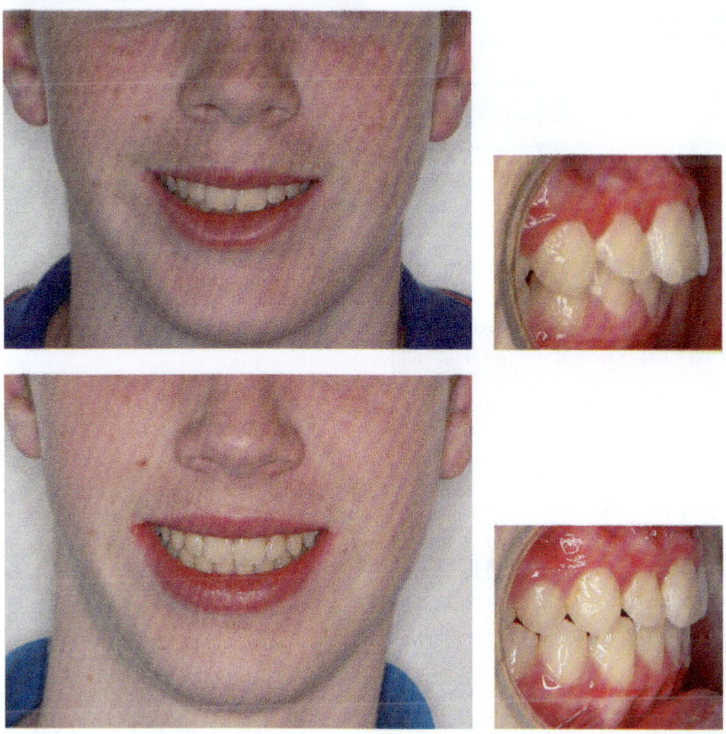

Fig. 18.49 Pretreatment and final smile and overjet.

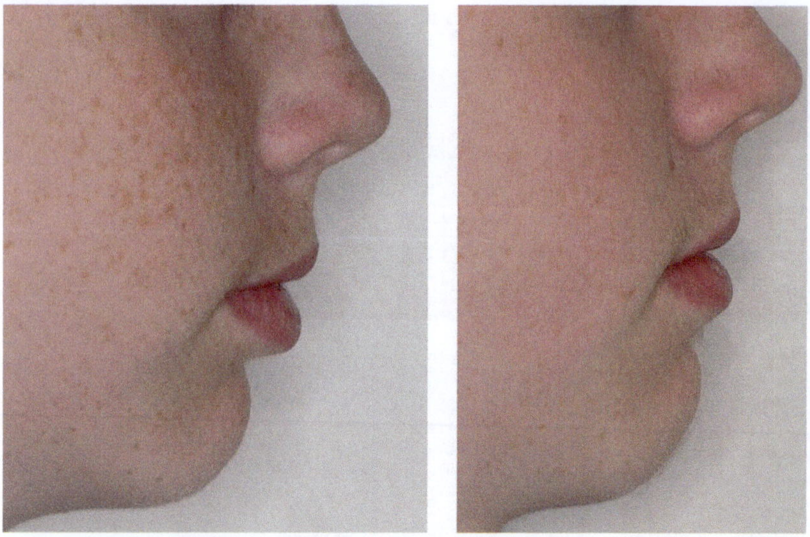

Fig. 18.50 Initial and final profiles.

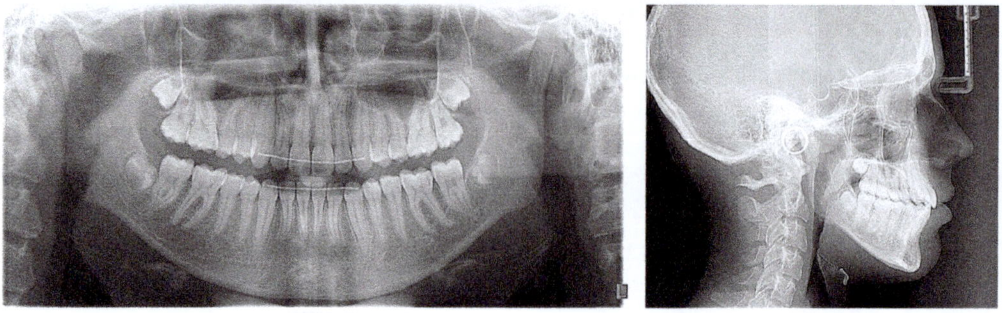

Fig. 18.51 Final panoramic and lateral X-rays.

18.2.2 Class II Treated with Comprehensive Treatment

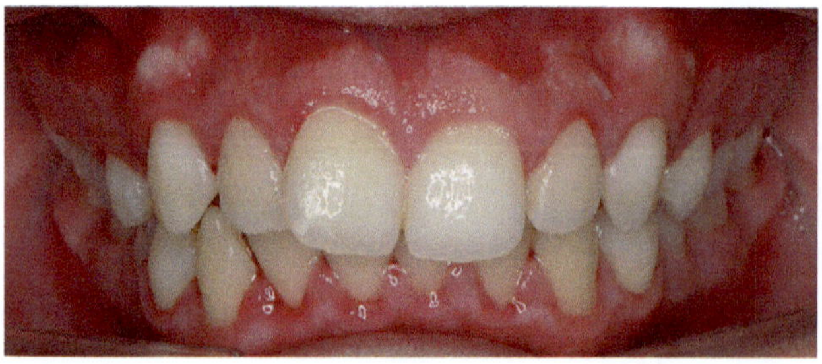

Fig. 18.52 Initial intraoral picture.

Diagnosis

A 16-year-old patient with normodivergent skeletal class II presented with maxillary prognathism and lower crowding with labial tipping of lower incisors.

Treatment Plan

- Upper and lower expansion and simultaneous retraction of upper and lower incisors
- IPR between 33 and 43 to upright lower incisors
- Class II to be corrected using class II elastics

Requirements for the Technician

- Apply lingual root torque to the upper incisors during all the retraction movement.
- A virtual jump at the end of the treatment to simulate the mesial movement of the lower dental-arch using the elastics.
- Provide an overjet of 1.5 mm after the virtual jump simulation in order to ensure no premature contact in the anterior zone at the end of the treatment.

Treatment Summary

- Total treatment time was 19 months.
- The patient was asked to wear every aligner on 10-day change intervals; the first set of aligners were 34 (12 months).
- After the first set of aligners, additional aligners were requested that were changed on a 1-week interval protocol as the class I canine had already been achieved during the first set of aligners.
- Full-time wearing of the elastic was essential for a successful outcome.
- Patient compliance was excellent and a bilateral class I with both midlines centred was obtained; we corrected upper diastemas maintaining upper incisors torque during all retraction movements.

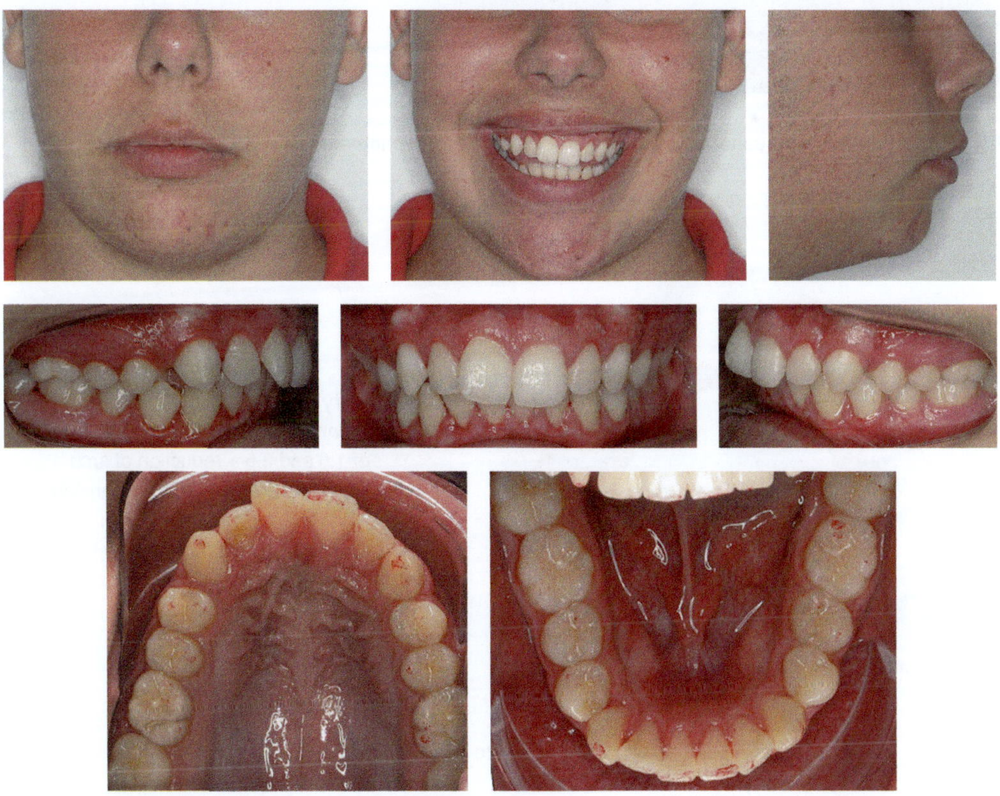

Fig. 18.53 Pretreatment views.

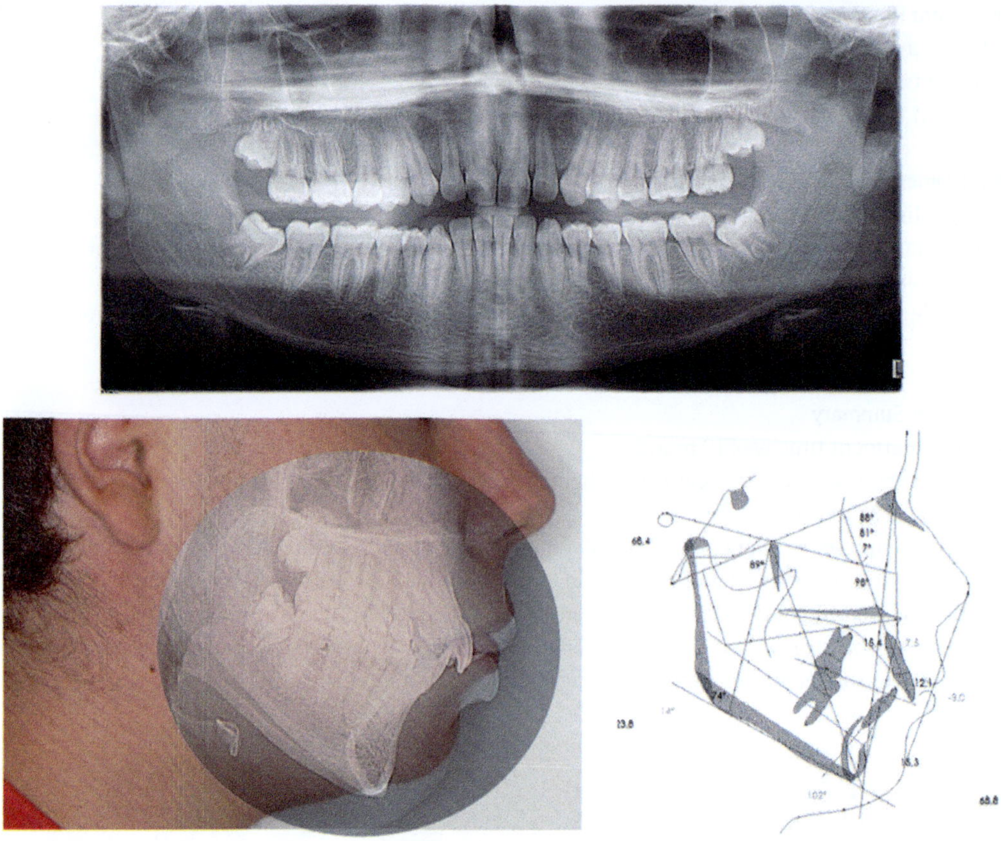

Fig. 18.54 Pretreatment panoramic X-ray, teleradiograph and cephalometry.

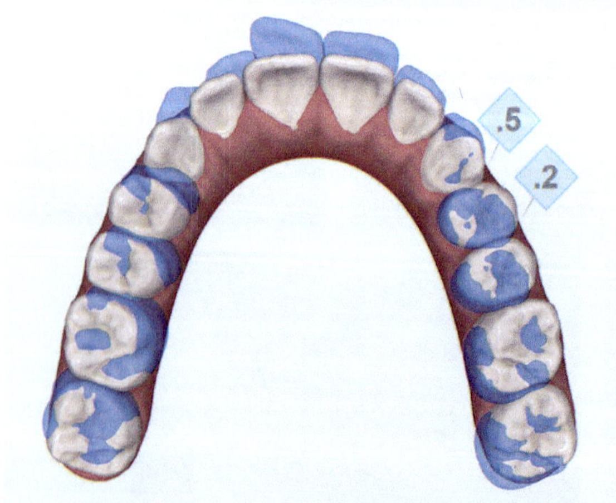

Maxillary:
- Expansion + mesial-out rotation of 1.6 and 2.6 + reduction of arch length simultaneously to expansion
- Use the space gained by expansion to move distally upper teeth.

Fig. 18.55 Upper CC superimposition and instructions to CAD designer.

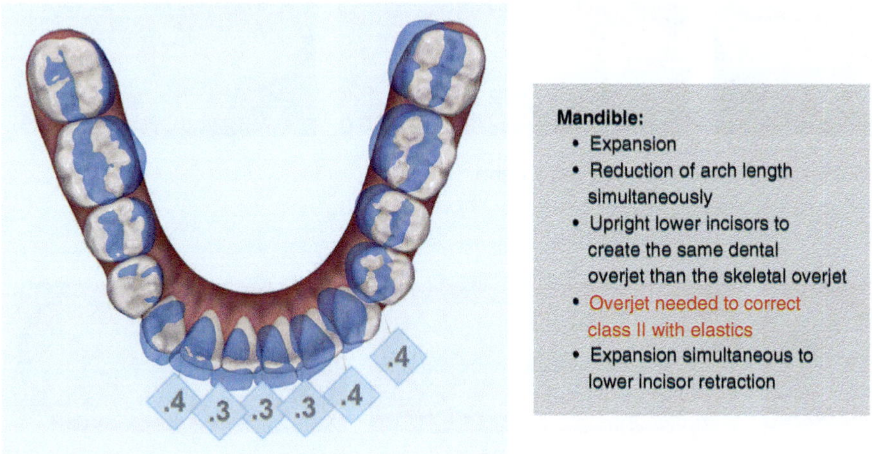

Fig. 18.56 Lower CC superimposition and instructions to CAD designer.

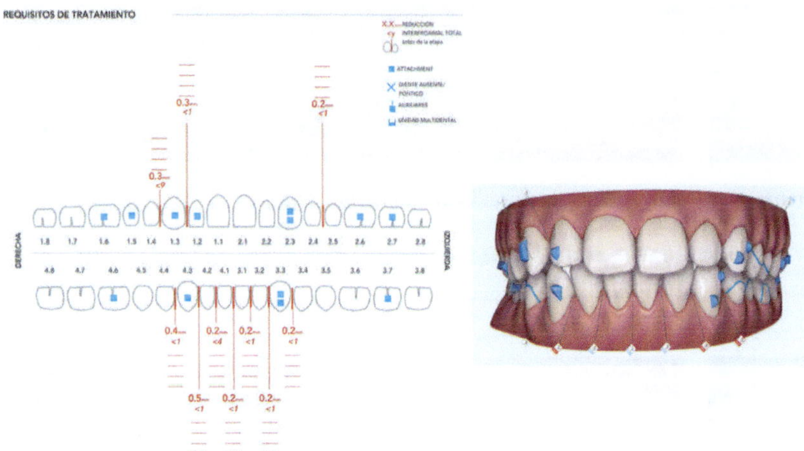

Fig. 18.57 Interproximal reduction necessary to upright lower incisors before virtual jump.

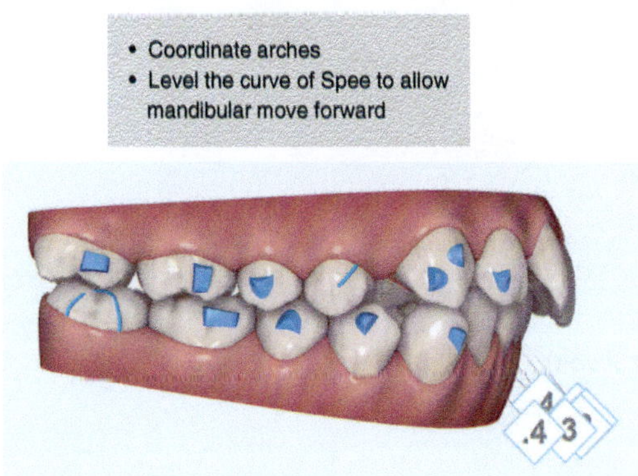

Fig. 18.58 Right ClinCheck view, initial situation.

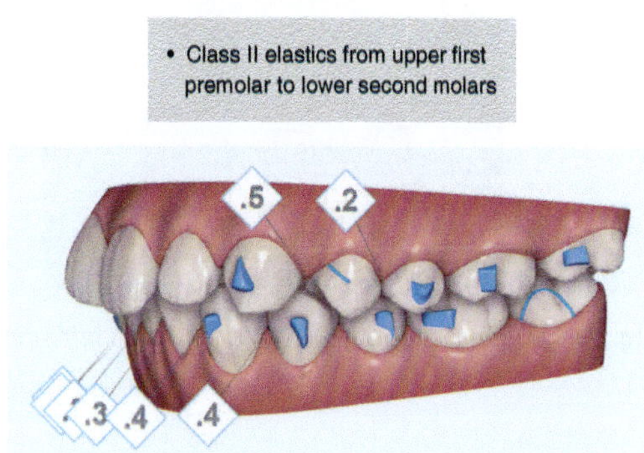

Fig. 18.59 Left ClinCheck view, initial situation.

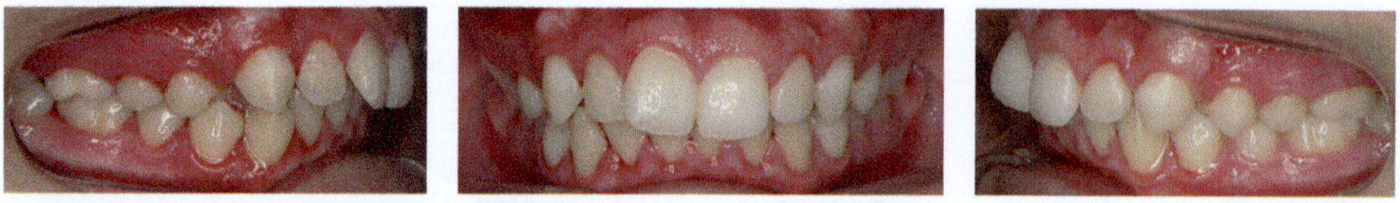

Fig. 18.60 Pretreatment intraoral views (left, front, right).

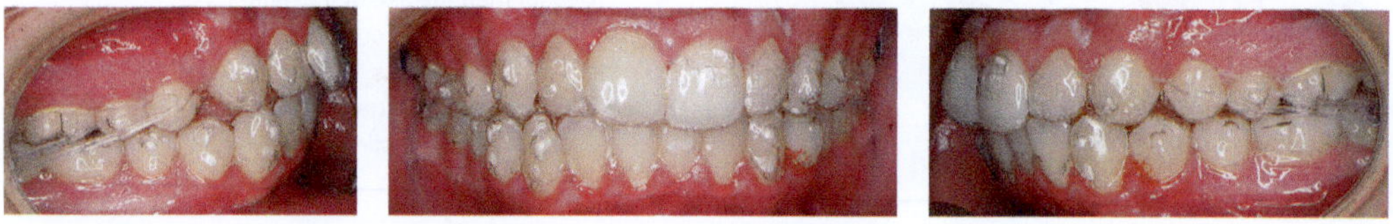

Fig. 18.61 Month 6 of evolution: intraoral views (left, front, right).

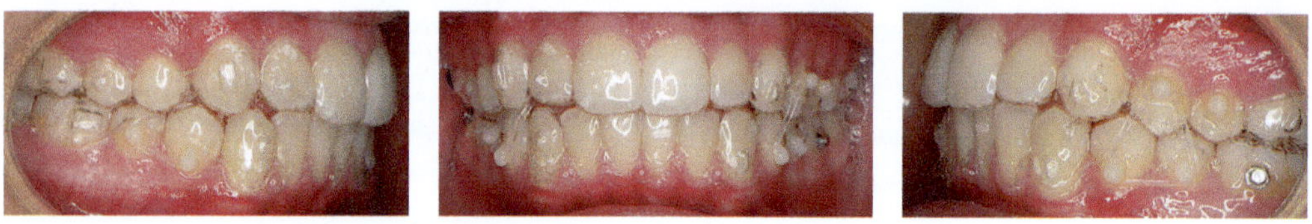

Fig. 18.62 Refinement: month 15 of evolution; intraoral views (left, front, right).

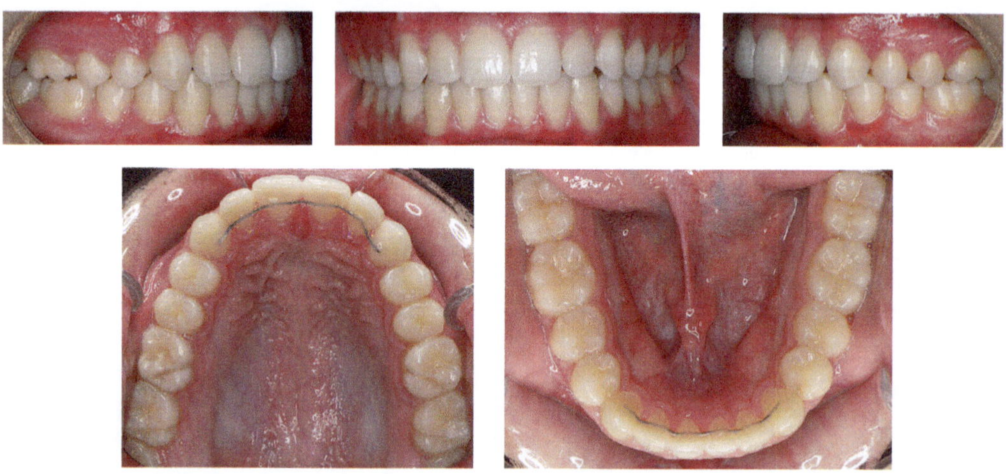

Fig. 18.63 Final intraoral views (right, front, left, upper, lower).

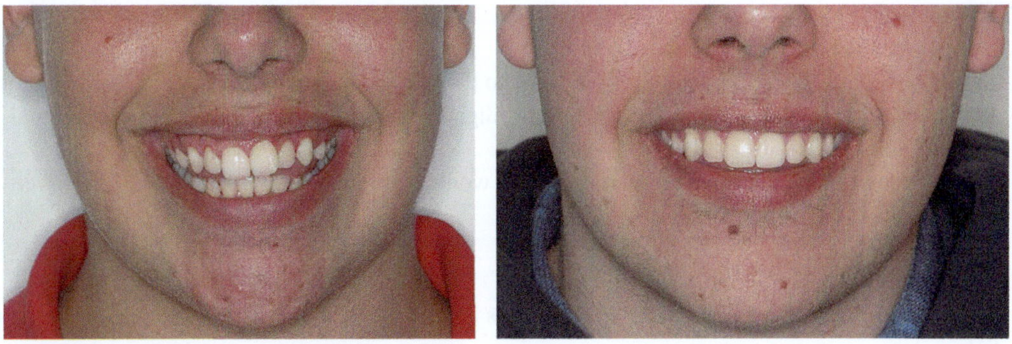

Fig. 18.64 Pretreatment and final smile.

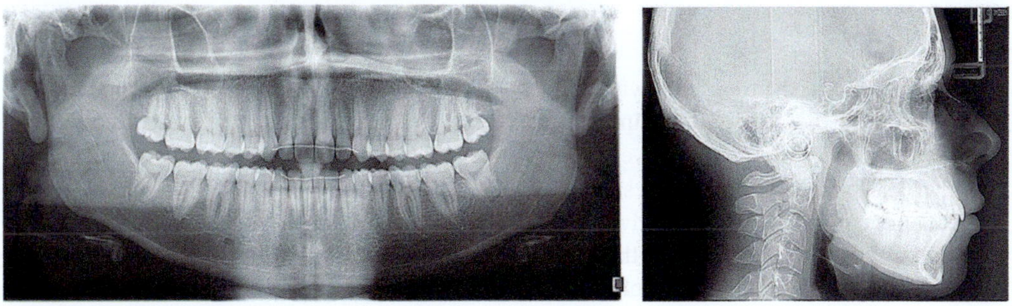

Fig. 18.65 Final panoramic and lateral X-rays.

18.2.3 Class III with Impacted Canine

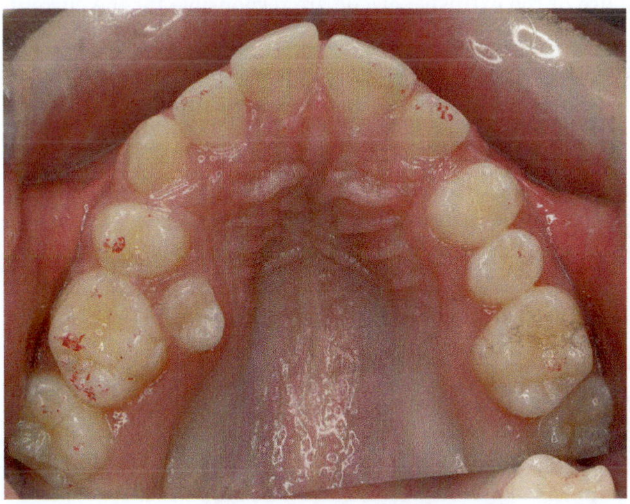

Fig. 18.66 Class III growing patient with comprehensive treatment, with 23 included.

Diagnosis

A 15-year-old hypodivergent skeletal class III patient presented with a maxillary compression, ectopic eruption of 15 and 23 included by labial, lower crowding and a benign cyst in 35 with third upper and lower molars included. They had a narrow smile and prognathic profile.

Treatment Plan

- Upper expansion to open space for 15 and 23
- 15 was not going to be included in the aligners, so the technician was asked not to eliminate the 15 in the ClinCheck but to eliminate it from the aligners as auxiliary techniques with a sectional wire would be used to bring it to labial
- The labial and lingual surface of microdontic 15 would not have enough retention to be driven to a labial position only with the aligners

Requirements for the Technician

- Apply simultaneous distalization to 16 and 17 as auxiliary technique with Locatelli was going to be used
- Protrude upper incisors and move the upper midline to the right to create space for the eruption of 23

Treatment Summary

- The patient started the treatment with aligners that did not cover 15, so space was made for 15 with a Locatelli that assisted the simultaneous distalization of 16 and 17 achieved with a sectional wire placed by lingual to drive the 15 to labial
- Another Locatelli was used to open space for the included 23, in order to force appearance of the upper canine in the mouth after driving the 15 to labial so that we did not need to ask twice for additional aligners (one to include the 15 and another to include the 23)
- In the 16 aligner the upper left canine erupted labially, at that time we removed the sectional wire on 15 and made a gingivectomy in order that the aligners could wrap the premolar
- The patient actually has finished this set of aligners, is in month 18 of treatment and now needs a second set of additional aligners to correct the posterior crossbite in 23 and 24
- 23 has been driven to the occlusal plane with the use of vertical elastic with a class II component; its high position in the gum and the use of the extrusive elastic are responsible for the current lingual torque of 23 that now has to be corrected
- After 18 months the patient has an erupted 23 and the ectopic 15 in place, she has a class I relationship and her smile has considerably improved thanks to the upper expansion

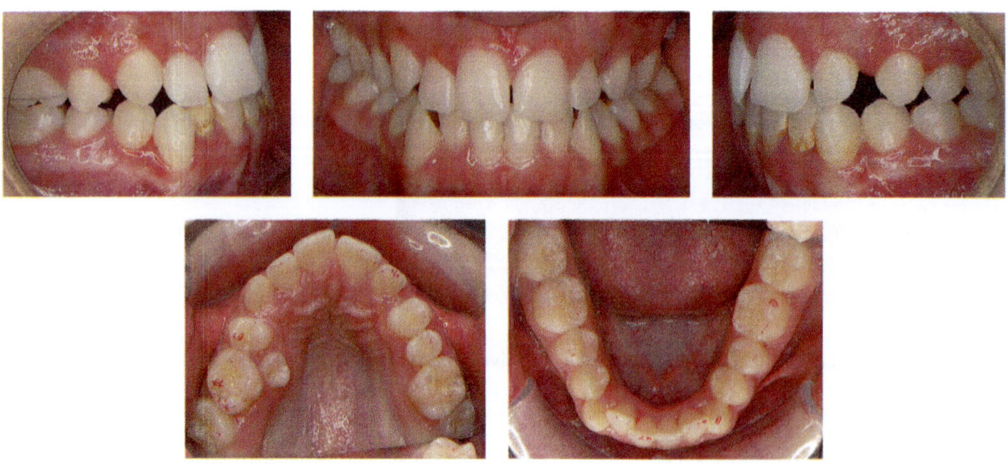

Fig. 18.67 Intraoral views (right, front, left, upper, lower).

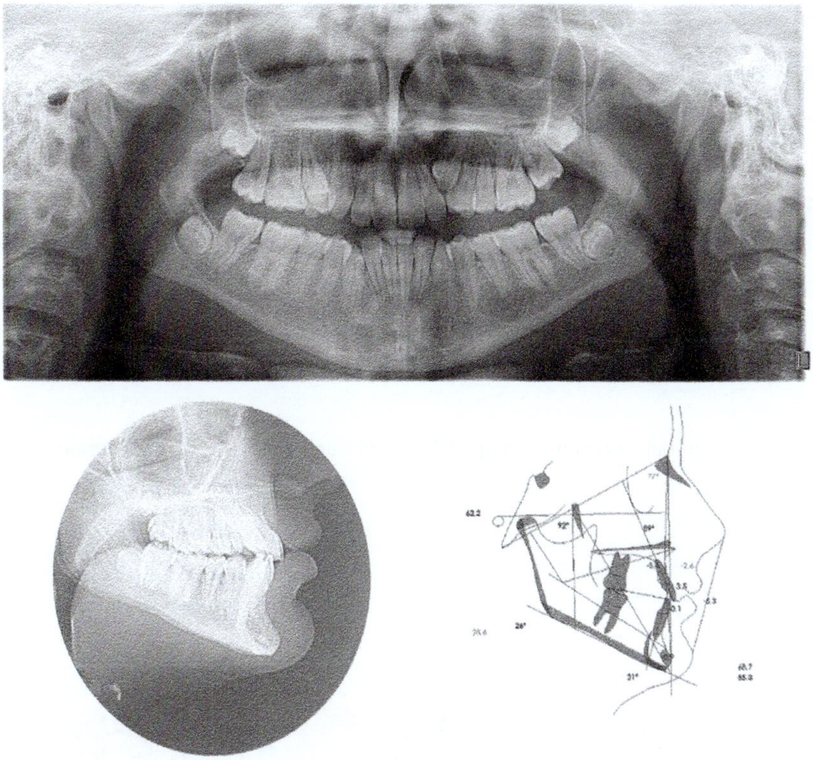

Fig. 18.68 Panoramic X-ray, teleradiograph, cephalometry.

Maxillary staging:
EXPANSION simultaneously to premolar rotation and distalization of 1.7 and 1.6
- Round tripping of 2.2 and 2.4 to open space for 2.3

Mandibular staging:
- Expansion and simultaneous proclination
- IPR + retraction + lingual root torque to lower incisors

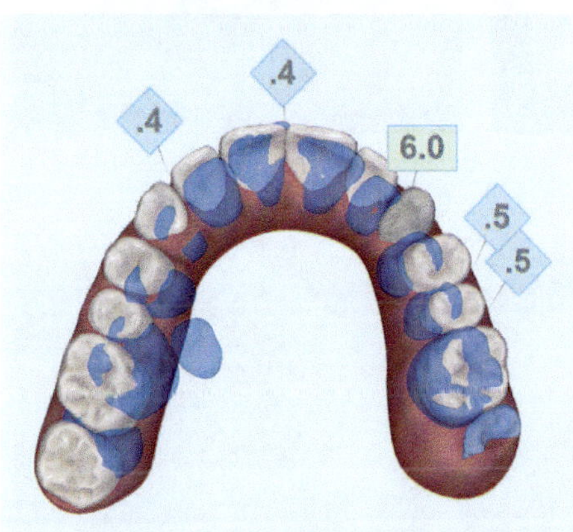

Fig. 18.69 Upper CC superimposition and instructions to CAD designer.

- Upper expansion with torque control + criss-cross elastics
- Anchorage gingival bevelled attachment
- HBG U4 and U6
- Optimized attachments in canines
- Lower IPR
- Locatelli to open space for 2.3 and 1.5
- Lingual sectional wire to pull 1.5 to labial

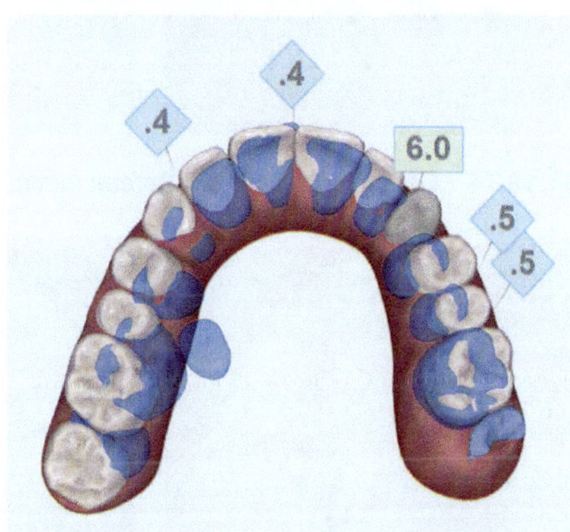

Fig. 18.70 Lower CC superimposition and instructions to CAD designer.

Maxillary:
- Correct by expansion and proclination
- Labial simulation movement in CC for 1.5.
- But do not include it in the aligner

Mandible:
- Expansion + proclination
- IPR + retraction + lingual root torque of lower incisors

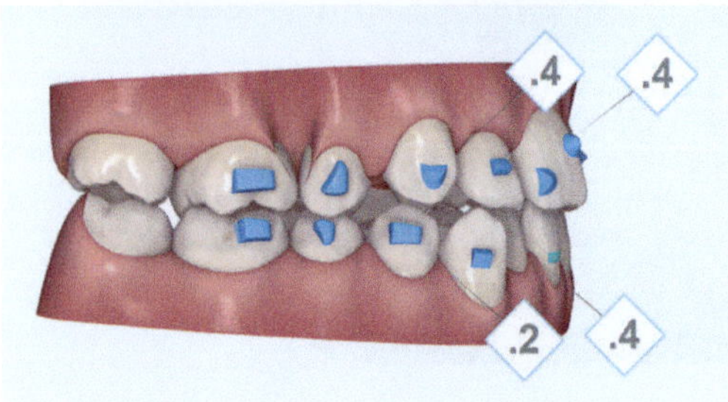

Fig. 18.71 Right ClinCheck view, initial situation.

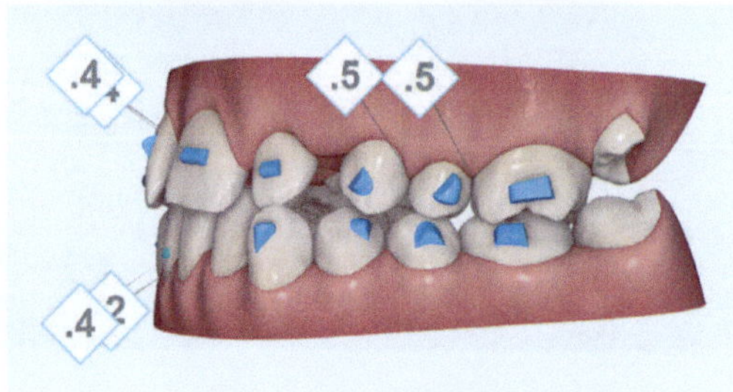

Fig. 18.72 Left ClinCheck view, initial situation.

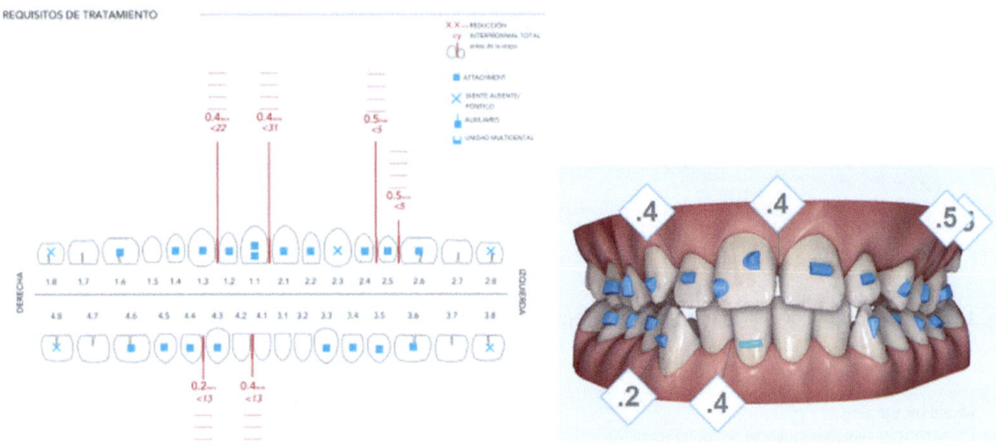

Fig. 18.73 Interproximal reduction in lower arch to create positive overjet.

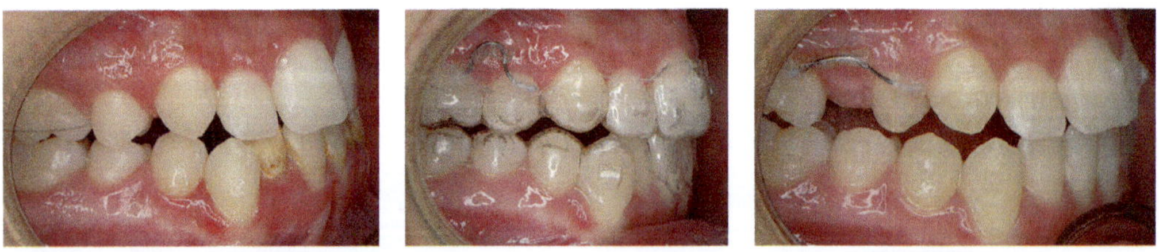

Fig. 18.74 Opening space for 15 (lateral view).

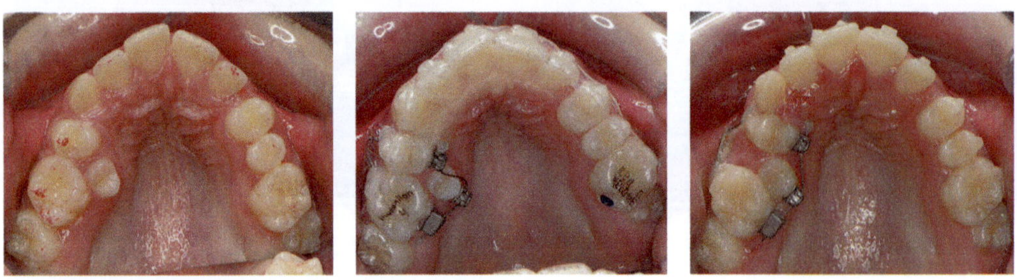

Fig. 18.75 Opening space for 15 (occlusal view).

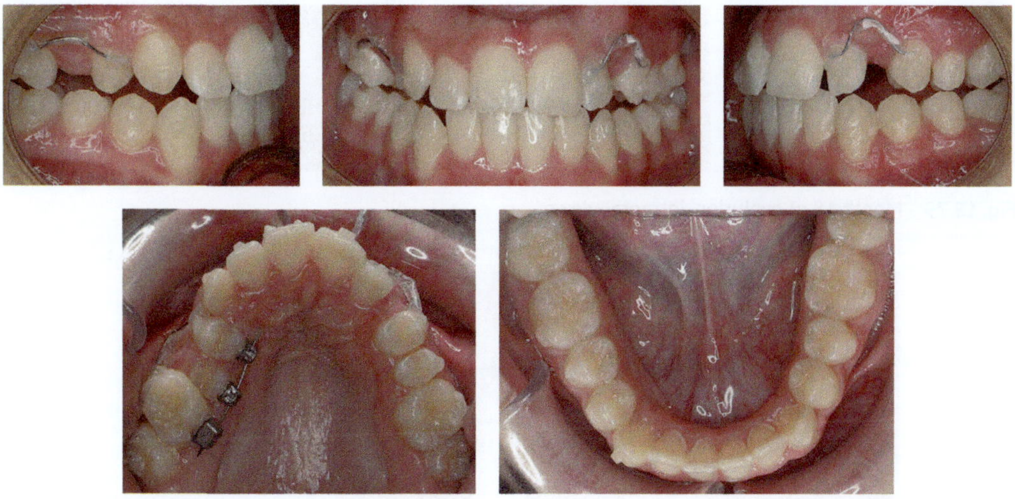

Fig. 18.76 Locatelli to open space for 15 and 23.

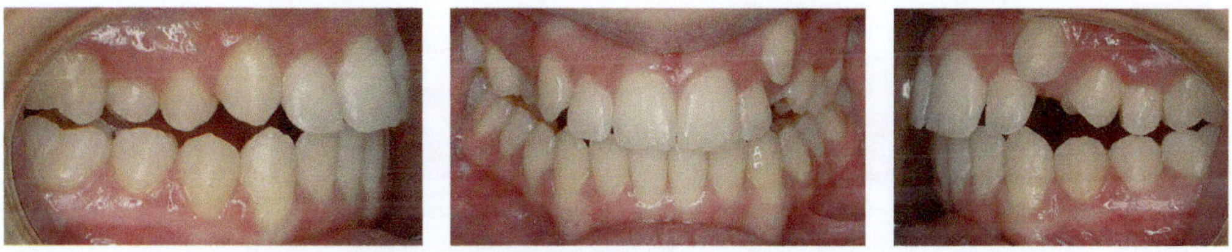

Fig. 18.77 Situation at the end of first set of aligners.

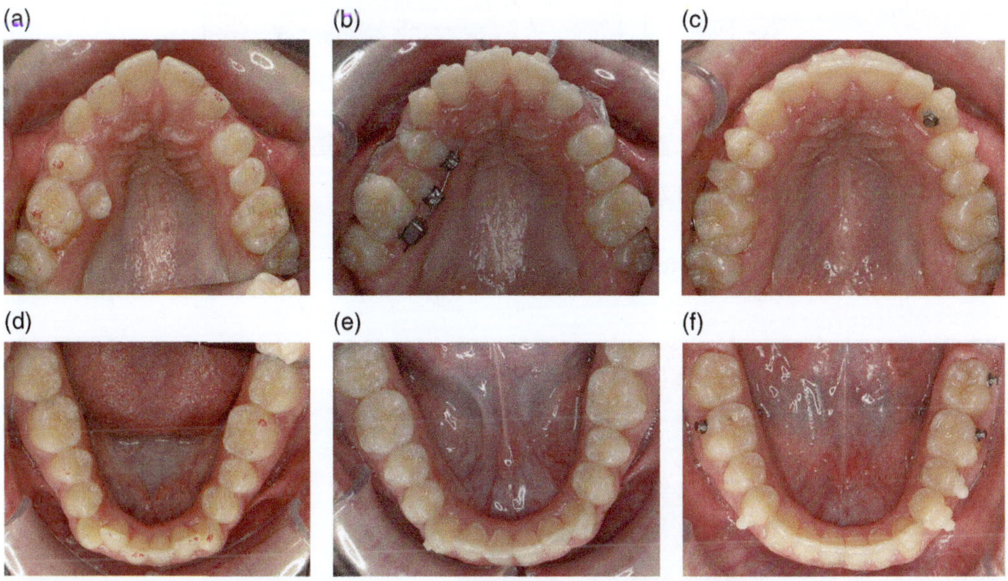

Fig. 18.78 (a–f) Transversal development of the arches.

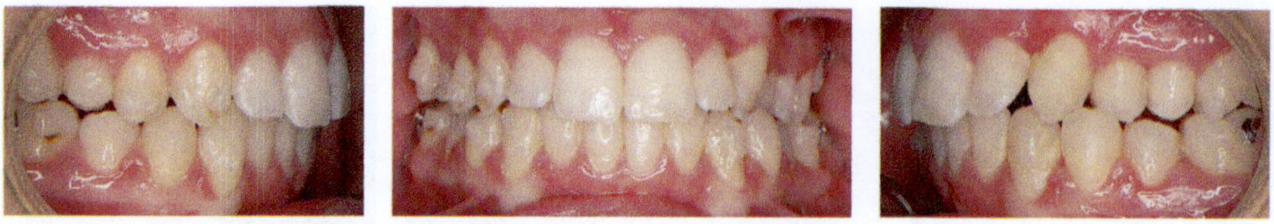

Fig. 18.79 Month 18 of evolution, intraoral views.

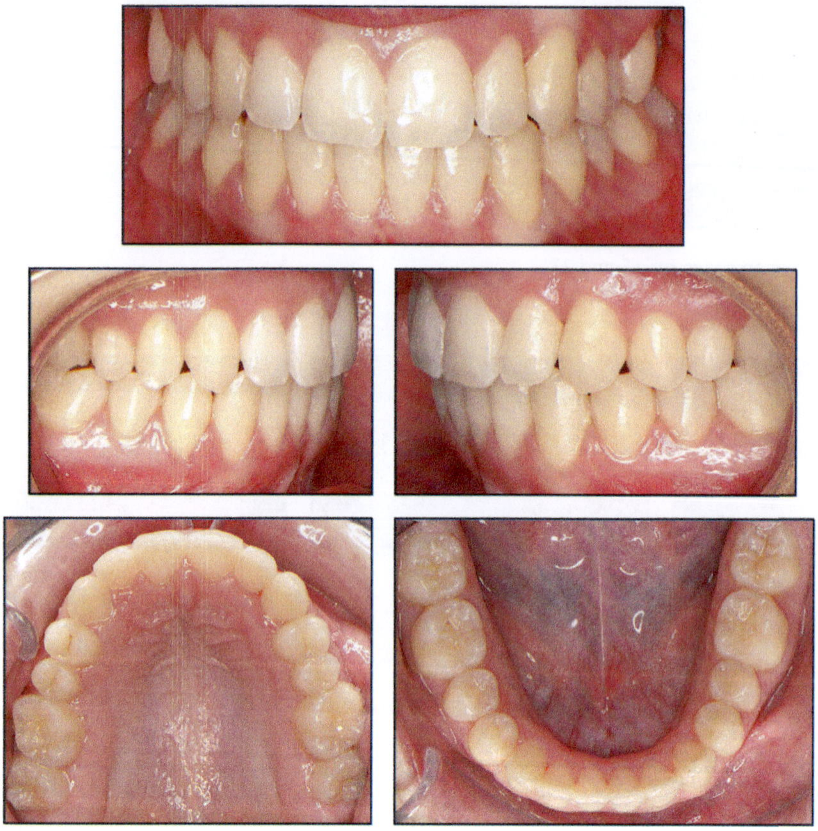

Fig. 18.80 Final views with 15 and 23 in place.

18.2.4 Traditional Technique for Impacted Canine Traction

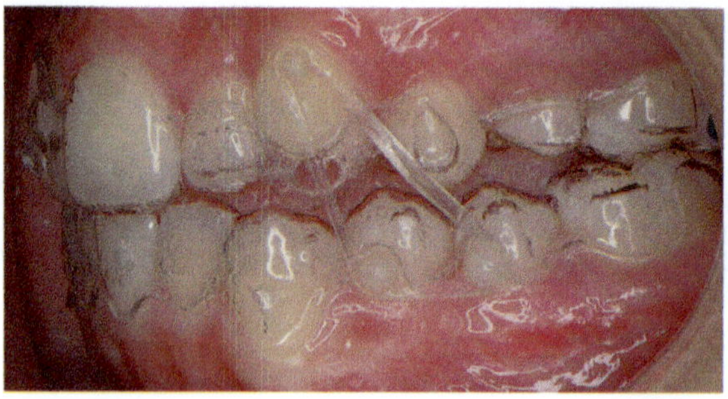

Fig. 18.81 By labial.

Fig. 18.82 By lingual.

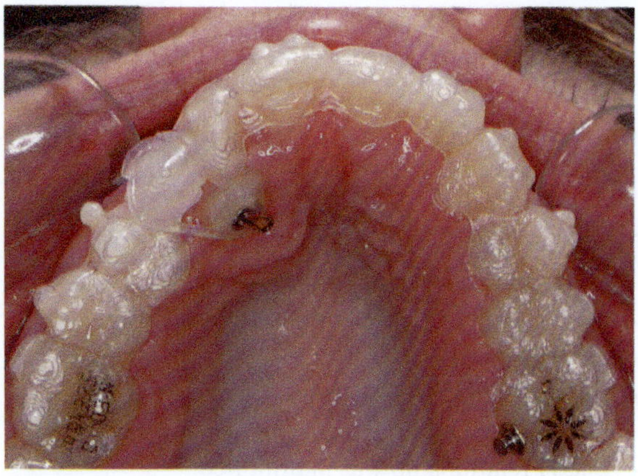

18.2.5 Deep Bite Lite Treatment in a Teenager

Fig. 18.83 Class I deep bite Lite treatment.

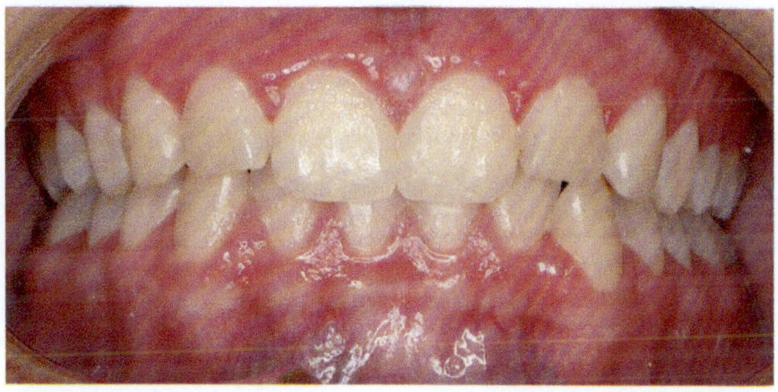

Diagnosis

A 17-year-old girl with hypodivergent skeletal class I presented with deep bite and minor lower crowding, lingual tipping of upper and lower incisors, facial competence and gummy anterior smile. She had a TMJ disorder resulting from a forced posterior position of the mandible, caused by the lingual tipping of the upper incisors and the deep bite anterior occlusion.

Treatment Plan

- Patient had posterior stable occlusion in class I, so a Lite treatment was planned, correcting the deep bite by proclination of upper and lower incisors (relative intrusion) and upper and lower incisors intrusion as the patient had gummy anterior smile
- As soon as the overjet was increased, the condyle could move to CR position and the symptomatology in the TMJ would be reduced

Requirements for the Technician

- Do not move upper and lower molars, as posterior anchorage is needed to correct the incisors inclination

- Expand from second premolar to second premolar in the upper and lower arches and to procline upper and lower incisors to remove the root from the cortical bone before starting the absolute intrusion
- Intrusion in both upper and lower incisors to correct the anterior gummy smile and to level the lower curve of Spee

Treatment Summary
- Treatment time was 14 months.
- Patient used 14 aligners in the first phase in 2-week change intervals and another set of 14 additional aligners.
- Patient used class II elastics, which were also worn at night to increase the anchorage during correction of incisor torque.
- Class I relationship was maintained.

Deep bite was corrected through incisor proclination (shown in the final lateral radiograph; Fig. 18.87) and incisors intrusion and the symptomatology of the TMJ disappear.

- We corrected the gummy anterior smile and the appearance improved considerably.

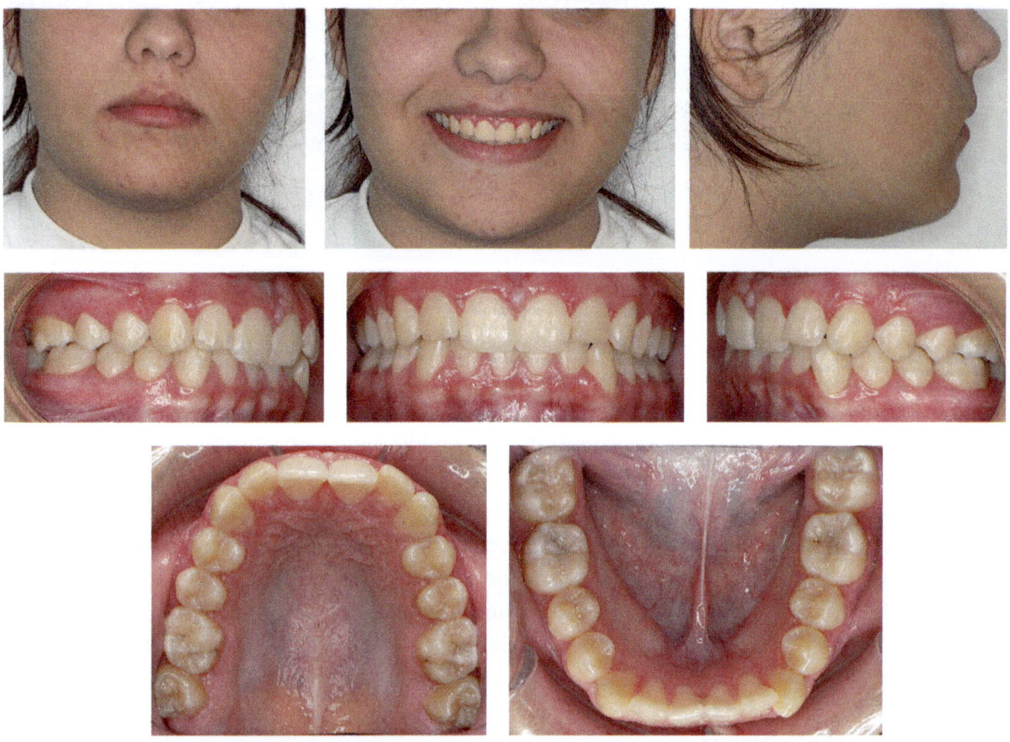

Fig. 18.84 Pretreatment views (right, front, left, upper, lower).

Maxilla:
- Expansion 1.5 to 2.5
- Proclination and lingual root torque of upper incisors
- Correct deep bite by relative intrusion (proclination) + intrusion

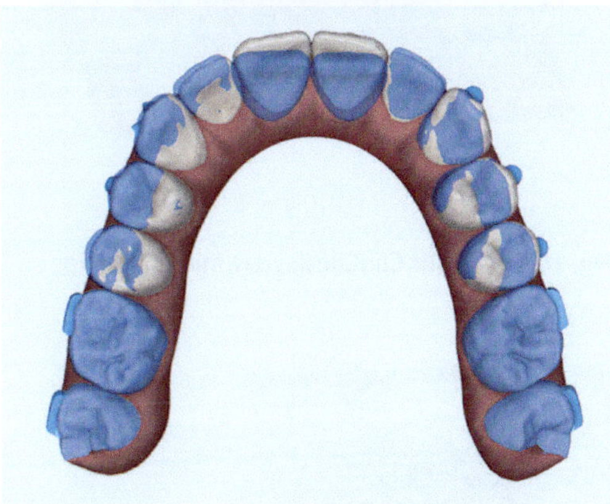

Fig. 18.85 Upper CC superimposition and instructions to CAD designer.

Expansion 3.5 to 4.5 + proclination of lower incisors (anterior limit: mesial surface of lower canines)
- Anchorage Attachment: HBO U4 / U5 / U6 + optimized AT in U3
- Do not move molars to increase anchorage to correct deep bite

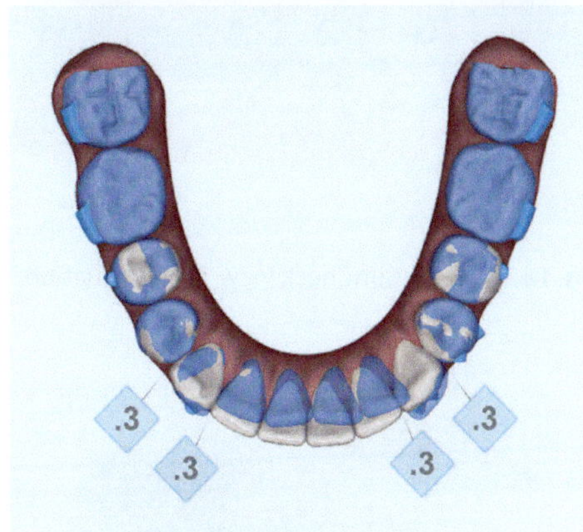

Fig. 18.86 Lower CC superimposition and instructions to CAD designer.

Correct deep bite
Level the curve of Spee

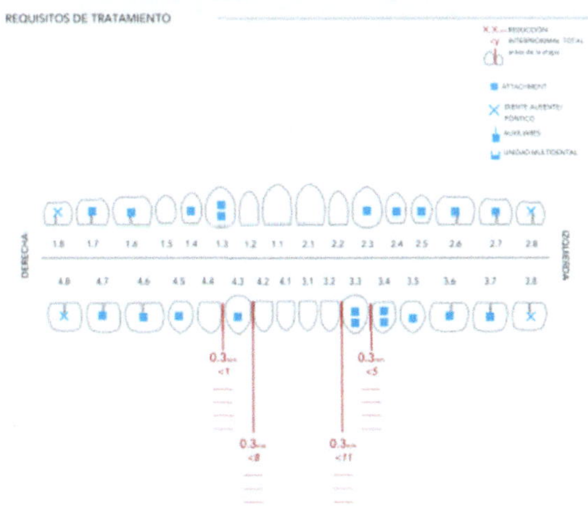

- Expansion 5 to 5 + proclination + upper intrusion
- Do not move molars and class II elastic night wear (anchorage)

Crowding and deep bite correction by expansion 5 to 5 and anterior torque correction combined with incisor intrusion 72

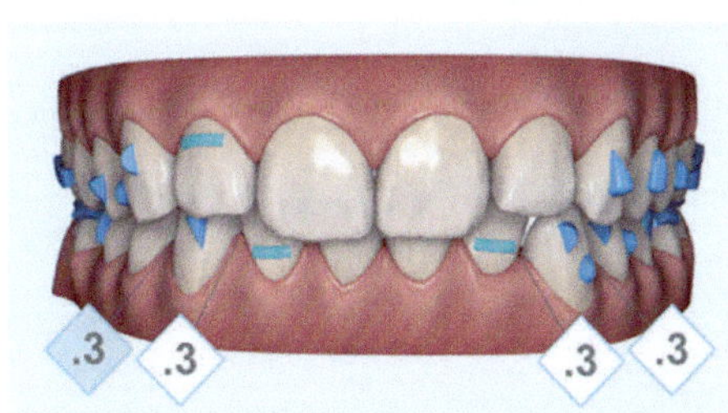

Fig. 18.87 Attachments and IPR can be seen in several areas of the ClinCheck software.

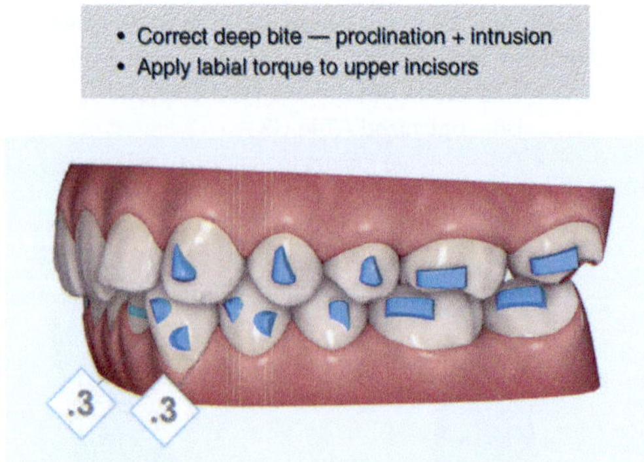

Fig. 18.88 Left ClinCheck view, initial situation.

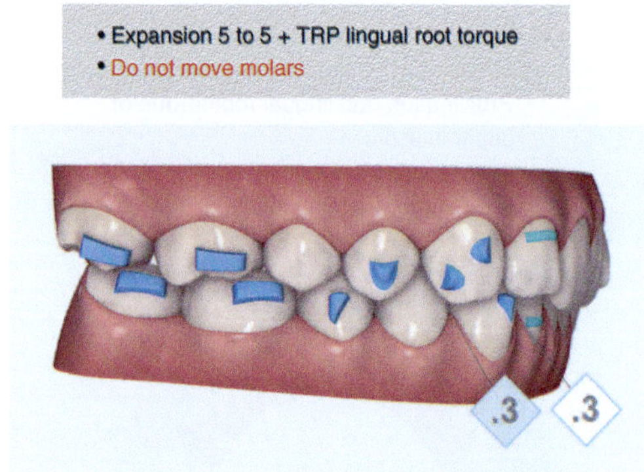

Fig. 18.89 Right ClinCheck view, initial situation.

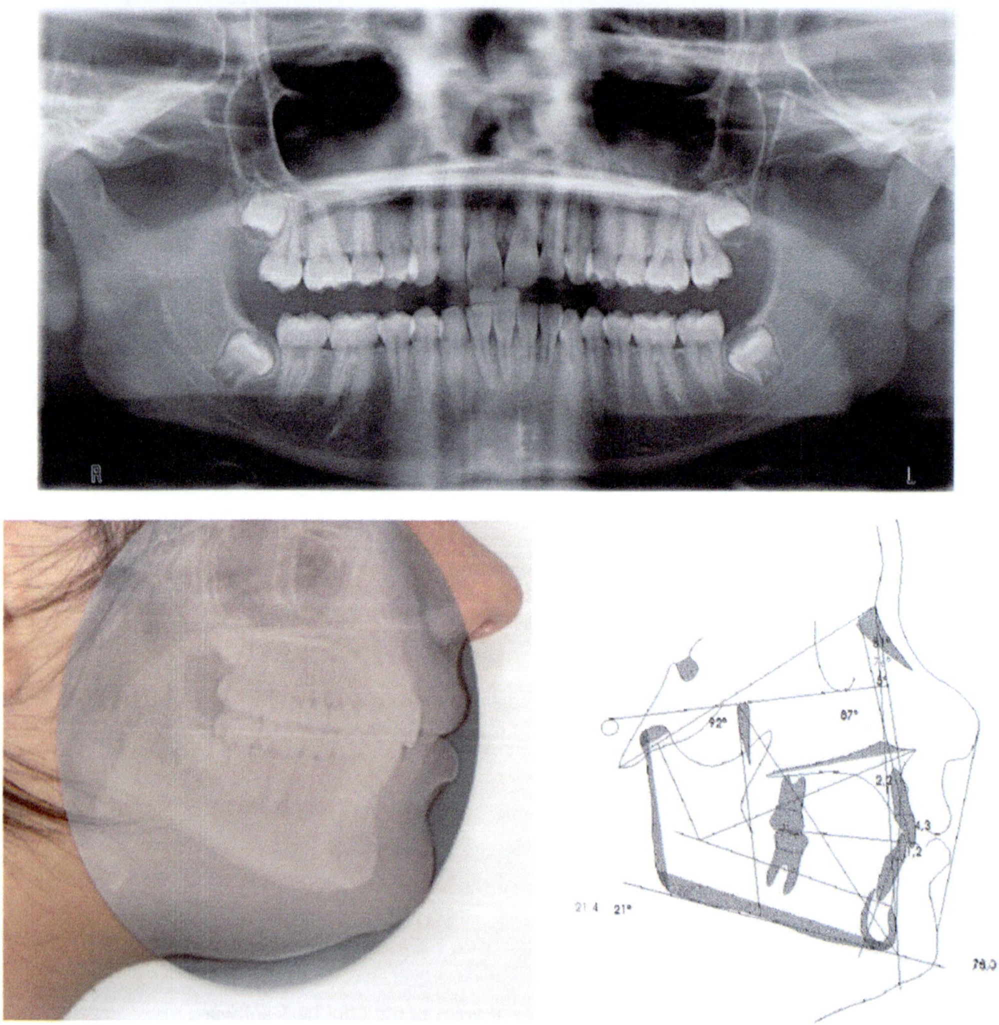

Fig. 18.90 Pretreatment panoramic X-ray, teleradiography and cephalometry.

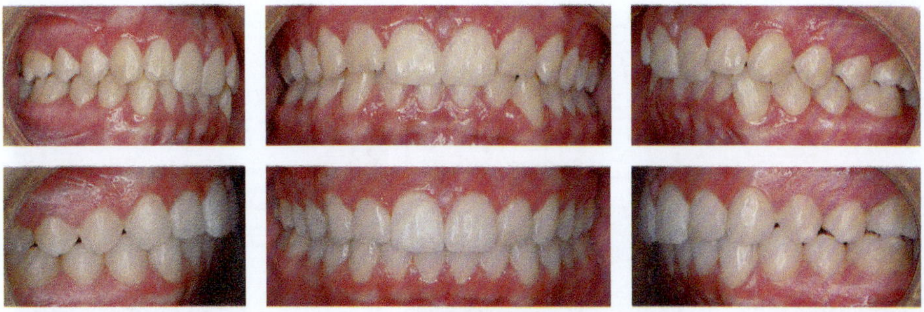

Fig. 18.91 Pretreatment (upper) and final (lower) results.

Fig. 18.92 Initial and final occlusal (upper and lower).

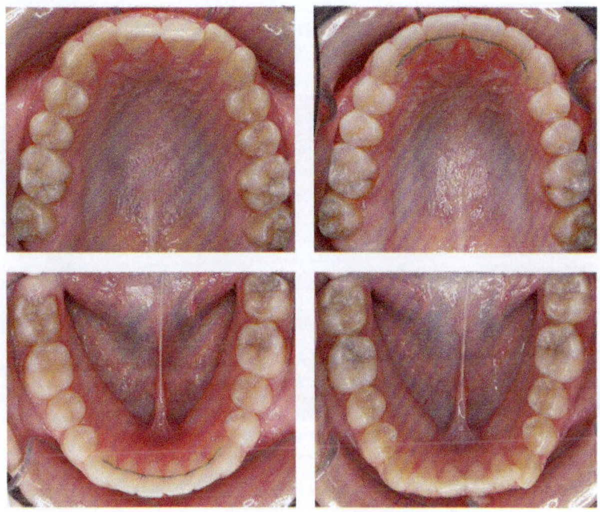

Fig. 18.93 Pretreatment and final smiles and overjets.

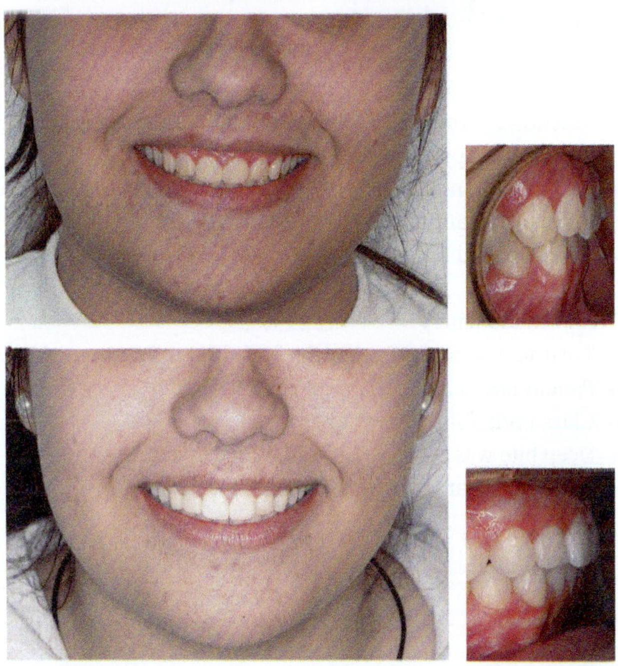

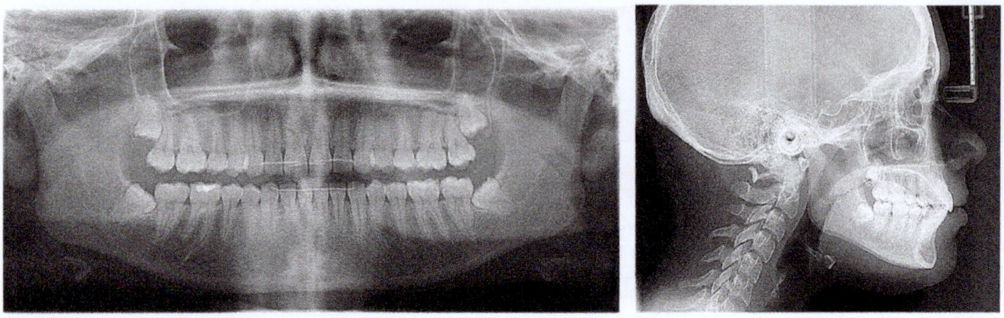

Fig. 18.94 Final panoramic and lateral X-rays.

18.2.6 Ectopic Palatal Canine

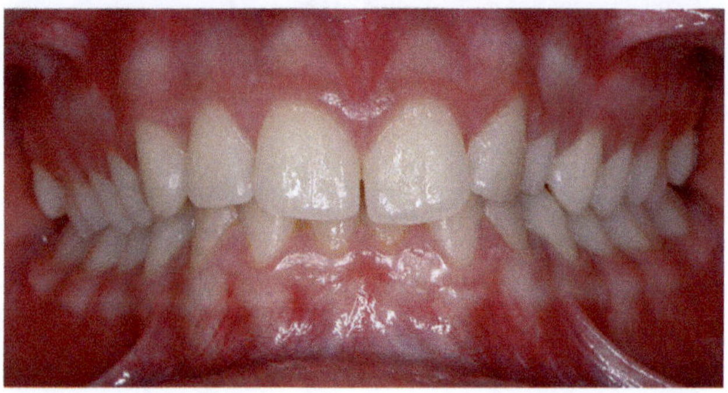

Fig. 18.95 Ectopic palatal canine.

Diagnosis

A 13-year-old girl with skeletal class I presented with deep bite and minor lower crowding. She had a gummy smile, bilateral mild dental class II and an ectopic palatal canine, 23.

Treatment Plan

- Traction 23 from transpalatal bar, changing force vectors in order to get it in the best position for aligner therapy
- Second quadrant mesialization occurred after traction, causing a class II on the left side and a midline deviation that had to be addressed
- Space opened for 23 with aligners

Treatment Summary

- Treatment time was 9 months for initial traction and 15 months for aligners therapy
- Patient used class II elastics, worn at night
- Class I relationship was achieved
- Deep bite was corrected through incisor intrusion
- The gummy anterior smile was corrected

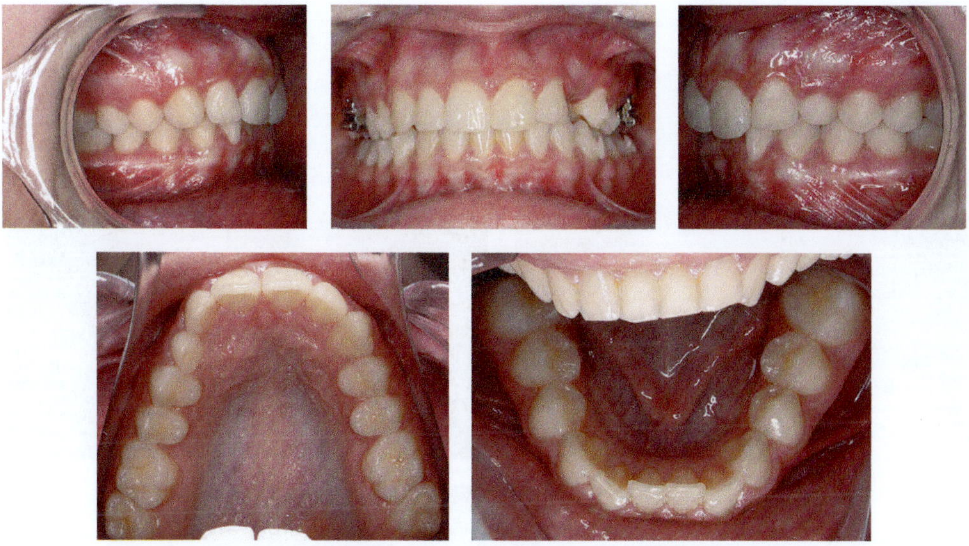

Fig. 18.96 Initial intraoral views (right, front, left, upper, lower).

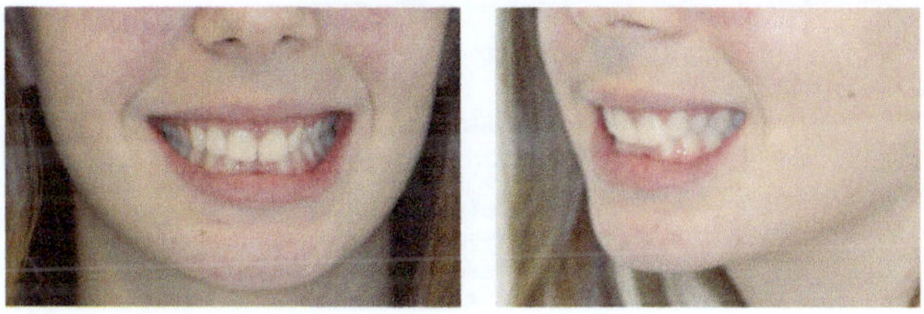

Fig. 18.97 Initial extraoral views.

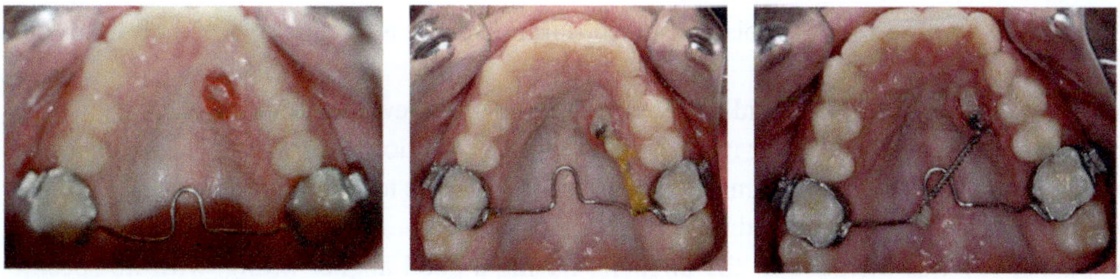

Fig. 18.98 Initial intraoral views: traction 1, 2, 3.

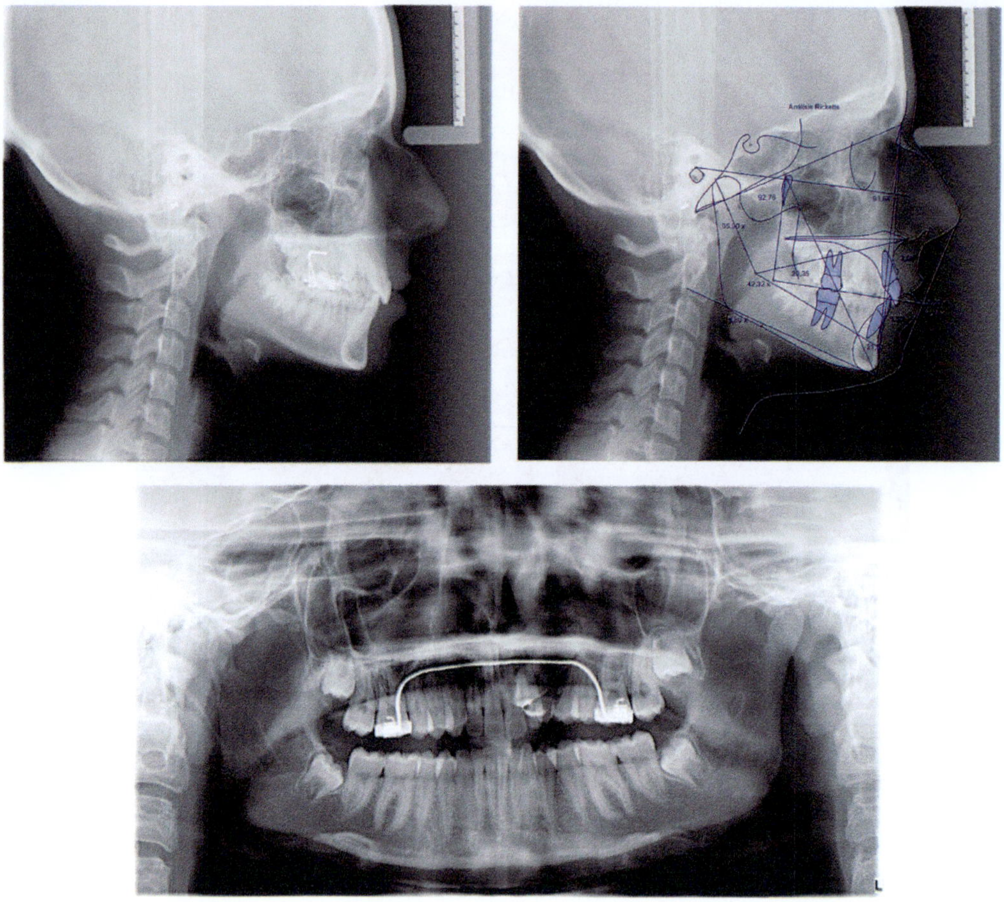

Fig. 18.99 Initial lateral and panoramic X-rays.

ClinCheck 1: Requirements for the Technician

- Do not move upper and lower molars, as posterior anchorage is needed to correct the incisors inclination
- Expand both arches and centre midlines at the same time by deviating upper one to the right
- Intrusion in both upper and lower incisors to correct the anterior gummy smile and to level the lower curve of Spee (For this, optimized deep bite attachments to be placed on premolars.)
- No class II correction was intended in this first set of aligners
- Transpalatal bar was included in the aligners, having a good aligner fitting, with no specific requirement for the technician
- During alignment, the powerchain to be linked to a button bonded to the surface of the canine

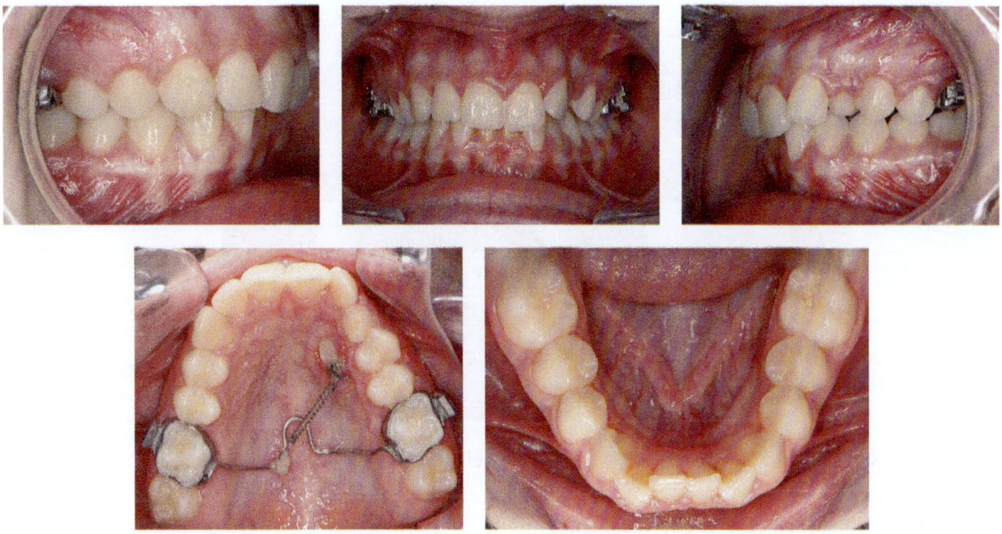

Fig. 18.100 Refinement: intraoral views (right, front, left, upper, lower).

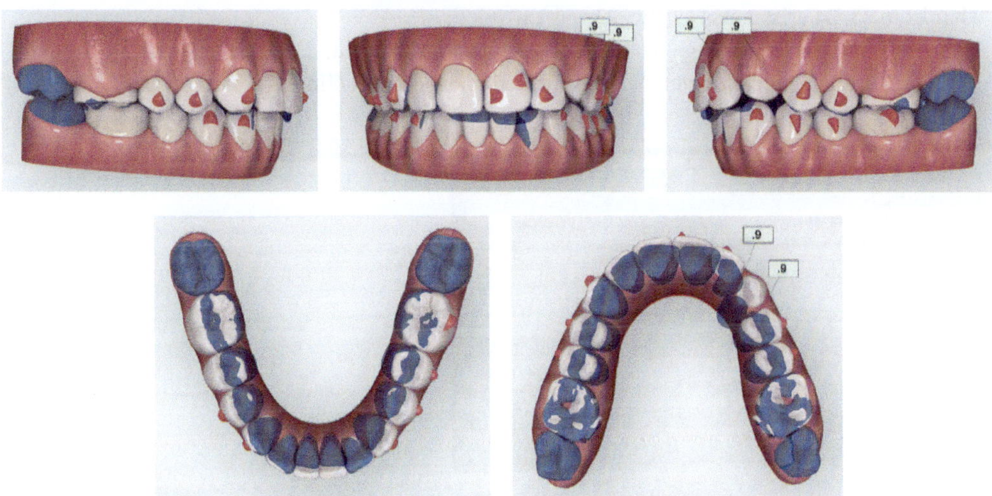

Fig. 18.101 ClinChecks: right, front, left, upper, lower.

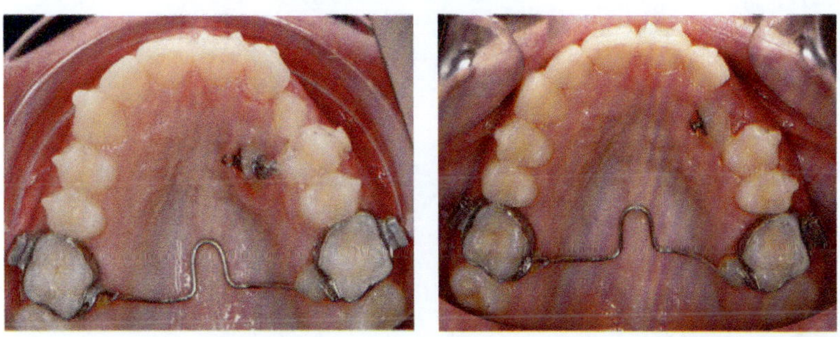

Fig. 18.102 Traction 4 and 5. Initial traction was delivered with constant forces delivered from a Powerchain bonded to a button on 24. After that the patient wore an elastic to a third quadrant button to create an extrusion force vector.

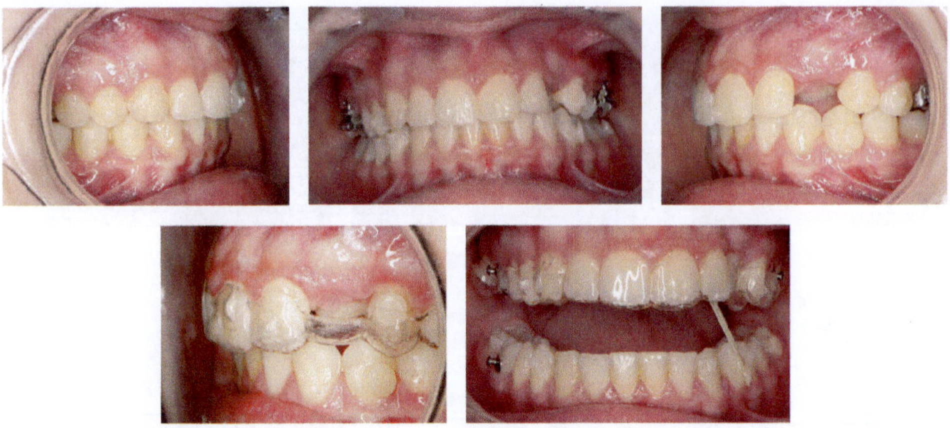

Fig. 18.103 Refinement 2: intraoral views (right, front, left, upper, lower).

ClinCheck2: Communications to the Technician

- After initial set of aligners, as a result of incisor protrusion, distalization of second quadrant happened, so no more distalization was needed.
- Thanks to 23–34 criss-cross elastic, 23 was extruded.
- Open the space for 23 adding 20% additional space than needed.
- Before scanning, a gingivectomy was performed to expose full clinical crown of 23.

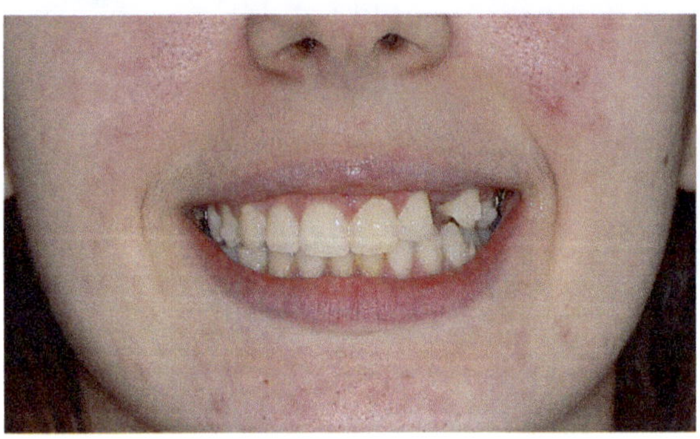

Fig. 18.104 Smile at refinement 2.

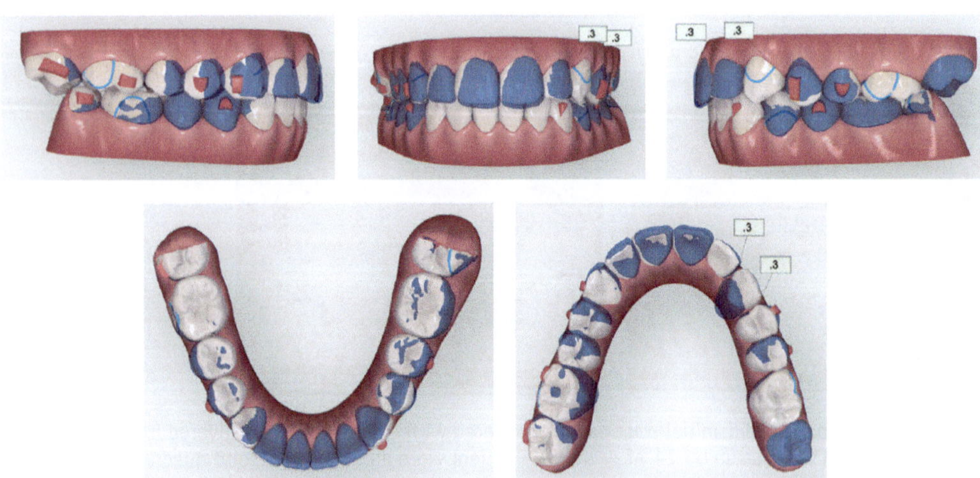

Fig. 18.105 Refinement 2 ClinChecks (right, front, left, upper, lower).

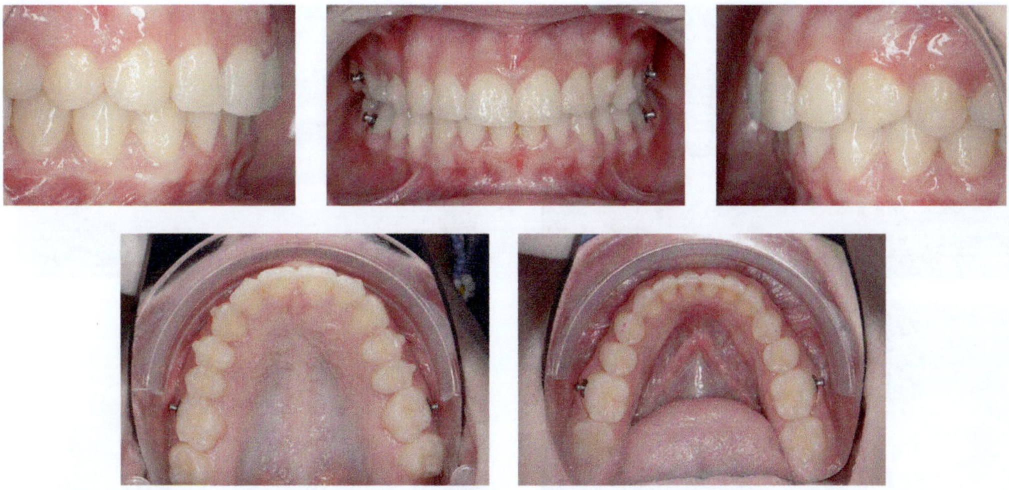

Fig. 18.106 Final intraoral views.

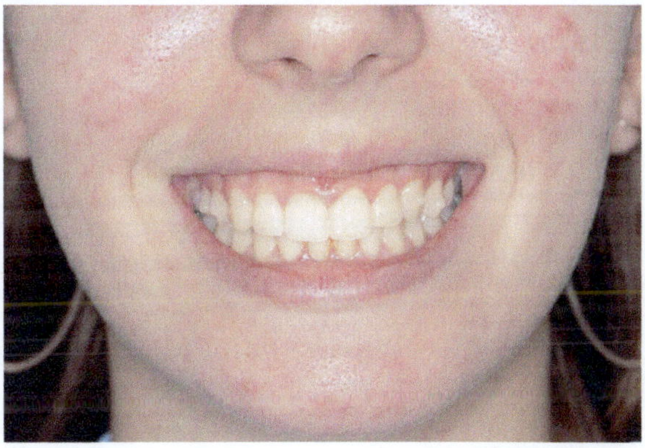

Fig. 18.107 Final smile view.

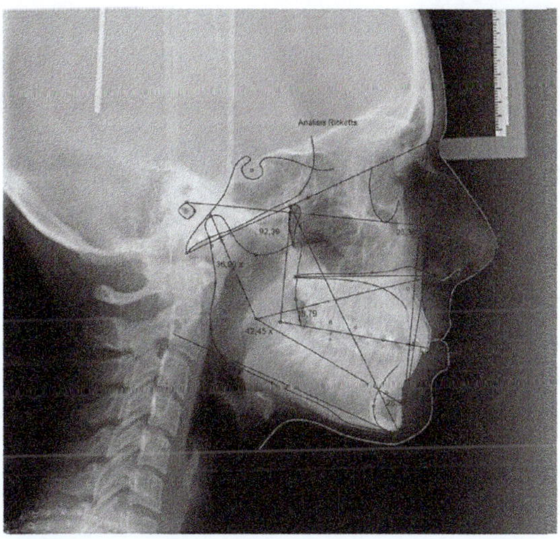

Fig. 18.108 Current cephalometric measurements.

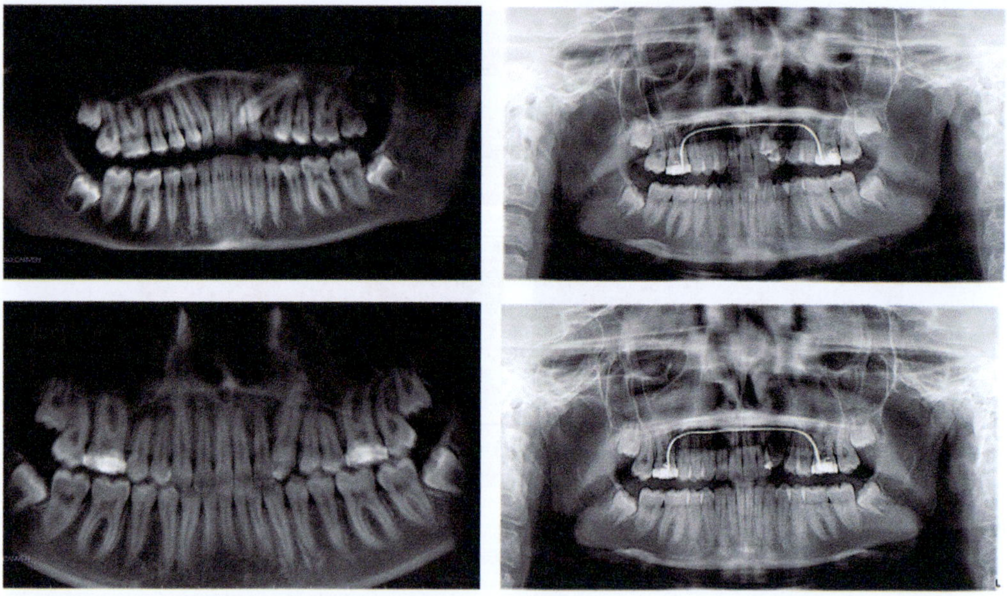

Fig. 18.109 Ortopantomographs (OPG) 0, 1, 2, 3. Evolution of the canine with OPGs and 2D cone beam computed tomography reconstruction.

18.2.7 Temporary Tooth Management

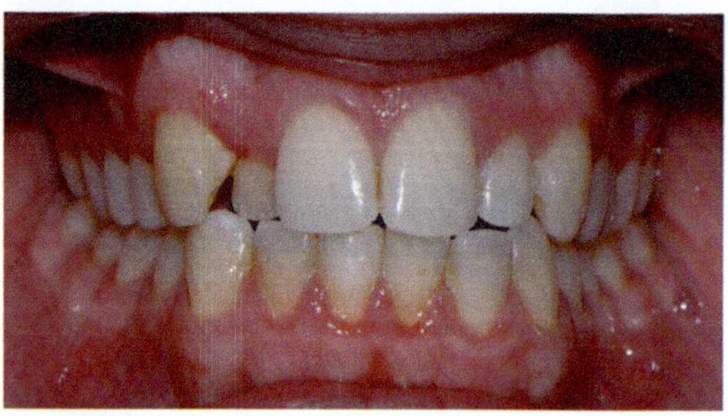

Fig. 18.110 Temporary 52.

Diagnosis

A 17-year-old boy with skeletal class I presented with open bite tendency. He had posterior compression, right half cusp class II, 18 was present, but not extracted to distalize, 12 was absent, 52 on crossbite.

Treatment Plan

- Distalize sequentially first quadrant, when there is space for 52, move it to its ideal position
- Lower IPR to compensate upper lateral incisors Bolton discrepancy
- Improve vertical anterior relationship by posterior expansion

Treatment Summary

- Treatment time was 15 months with two sets of aligners
- Patient used class II elastics 24/7
- A class I relationship was achieved
- A composite veneer was bonded to 52 at the end of treatment

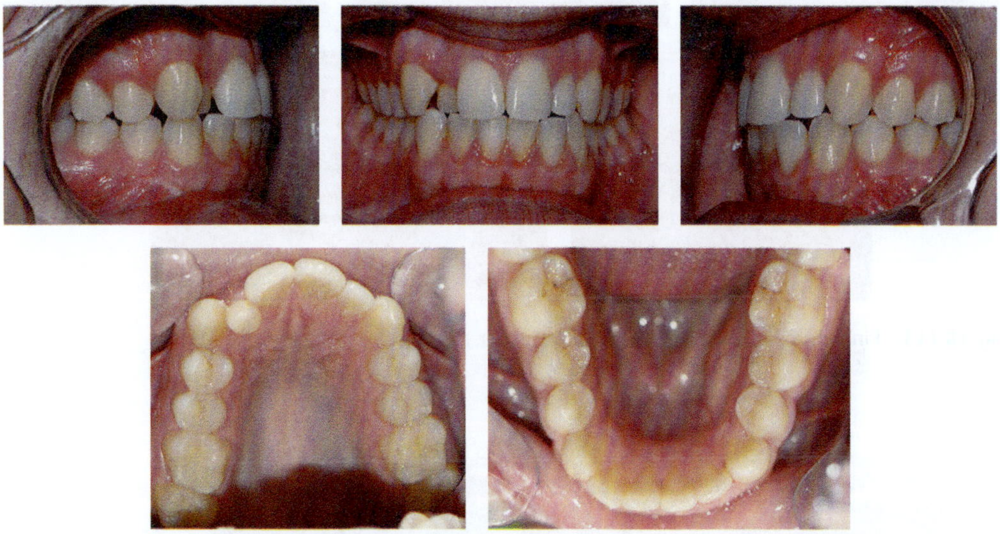

Fig. 18.111 Initial intraoral views (right, front, left, upper, lower).

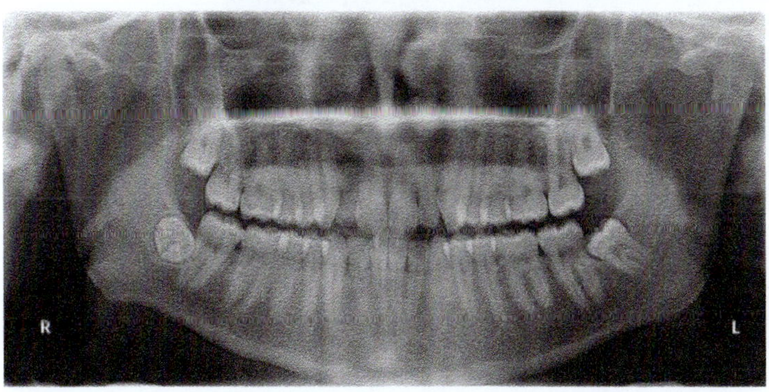

Fig. 18.112 Pretreatment panoramic X-ray with wisdom teeth present.

ClinCheck 1: Requirements for the Technician

- Distalize while expanding both sides of the patient, more on the right side of the patient as it was more compressed.
- Do not move 52 until there is enough for it.
- Perform lower IPR and add extra lingual root torque to 32–42 while retruding to create an 'en masse' movement.
- In this case, we did not ask for class II precision cuts, so they were made manually and patient wore 24/7 class II elastics.

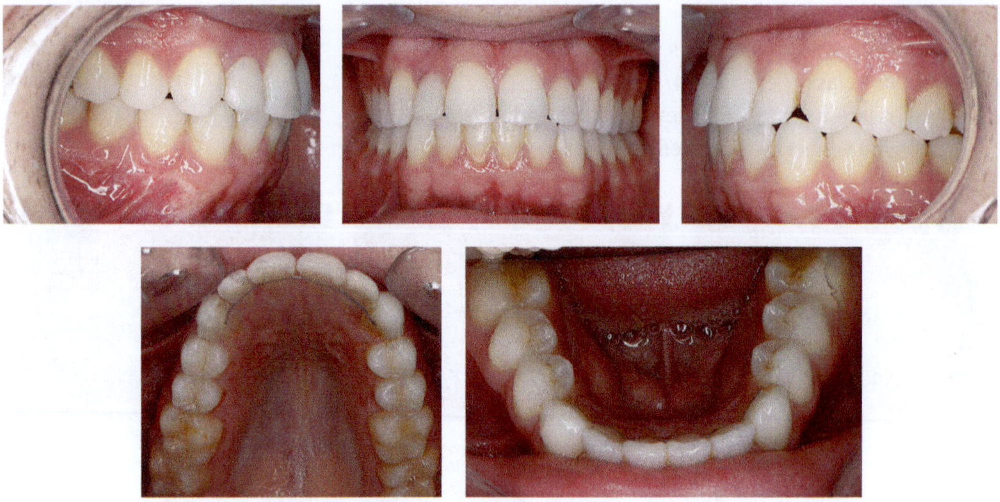

Fig. 18.113 Final intraoral views (right, front, left, upper, lower).

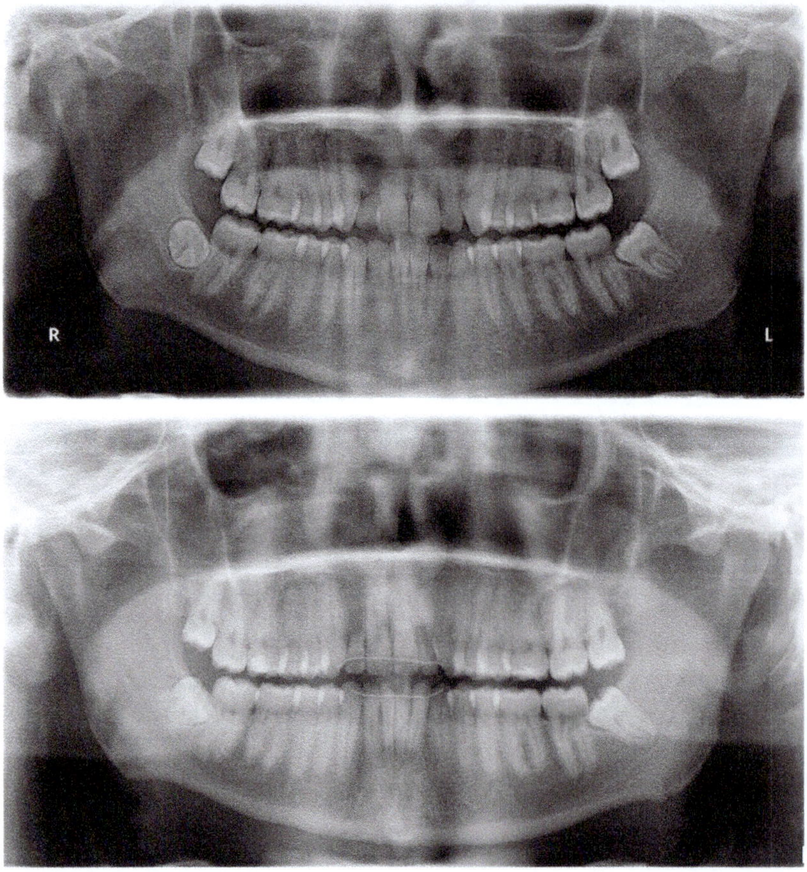

Fig. 18.114 Initial and final panoramic X-rays. Right class I was achieved even with the wisdom tooth present, as it was in a growing patient; 52 could be kept during the whole treatment and there was no need for replacement at the end.

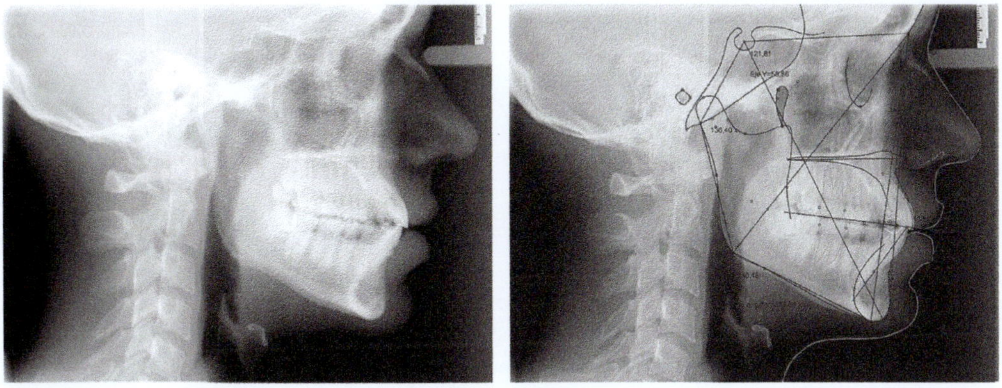

Fig. 18.115 Final lateral X-ray and cephalometric analysis.

19

Transversal Problems: Symmetric and Asymmetric Expansion

It is commonly accepted that, in the transverse dimension, normal occlusion is when the palatine cusps of the upper molars and premolars occlude in the fossa of lower molars and premolars.

This is also related to arch expansion, which is mostly defined by the patient's skeletal condition, and is one of the key factors in success with aligners, as it is possible to expand asymmetrically with the archform tool – something that has never been possible with standard preformed NiTi archwires.

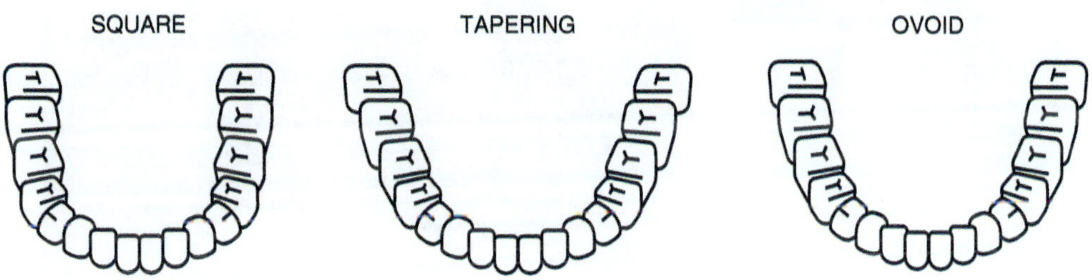

Fig. 19.1 Classic NiTi archwires were only available on standard sizes and shapes, now, with aligners, we can define exactly the best archform for every patient.

This is especially important in order to avoid gingival recessions associated with excessive dental expansions, and this is the reason why it is so important to use the archform tool to decide whether to have a regular expansion or more posterior/anterior sector one.

Aligner Techniques in Orthodontics, First Edition. Susana Palma Moya and Javier Lozano Zafra.

Companion website: www.wiley.com/go/lozano-zafra/aligner-techniques

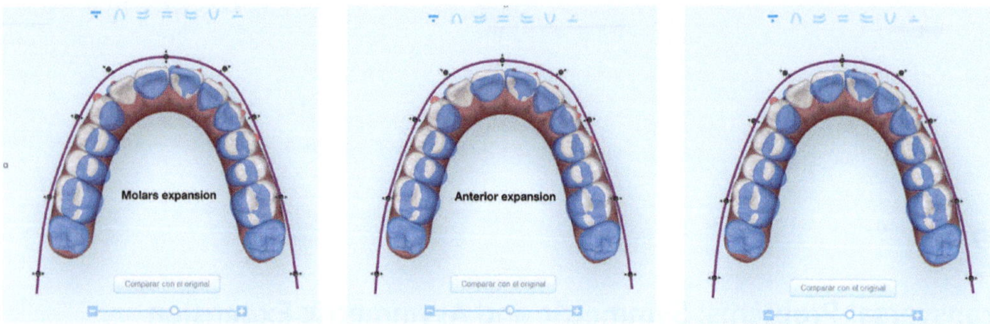

Fig. 19.2 Expansion can be defined in a precise way, with the decision about whether it is more or less anterior/posterior made according to patient's available bone.

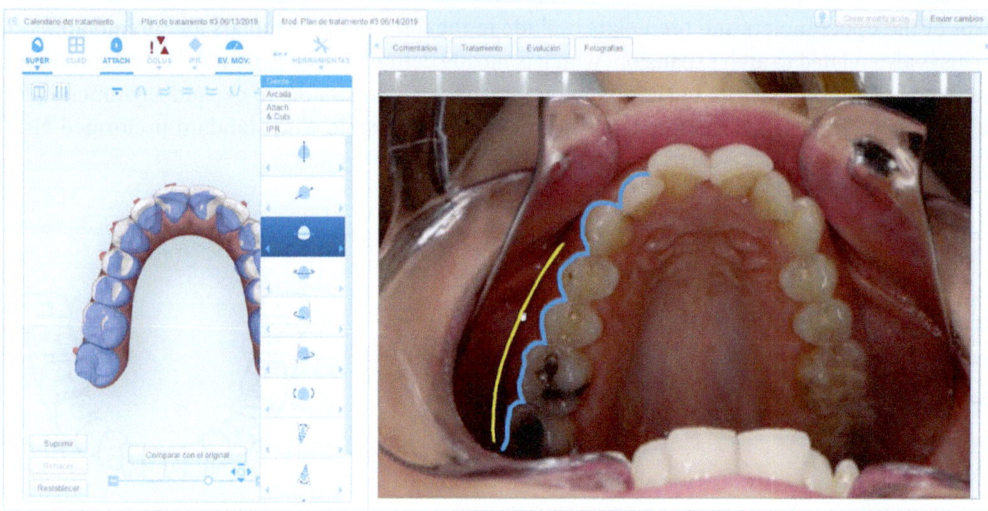

Fig. 19.3 Expansion with aligners can be defined in between Fa point (blue line) and Wa point (yellow line).

That said, a crossbite is a commonly seen discrepancy in the buccolingual relationship of the upper and lower teeth, when the lower teeth are in a buccal or labial position with regards to the upper teeth, in a unilateral, bilateral, anterior and/or posterior manner.

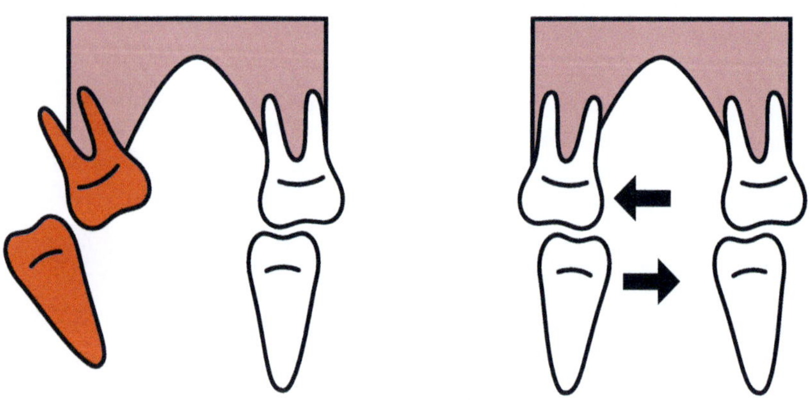

Fig. 19.4 Dentoalveolar expansion can be achieved with aligners, as with braces and wires, to solve crossbites.

Crossbite malocclusion can have a skeletal or dental component or a combination of both. For this reason, when facing transversal problems, the first thing needed is a careful diagnosis, in order to determine the protocol to follow:

- Checking the occlusal view with the occlusal grid if there is a symmetric arch in shape, torque and size.
- In the frontal view, check the posterior lateral torques to see if torque in both sides is symmetric or asymmetric.

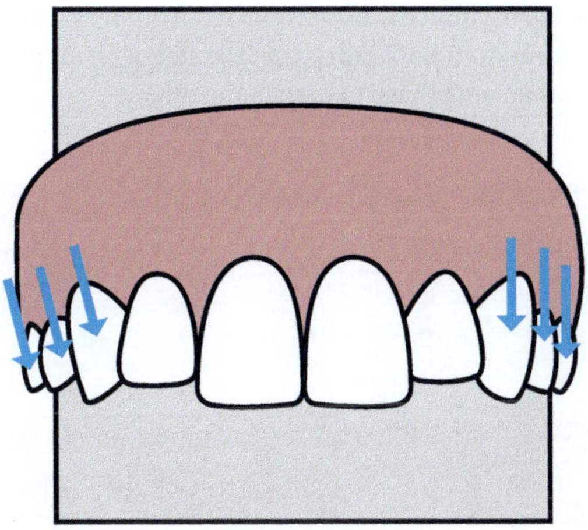

Fig. 19.5 In this situation, if we ask for the same amount of expansion in both sides, the left side with correct torque at the beginning will end up with premolars and molars tipped to labial and the labial cusp of those teeth would rise altering the Wilson curve.

- Smile analysis: check if the patient displays more gum on one side than on the other. Normally, if there is a side with less torque it will be accompanied by an increase in gum exposure on the same side.

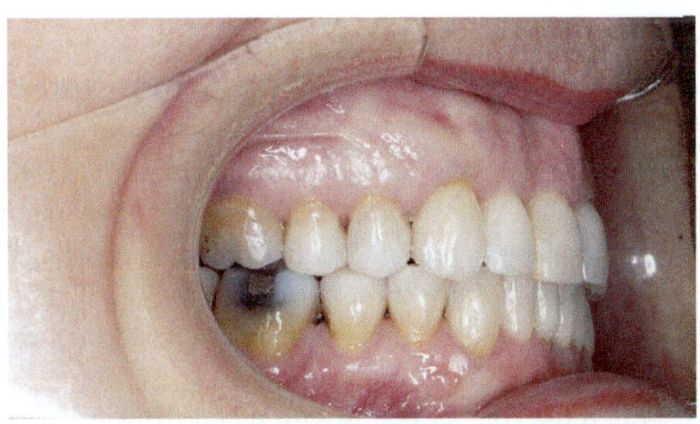

Fig. 19.6 Check smile. In unilateral masticatory side the patient will expose more gummy posterior smile in the non-masticatory side. We will need to achieve a final alternate bilateral mastication and to make the torque of posterior teeth equal at the end of the treatment.

- For symmetric expansion ask for labial crown torque to the laterals, canines, premolars and molars until they become perpendicular to the bone (0 degrees of final torque).

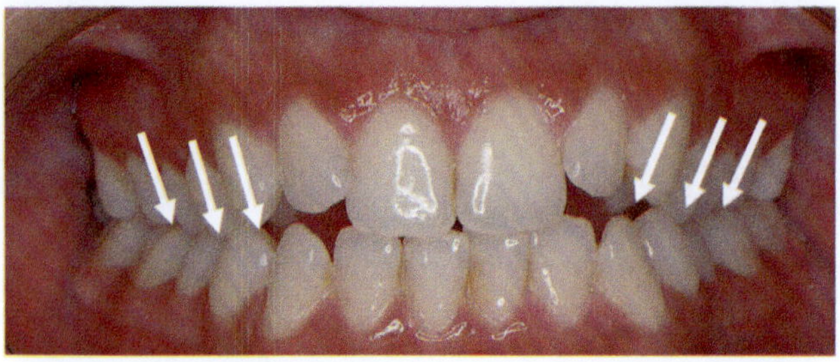

Fig. 19.7 Asymmetric expansion.

- For asymmetric expansion: teeth on the side with correct torque in the posterior area should not be moved until correcting the side with altered torque. In this way, one hemiarch is being used as an anchorage to correct the other.

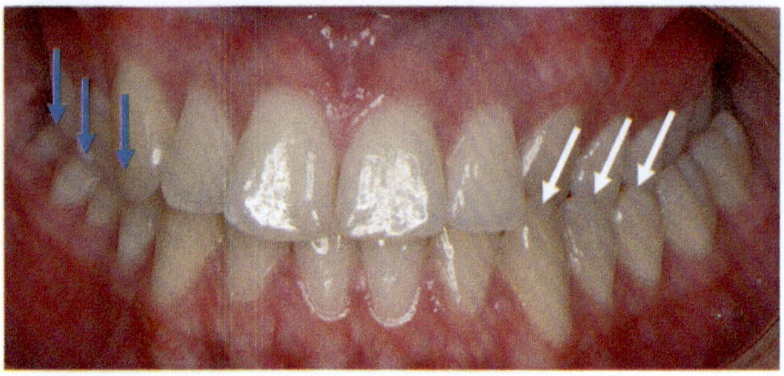

Fig. 19.8 Blue arrows indicate proper posterior torque, white ones show arch to be developed transversally.

- If patients need asymmetric expansions they should be informed that a final open bite in the posterior zone will require using intermaxillary elastics to close it.
- Protrusion: in patients with upper protrusion, in order to get a bigger expansion, the clinician should request the technician to apply a simultaneous movement of expansion and arch length reduction. In that way, retracting the incisors at the same time as expanding will provide us with very predictable and very effective transversal development of the arches.

19.1 Things to Consider in Expansion Cases

1. Plan ahead for anchorage attachments to provide labial root torque to the premolars and molars during the expansion. AT HBG bevelled attachment to gingival of 4 mm in first premolars and first molars provide an effective anchorage during the expansion.
2. Maintain third upper molars if possible and do not move them during the expansion.
3. If second and third molars are not in posterior crossbite, for better posterior anchorage, do not move them during the expansion.
4. Soften the contact points with metal strips if posterior contact points are tightened before the expansion.
5. Consider how much overjet there is before doing the expansion: if there is not enough overjet, the moment the expansion is made, even if we do not see the retraction in the ClinCheck, the incisors will move backward (pearl necklace effect).

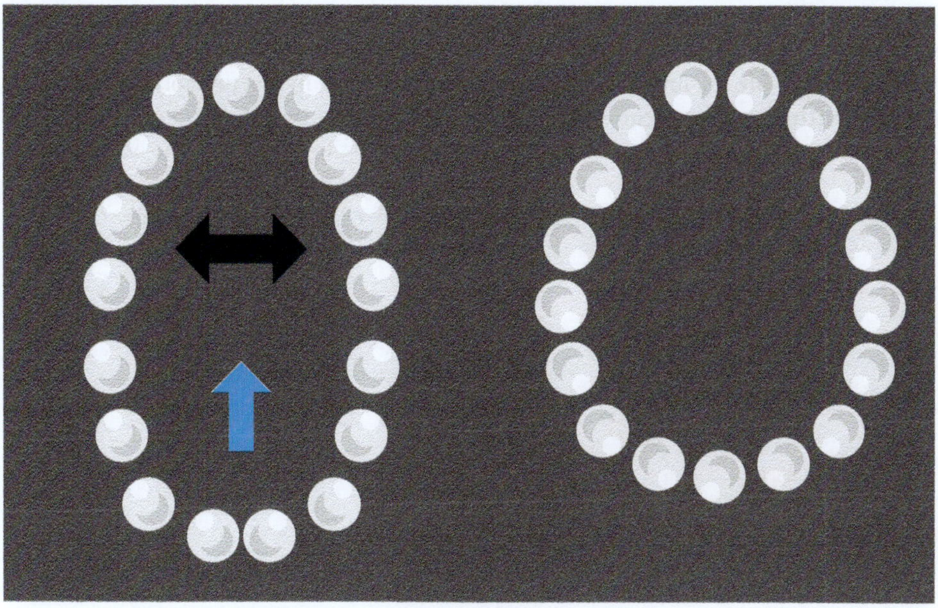

Fig. 19.9 Pearl necklace effect.

6. For staging:
   - Define staging
   - Expansion and rotation corrections: move simultaneously
   - Symmetric expansion: move simultaneously both sides
   - Asymmetric expansion: sequential movement, first the side with negative torque or posterior crossbite and then the anchorage side.
7. **In the posterior view** check in the final position of the ClinCheck that the palatal upper cusp of the molars occludes in the fossae of the lower molars.

The key to effective transversal development of the arches is the staging of movements:

1. Symmetric expansion and provide a parabolic arch: this movement can be done simultaneously to
   - Incisor retrusion (arch length reduction)
   - Rotation of molars and premolars
   - Minor corrections of molars through distalization
2. Proclination
3. Vertical goals: extrusion or intrusion of incisors.

If we need to expand and distalize, we can make at the same time the expansion, the mesial-out rotation of first molars and the sequential distalization.

If we need to expand and procline: first expand (transversal compensation), second procline (sagittal compensation) and third, intrude or extrude (vertical compensation).

4. Attachments: in the asymmetric expansion the key attachments are on the anchorage side, which is the side that is not going to move until the posterior crossbite on the contralateral side is corrected.
   - In the **anchorage side** ask for *rectangular attachments of 4 mm* in first premolars and molars.
   - In the **side with negative torque or with posterior crossbite** ask for *horizontal attachments bevelled to gingival* that provide a labial root torque to the root during the expansion.

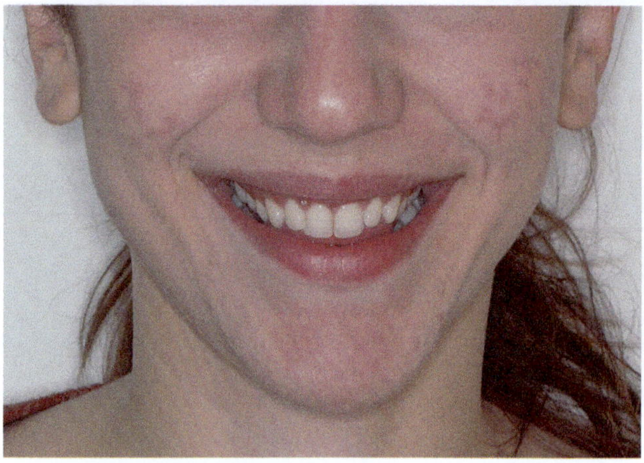

Fig. 19.10 Smile picture.

19.2 Symmetric Expansion

19.2.1 Symmetric Compression Causing Anterior Open Bite

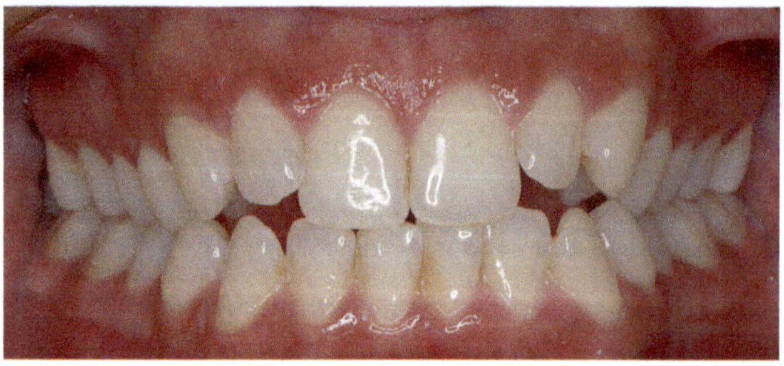

Fig. 19.11 Symmetric compression causing anterior open bite.

Diagnosis

A 26-year-old woman with a normodivergent skeletal class I presented with narrow arches and symmetric compression. She had a class I relationship with negative torque of posterior canines, premolars and molars, wisdom teeth erupted, labially flared maxillary lateral incisors and mild lower crowding, with a posterior gummy smile resulting from the inadequate posterior torque.

Treatment Plan

- Open space by upper expansion and sequential distalization
- In the lower arch, as the initial dental relationship was a class I, a sequential lower distalization was also planned
- All four wisdom teeth were extracted 2 weeks before the start of treatment

Requirements for the Technician

- *In the upper arch*, make a symmetric expansion by changing torque applying labial crown torque to canines and premolars simultaneously to the sequential upper distalization of 1.5 mm.
- Sequence the movement on the incisors, first proclining 11 and 21 to make torque equal to 12 and 22 and to make space for the correction of the upper lateral and then making an IPR and applying a simultaneous movement of distal-tipping of the crown in 12 and 22 and retrusion (relative extrusion). Horizontal attachments to be placed on the lateral incisors for better control.
- *In the lower arch*, make a sequential distalization, maintaining the class I molar relationship during the treatment.

Treatment Summary

- The total treatment was 18 months.
- The patient wore a set of 38 aligners used in a 10-day change interval protocol.
- An additional aligners set was planned to settle the posterior occlusion.
- A final bilateral class I was obtained with adequate overbite and overjet, after uprighting posterior teeth, which provided the patient with a final beautiful smile and a stable occlusion.

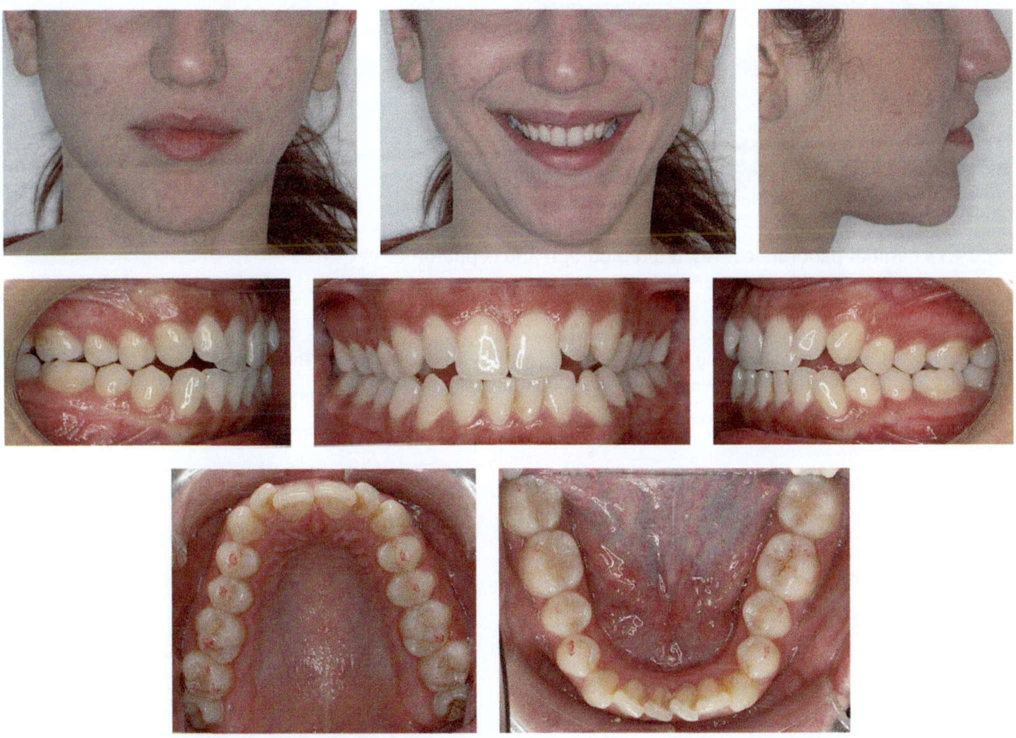

Fig. 19.12 Pretreatment extraoral and intraoral views.

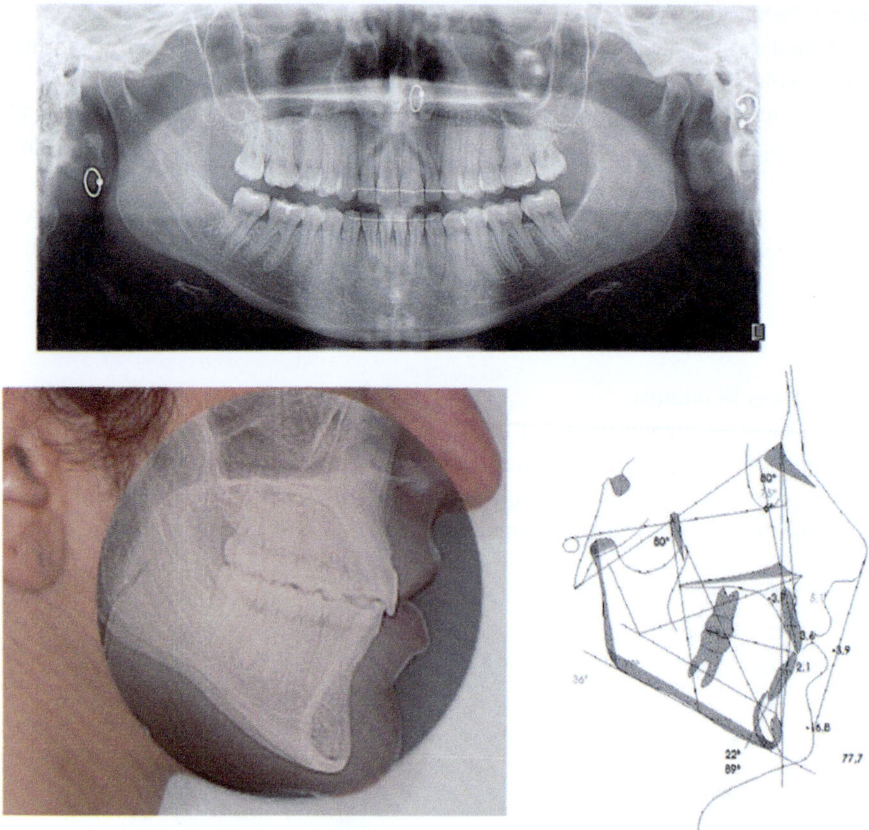

Fig. 19.13 Initial panoramic X-ray, teleradiograph and cephalometry.

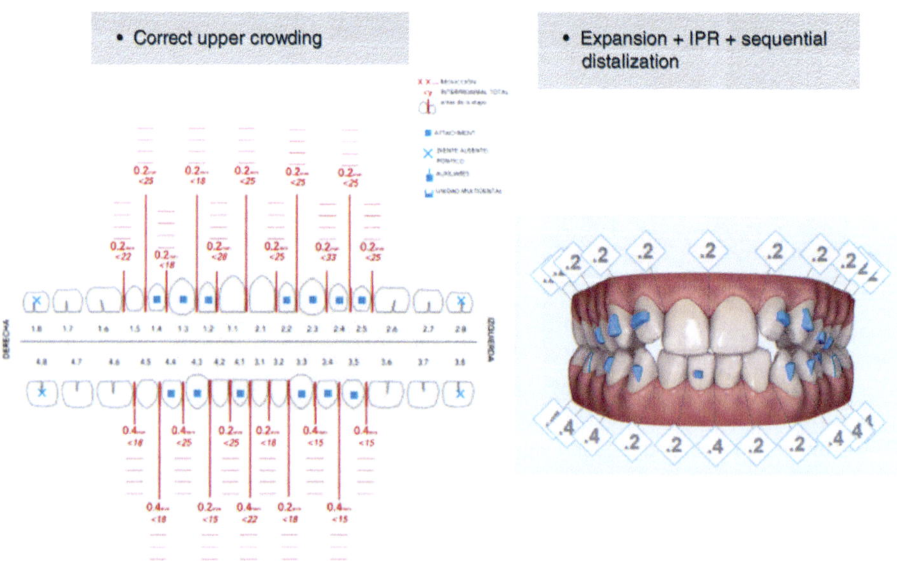

Fig. 19.14 Interproximal reduction.

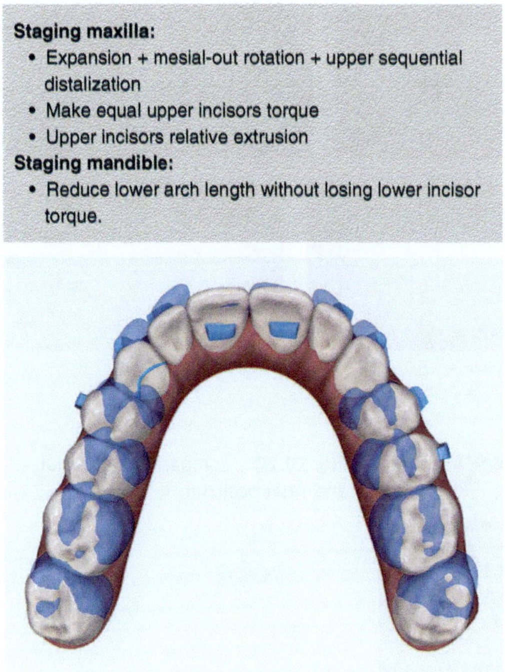

Fig. 19.15 Upper superposition.

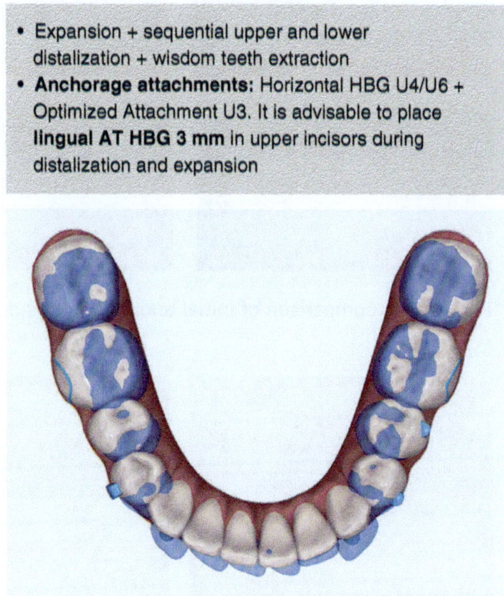

Fig. 19.16 Lower superposition.

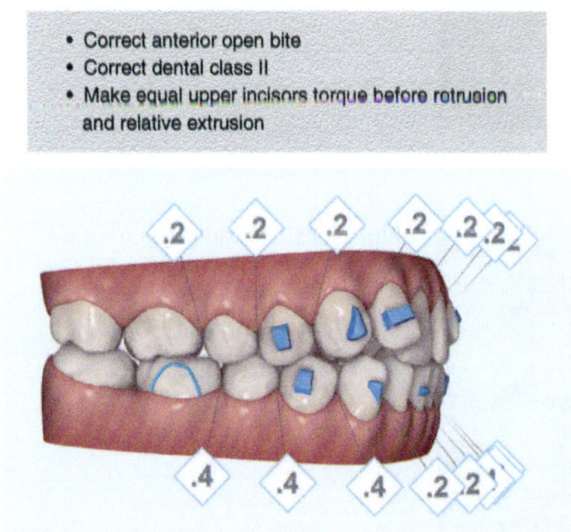

Fig. 19.17 Initial right ClinCheck view, with CAD designer instructions.

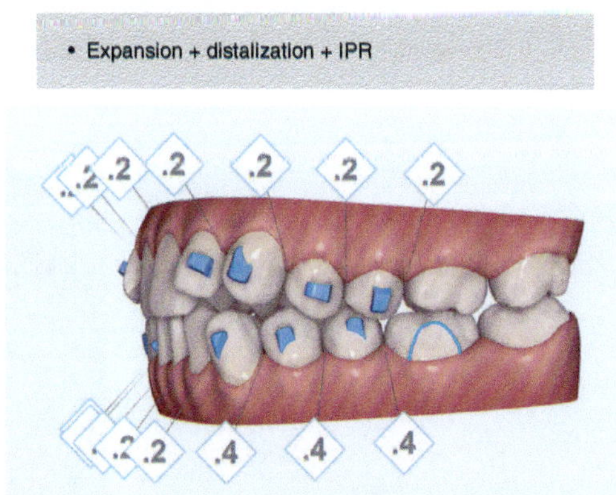

Fig. 19.18 Initial left ClinCheck view, with CAD designer instructions.

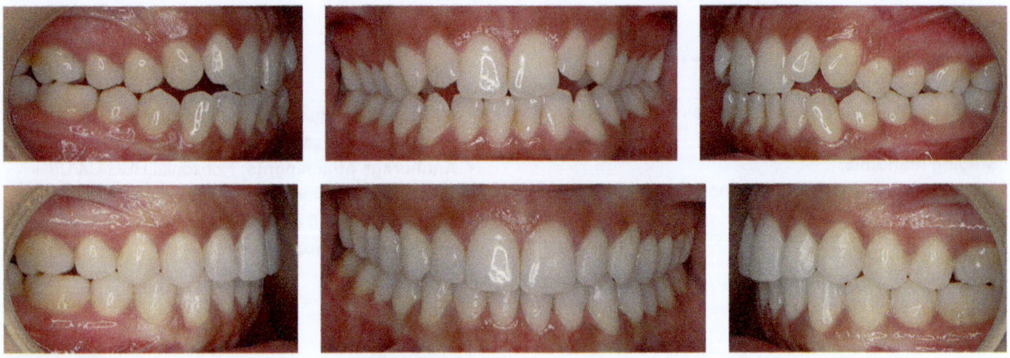

Fig. 19.19 Comparison of initial and final occlusion.

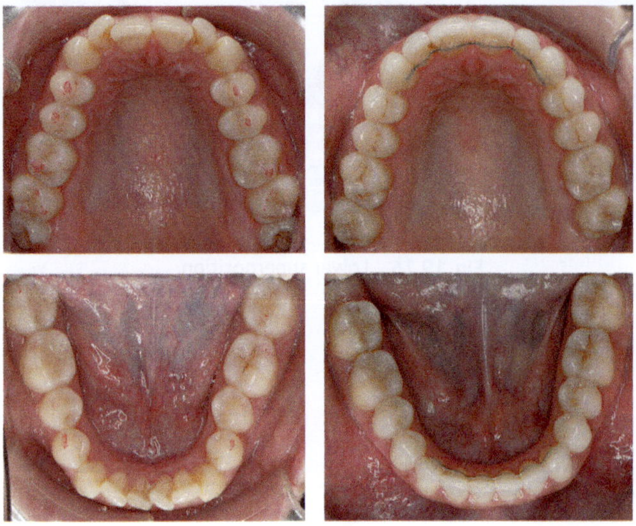

Fig. 19.20 Comparison of initial and final occlusal.

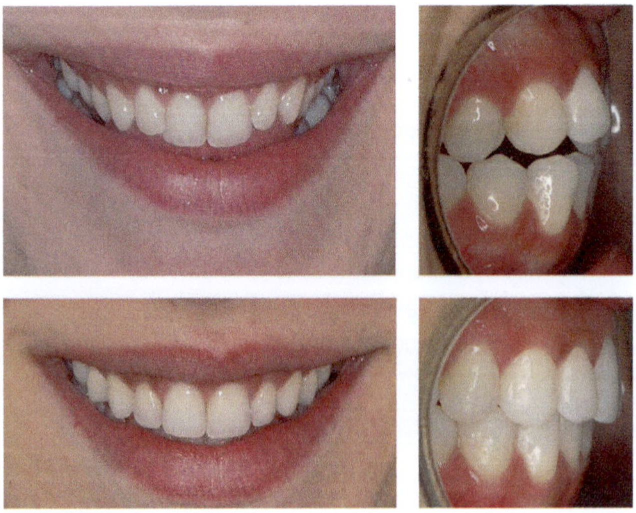

Fig. 19.21 Comparison of initial and final smile overjets.

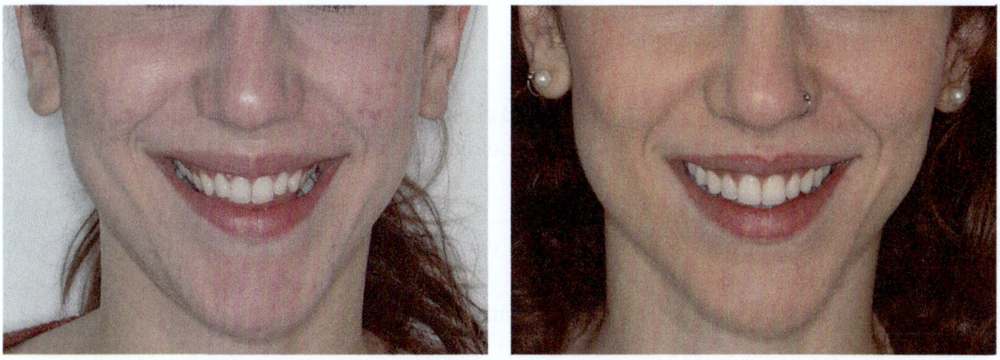

Fig. 19.22 Comparison of initial and final smiles.

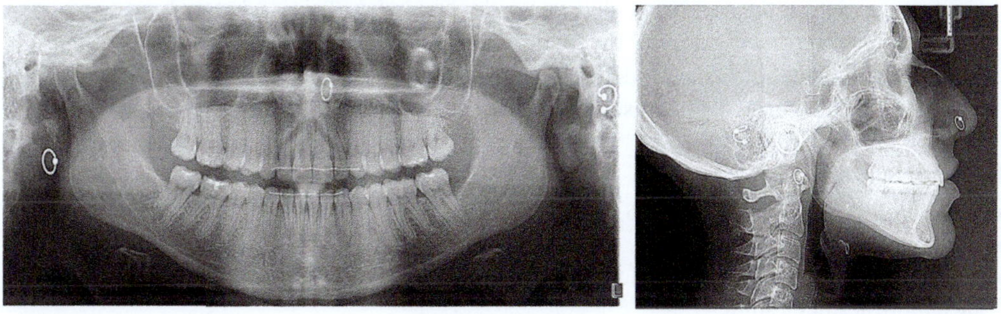

Fig. 19.23 Final panoramic X-ray and teleradiograph.

19.2.2 Symmetric Compression with Edge to Edge Bite

Fig. 19.24 Edge to edge bite with open bite tendency.

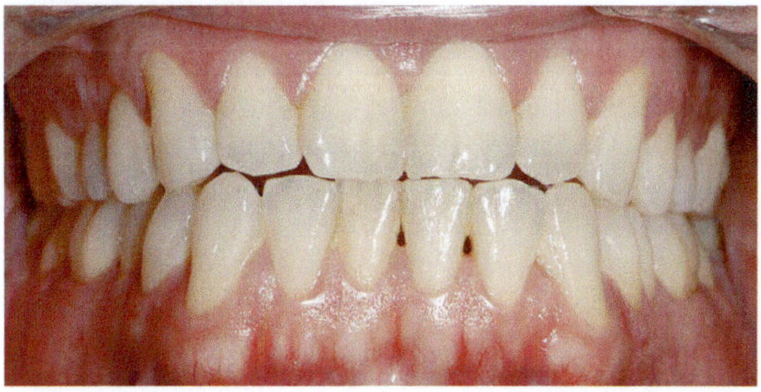

Diagnosis

A 33-year-old man with skeletal class I presented with narrow arches and symmetric compression. He had class I relationship with negative torque of posterior canines, premolars and molars, short display causing 'old' smile and edge-to-edge bite resulting from an upper laterals Bolton discrepancy.

Treatment Plan

- Space opening by upper expansion.
- Anchorage based on wisdom teeth.
- Anterior lower IPR to avoid black triangles and create overjet despite the Bolton discrepancy.
- All four wisdom teeth to be extracted 2 weeks before the start of treatment.

ClinCheck 1: Requirements for the Technician

- In the upper arch: make an incisors extrusion with optimized extrusion attachments on 12-22 after torque correction
- In the lower arch: make a bilateral expansion with anterior lower IPR, adding lingual root torque to 32–42 to create an 'en masse' movement after space closure. IPR to be done after proclination to create good position for incisors to have the IPR done

This, so-called 'round tripping' in the lower arch is usually avoided, but was considered to be more appropriate as the number of aligners would remain low. This is what we have done in the past with brackets and wires, after the first round NiTi aligned every tooth, so we consider it is not to be forbidden but to be avoided whenever possible. This allowed creation of both overjet with retrusion and overbite as a result of relative extrusion.

Treatment Summary

- The total treatment was 17 months
- We planned two sets of aligners
- We obtained a final bilateral class I with adequate overbite and overjet, improving display to create a more aesthetic smile

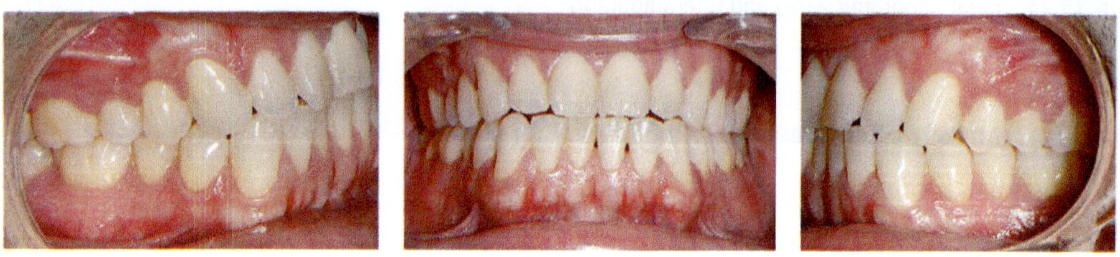

Fig. 19.25 Pretreatment intraoral views (right, front, left, upper, lower).

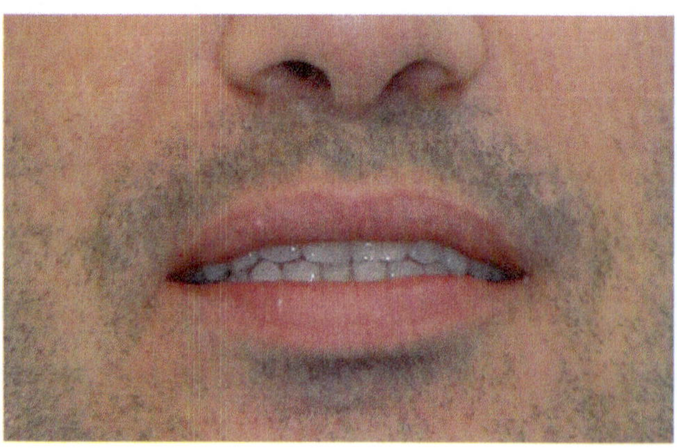

Fig. 19.26 Initial extraoral view: short display.

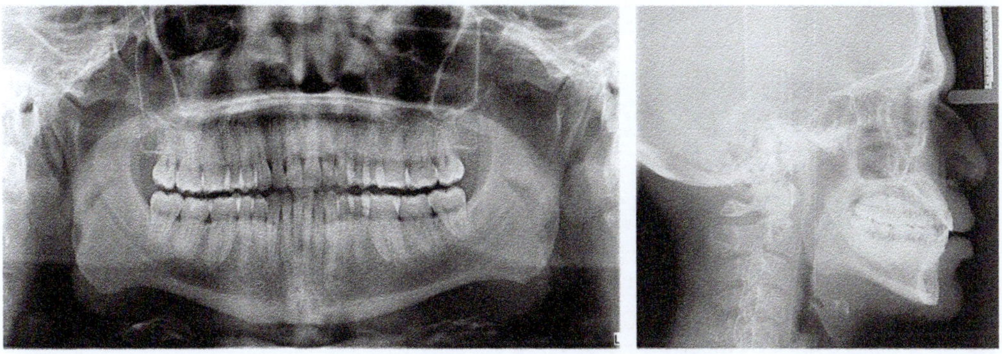

Fig. 19.27 Pretreatment panoramic and lateral X-rays.

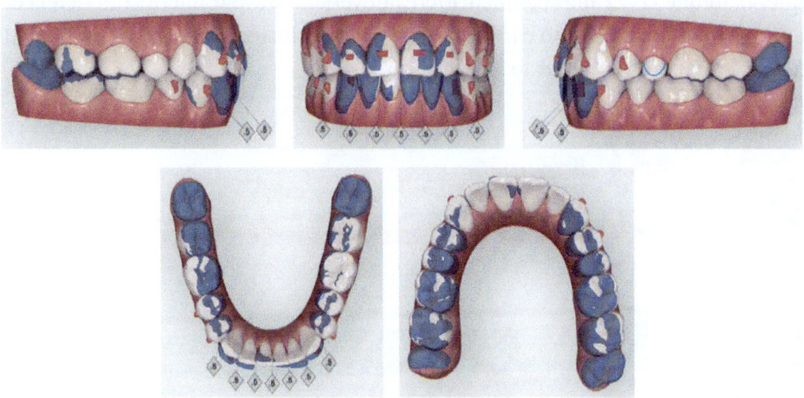

Fig. 19.28 Pretreatment ClinChecks (right, front, left, upper, lower).

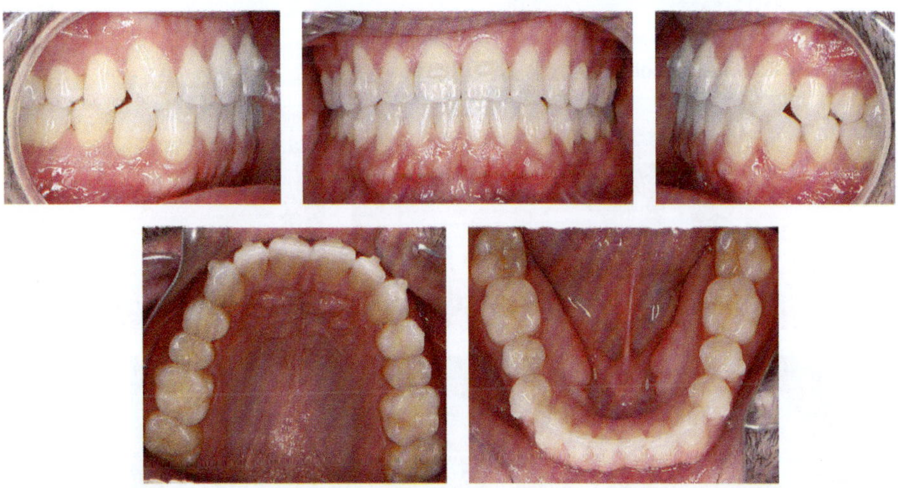

Fig. 19.29 Refinement intraoral views (right, front, left, upper, lower).

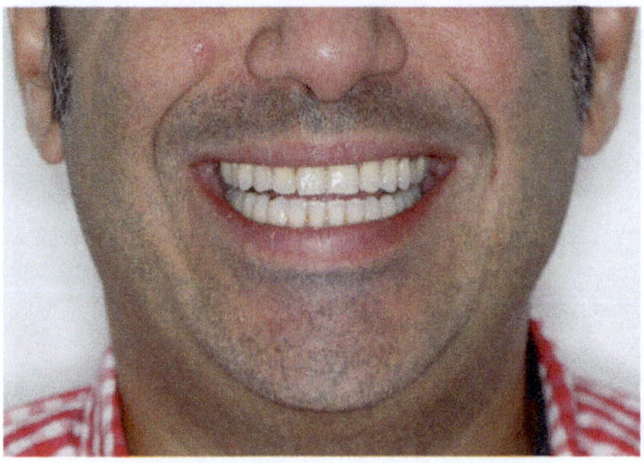

Fig. 19.30 Refinement smile.

ClinCheck 2: Requirements for the Technician

- In the upper arch: anterior torque 12–22 and alignment to create overjet and avoid anterior interferences
- In the lower arch: extra IPR added distal to canines to improve occlusion and slightly expanded posterior sectors to lose arch depth in order to increase overjet

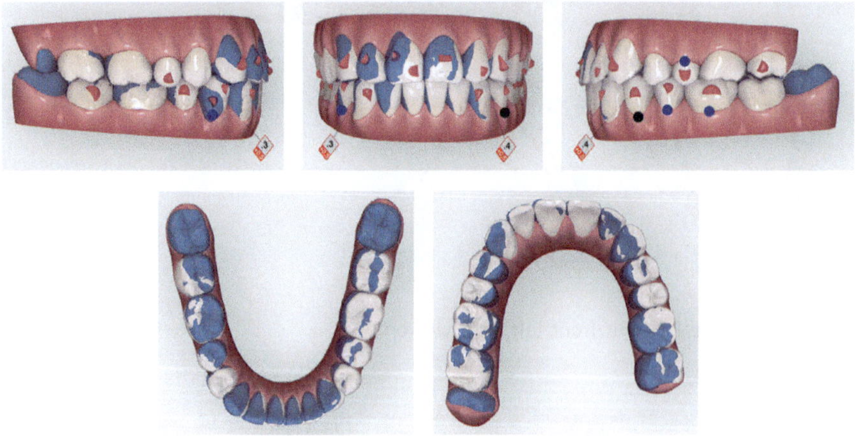

Fig. 19.31 Refinement ClinChecks (right, front, left, upper, lower).

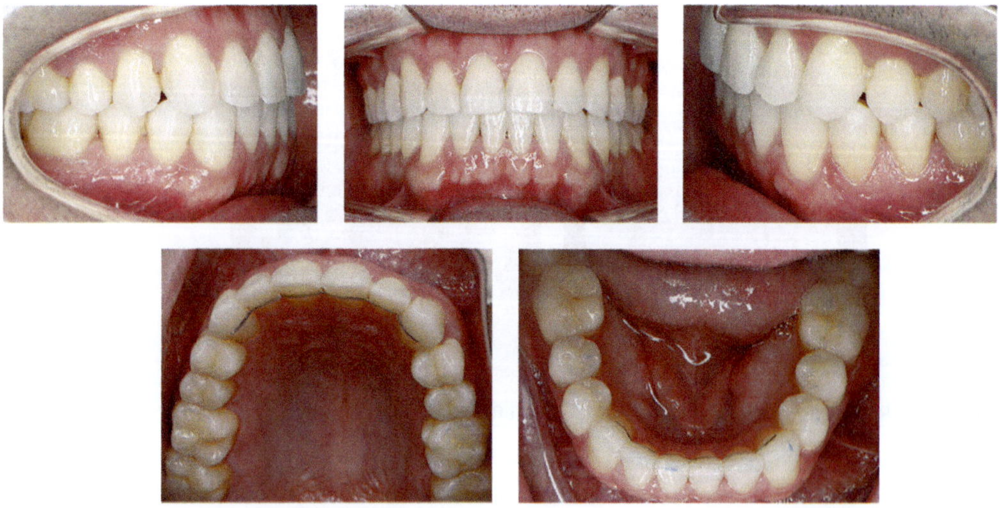

Fig. 19.32 Final intraoral views (right, front, left, upper, lower).

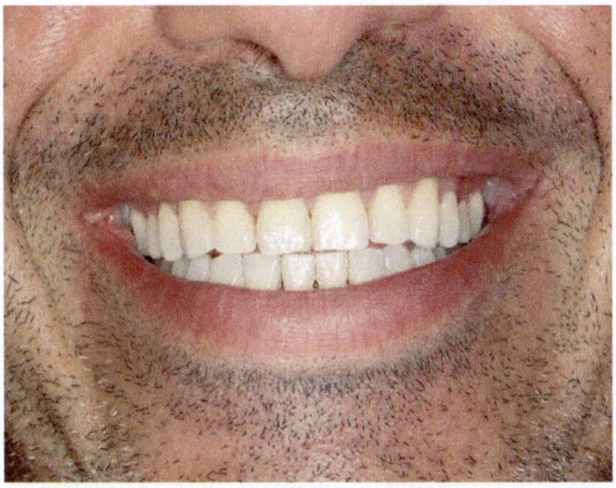

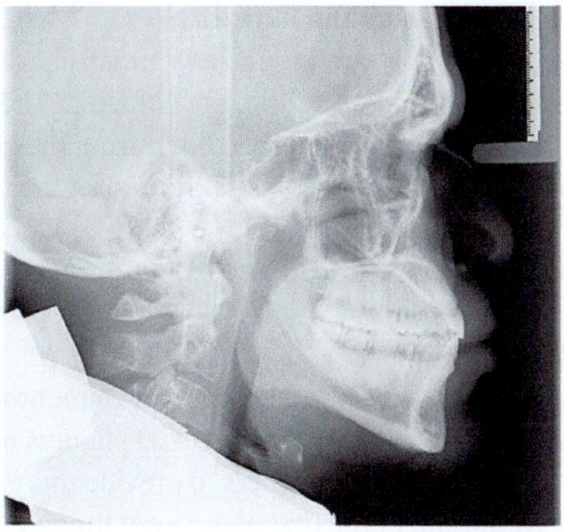

Fig. 19.33 Final smile picture and lateral X-ray.

19.2.3 Symmetric Compression Combined with Skeletal Class III

Fig. 19.34 Symmetric compression.

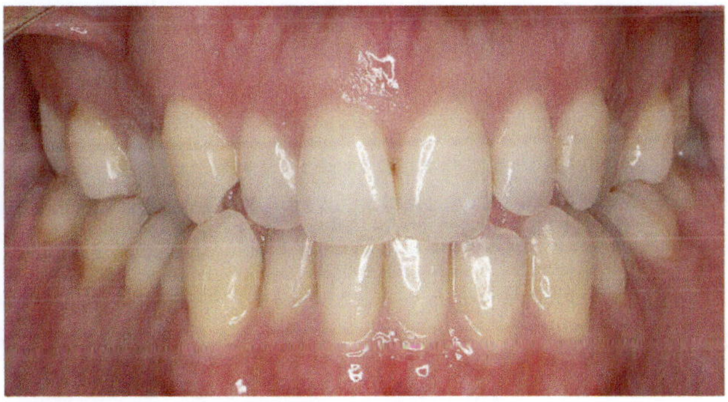

Diagnosis

A 42-year-old patient with hyperdivergent skeletal class III presented with symmetric compression. He had a posterior gummy smile caused by posterior negative torque, upper midline cantered, mild lower crowding with prominent nasolabial folds, a prognathic profile and an opened nasolabial angle.

Treatment Plan

- Plan consisted of upper symmetric expansion, but as there was not enough overjet and the patient presented with lower crowding, we needed to distalize the lower arch in order to provide positive overjet before the upper expansion
- The patient did not want extraction of the lower third molar on the left side so IPR was planned in that quadrant and the space used to distalize lower teeth

Requirements for the Technician

- In the upper arch make a symmetric expansion and do not move the second and third upper molars to have posterior anchorage. AT horizontal bevelled to gingival used to provide labial root torque to the lateral segment during the expansion
- In the lower arch, make IPR to solve the crowding and to apply lingual root torque to the lower incisors
- Class III elastic to be used after uprighting the lower incisors

Treatment Summary

- The total time of treatment was 26 months
- The patient used a first set of 33 aligners in a 2-week change interval protocol, and needed a new set of additional aligners to provide more overjet
- At the end of the first phase even though we asked for retraction of the lower incisors the overjet was not enough and the patient presented with premature anterior contacts and a posterior open bite
- To settle the occlusion in the additional aligners, we had to request further labial crown torque to the upper incisors and more IPR and retrusion of the lower incisors
- At the end of the treatment, the patient achieved a bilateral class I relationship with normal overbite and overjet and a smile improved considerably as a result of the arch expansions

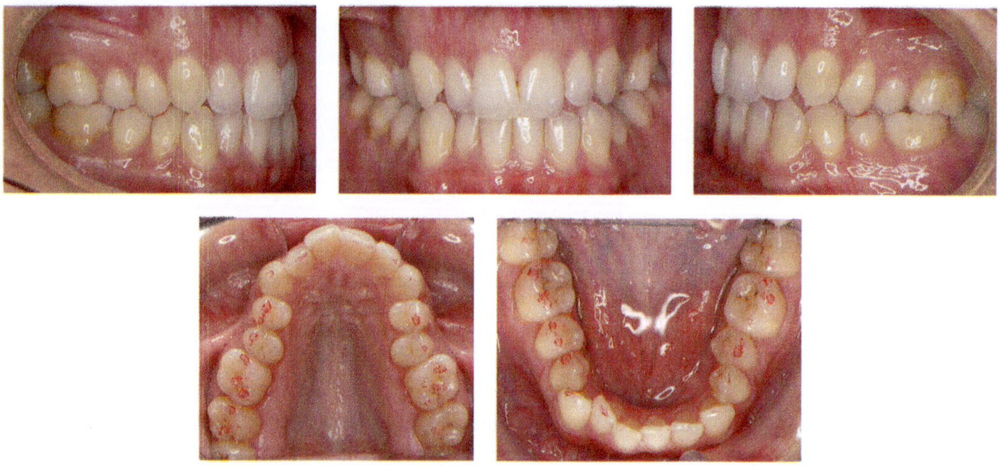

Fig. 19.35 Pretreatment intraoral views (right, front, left, upper, lower).

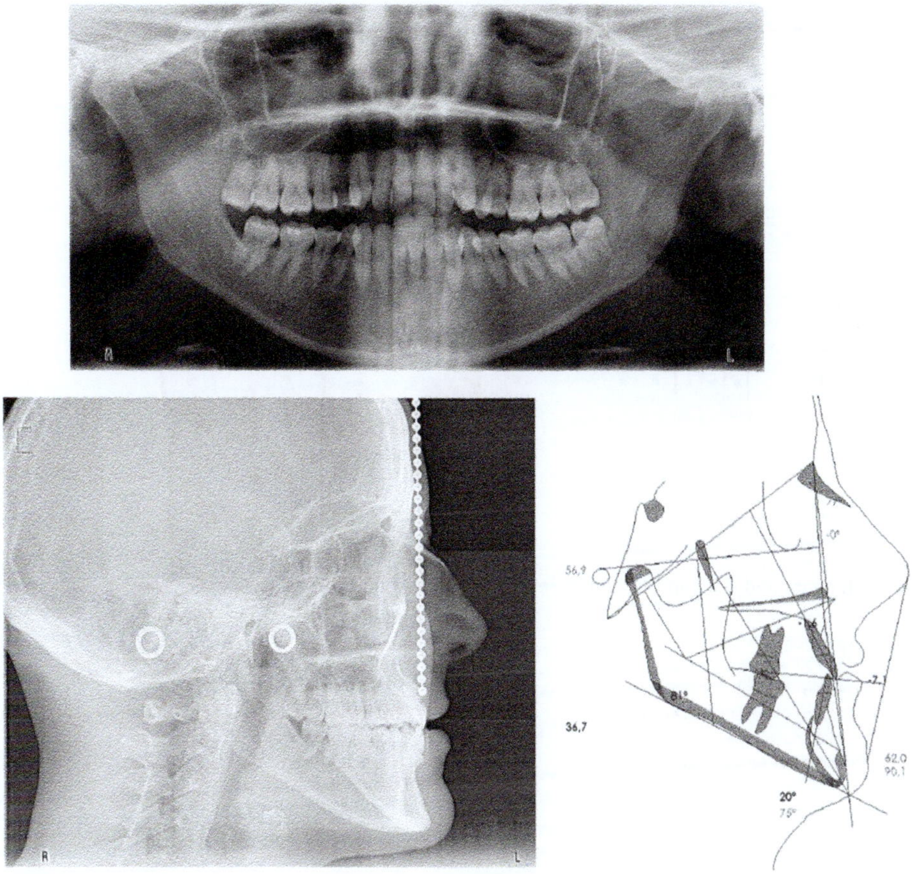

Fig. 19.36 Pretreatment panoramic X-ray, teleradiograph and cephalometry.

Symmetric upper expansion:
- Do not move 17/ 18 / 27 and 28
- AT HBG 4 mm U4 / U6

- IPR and sequential lower distalization using the space of the IPR (she did not want 38 extracted)
- Class III elastics

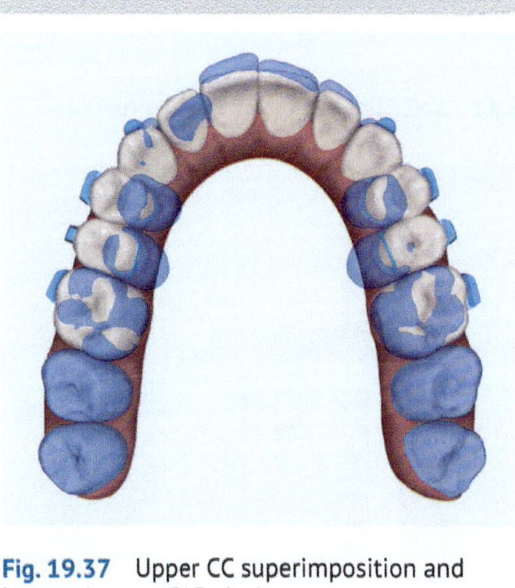

Fig. 19.37 Upper CC superimposition and instructions to CAD designer.

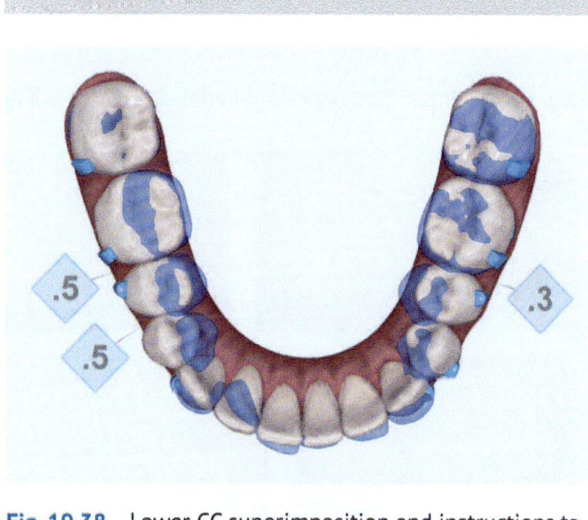

Fig. 19.38 Lower CC superimposition and instructions to CAD designer.

Correct class III and anterior edge to edge occlusion

• Expansion + IPR + class III elastics

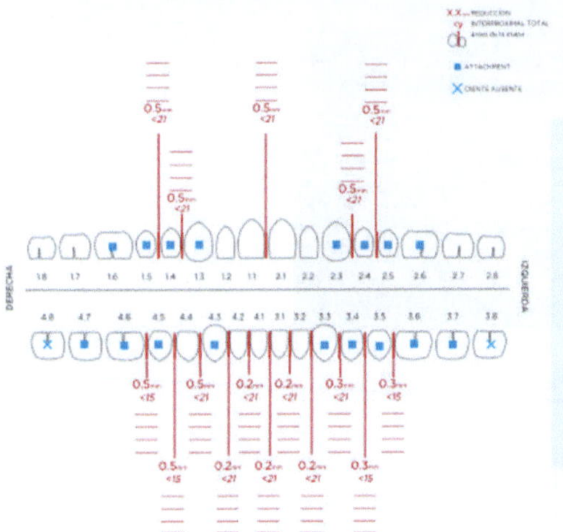

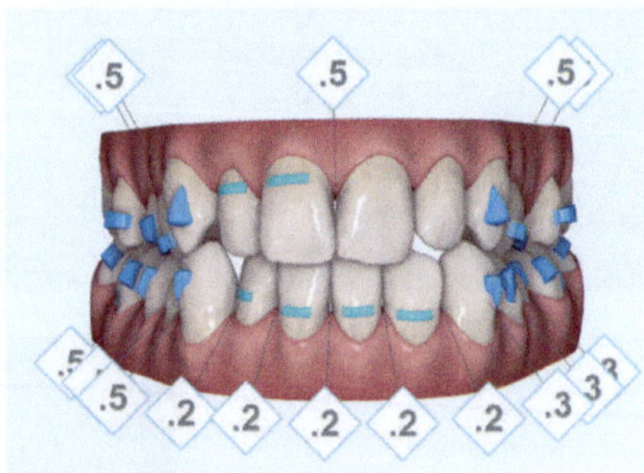

Fig. 19.39 Attachments and IPR can be seen in several areas of the ClinCheck software.

Symmetric upper expansion:

- Do not move 17/ 18 / 27 and 28
- AT HBG 4 mm U4 / U6

Take care with the reduction of upper arch length during expansion. Provide lingual root torque upper incisors and IPR + retrusion of lower incisors to create positive overjet.

- IPR and sequential lower distalization using the space of the IPR
- Class III elastic

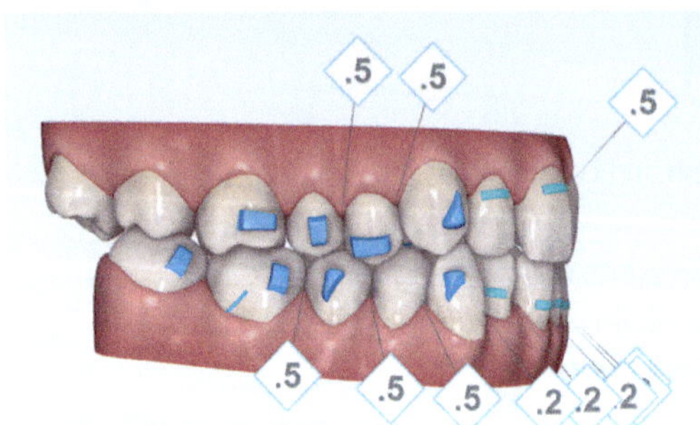

Fig. 19.40 Right ClinCheck view, initial situation.

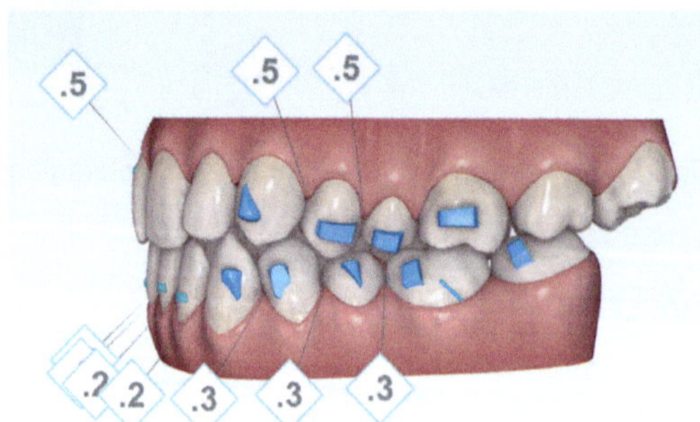

Fig. 19.41 Left ClinCheck view, initial situation.

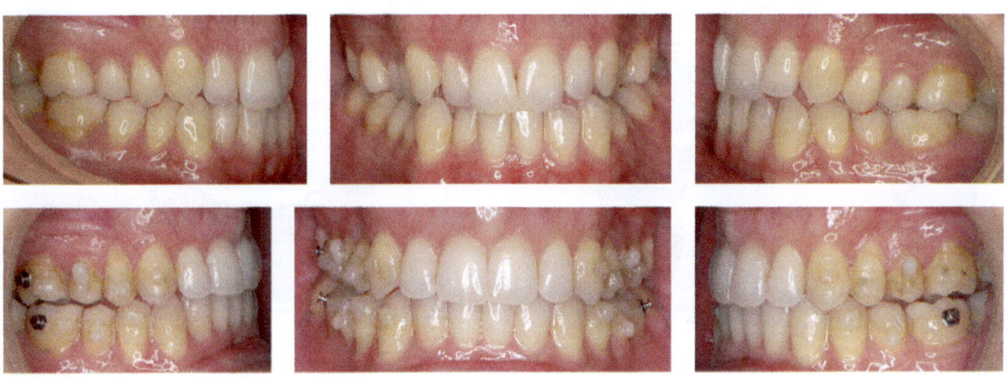

Fig. 19.42 Views before starting refinement.

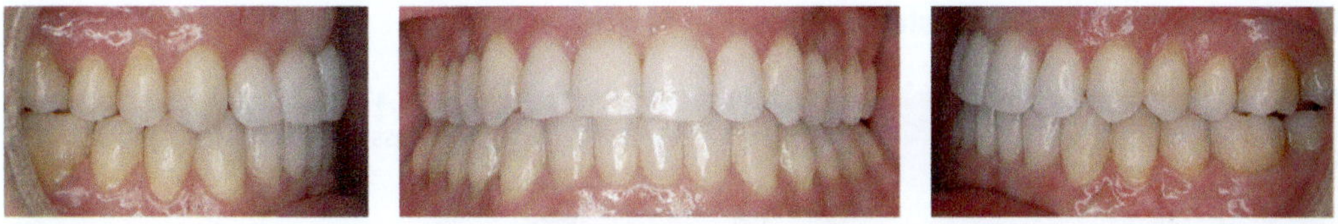

Fig. 19.43 Final views.

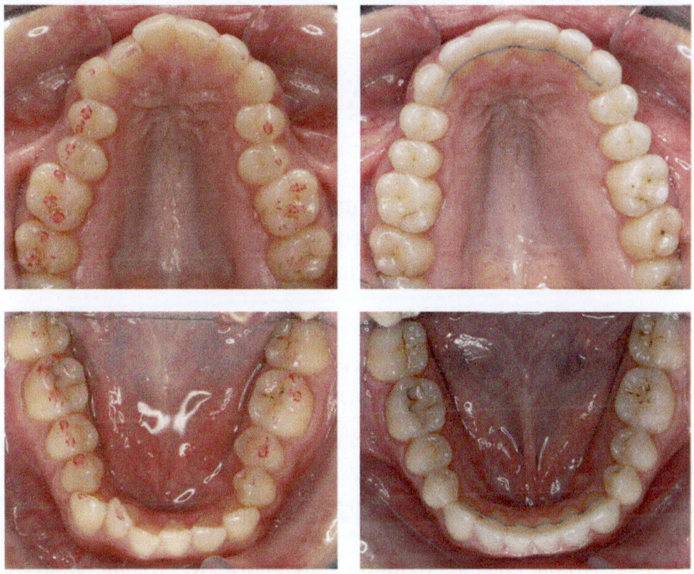

Fig. 19.44 Comparison of initial and final occlusal (upper and lower).

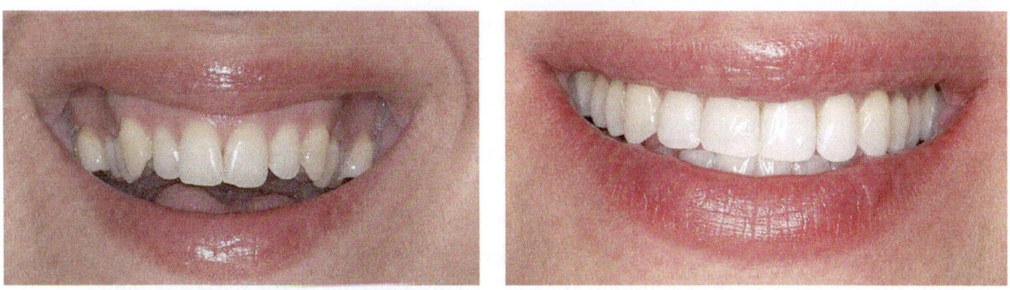

Fig. 19.45 Final expansion reducing buccal corridors.

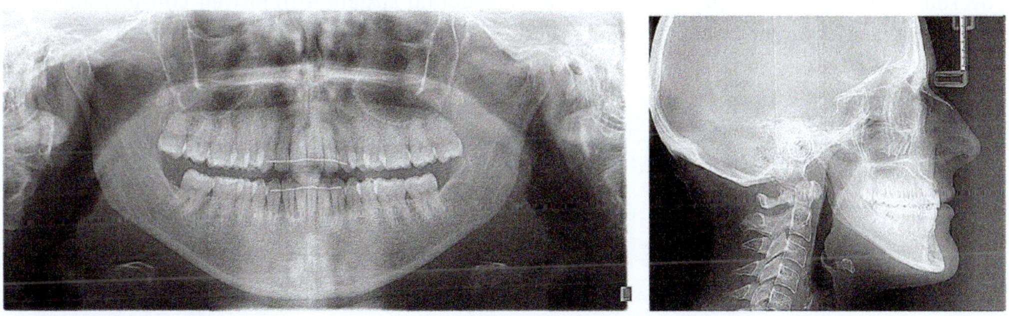

Fig. 19.46 Final Panoramic X-ray and teleradiography.

19.2.4 Symmetric Compression with Loss of Attachment

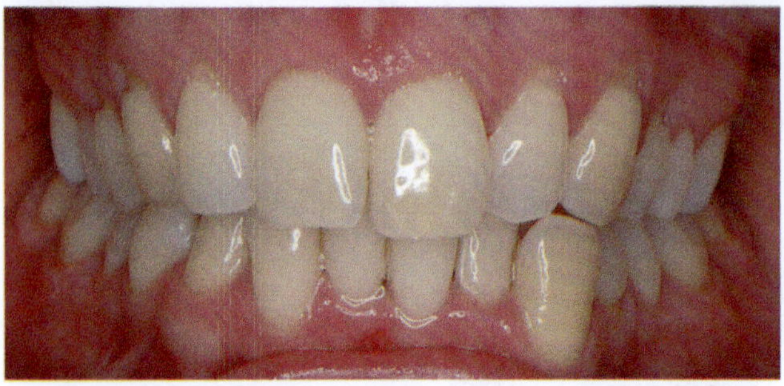

Fig. 19.47 Symmetric compression with loss of attachment.

Diagnosis

A 33-year-old patient with a normodivergent skeletal class I presented with symmetric compression and loss of attachment caused by negative torque in lateral zone. He had left-side deviation of lower midline, mild lower crowding, labial competence and opened nasolabial angle.

Treatment Plan

- Upper symmetric expansion at the same time as sequential upper distalization
- The expansion has to be performed by labial crown torque, with no movement of the roots

Requirements for the Technician

- In the upper arch make a symmetric expansion at the same time that the upper teeth move distal every four aligners
- AT horizontal bevelled to gingival to be used to provide labial root torque to the lateral segment during the expansion
- In the lower arch, make IPR to solve the crowding and to apply lingual root torque to the lower incisors

Treatment Summary

- The total time of treatment was 18 months
- The patient used a first set of 40 aligners in a 7-day change interval protocol and needed a new set of additional aligners to settle the occlusion
- At the end of the first phase, even though we asked for IPR and retraction of the lower incisors, the overjet was not enough and the patient presented premature anterior contacts
- To settle the occlusion in the additional aligners, we used elastics in the posterior zone
- At the end of the treatment, the patient achieved a bilateral class I relationship with normal overbite and overjet and the smile and the periodontal situation improved considerably as a result of the arch expansions

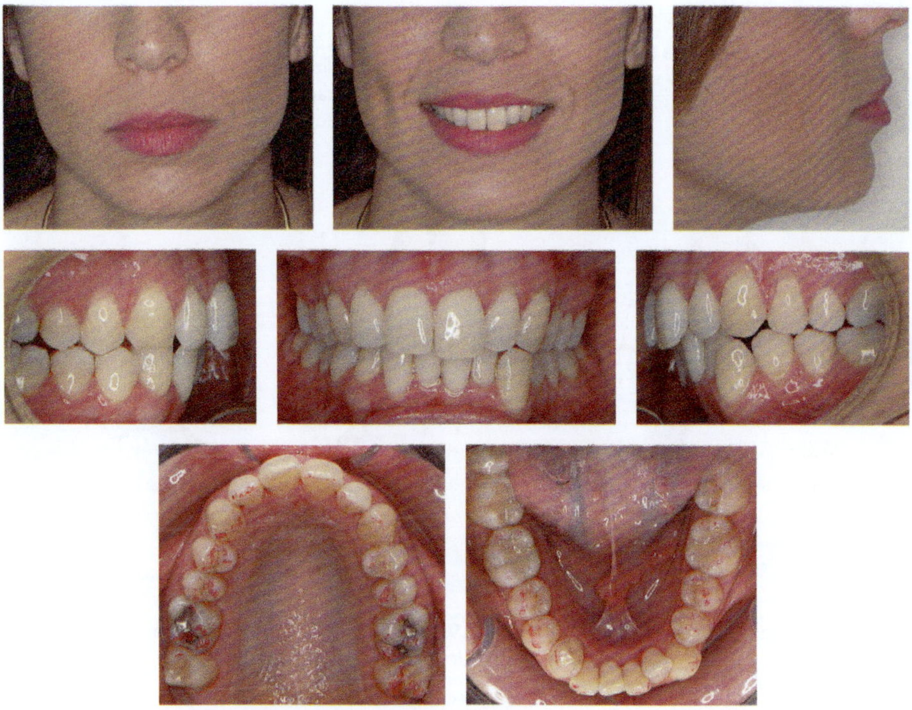

Fig. 19.48 Pretreatment extraoral and intraoral views.

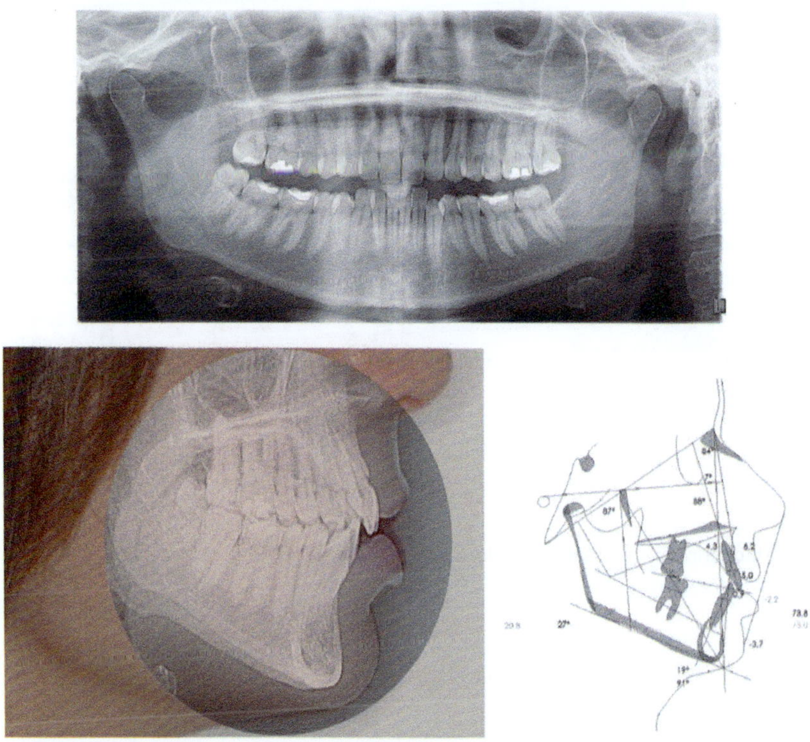

Fig. 19.49 Pretreatment panoramic X-ray, teleradiograph and cephalometry.

Maxilla:

- Symmetric expansion by changing torque (labial crown torque to premolars and canines)+ sequential distalization

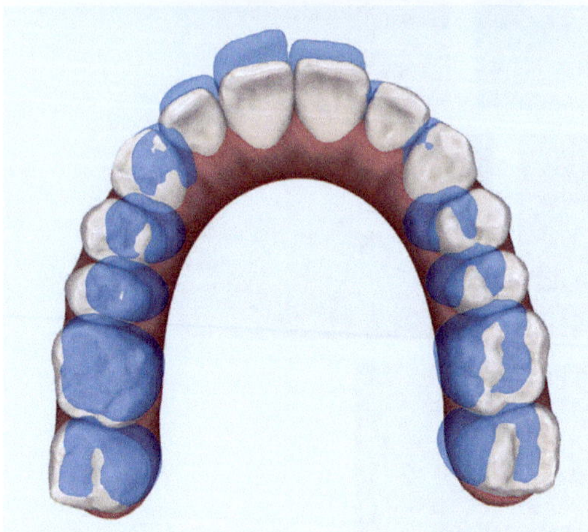

Fig. 19.50 Upper CC superimposition and instructions to CAD designer.

- Expansion + distalization + IPR
- Lower incisors retraction simultaneous with centring the lower midline to the right

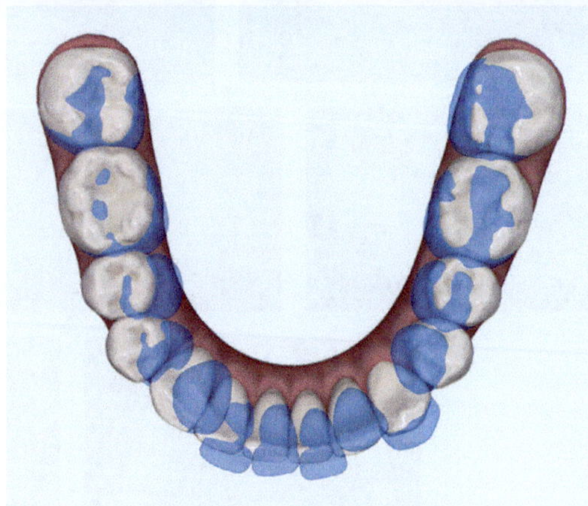

Fig. 19.51 Lower CC superimposition and instructions to CAD designer.

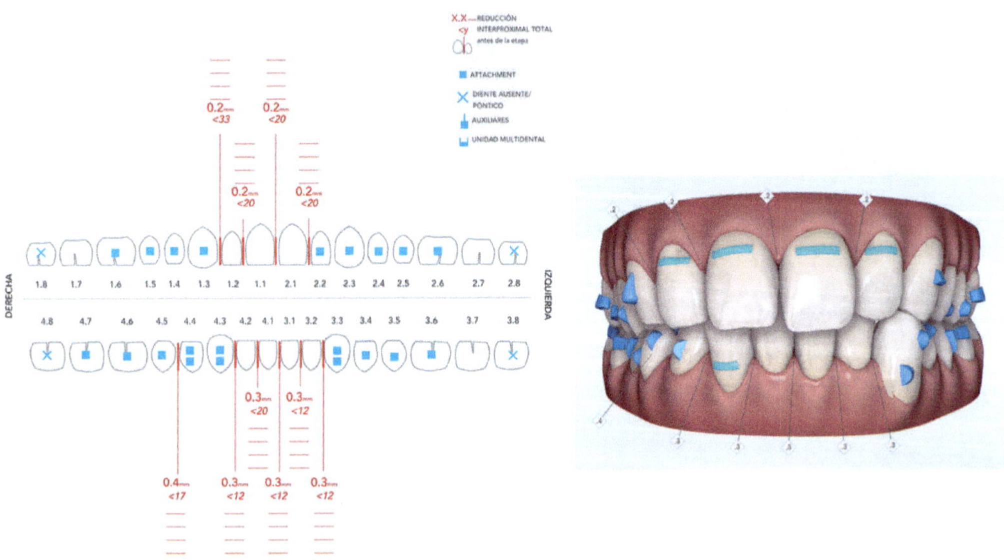

Fig. 19.52 Interproximal reduction is necessary to upright lower incisors.

Upper and lower sequential distalization
Upper symmetric expansion by changing torque of premolars and canines **IPR**

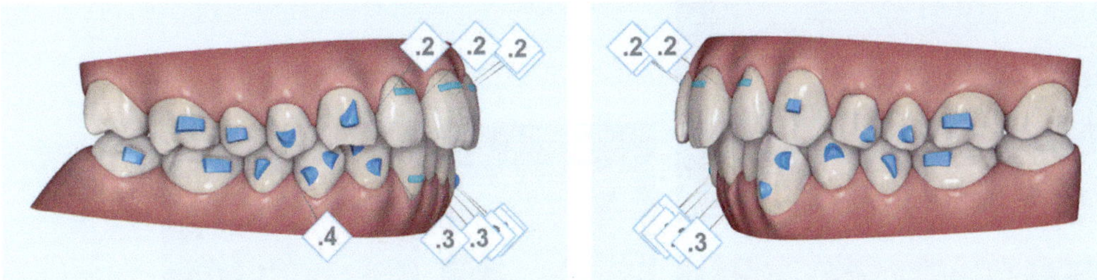

Fig. 19.53 Right and left ClinCheck view, initial situation.

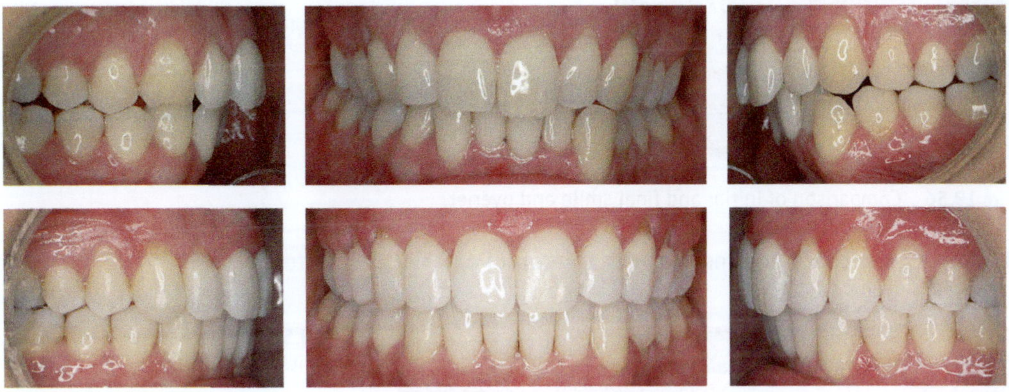

Fig. 19.54 Comparison of pretreatment (upper) and final (lower) views.

Fig. 19.55 Comparison of initial and final occlusal.

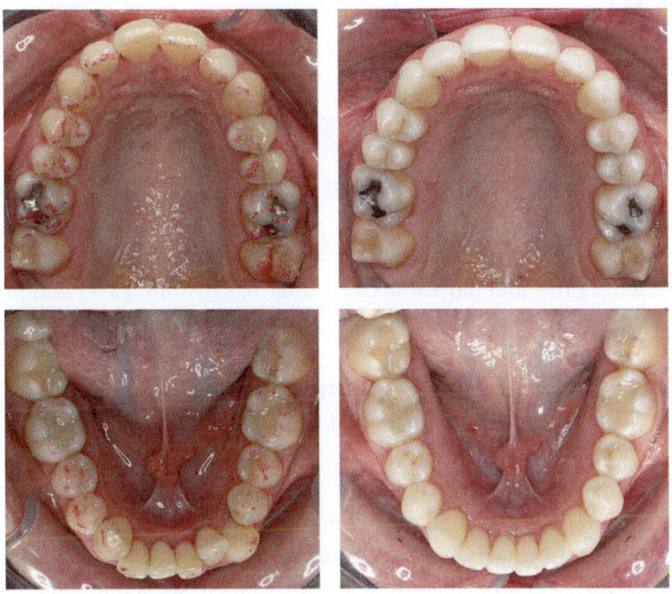

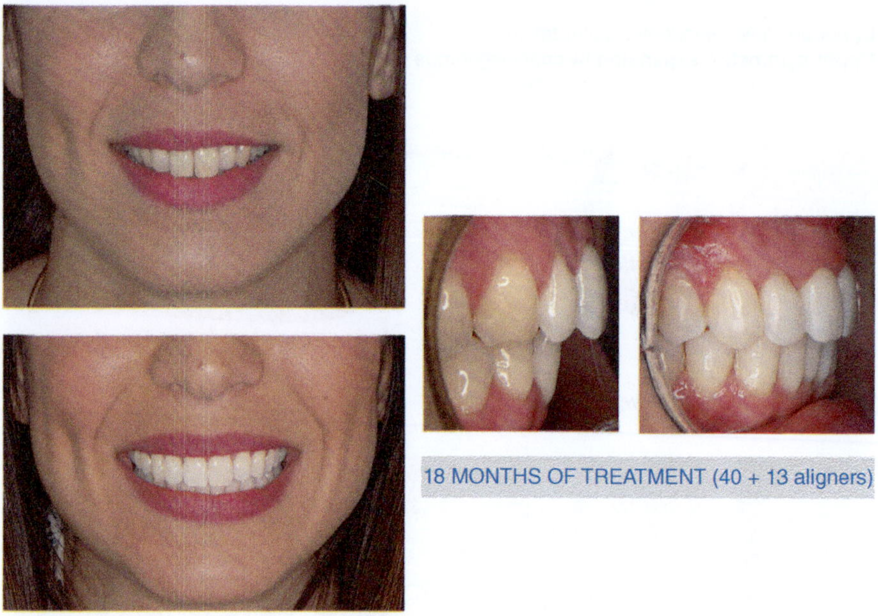

Fig. 19.56 Comparison of initial and final smile and overjet.

19.2.5 Symmetric Compression with Bilateral Posterior Crossbite

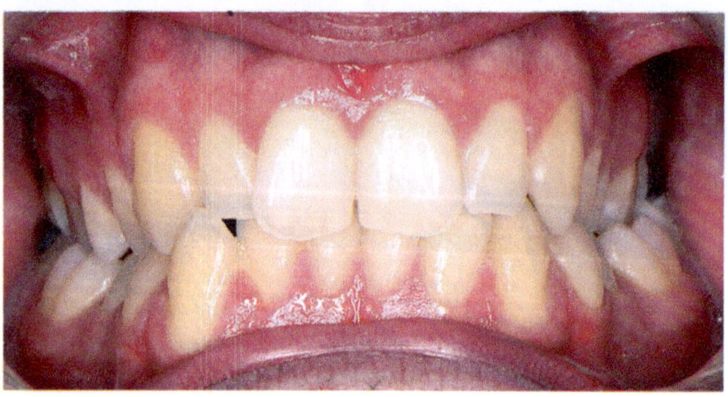

Fig. 19.57 Posterior bilateral crossbite.

Diagnosis

A 28-year-old patient presented with a symmetrical compression on both sides with posterior gummy smile and narrow arches, anterior crossbite 13-43 and mild lower crowding.

Treatment Plan

- Plan consisted of upper symmetric expansion at the same time as lower compression
- The expansion to be performed by labial crown torque, with no movement of the roots

Requirements for the Technician

- In the upper arch make a symmetric expansion
- Horizontal attachments on molars to provide anchorage during expansion
- In the lower arch, align first lower molars to second molars

Treatment Summary

- The total time of treatment was 12 months
- The patient used three sets of 14 aligners in a 7-day change interval protocol, under a Lite portfolio
- Patient used criss-cross elastics from day 1 to solve posterior crossbite. No anterior elastics were needed

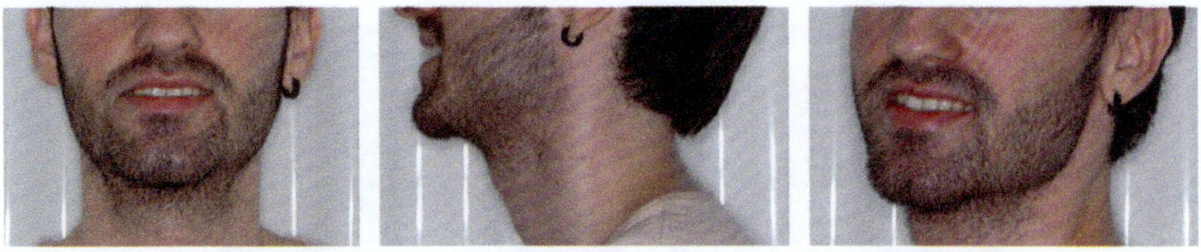

Fig. 19.58 Initial extraoral views.

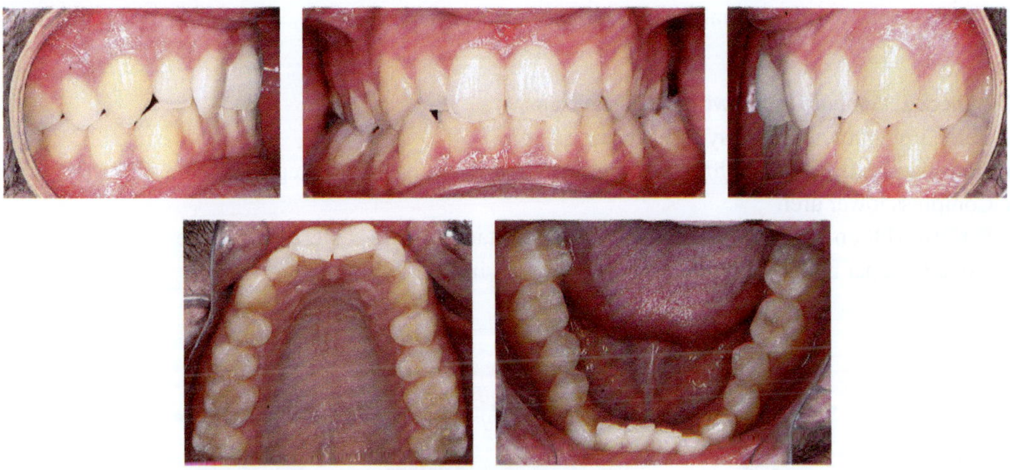

Fig. 19.59 Initial intraoral views (right, front, left, upper, lower).

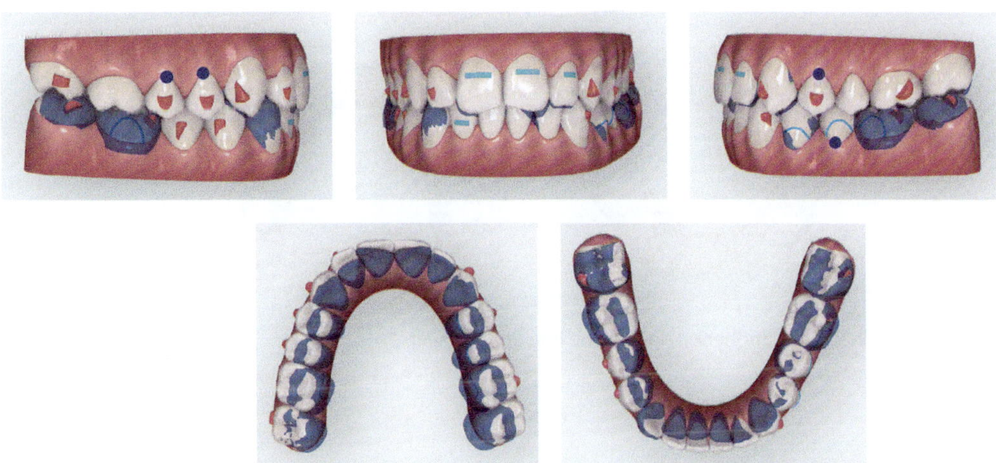

Fig. 19.60 Pretreatment ClinChecks: right, front, left, upper, lower.

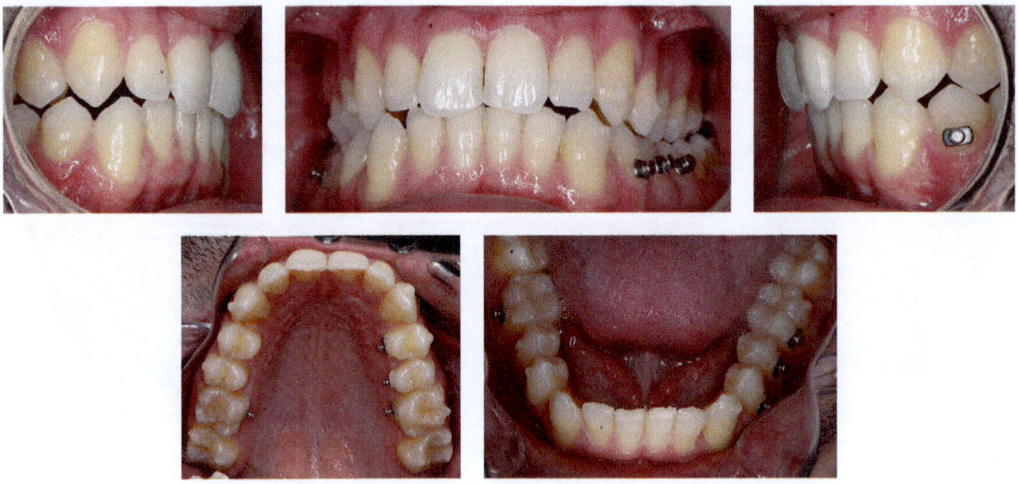

Fig. 19.61 Refinement: intraoral views (right, front, left, upper, lower).

ClinCheck 2: Communication with the Technician

- In the upper arch make a symmetric expansion
- Optimized extrusion attachments on molars to prevent flaring during expansion
- Compress lower arch
- Perform IPR on lower arch to avoid anterior contact causing posterior crossbite
- Extrude upper molars palatal cusps with a final virtual jump

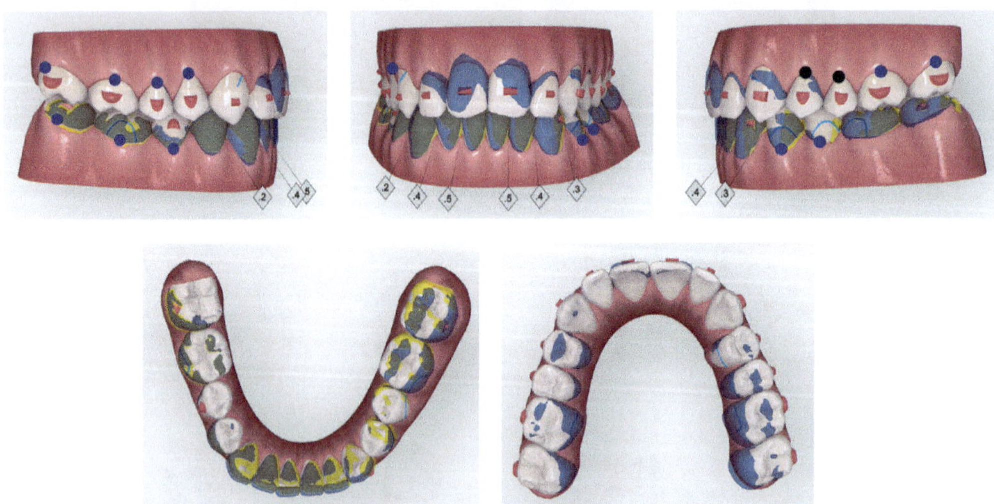

Fig. 19.62 Refinement ClinChecks: right, front, left, upper, lower.

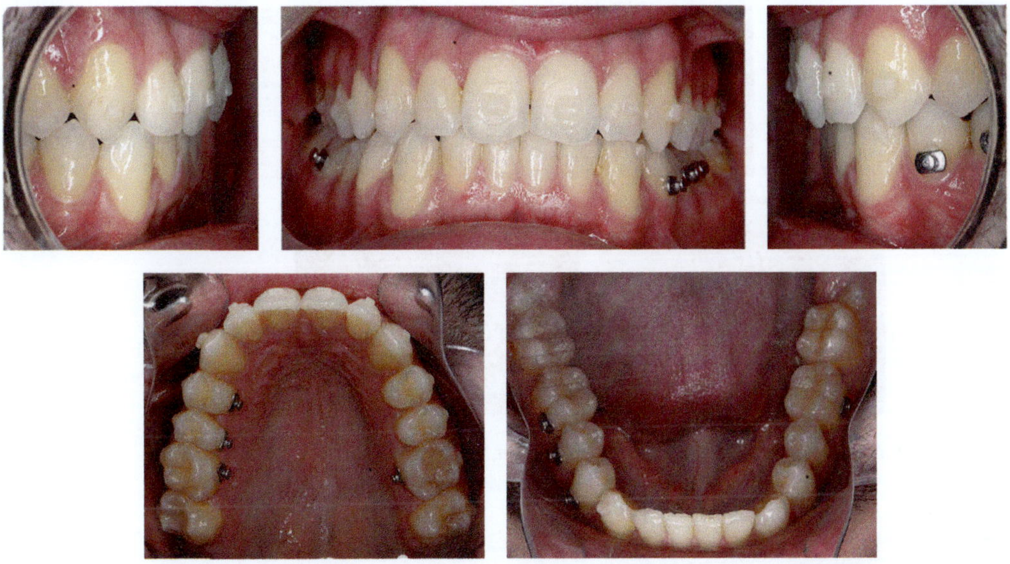

Fig. 19.63 Refinement 2: intraoral views (right, front, left, upper, lower).

ClinCheck 3: Communication with the Technician

- Extrude buccal cusps of molars
- Precision cuts for vertical elastics
- Anterior torque correction with power ridges

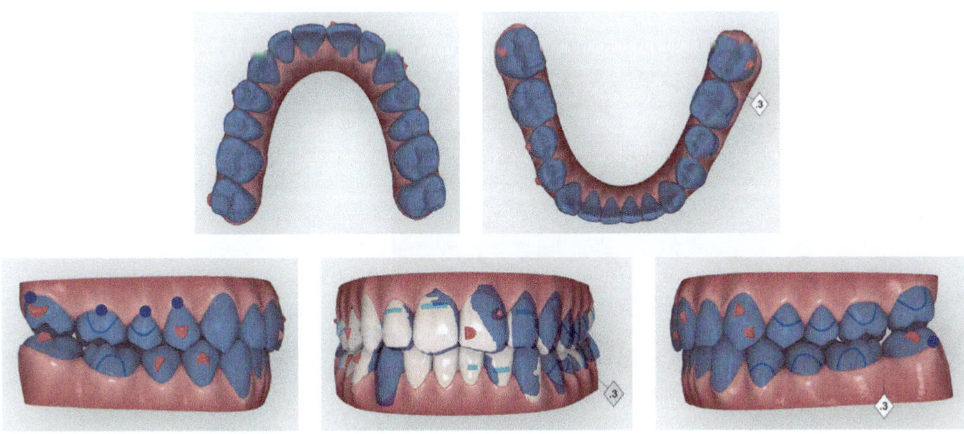

Fig. 19.64 Refinement 2 ClinChecks: right, front, left, upper, lower.

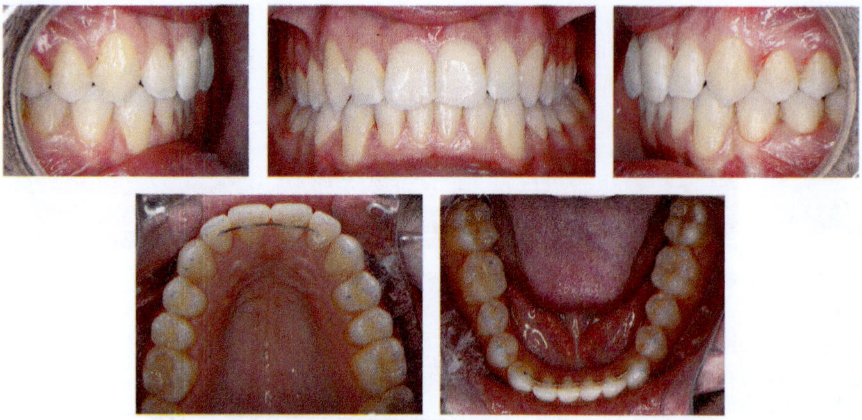

Fig. 19.65 Final intraoral views (right, front, left, upper, lower).

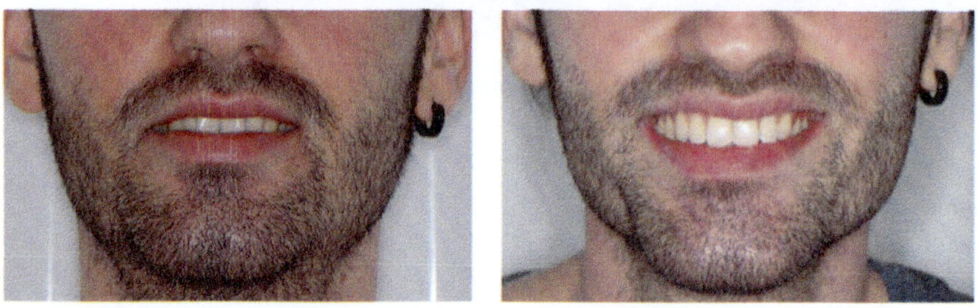

Fig. 19.66 Pretreatment and final smile.

19.2.6 Symmetric Compression with Class II and Gummy Smile

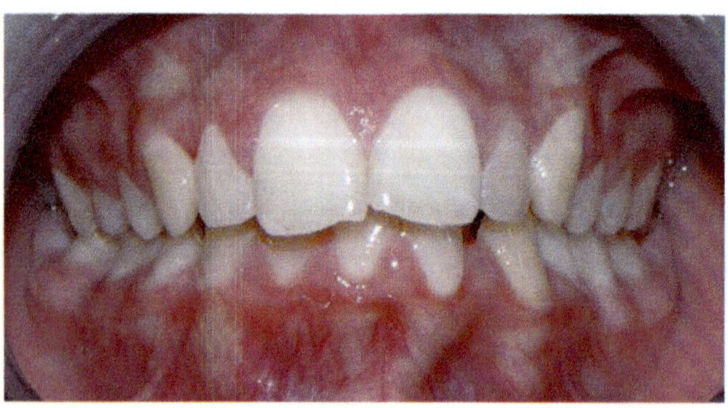

Fig. 19.67 Posterior bilateral compression.

Diagnosis

A 13-year-old patient presented with a symmetric compression on both sides with gummy smile and narrow arches, protrusion, deep bite, moderate lower crowding and lip incompetence.

Treatment Plan

- Upper symmetric expansion on both lower and upper arch
- Initial plan to solve class II was sequential distalization and expansion to lose arch depth without elastics, but no results were obtained so we had to change to elastics
- The expansion needed to be performed by labial crown torque with no movement of the roots
- Lower arch needed intrusion with attachments bevelled to gingival on posterior sectors

ClinCheck 1: Requirements for the Technician

- In the upper arch make a symmetric expansion to lose arch depth and solve class II
- Extrusion attachments on premolars to provide anchorage during anterior intrusion
- Sequential distalization

Treatment Summary

- The total time of treatment was 20 months
- The patient used three sets of aligners in a 7-day change interval protocol
- Patient used upper canine to lower molar elastics to help resolve class II
- Second and third refinement increased posterior expansion

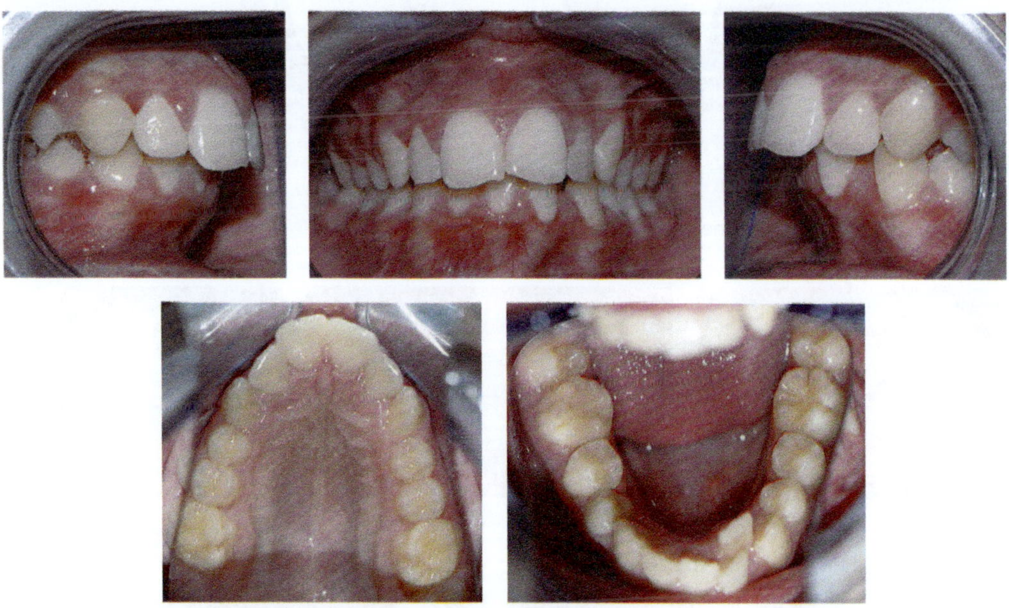

Fig. 19.68 Initial intraoral views (right, front, left, upper, lower).

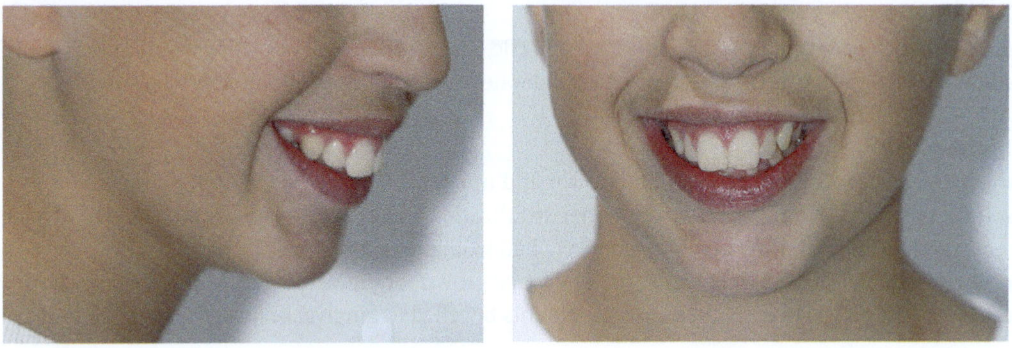

Fig. 19.69 Initial extraoral views: profile, front smile.

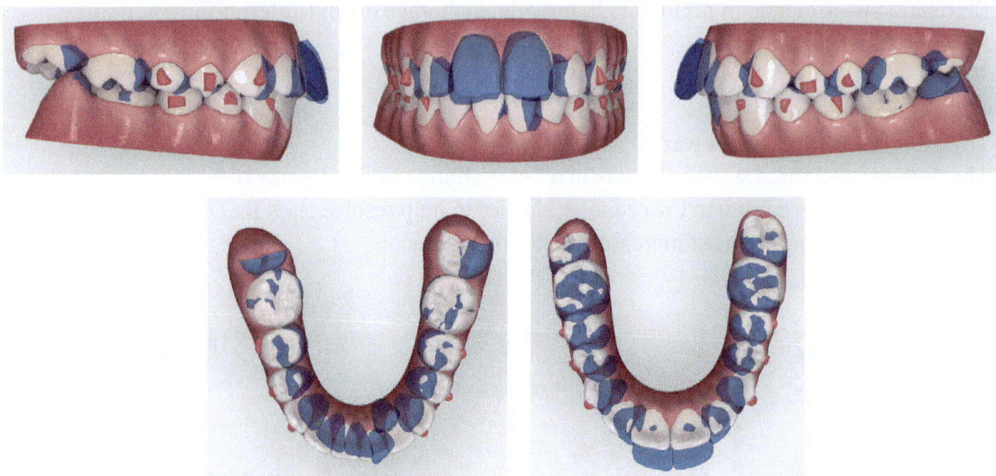

Fig. 19.70 Pretreatment ClinChecks: right, front, left, upper, lower.

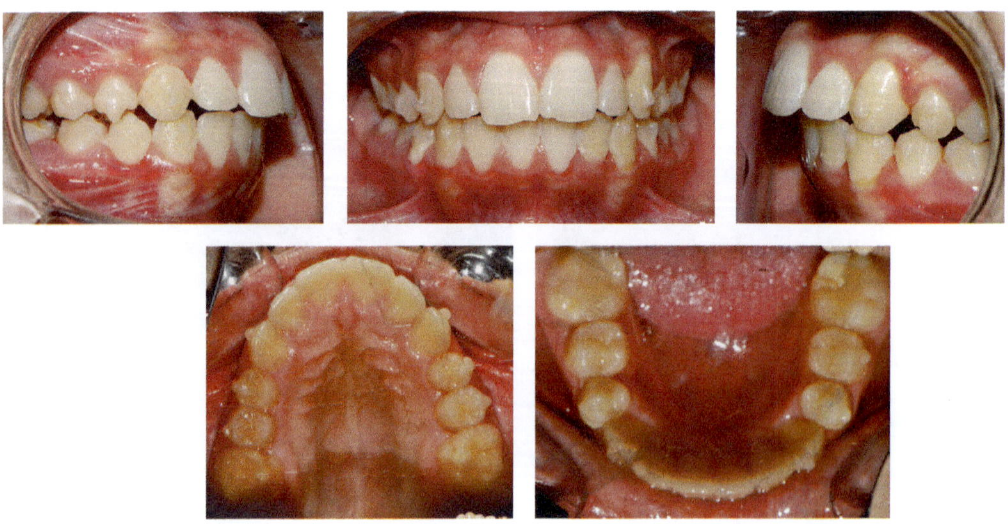

Fig. 19.71 Refinement: intraoral views (right, front, left, upper, lower).

ClinCheck 2: Requirements for the Technician

As alignment was achieved in both upper and anterior intrusion in the first ClinCheck, goals for the second were saggital and so the following goals were established for the technician:

- In the upper arch make a symmetric expansion to lose arch depth and solve class II
- Plan upper hooks to reduce overjet and lower button cutouts for class II elastics 24/7

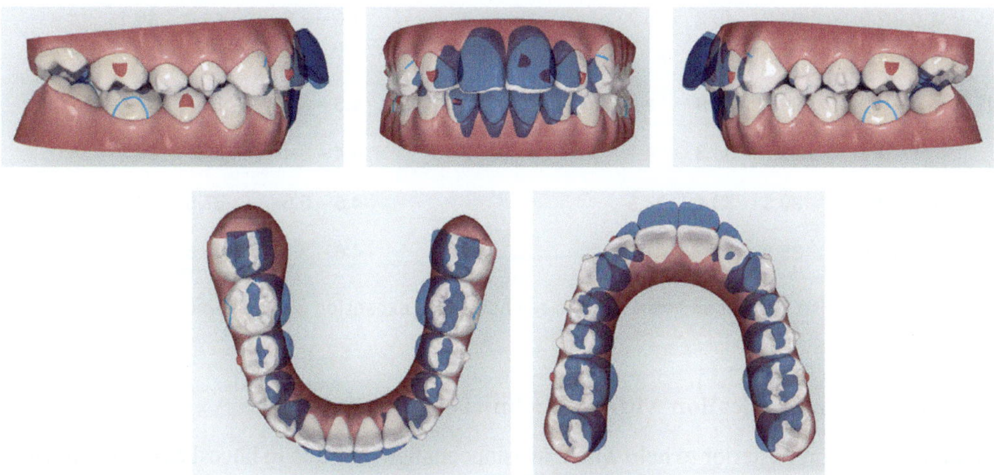

Fig. 19.72 Refinement ClinChecks: right, front, left, upper, lower.

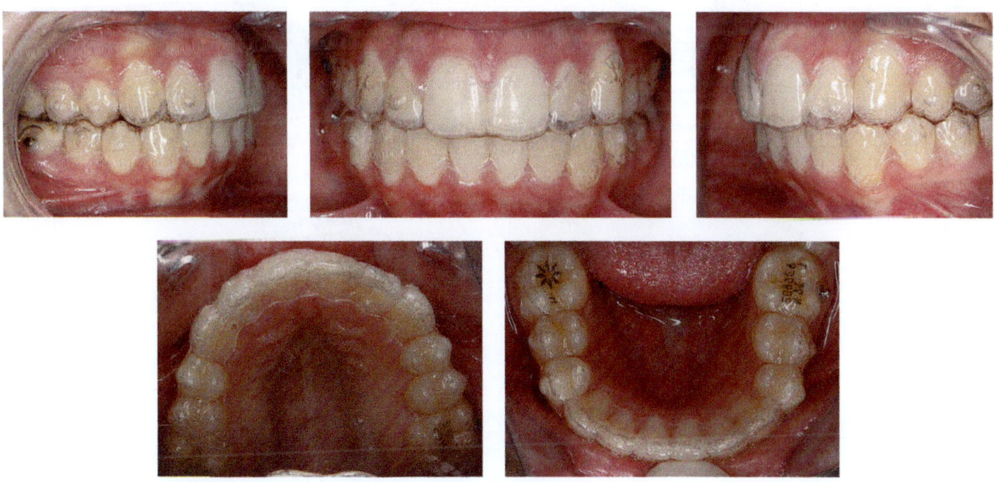

Fig. 19.73 Refinement 2: intraoral views (right, front, left, upper, lower).

CLINCHECK 1

Arch width (mm) -

	Teeth—	Initial	Final	Stage 0
SUP	1.3 – 2.3	30.3	35.5	30.3
	1.4 – 2.4	30.7	35.0	30.7
	1.5 – 2.5	35.4	37.8	35.4
	1.6 – 2.6	39.2	40.2	39.2
INF	4.3 – 3.3	22.2	27.9	22.2
	4.4 – 3.4	25.7	30.8	25.7
	4.5 – 3.5	30.5	33.4	30.5
	4.6 – 3.6	35.3	35.9	35.3

CLINCHECK 3

Arch width (mm) -

	Teeth—	Initial	Final	Stage 0
SUP	1.3 – 2.3	38.9	38.9	38.9
	1.4 – 2.4	39.4	40.0	39.4
	1.5 – 2.5	42.3	43.3	42.3
	1.6 – 2.6	44.9	46.1	44.9
INF	4.3 – 3.3	30.7	29.4	30.7
	4.4 – 3.4	36.0	34.7	36.0
	4.5 – 3.5	37.5	38.2	37.5
	4.6 – 3.6	40.6	42.4	40.6

Fig. 19.74 Check first column on both charts to see how much expansion was achieved on just two sets of aligners.

ClinCheck 3: Communication with the Technician

- Button cutouts on posterior to help with extrusion, changing torque to buccal cusps and intruding palatal ones
- Extrusion attachments on laterals to help with central incisors intrusion as a countermovement

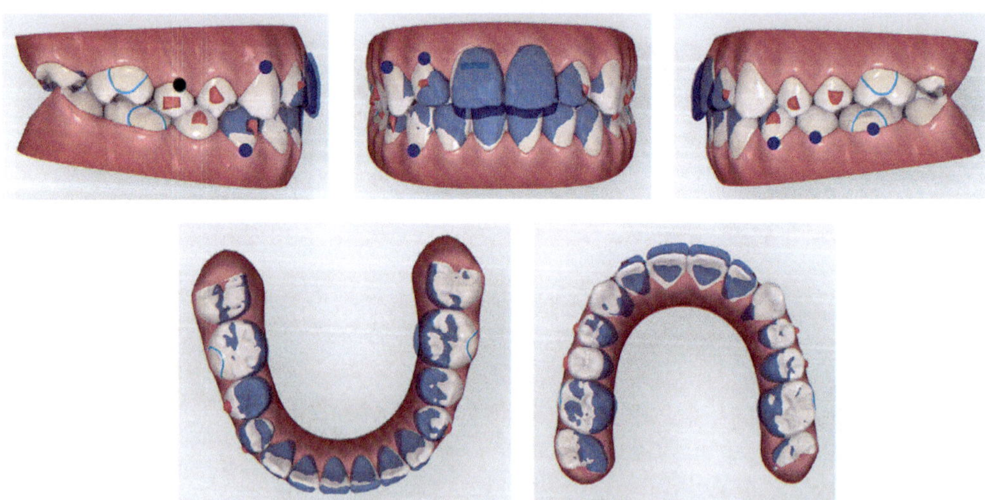

Fig. 19.75 Refinement 2 ClinChecks: right, front, left, upper, lower.

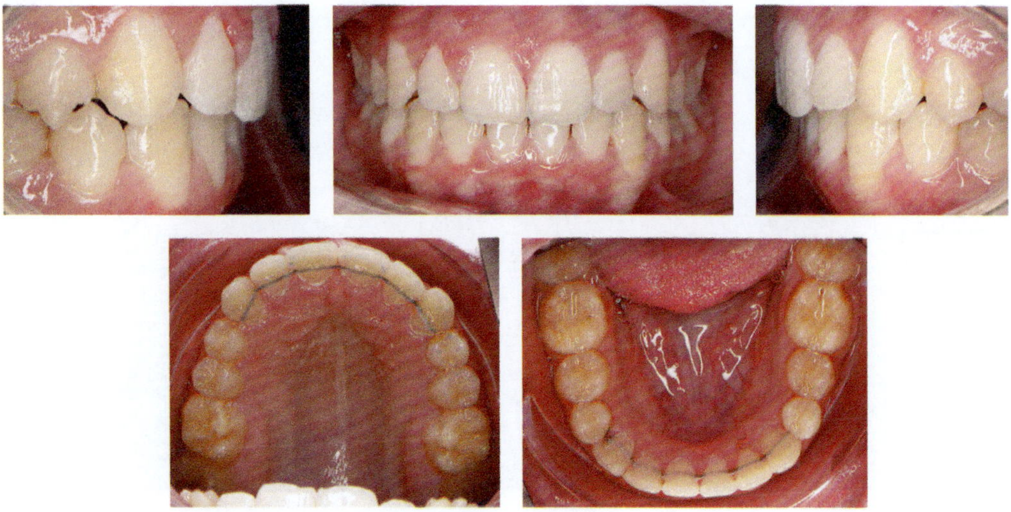

Fig. 19.76 Final intraoral views: right, front, left, upper, lower.

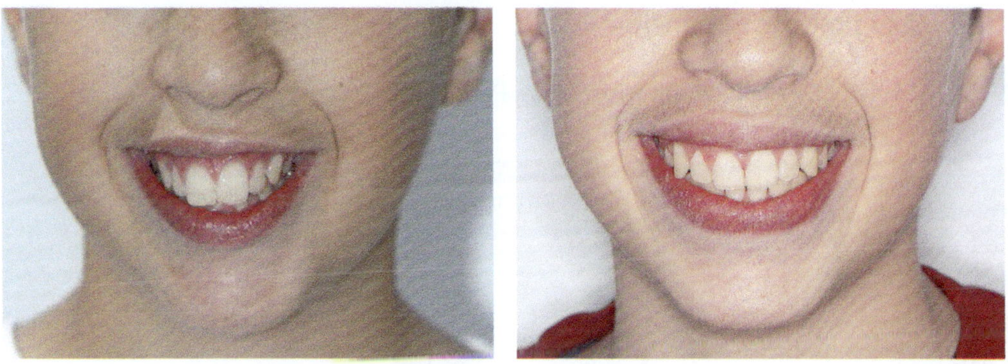

Fig. 19.77 Pretreatment and final smile.

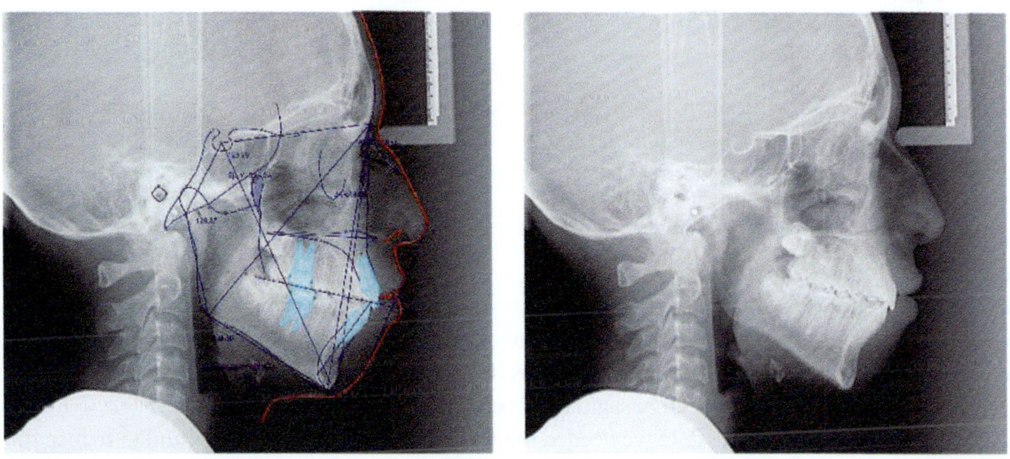

Fig. 19.78 Final lateral, cephalometric analysis and panoramic X-ray.

(Continued)

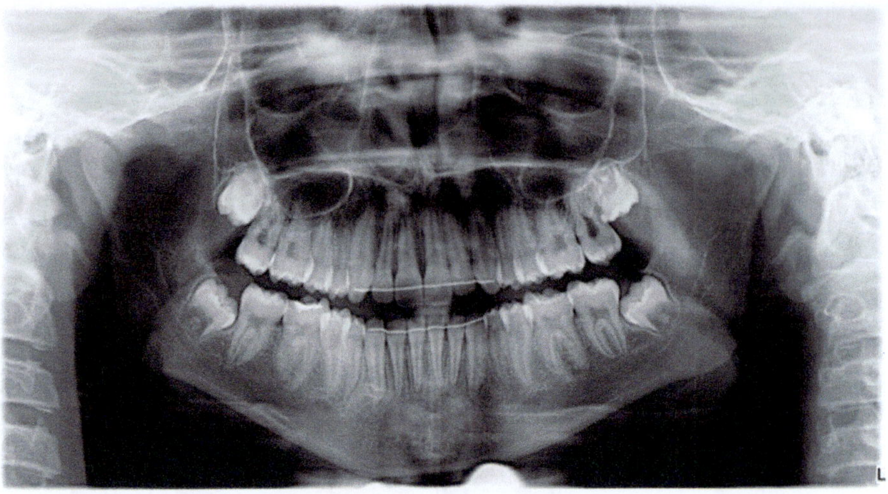

Fig. 19.78 (Cont'd)

19.3 Asymmetric Expansion

19.3.1 Skeletal Class III Patient with Severe Periodontal Disease

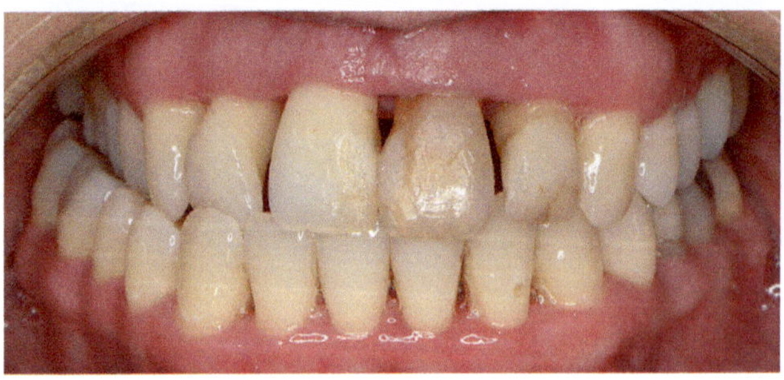

Fig. 19.79 Patient with severe periodontal disease.

Diagnosis

A 37-year-old woman with normodivergent skeletal class III presented with a maxillomandibular protrusion. She had class III division on the right side with unilateral posterior crossbite, anterior crossbite (12), advanced periodontal disease and anterior occlusal trauma.

Treatment Plan

- Eliminate fremitus on upper incisors
- Correct anterior crossbite (12)
- Eliminate the anterior occlusal trauma to help improve periodontal disease
- Correct posterior crossbite and the buccal class III relationship on the right side without making the periodontal teeth suffer a large sagittal movement
- To correct the posterior crossbite we needed to increase the upper dental mass and to reduce the lower dental mass. We therefore asked the technician to open up space for a second upper left canine, to place an implant for a second 13, with the goal of increasing the upper dental mass

and avoiding sagittal translation of the periodontal affected teeth. This implant would provide support to 12 and would help us to expand the upper arch correcting the posterior crossbite
- In the lower arch, IPR was requested to reduce dental mass

Requirements for the Technician
- Make an asymmetric expansion
- Do not move the teeth on the left side to use them as anchorage to correct the unilateral crossbite on the right side
- Open a space of 8 mm for a second canine and place two vertical attachments on 13 and 12 to control the tipping of those teeth while opening up space for the implant
- Compress lower right quadrant to assist the correction of the posterior crossbite
- Plan IPR to reduce the lower mass in lower arch, approximating the roots of the lower incisors to reduce black triangles

Treatment Summary
- Total treatment time was 22 months
- In periodontally compromised teeth the attachments were softened with a handpiece to make them less retentive; the aligner one-third in the gingival zone was also trimmed
- To correct posterior crossbite, the patient used criss-cross elastic (night use) on the right side
- The first set of aligners were 46 with a 10-day change interval protocol
- The patient needed a new set of additional aligners
- After the treatment the patient had aesthetic composite veneers done together with a Michigan bruxism splint

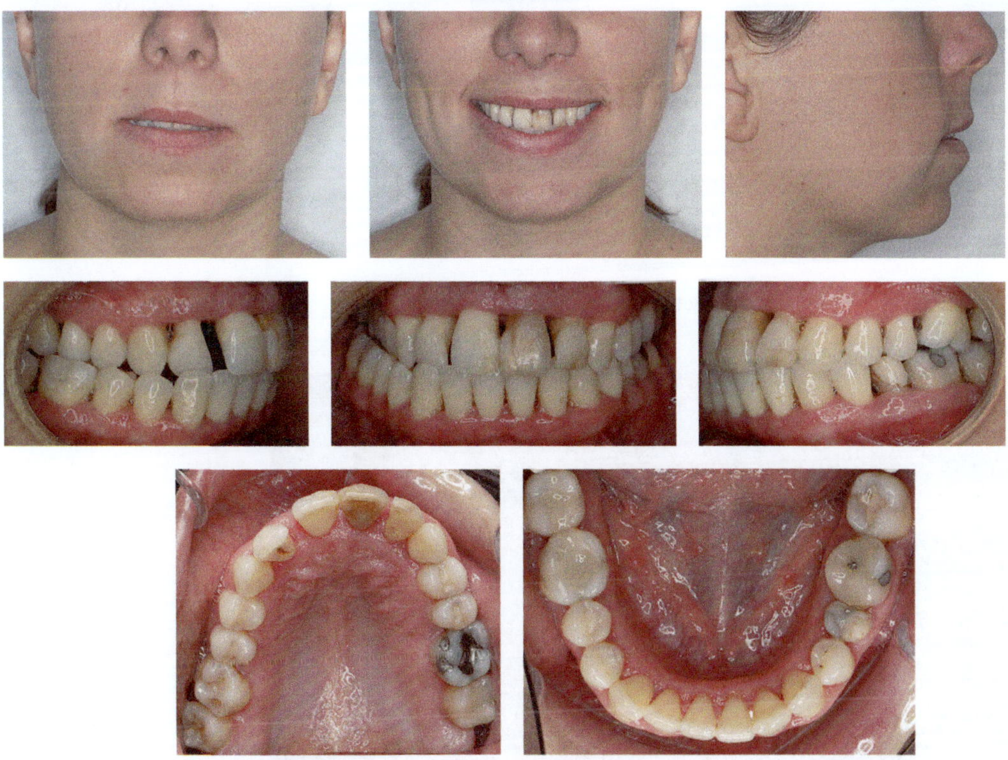

Fig. 19.80 Pretreatment views. Note the critical periodontal situation of upper incisors.

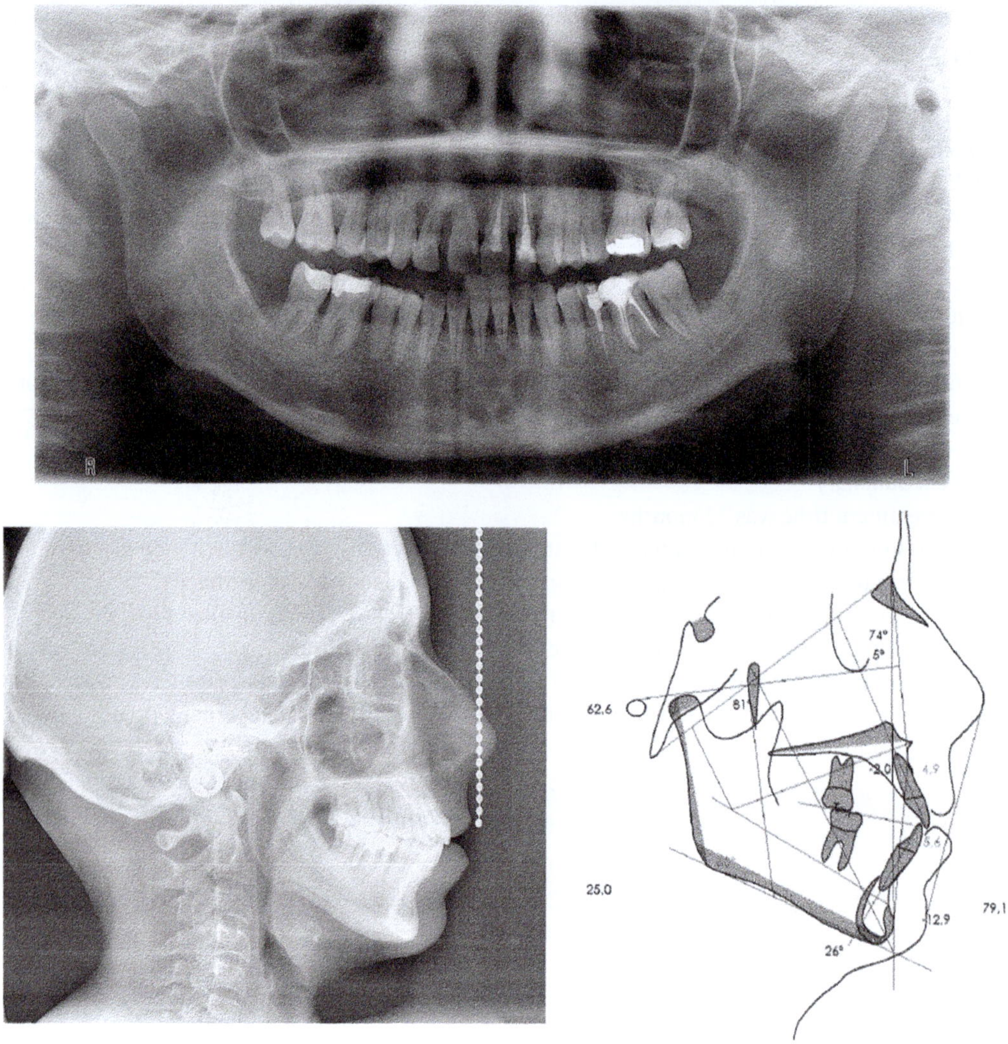

Fig. 19.81 Initial panoramic X-ray, teleradiograph and cephalometry.

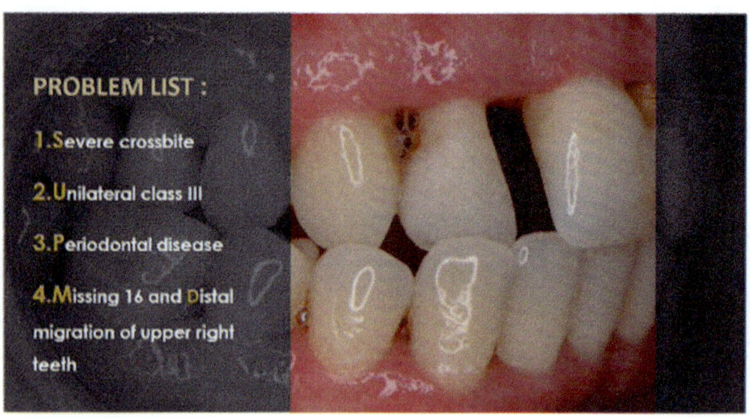

Fig. 19.82 Problem list.

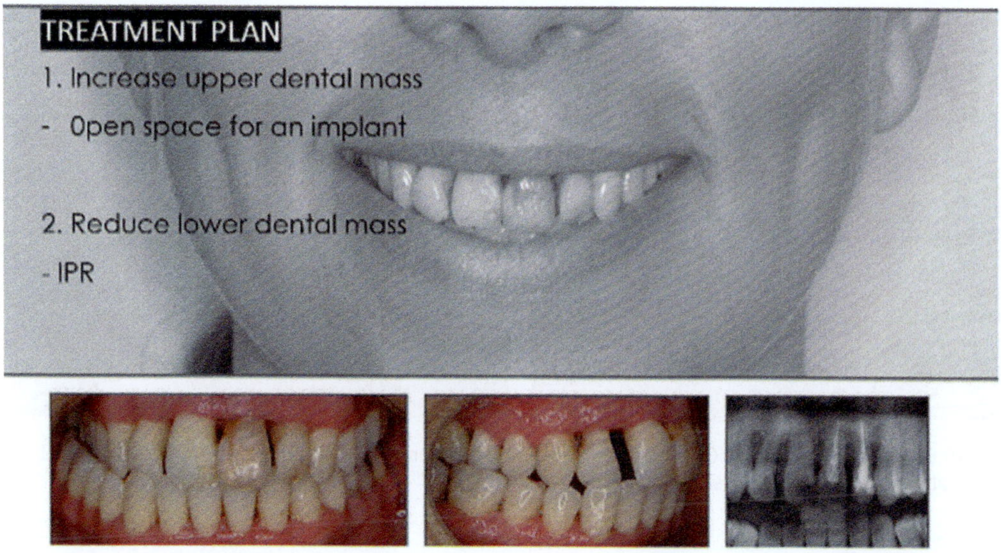

Fig. 19.83 Treatment plan.

Periodontal patients get benefit from a large amount IPR to make the root become closer and reduce black triangles

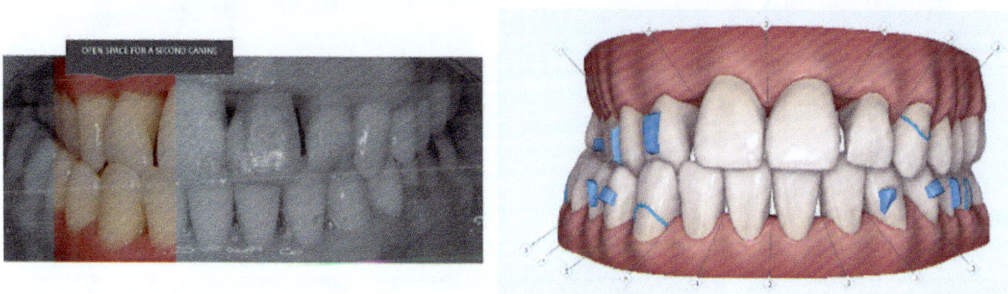

Fig. 19.84 It is important to relate clinical view to the ClinCheck.

Unilateral maxillary expansion + IPR + criss-cross elastic on the right side (night wear)

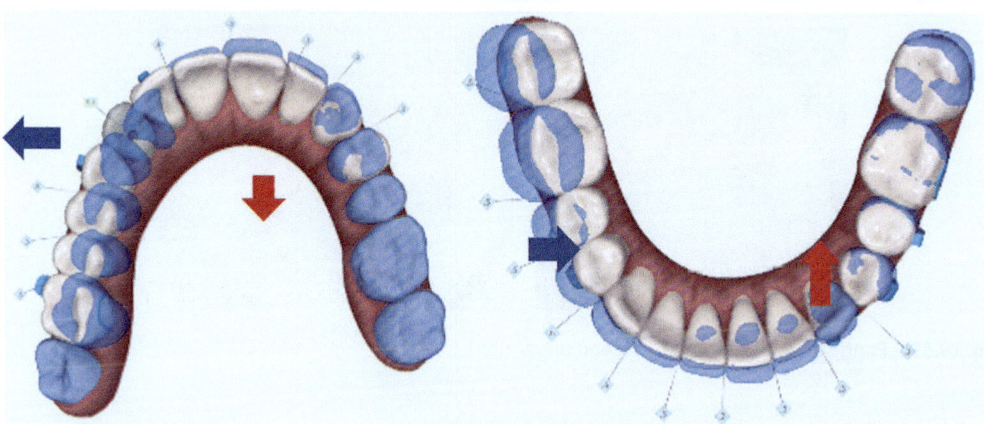

Fig. 19.85 Upper and lower CC superimposition and instructions to CAD designer.

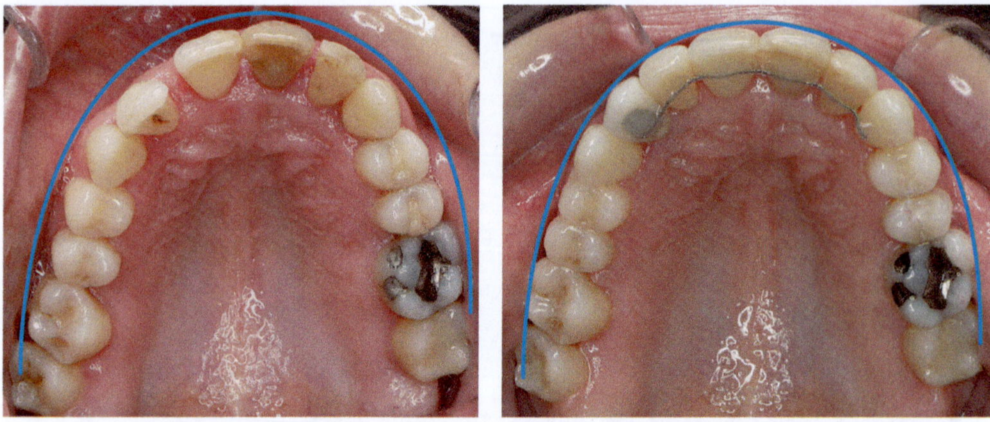

Fig. 19.86 Goal of treatment. Open space by asymmetric upper expansion on the right side, from initial occlusal (left) to final occlusal situation (right).

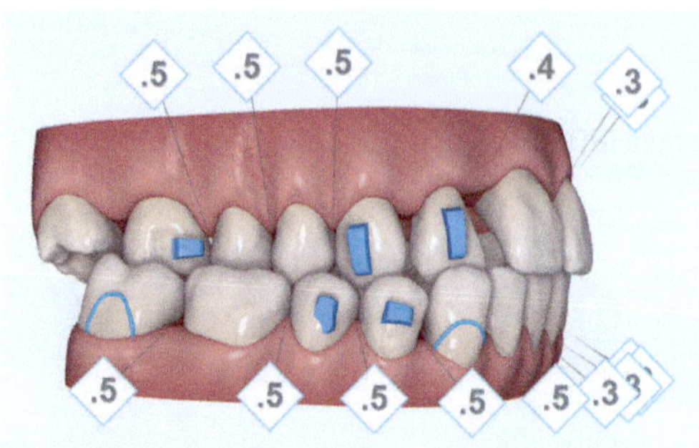

Fig. 19.87 Right ClinCheck view, initial situation.

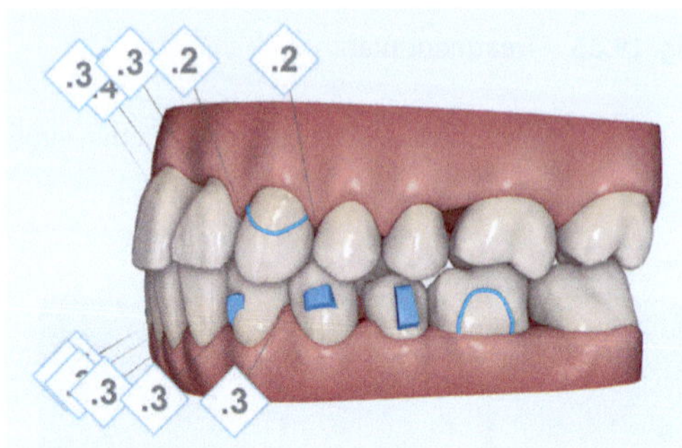

Fig. 19.88 Left ClinCheck view, initial situation.

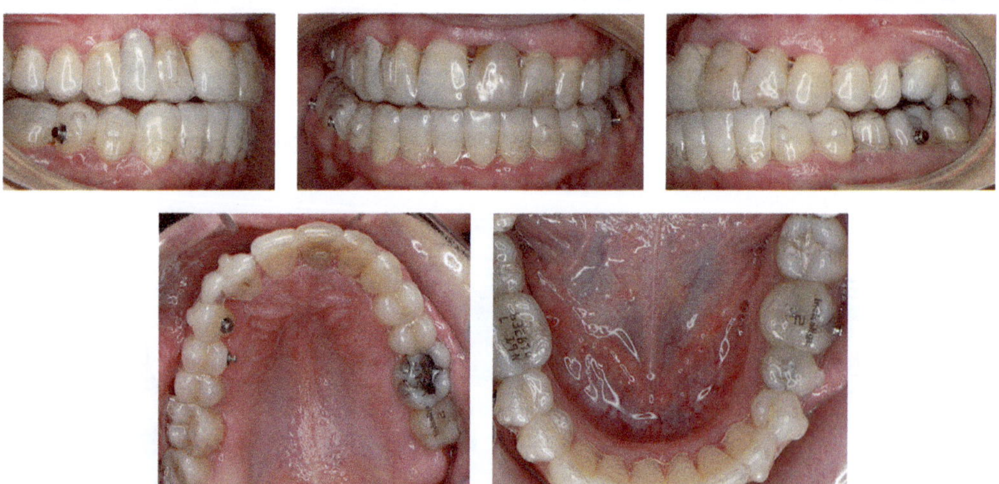

Fig. 19.89 Pontic to open space for a second upper right canine.

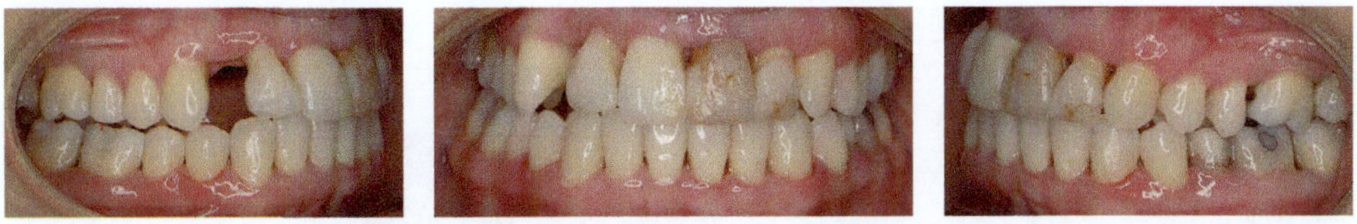

Fig. 19.90 Views before refinement.

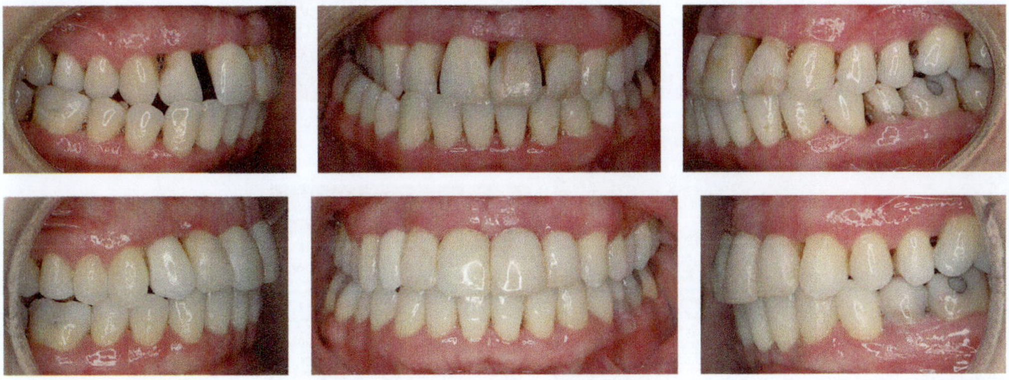

Fig. 19.91 Comparison of initial (upper) with final (lower) occlusion. Composite veneers in upper incisors and implant for 13.

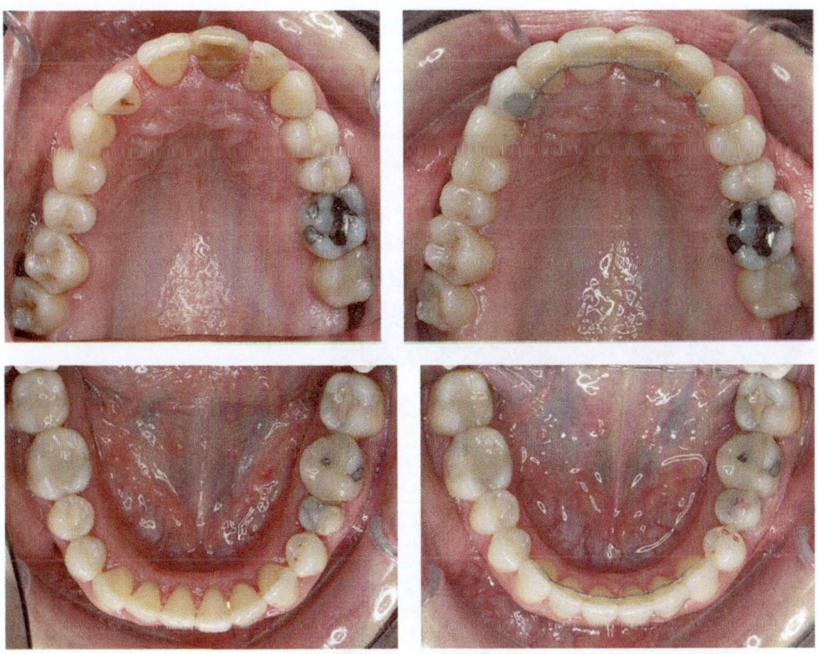

Fig. 19.92 Comparison of initial and final occlusal.

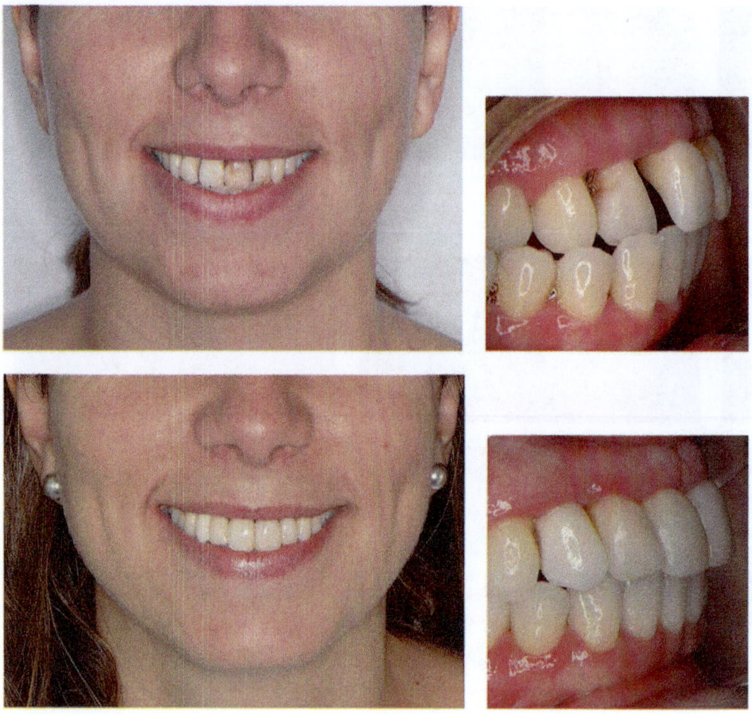

Fig. 19.93 Comparison of initial and final smile and overjet.

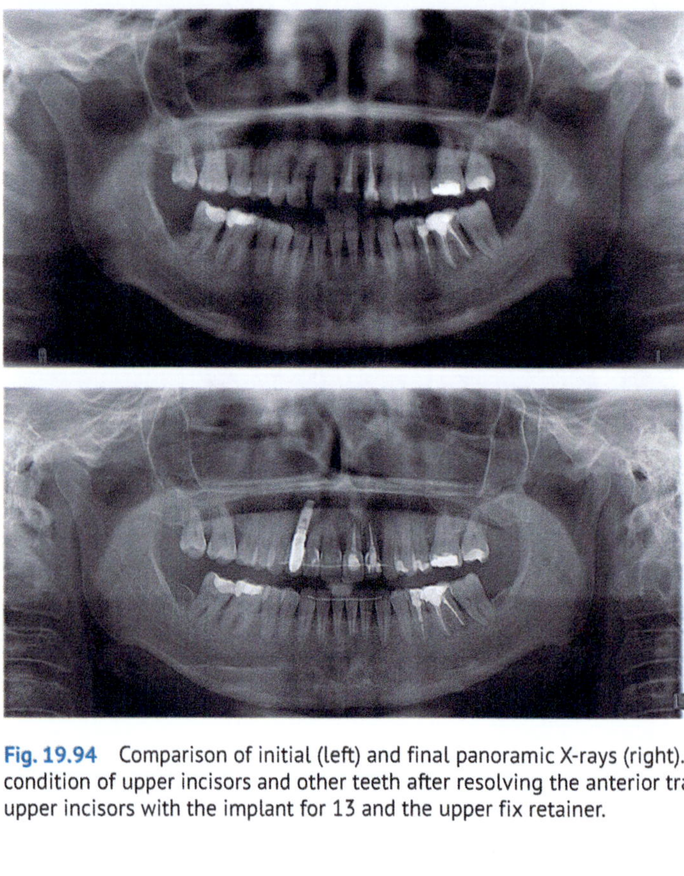

Fig. 19.94 Comparison of initial (left) and final panoramic X-rays (right). Improvement in the periodontal condition of upper incisors and other teeth after resolving the anterior trauma and providing support to the upper incisors with the implant for 13 and the upper fix retainer.

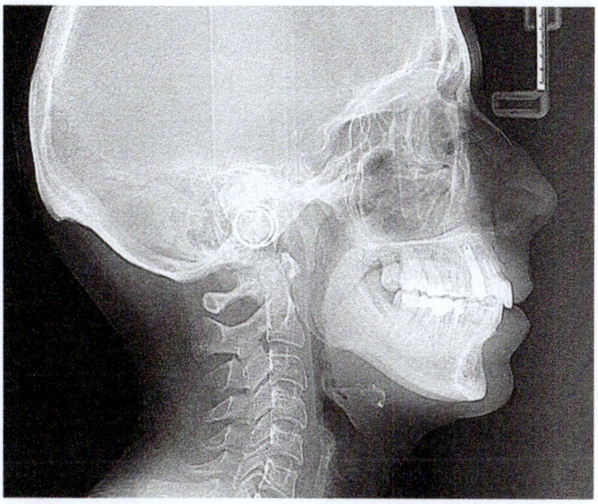

Fig. 19.95 Final teleradiograph.

19.3.2 Asymmetric Compression with Unilateral Posterior Crossbite from Canine to Second Molar

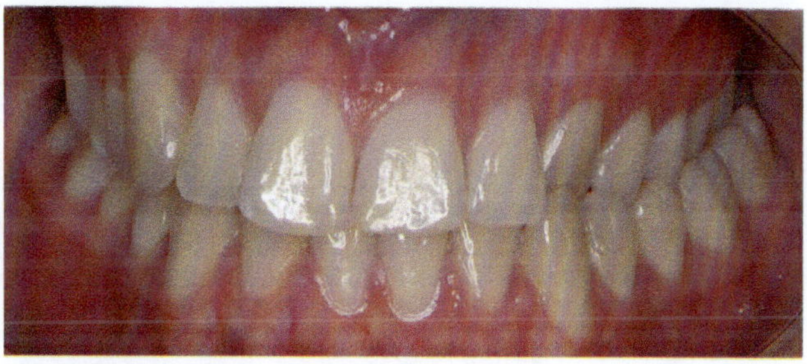

Fig. 19.96 Asymmetric compression.

Diagnosis

A 23-year-old woman with normodivergent skeletal class III presented with dental class I, left unilateral posterior crossbite and right tipping of upper midline, TMJ disorder and a left side deviation of lower jaw.

Treatment Plan

- Correct posterior crossbite by asymmetric upper expansion and asymmetric lower compression to reduce dental mass
- IPR was requested in the lower arch
- The treatment plan included centring both midlines at the end of the treatment and reducing premature contact to improve the TMJ disorder

Requirements for the Technician

- Make an asymmetric expansion, first expand upper left from canine to first molar without moving anything on the right side in order to have enough anchorage
- After correcting crossbite from 23 to 26, expand right side and 27, not moving in that moment from 23 to 26 and not moving 28 either, in order to provide enough differential anchorage
- Compress lower left quadrant to assist the correction of the posterior crossbite, applying lingual root torque during all the compression movements
- Plan IPR to reduce the lower mass in lower arch

Treatment Summary

- Total treatment time was 26 months
- To correct posterior crossbite, the patient used criss-cross elastic (night use) on the left side.
- The first set of aligners were 46 with a 10-day change interval protocol
- Patient needed a new set of additional aligners to settle the occlusion as, after correcting the posterior crossbite, they presented with a posterior open bite on the left side
- To settle the occlusion in the additional aligners, we used elastics in the posterior zone
- At the end of the treatment, the patient achieved a bilateral class I relationship with normal overbite and overjet, the unilateral posterior crossbite was solved, both midlines were centred and the symptomatology in the TMJ improved
- After the treatment the patient had a Michigan bruxism splint as a retention

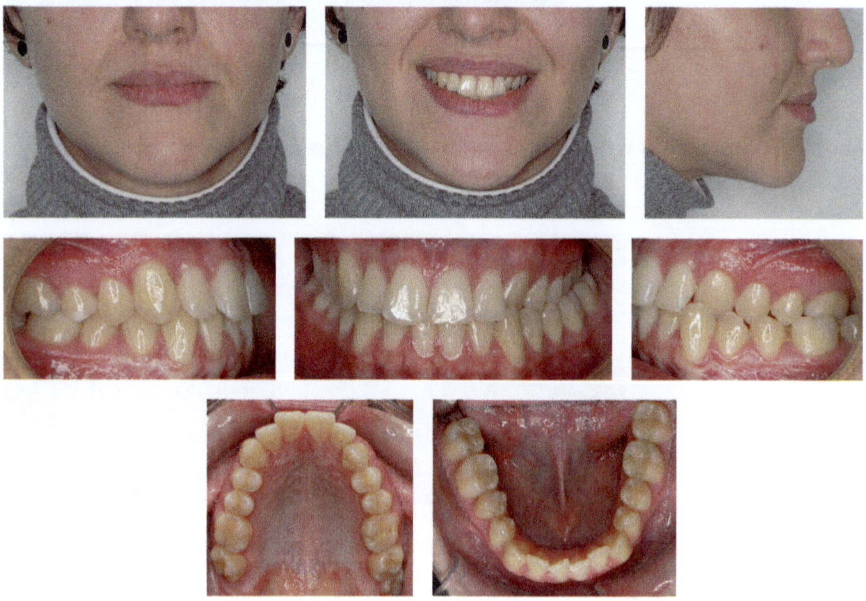

Fig. 19.97 Pretreatment views.

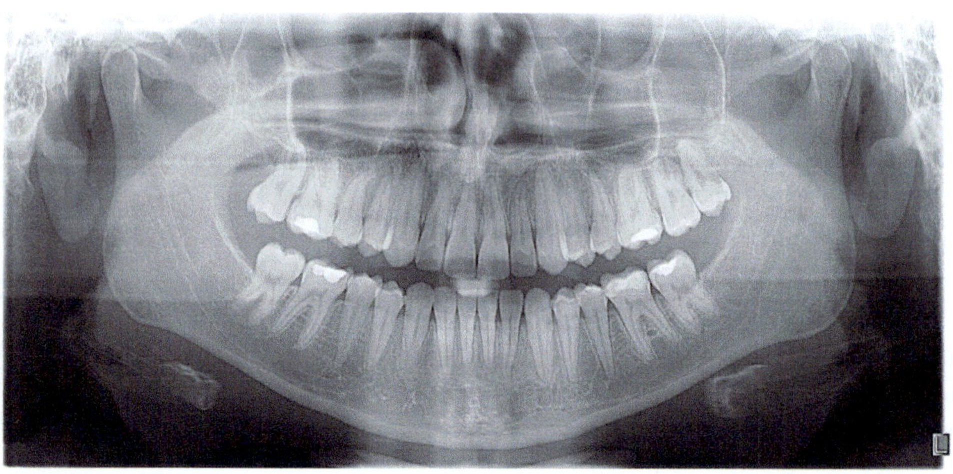

Fig. 19.98 Initial panoramic X-ray, teleradiograph and cephalometry.

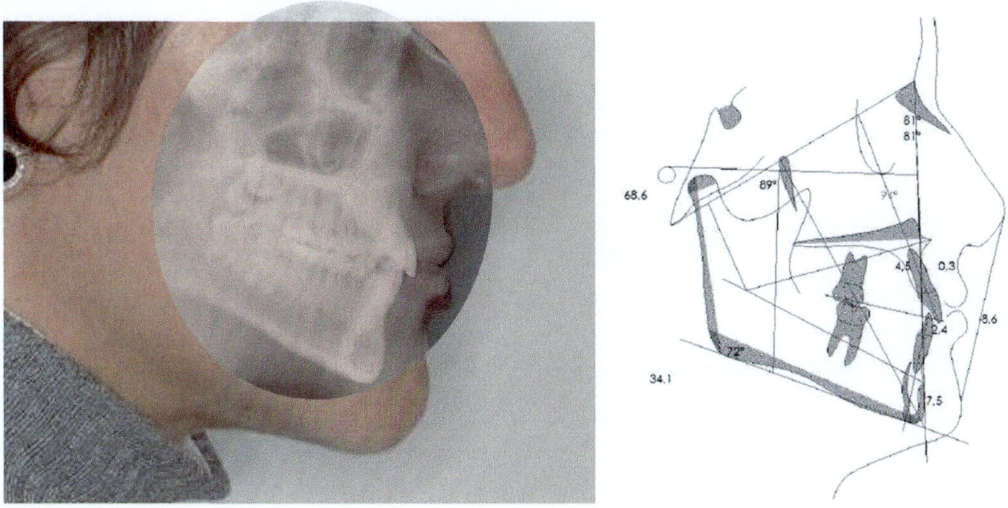

Fig. 19.98 (Cont'd)

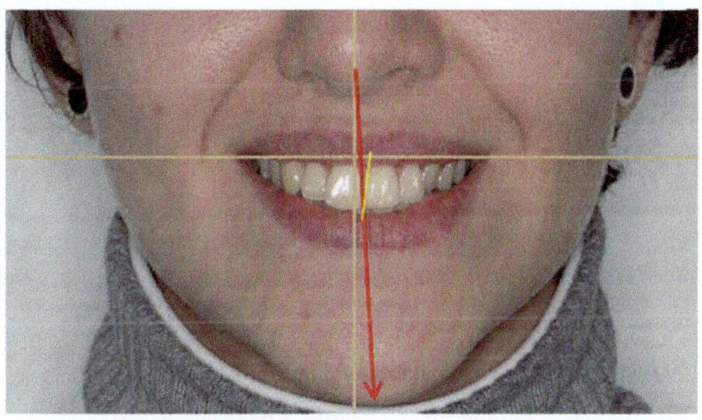

Fig. 19.99 Left-side deviation of lower jaw.

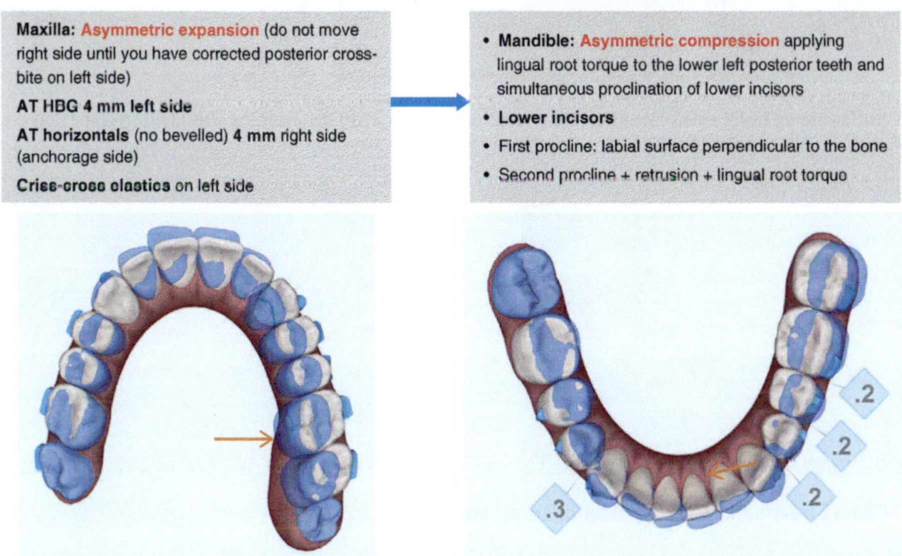

Fig. 19.100 Upper and lower CC superimposition and instructions to CAD designer.

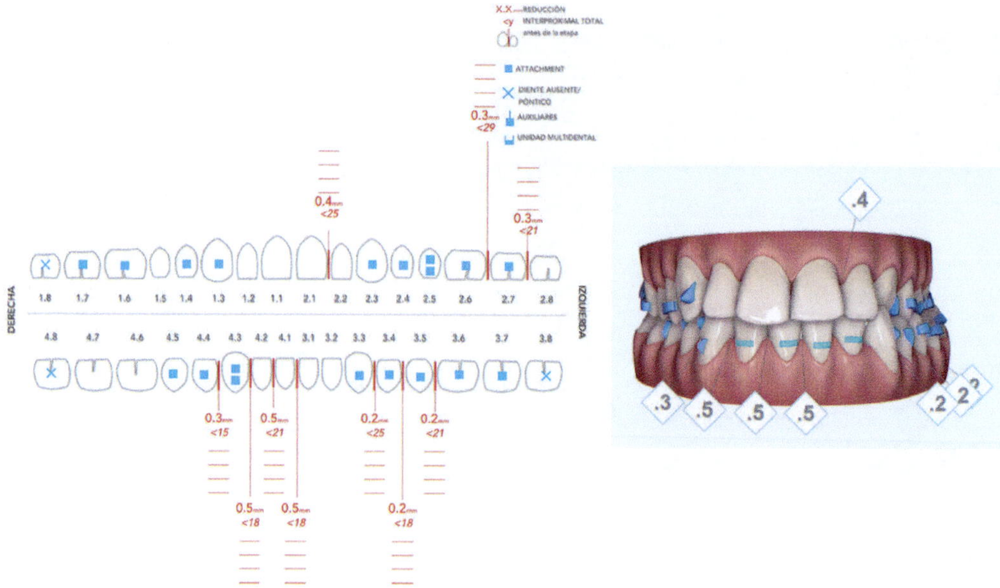

Fig. 19.101 Interproximal reduction is necessary to reduce the lower dental mass.

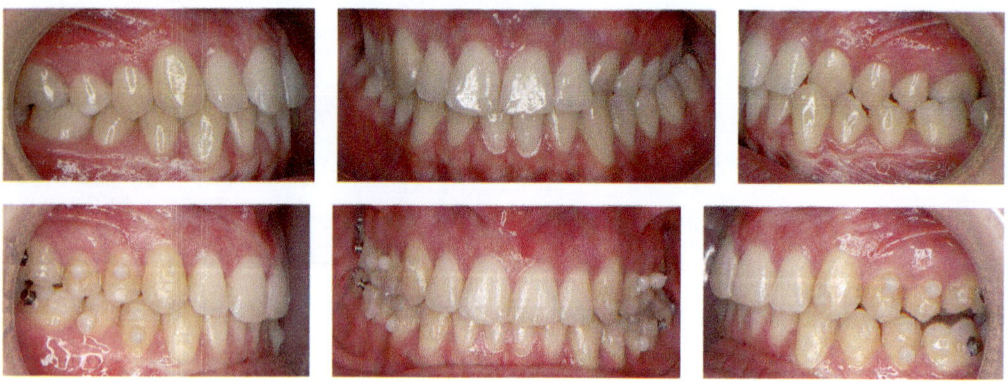

Fig. 19.102 Initial views before refinement. The posterior open bite on left side needed triangular elastics during refinement.

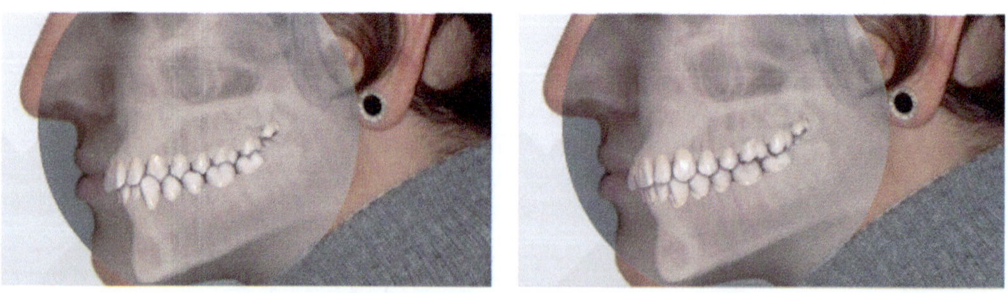

Fig. 19.103 Goal of treatment: correct posterior crossbite from 23 to 27.

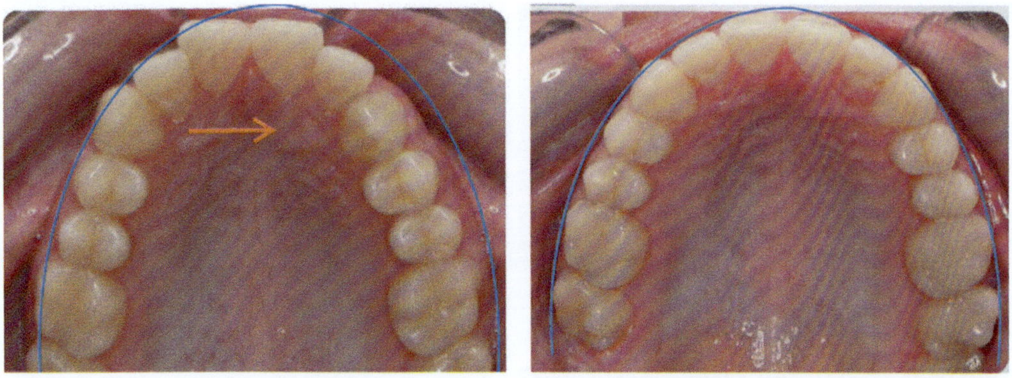

Fig. 19.104 Initial and final design of the asymmetric expansion of the upper arch.

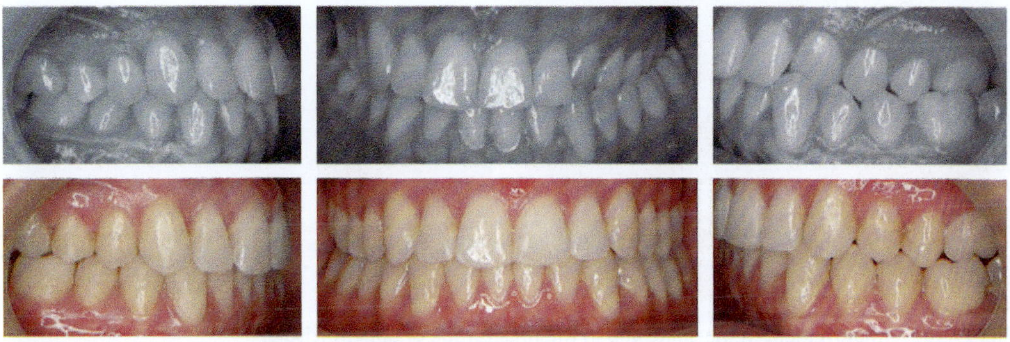

Fig. 19.105 Comparison of initial and final occlusion.

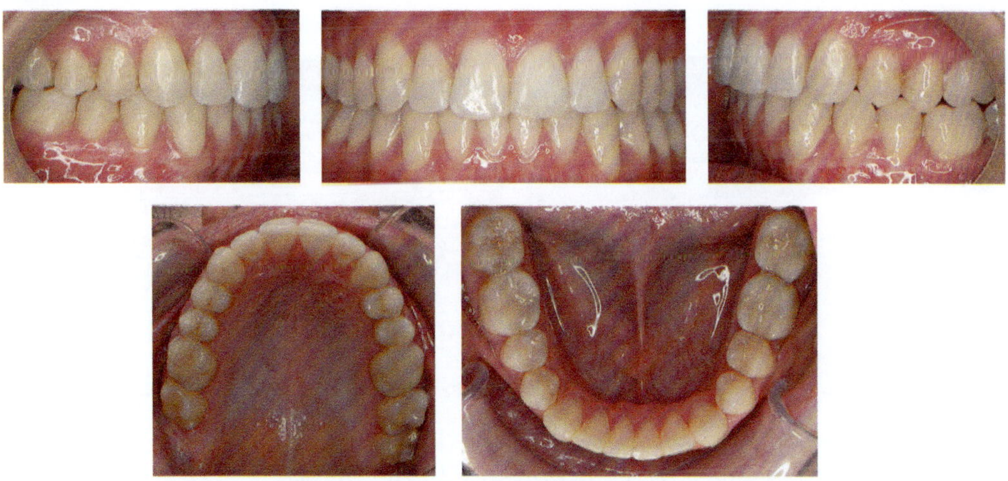

Fig. 19.106 Final occlusion. Both midlines centred. Unilateral posterior crossbite on left side.

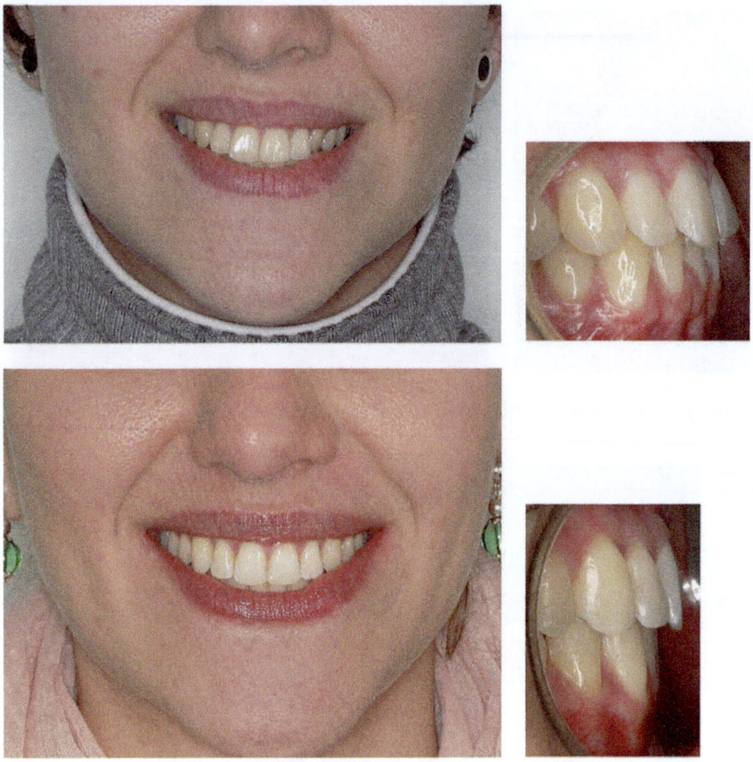

Fig. 19.107 Improvement in the smile and in the final torque of upper incisors.

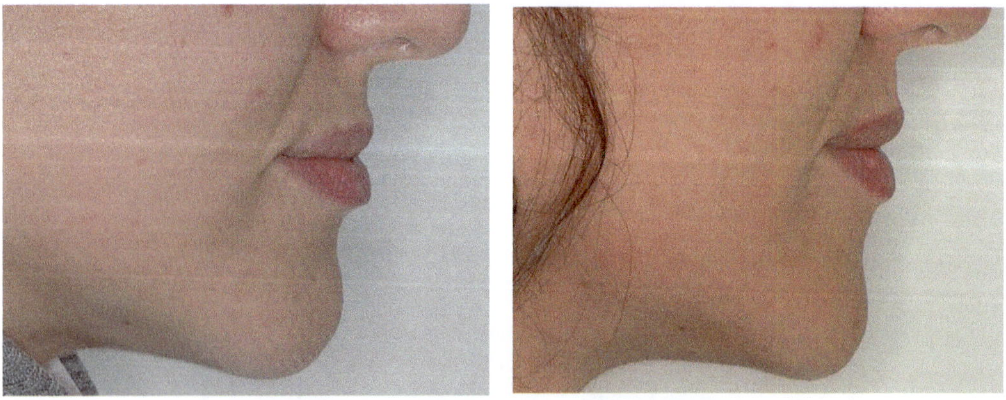

Fig. 19.108 Improvement in the profile by clockwise rotation of the mandible.

19.3.3 Asymmetric Compression with Unilateral Posterior Molar Crossbite: a Two-stage Approach

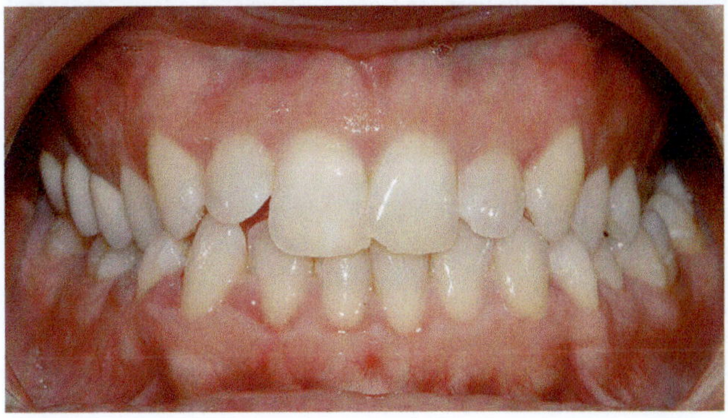

Fig. 19.109 Posterior crossbite with anterior crowding.

Diagnosis

A 33-year-old woman with normodivergent skeletal class III presented with dental class I with left unilateral posterior crossbite, a TMJ disorder and a thin gingival biotype.

Treatment Plan

- First stage: anterior alignment and expansion having posterior sectors as anchorage
- Buttons on 12-22 were bonded after manual precision cuts on both buccal and palatal surface in order to use an elastic over the aligner for extrusion
- Second stage: anterior anchorage and posterior expansion with extra BRT to 26–27, anchoring on 28 to create a 'hinge' movement

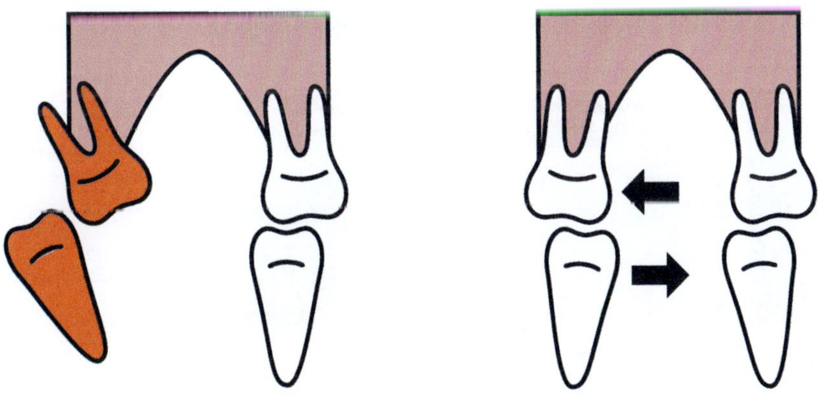

Fig. 19.110 Careful diagnosis of the crossbite origin will lead to a great result.

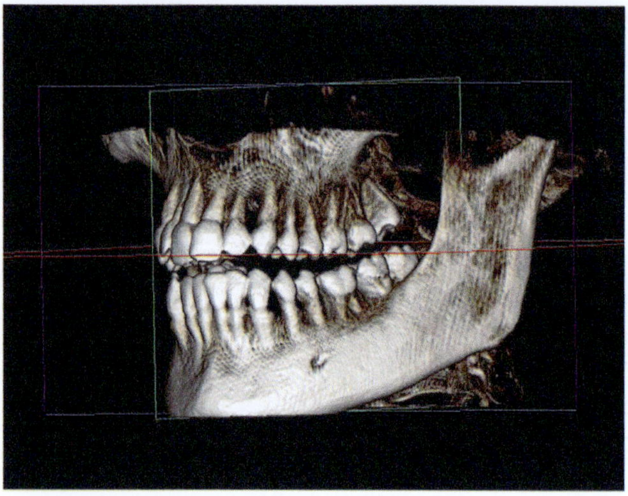

Fig. 19.111 Cone beam computed tomography: 3D radiological examination is mandatory when large transverse discrepancies are detected.

ClinCheck 1: Requirements for the Technician

First phase

- Make a symmetric expansion on anterior sector, having molars as anchorage
- On lower arch, level Spee curve with conventional protocols (extrusion attachments on premolars) and sequencing of lower incisor movement (protrusion, intrusion, retrusion); IPR to be able to compress the lower arch

Treatment Summary

- Total treatment time was 16 months.
- Patient used criss-cross elastics at the beginning and buccal extrusion attachments on the affected molars at the end of treatment.
- Weekly change of aligners.
- At the end of the treatment, the patient achieved a proper occlusion with symmetrical posterior expansion.

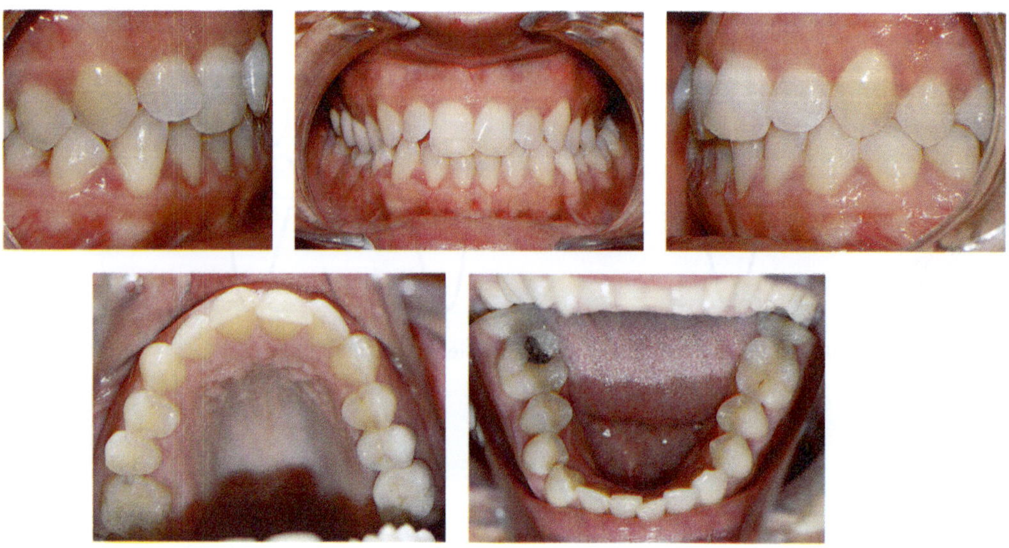

Fig. 19.112 Pretreatment intraoral views (right, front, left, upper, lower).

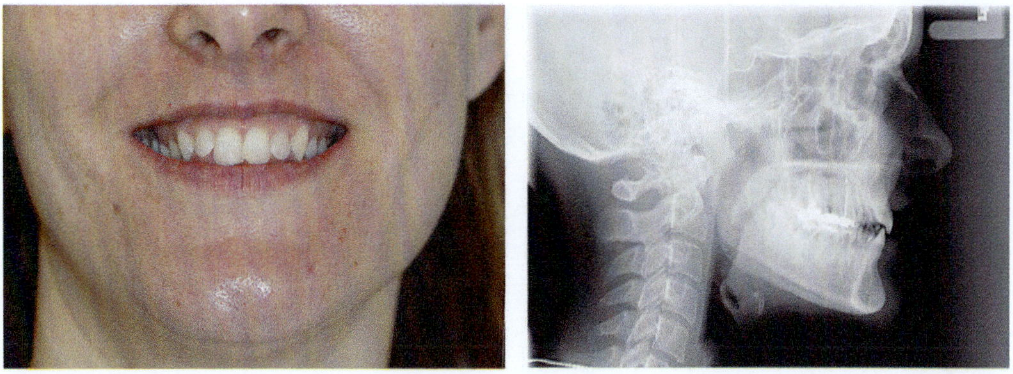

Fig. 19.113 Pretreatment smile and lateral X-ray.

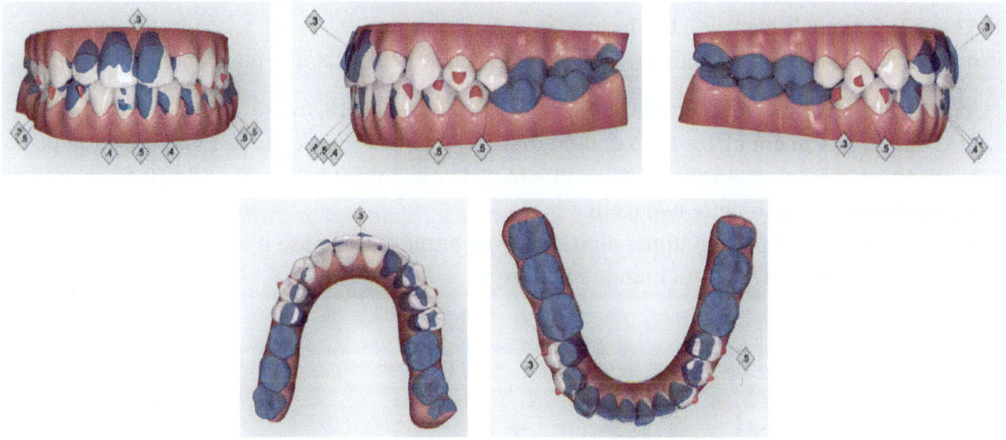

Fig. 19.114 Pretreatment ClinChecks: right, front, left, upper, lower.

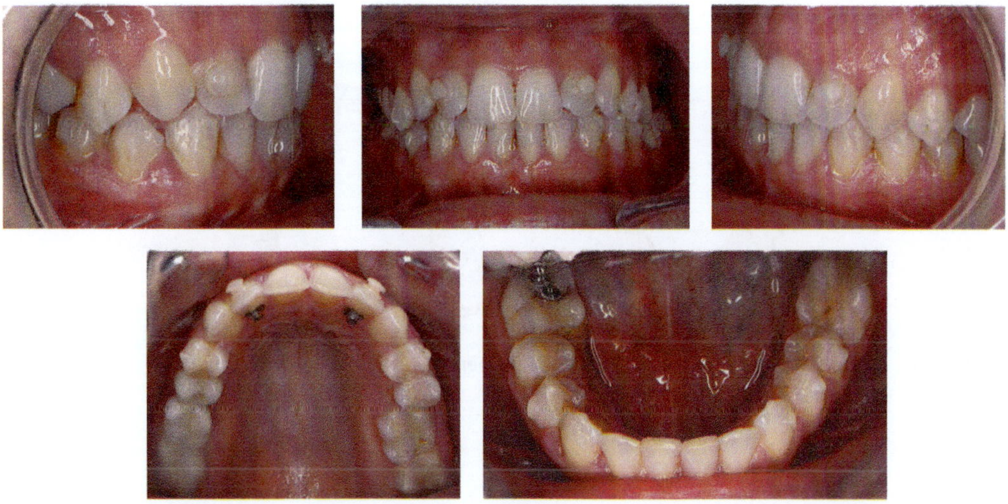

Fig. 19.115 Refinement: intraoral views (right, front, left, upper, lower).

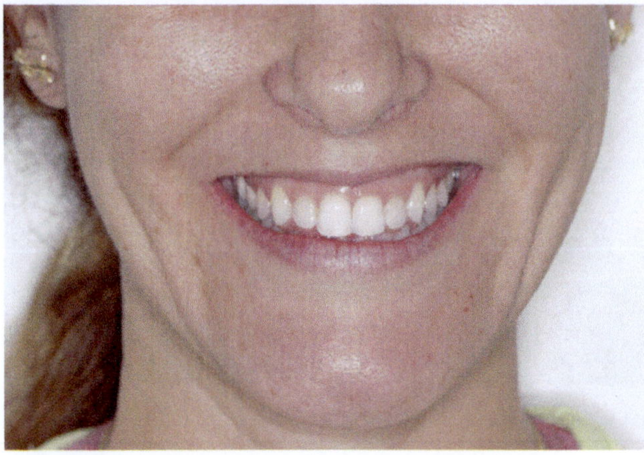

Fig. 19.116 Smile after first set of aligners.

ClinCheck 2: Communication with the Technician

Second phase, with additional aligners, after reviewing bone availability on a CBCT

- Upper arch: set first quadrant molars as unmovable, as well as 18, to use it as anchorage and create a 'hinge' movement of 16–17 to uncross bite. Horizontal bevelled to gingival attachments to ensure an 'en masse' expansion movement, not just crown positive torque. Add 10 degrees extra of buccal root torque to these two teeth.
- Coordinate the lower arch to upper arch. Set 38 as unmovable to use it as anchorage, compress 36 and 37, add 10 degrees extra lingual root torque.

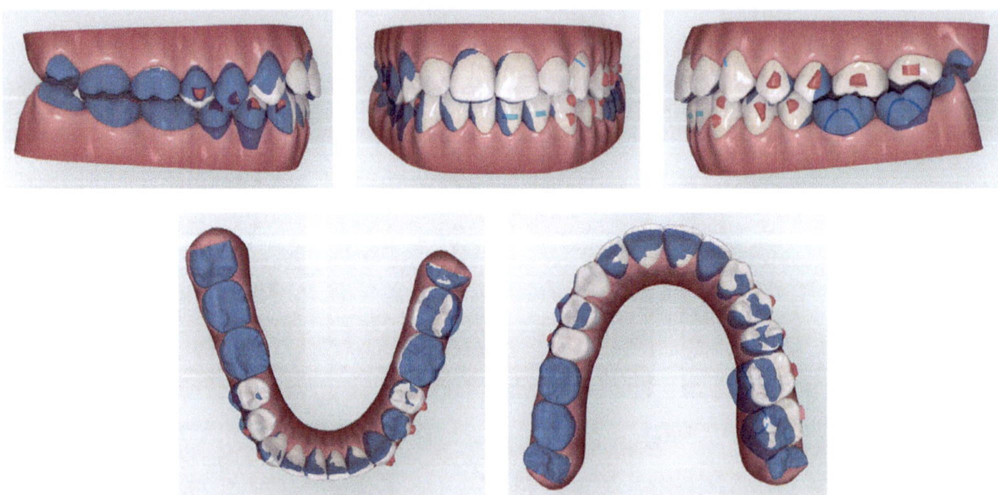

Fig. 19.117 Refinement ClinChecks: right, front, left, upper, lower.

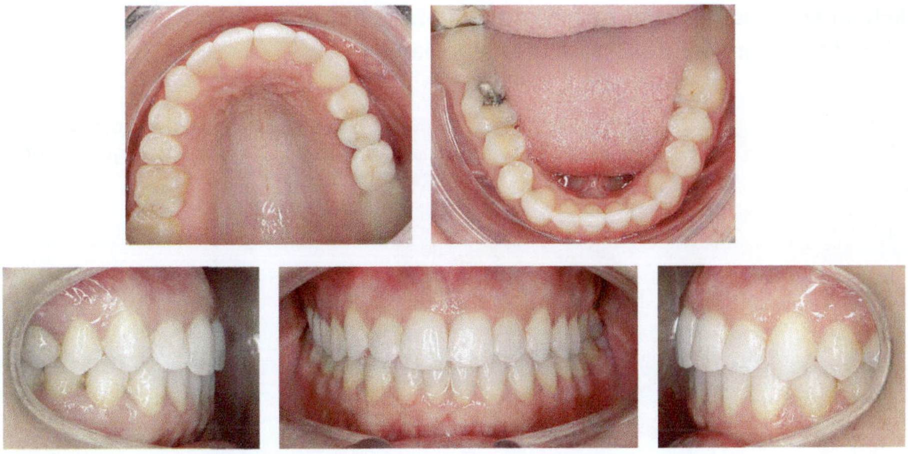

Fig. 19.118 Final intraoral views: right, front, left, upper, lower.

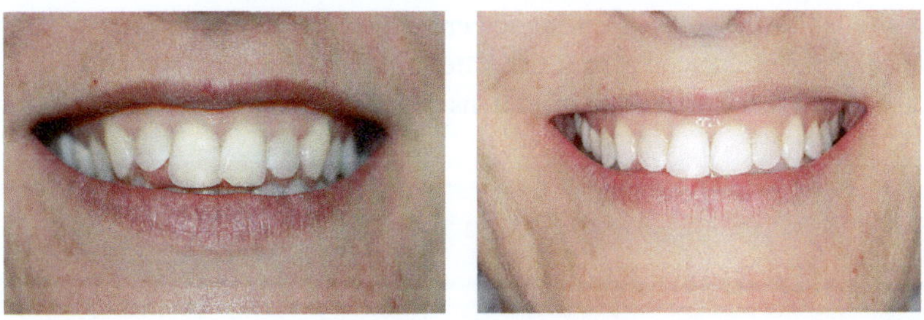

Fig. 19.119 Pretreatment and final smile: we can observe how posterior expansion has improved smile aesthetics.

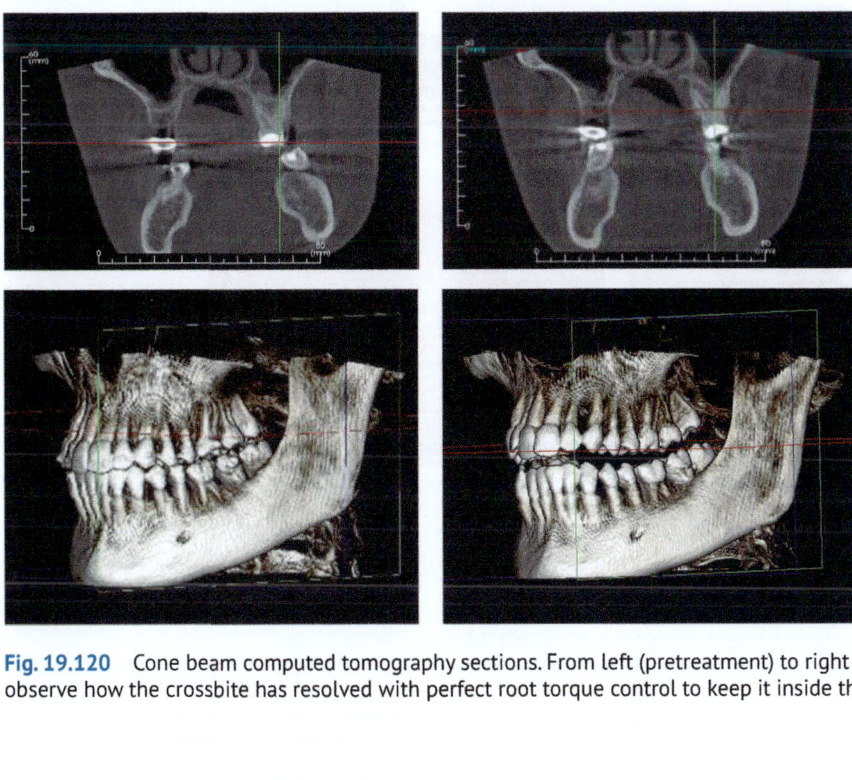

Fig. 19.120 Cone beam computed tomography sections. From left (pretreatment) to right (final), we can observe how the crossbite has resolved with perfect root torque control to keep it inside the cortical bone.

19.3.4 Skeletal Asymmetric Compression with Unilateral Posterior Molar Crossbite: Use of Maxillary Assisted Rapid Palatal Expander

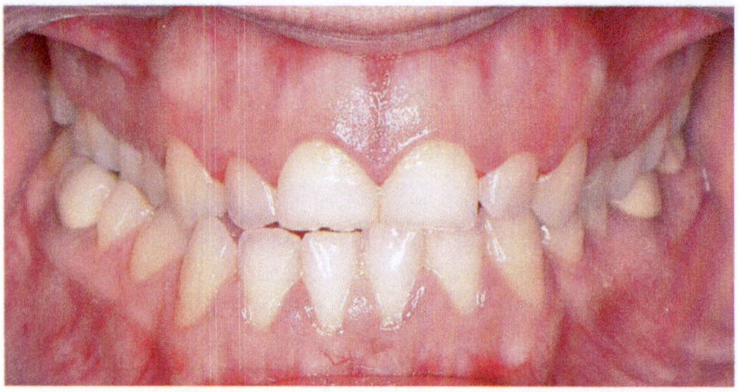

Fig. 19.121 Posterior crossbite, with anterior crossbite and edge-to-edge occlusion.

Diagnosis

A 30-year-old woman presented with a skeletal posterior crossbite. The second molars with a proper transverse relationship suggested good prognosis. Anterior teeth wear was associated with edge-to-edge pathological occlusion and short clinical crowns derived from attrition.

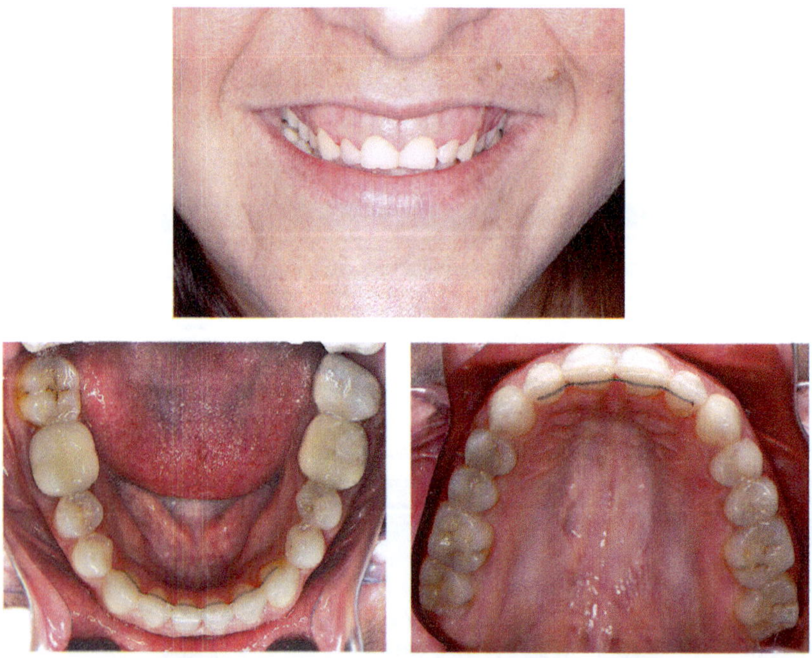

Fig. 19.122 Smile and upper and lower arch view.

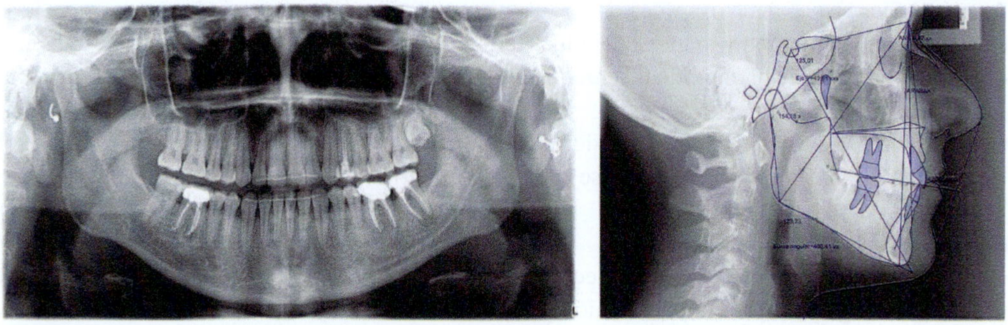

Fig. 19.123 Panoramic and lateral X-rays.

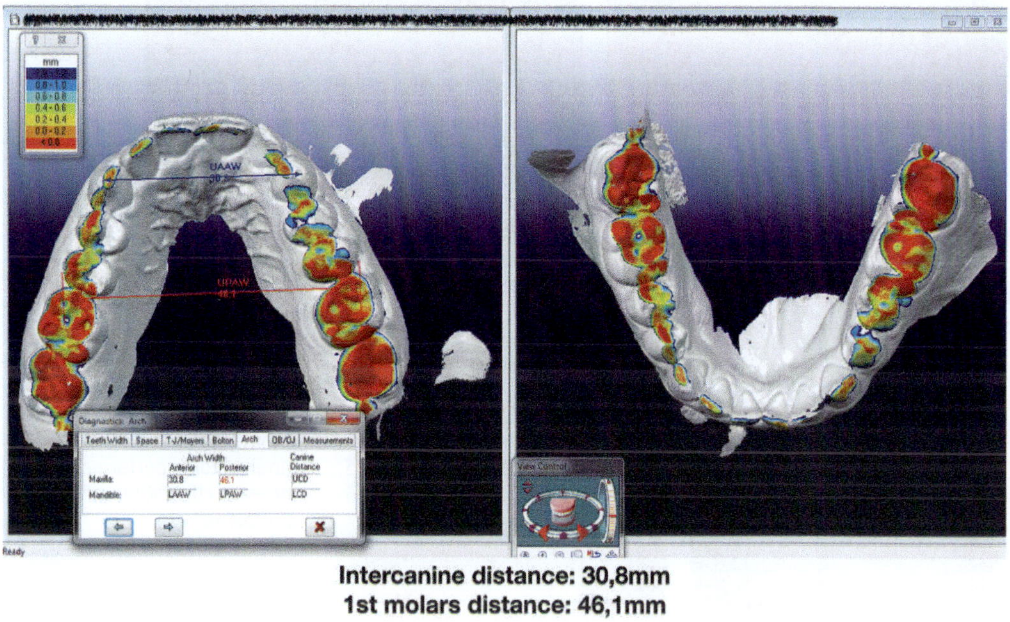

Fig. 19.124 Measurements were performed after iTero scanning and OrthoCad software analysis.

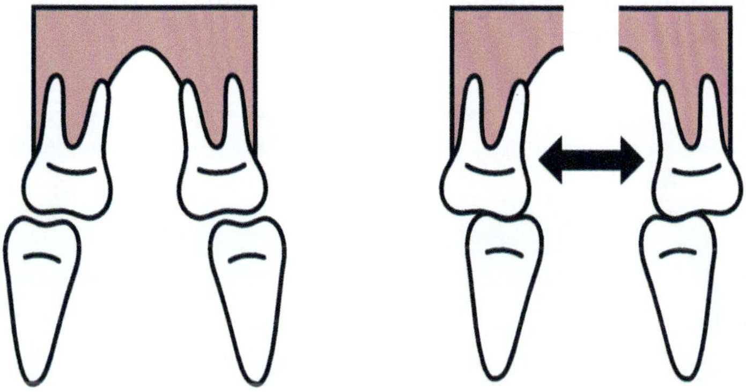

Fig. 19.125 Skeletal compression has to be approached with a surgical procedure such as a miniscrew-assisted rapid palatal expander (MARPE).

Treatment Plan

- First phase: gingivectomy to increase clinical crown surface.
- Second phase: MARPE, modified technique without bands, to break palatal suture and perform a skeletal disjunction.
- Third phase: immediately after expansion treat the case as a spacing case: optimized root control attachments on central incisors to close space and posterior torque correction.

Phase 1: Gingivectomy

Gingivectomy was performed with an electrical scalpel and the patient had a second appointment for MARPE surgery 2 weeks later, in which the soft tissue was fully recovered.

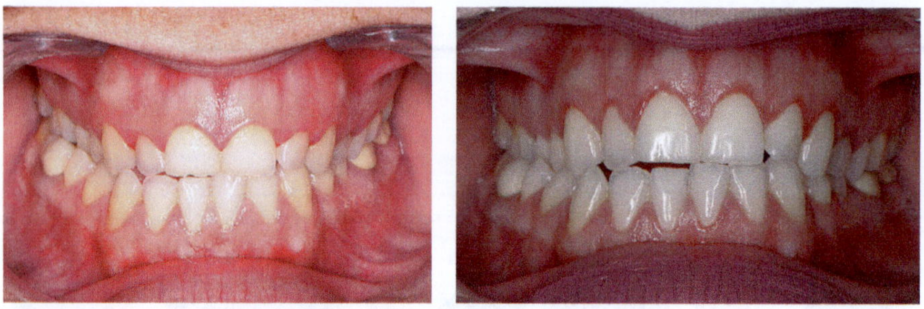

Fig. 19.126 First phase: initially, the patient had a gingivectomy performed to increase clinical length of crowns.

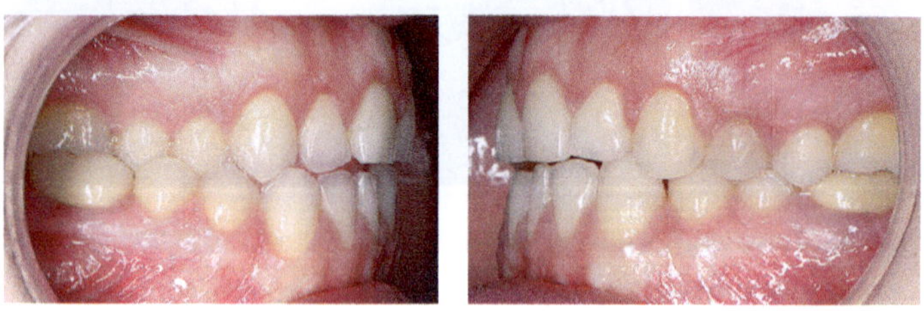

Fig. 19.127 First phase: initially, the patient had a gingivectomy performed to increase clinical length of crowns.

Phase 2: MARPE

A MARPE surgery was performed with local anaesthesia, and patient was instructed to make four screw activations every day until the screw (8 mm) was totally opened.

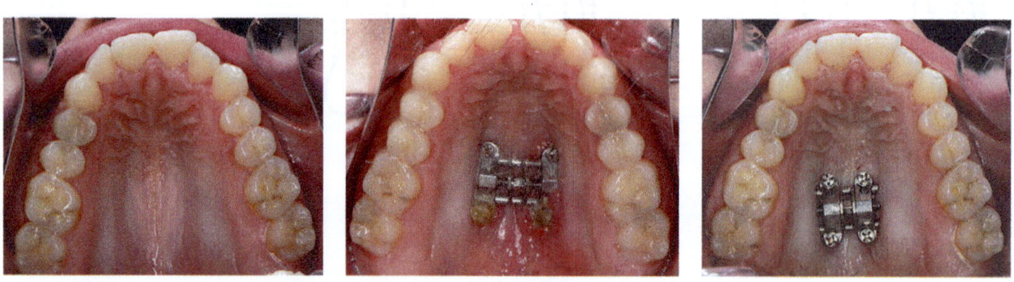

Fig. 19.128 Upper pre-miniscrew-assisted rapid palatal expander (MARPE): post MARPE surgery, post MARPE opening. The arch was developed with no dental anchorage.

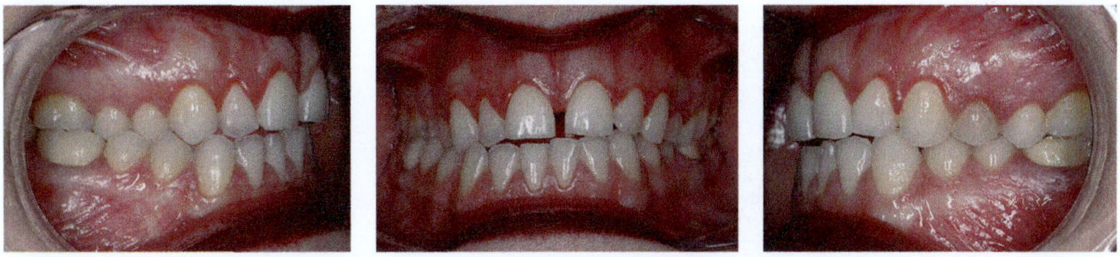

Fig. 19.129 Right, front, left post-miniscrew-assisted rapid palatal expander opening. Greater expansion was achieved on left side as a result of the crossbite on the right.

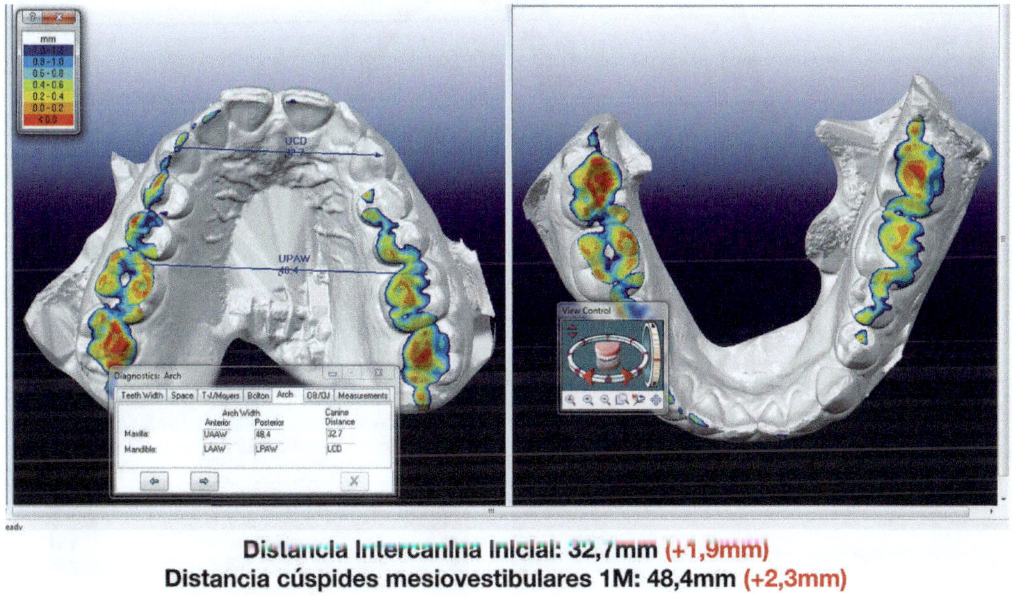

Fig. 19.130 Second phase. Measurements were performed after iTero scanning and OrthoCad software analysis, resulting in correct skeletal expansion with just the miniscrew-assisted rapid palatal expander.

ClinCheck 1, Communication with the Technician

- Set second molars as unmovable, in order to use them as anchorage
- Expand first quadrant more than second, asymmetrically
- Centre midline with space closure by 21 mesialization. Add optimized root control attachment to this to create an 'en masse' movement.
- Perform lower IPR to create overjet
- Add extra buccal root torque to 12–22

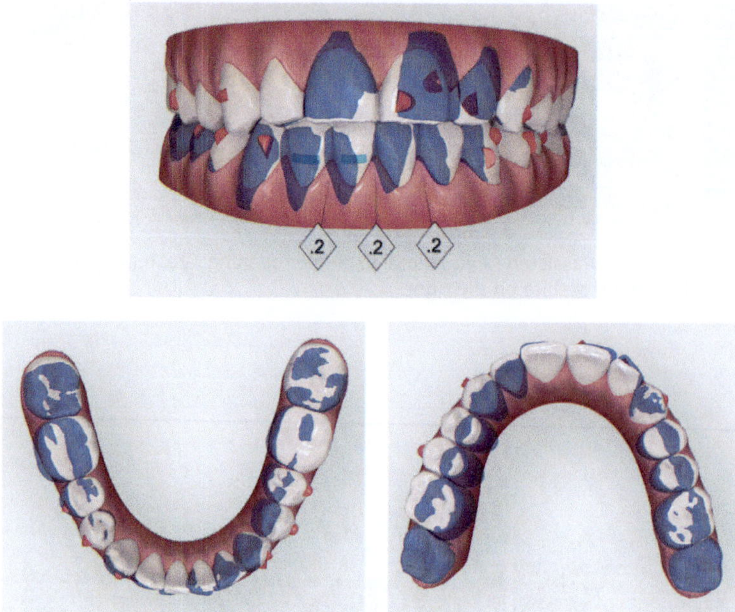

Fig. 19.131 Second phase ClinChecks (front, upper, lower).

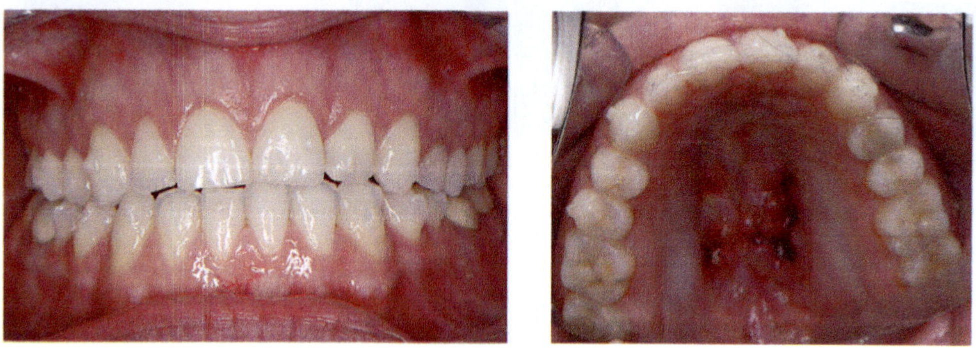

Fig. 19.132 Third phase: intraoral views (front and upper).

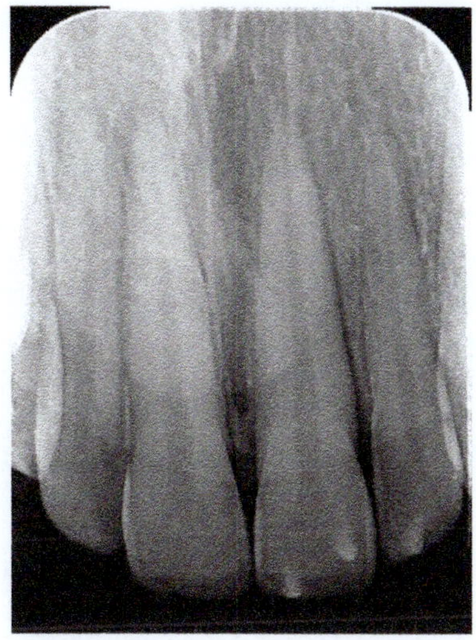

Fig. 19.133 After 16 aligners space was closed, palatal suture was still open in the X-ray, and the miniscrew-assisted rapid palatal expander was removed.

ClinCheck 2, Communication with the Technician

- Set upper second molars as unmovable, in order to use them as anchorage
- Expand first quadrant more than second, asymmetrically
- Centre midline with space closure by arch development
- Perform lower IPR to improve the premolar final occlusion as a Bolton discrepancy was detected
- Add extra buccal root torque to 12–21
- Precision cuts for buttons and elastics to help with posterior extrusion

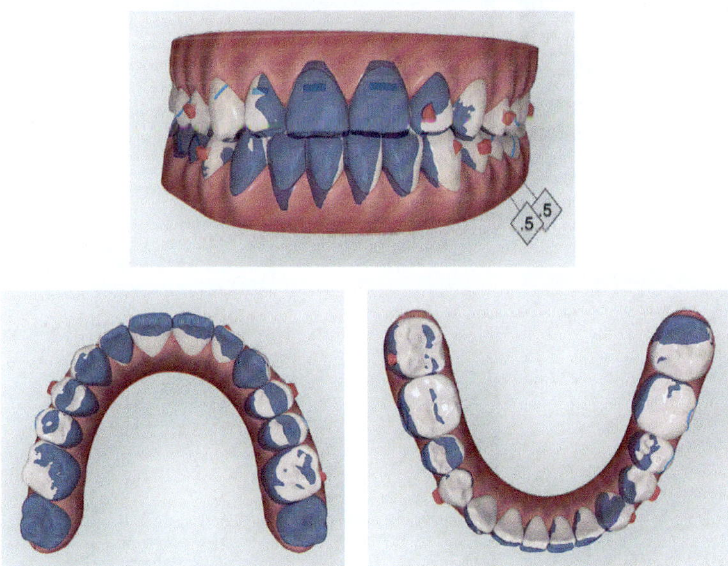

Fig. 19.134 Third phase ClinChecks (front, upper, lower).

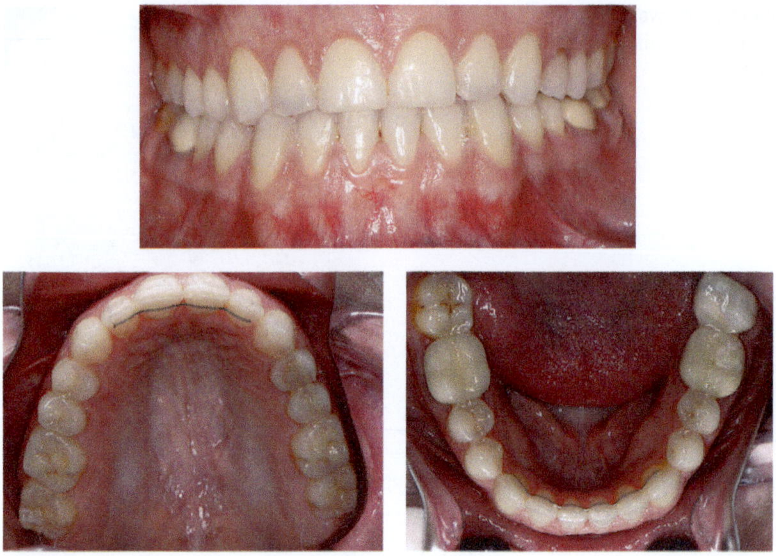

Fig. 19.135 Final intraoral views: front, upper, lower.

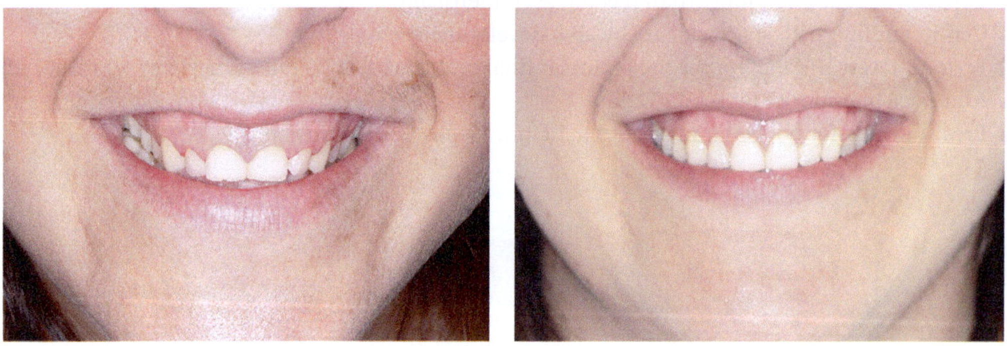

Fig. 19.136 Pretreatment and final smile.

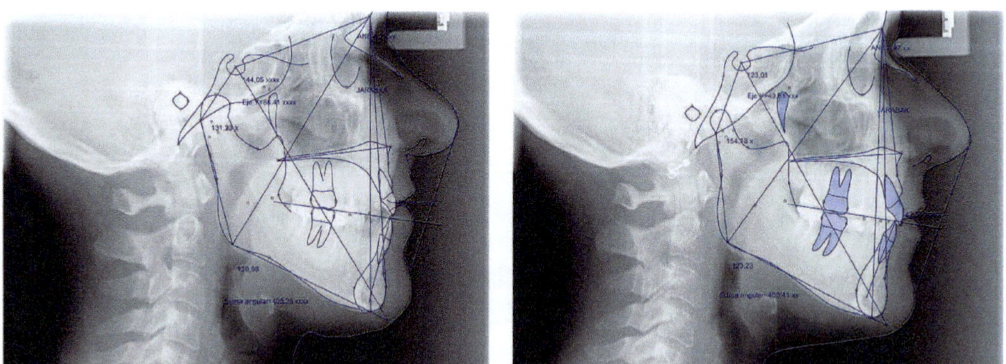

Fig. 19.137 Initial and final cephalometric measurements, with the final position of the upper lip improved thanks to anterior torque correction and creation of overjet.

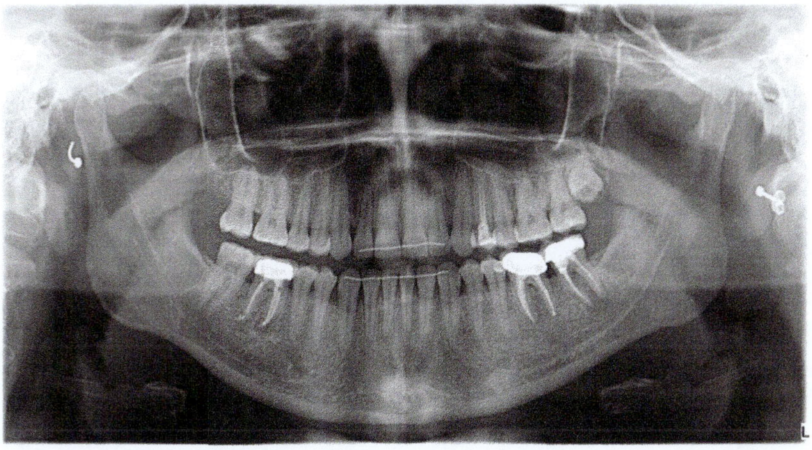

Fig. 19.138 Final panoramic X-ray. Patient smile was widened and skeletal bases were properly related as a result of surgical expansion.

19.4 Tips for Transversal Arch Compensation

- Always analyse whether there is a symmetric or an asymmetric expansion, checking the occlusal view, the frontal intraoral view and the gum posterior exposition in the smile.
- Ask the technician to provide symmetric arches at the end of the treatment, both in shape (we suggest parabolic) and torque.
- Do not simultaneously expand both sides in asymmetric compressions, posterior crossbites and asymmetric posterior torque.
- The only simultaneous movement must be the expansion of one side and the change of torque in the other side.
- Consider the arch length reduction made as a secondary effect of every expansion; the bigger the expansion the more arch length reduction will occur. In cases with expansion and reduced overjet ask the technician for 5 degrees of extra labial crown torque to the upper incisors and IPR and retraction of lower incisors to provide enough overjet. This will avoid final premature contacts at the end of the treatment and an iatrogenic posterior open bite at the end of the expansion.
- Always correct the molars and premolars rotations at the same time as expansion is made. For example, ask the technician to rotate mesial-out the first molars until the mesiolabial cusp of first molars occlude with central line of the lower molars in class I.
- In severe compressions, soften molar contact points with a metal strip the same day as the attachments are bonded.
- Check in the ClinCheck posterior view that, after expansion, the palatal upper cusps of the molars occlude in the fossae pits of the lower molars. Ask the cad designer for extra labial root torque in molars during all expansion movement.
- In large expansions, in order to control posterior torque, use horizontal attachments bevelled to gingival of 4 mm in first premolars and molars in order to provide labial root torque during the expansion. Maintain the optimized attachments on canines. If expanding only on one side, on the anchorage side use non-bevelled horizontal attachments and reduce the movement in the other side to half speed.

20

Sagittal Discrepancies

Every time we face a sagittal discrepancy on a patient occlusion, a comprehensive treatment should be required to fully develop aligners capacity to achieve an ideal occlusion.

Several specific features have been developed by Align Technology for this purpose, which are summarized below.

Passive Aligners

Passive aligners designed for the arch with fewer movements, so as to make the number of aligners equal in both arches, in order to be able to use intermaxillary elastics. They are usually placed by default in all treatment options (shown in light blue in the staging bar in Fig. 20.1).

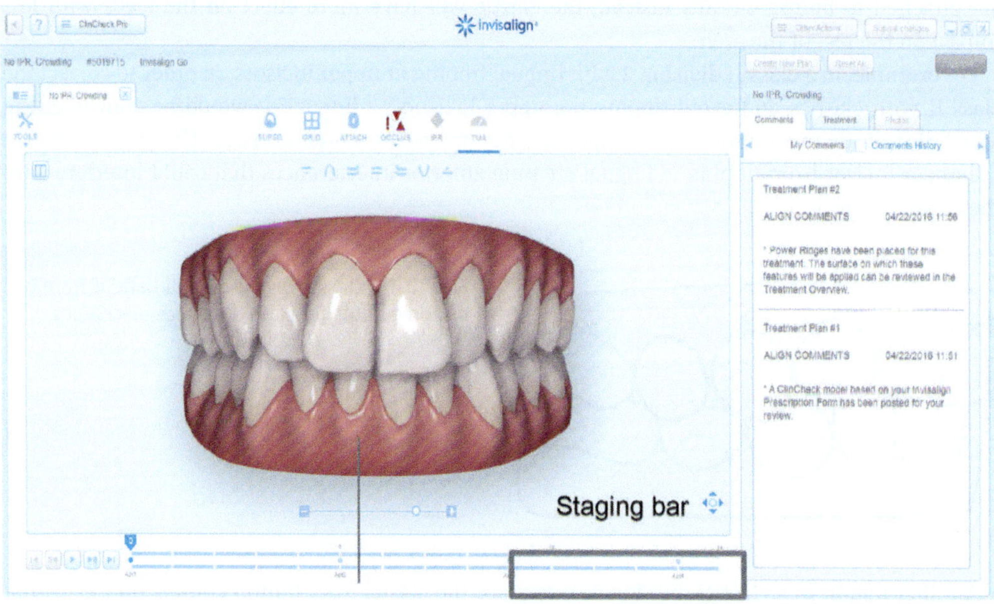

Fig. 20.1 Precision cuts and button cutouts: to hold the intermaxillary elastics.

Aligner Techniques in Orthodontics, First Edition. Susana Palma Moya and Javier Lozano Zafra.

Companion website: www.wiley.com/go/lozano-zafra/aligner-techniques

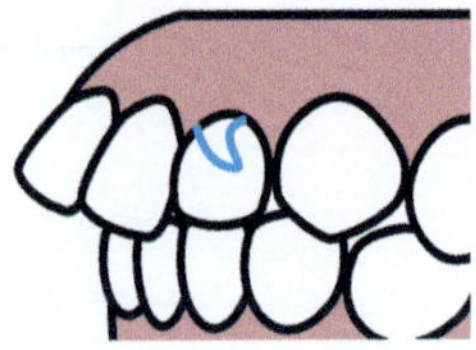

Fig. 20.2 Precision hooks would be equal to archposts in fixed appliances.

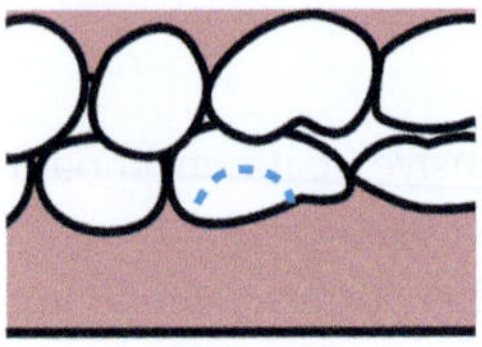

Fig. 20.3 Button cutouts allow bonding a metal/ceramic button.

Precision Cuts

- Class II: on upper canines
- Class III: on lower canines
- Default hook placement can be modified on Clinical preference #14
- Hooks can be prescribed on the buccal surfaces of canines, premolars and molars
- By default, in cases of incompatibility, optimized attachments will be prioritized based on clinical preference

Button Cutouts

- Class II: on lower first molars
- Class III: on upper first molars
- Default, button cutouts placement can be modified on Clinical preference #14
- Button cutouts can be prescribed on the buccal and palatal/lingual surfaces of canines, premolars and molars
- By default, in cases of incompatibility, optimized attachments will be prioritized based on clinical preference

Precision Cuts Versus Button Cutouts The difference between a precision cut and a button cutout is the effect they have on the rest of the teeth of that arch. The effect of the elastics, whenever they are held in a precision cut, will be on the tipping of the incisor of that arch, whereas if the elastics are attached to button cutouts instead, the elastic will have more effect on the teeth with less impact on the rest of the arch.

For example, in a class II division 2 with lingual tipping of upper incisors, in order to correct the class II with elastics and avoid tipping the upper incisors to lingual, it would be convenient to attach the elastic to a button on the upper canines instead of a precision cut. This would prevent the upper incisor from tipping to lingual creating anterior interferences that could interfere with the class II correction.

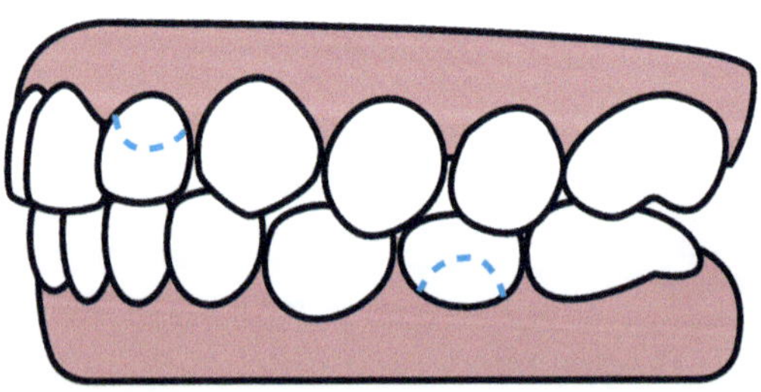

Fig. 20.4 Class II division 2 will benefit from two button cutouts for class II elastics mechanics.

Another option in a class II division 2, is to place the elastic from button cutouts on upper first premolars to button cutouts on second lower molar. If the force is moved to a more distal tooth in the arch, the effect on the upper incisors will be reduced.

In contrast, in a class II division 1 with labial tipping of upper incisors at the beginning of the treatment, the class II side effect of tipping the upper incisor to lingual would be beneficial, so for that purpose the class II elastic from precision cut would be placed on the upper canines to button cutouts on first lower molars.

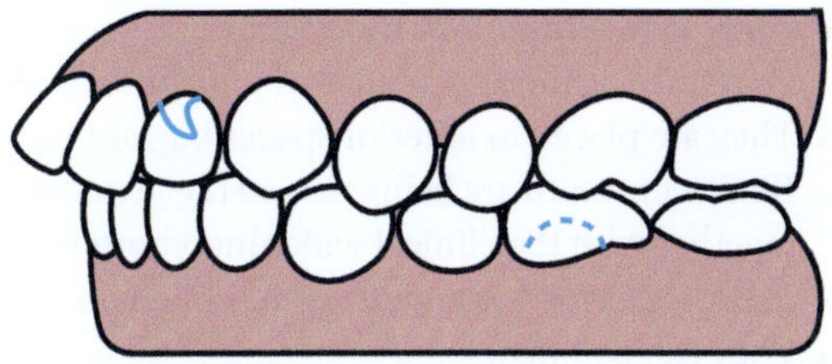

Fig. 20.5 Class II division 1 will benefit from canine hook and molar button for class II elastics mechanics.

Rotating Canines with Elastics For this very same reason, if at the beginning of a class II treatment, the upper canine is rotated mesial-out, instead of placing the aesthetic button on the labial surface of the upper canine, which would cause an increase in the rotation of the canine during the class II correction, it would be better placed on the lingual surface of the tooth: in this way canine rotation will be corrected at the same time as the class II correction.

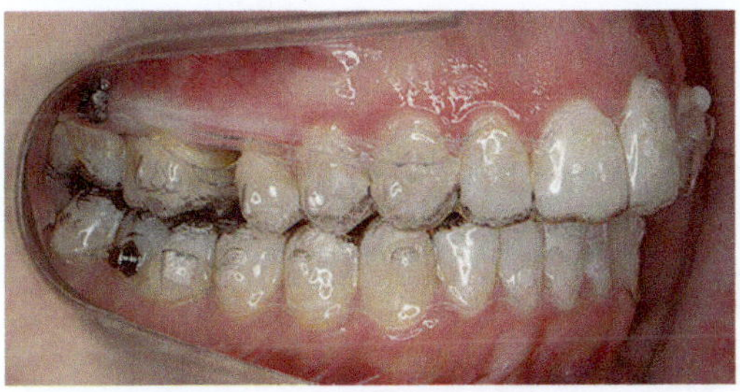

Fig. 20.6 Mesial-in rotation of the canine.

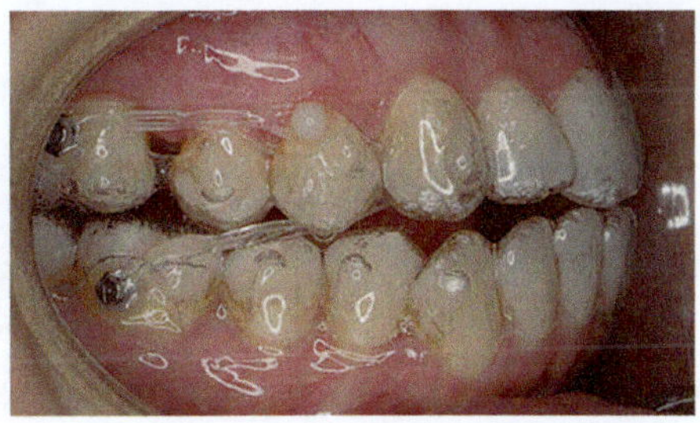

Fig. 20.7 Mesial-out rotation of the canine.

- If the upper canine is initially rotated mesial-in, place the precision cut from labial
- If the upper canine is initially rotated mesial-out, bond a button in the lingual surface of the upper canine and place the elastic from the lingual surface in order to provide a mesial-in rotation at the same time that the class II is corrected

Providing Labial Crown Torque to Upper Canine with the Elastics

- The same happens in narrow arches with 13 and 23 with lingual tipping of the crown
- At the same time that the class II is corrected with the intermaxillary elastic, if an aesthetic button is placed on the lingual surface of the upper canine, both canines can be provided with labial crown tipping and the smile widened at the same time

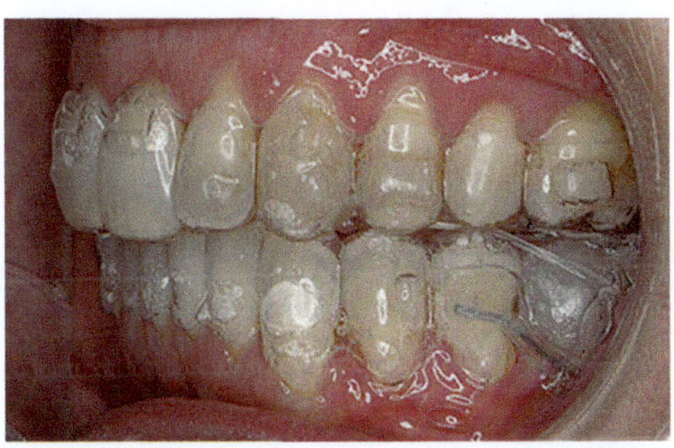

Fig. 20.8 Whenever a lingual button is placed on the lingual surface of the upper canines, class II elastics will be providing crown tipping and smile widening simultaneously.

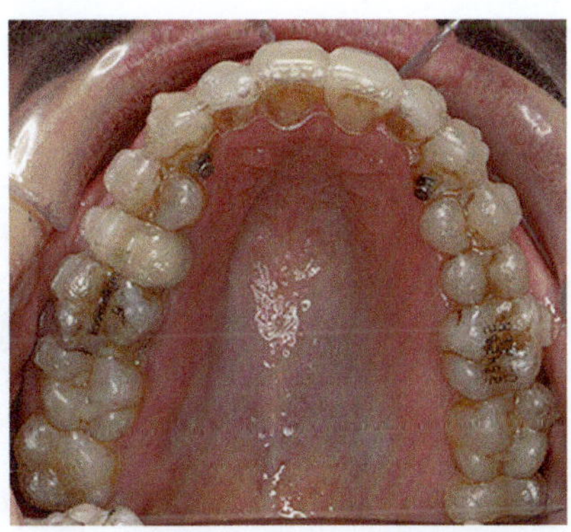

Fig. 20.9 Occlusal view of lingual buttons on upper canines.

Pontics: to Substitute a Missing Tooth

- To minimize the appearance of a missing tooth during treatment
- They are placed in anterior spaces bigger than 4 mm
- If adjacent teeth are being moved (i.e. extraction cases), pontics adjust their width automatically together with the clinical widening/shortening
- Preferences for pontics can be modified on Clinical preferences #6
- They can be filled:
- With temporary teeth resin (self-curing)
- With flow composite (cure the composite from the labial surface of the aligner and not from occlusal because the composite cures toward the light and would get detached from the aligner)
- With tooth-coloured dental wax

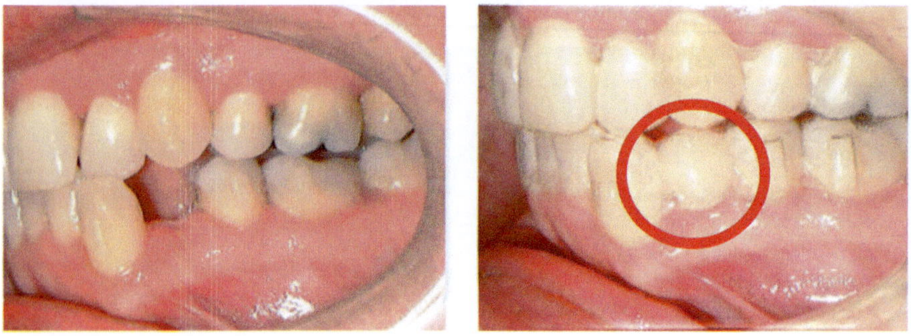

Fig. 20.10 Pontic to cover missing 34.

Pontic Selection Criteria

- In cases of extractions it is better to ask for a small pontic or no pontic at all so the aligner wraps around the teeth better and provides a better control of the root tipping. The clinician will need to fill all the aligners, as in this case there is no change to fill one in and ask the patient to use the resin for the whole set of aligners, due to the fact that it is reducing its size during the closure of the extraction space.
- If the missing tooth is a molar, and we have to upright the second molar, do not use a pontic and ask for a bar instead, this will enable the aligner to wrap the second molar by mesial and it will help upright the tipped molar.
- Included canines: semipontic by palatal.

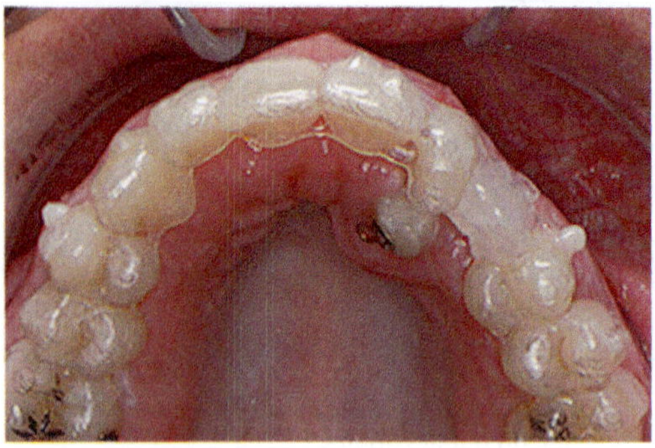

Fig. 20.11 Traction of impacted canine using elastic from button in canine to the aligner by labial.

- Ectopic canines: extract virtually and ask for a pontic with its cuspid parallel to occlusal plane, and a big one if it overlaps the lateral incisor.

20.1 Filling the Prescription form for Class II/III Patients

To do this, first define the treatment goal:

- Do you want to maintain the class II?
- Do you want to achieve canine class I?
- Do you want to achieve canine and molar class I?

With that in mind, click whether to maintain anterior–posterior relationship, improve canine relationship only, improve it up to 4 mm or correct to both molar and canine class I.

After this, if a class I is to be achieved, you will have to define how you want to do it.

For this the following options can be selected:

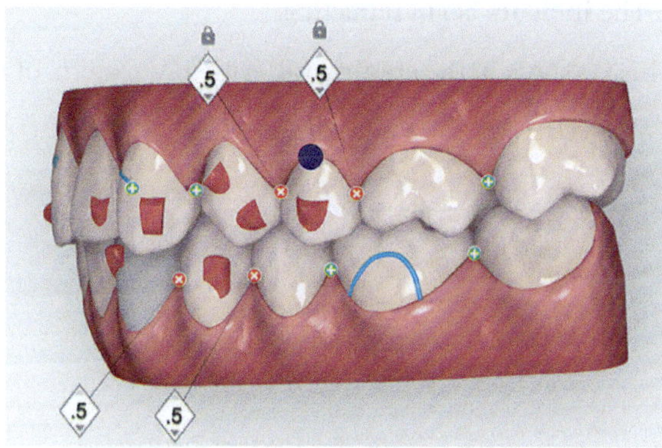

Fig. 20.12 Interproximal reduction can be performed on upper premolars to distalize, or in lower ones to mesialize posterior sector, after considering lower canine to be 'unmovable'.

- Posterior IPR: with a maximum value of 0.5 mm on each contact point from 3 to 6
- Class II or class III correction simulation (virtual jump) to simulate the effect of the intermaxillary elastics:
  - virtual jump will be shown at the end of the treatment in a single stage shift in the ClinCheck. The result should be shown to the patient in case compliance on the use of elastics is not enough
  - the technician could also be asked to simulate the virtual jump throughout the treatment, instead of doing it at the final stage

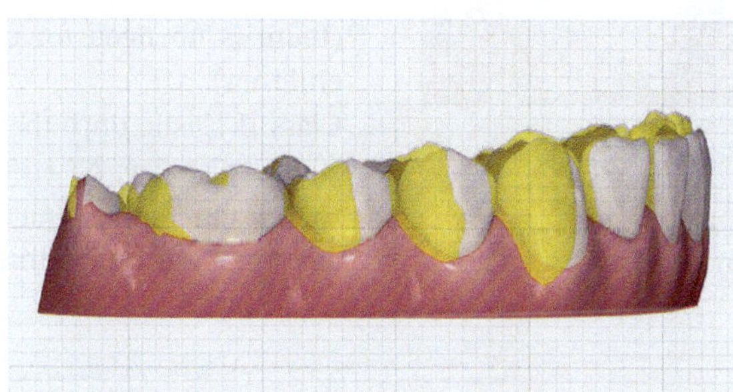

Fig. 20.13 With the use of class II or class III elastics, visualization will be shown throughout the treatment to simulate the simultaneous AP corrections.

- Sequential distalization: distalizing tooth by tooth the upper arch (class II) or the lower one (class III):
  - Especially indicated for adults with class II, with adequate torque in the posterior teeth or positive torque, with no constricted arches, without a torque problem in the upper canines or important rotation of first upper molars.
  - When the possibility of compensating part of the class II by transversal compensation and mesial-out rotation of the first molars is not available, sequential distalization is needed to correct the buccal relationship into a class I.

It is suggested that staging of sequential distalization should be moving towards the distal half of the total movement of the first tooth before starting distalization of the following one.

- The **upper 7s** begin distalizing and when they achieve half of their amount of distalization.
- The **upper 6s** begin distalizing and when they achieve half of their amount of distalization.
- The **upper 5s** begin distalizing and when they achieve half of their amount of distalization.
- The **upper 4s** begin distalizing and when they achieve half of their amount of distalization.
- The **upper 3s** begin distalizing and when they achieve half of their amount of distalization.
- The **incisors** begin retracting.

This is shown in the **staging tab** with a 'V pattern' of movements.

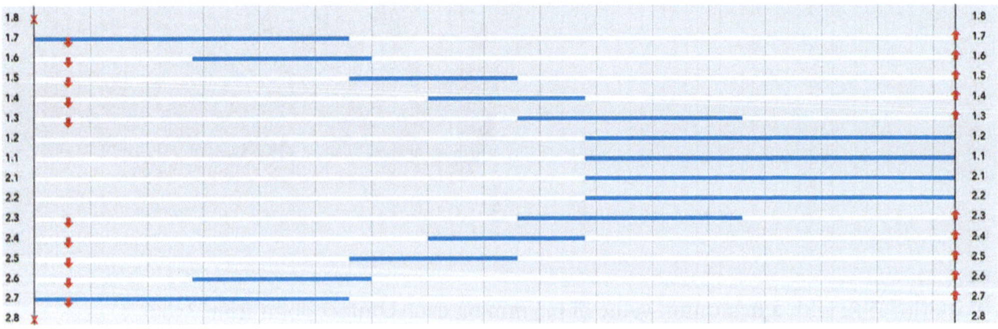

Fig. 20.14 From a 'left 90 degrees view' the sequential distalization is seen as a 'V'.

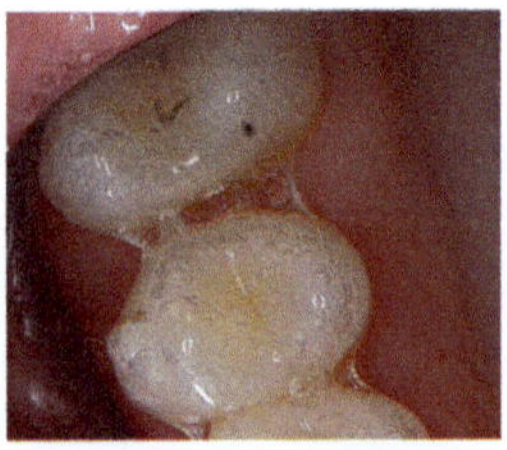

Fig. 20.15 Sequential distalization increases surface contact with molars on their mesial surface.

- The technician should be asked to apply lingual root torque to the upper incisors during all the retraction movement to compensate for the loss of upper torque during the retraction
- Extraction of upper (class II) or lower (class III) third molars (there is no need for extraction if they are still growing, as in children)
- Class II elastic until the moment that the second upper premolars start to distalize; AT HBG horizontal attachments bevelled to gingival of 3 mm in the lingual surface of upper incisors can provide extra anterior anchorage during the sequential distalization

Indications for Sequential Distalization

- *Teen*: full class II with normal or labial torque of premolars and molars (wide arches) where there is little or no possibility of transversal compensation
- *Adults*: incomplete class II (if patient has a full class II, simultaneous distalization using temporary attachment devices (TADs) can be an option to reduce the treatment time)

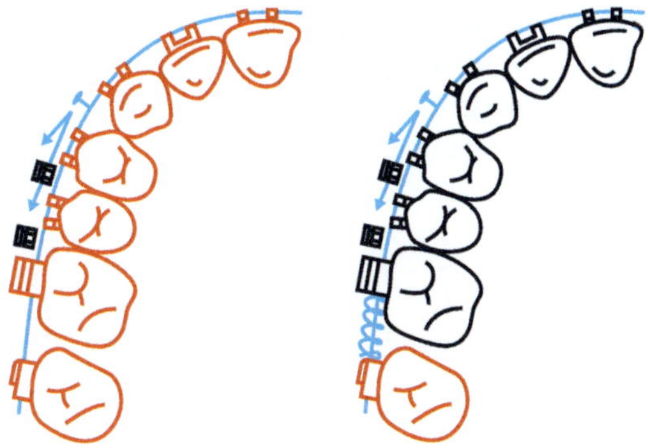

Fig. 20.16 Effect of a coil spring, opening space is similar to sequential distalization with aligners.

Considerations for Sequential Distalization

Sequential distalization would be equal to distalization of upper teeth with a coil spring mesial to those teeth.

With brackets and wires this would imply two side-effects:

- A lack of torque control
- Anterior protrusion effect

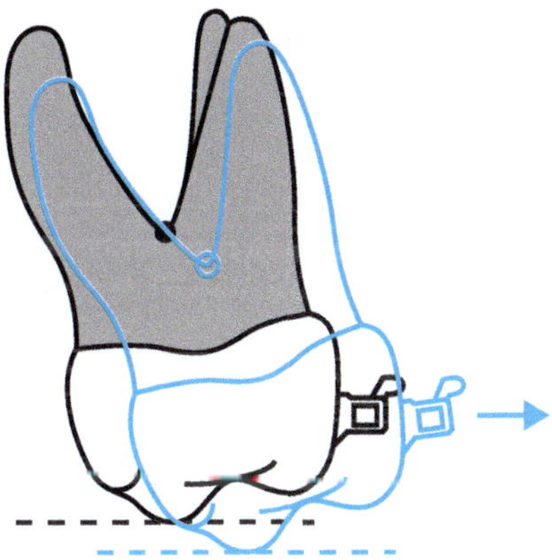

Fig. 20.17 Effect of a coil spring, opening space would lead to lack of torque control on adjacent teeth.

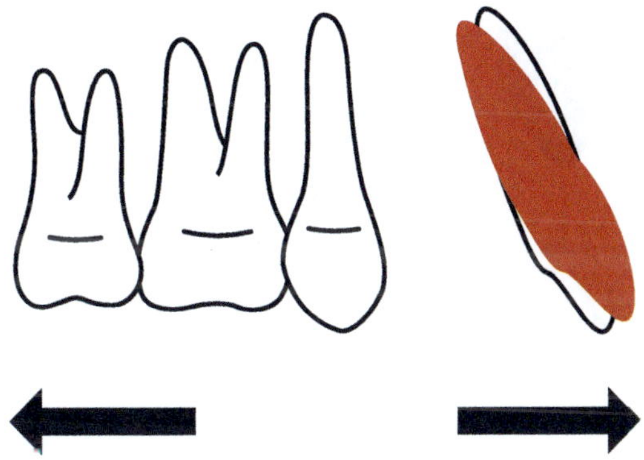

Fig. 20.18 Effect of a coil spring, opening space would lead to anterior proclination.

This last point would be the same with aligners: as aligners increase their 'size' every step of the treatment, there is a protrusion effect on anterior teeth, which will have to be considered in the sequential distalization mechanics.

Mandibular Advancement (MA)

This might be selected for growing patients with mandible hypoplasia, as it is one of the latest innovations developed by Align Technology to achieve the same results as functional appliances by advancing mandible position.

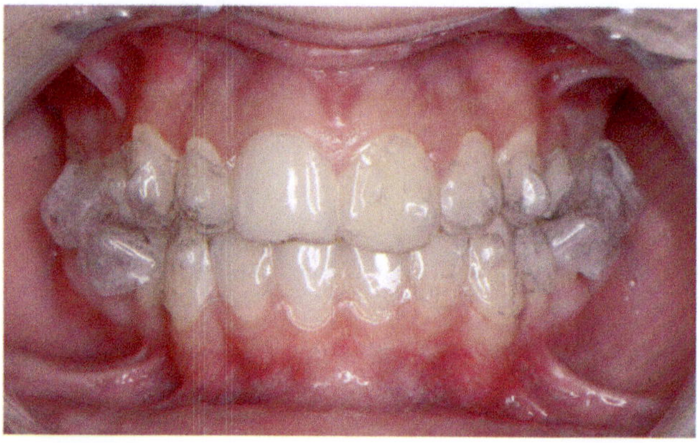

Fig. 20.19 Posterior power wings on aligner help advancing mandible on growing patients.

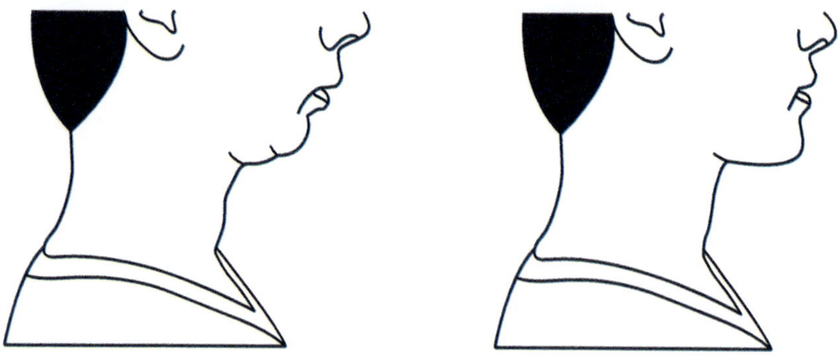

Fig. 20.20 Class II profiles will benefit from this feature.

Orthognathic Surgical Simulation

For surgical simulation, we will have visualization at the end of treatment unless requested at the beginning of treatment. It will also be shown as a single-stage shift in the ClinCheck model.

In which treatments are we going to need intermaxillary elastics?

When asking for correction of the class II with elastics so the technician makes a *virtual jump* to simulate the elastics effect:

- The clinician should start with the elastics as soon as possible, as in this type of correction the number of aligners is reduced by the virtual jump, so it is necessary to have a transversal development of the arches first and enough overjet to begin with the intermaxillary elastics.
- In sequential distalization:
  - the clinician should start with the elastics when the second premolars begin to distalize, at the latest.
- In MA cases during the advance phase, with night use,
  - this will help to hold the precision wings in place during the night, preventing the patient from opening his mouth and preventing the distortion of the precision wings due to the parafunctional movement of the mandible during the night.

20.2 Class II Cases

Class II malocclusion affects 12–32% of the population, a fact that has motivated the development of several treatment approaches during the last decades, involving removable or fixed appliances with or without teeth extractions.

Sagittal discrepancies are usually named according to Edward Angle's classification of malocclusions based on the relationship between the upper and lower permanent first molars. Angle's classification of class II subjects into division 1 and 2 groups is still commonly used.

The development of class II malocclusion might be linked to several factors; hence, accurate diagnosis is important for the selection of the corresponding treatment plan. Among these factors, mandibular retrognathia is considered a dominant one, which makes aligners the best treatment option on growing patients, as mandibular advancement might be performed at the same time as teeth alignment.

There are also several advantages linked to aligners for adults, such as sequential distalization with differential anchorage, which might be combined with the use of elastics, which is almost the only option for distalization with brackets and wires, which have a more limited range of treatment options.

20.2.1 Considerations for Class II Patients

- Favourable skeletal pattern for a class II correction will be a normodivergent or hypodivergent skeletal pattern
- Key to the correction of class II cases is the possibility of transversal compensation: the more constricted the arches are at the beginning, the better the prognosis
- The third upper molars usually need to be extracted if the correction is going to be prescribed by sequential upper distalization
- Appropriate torque of the upper and lower incisors must be ensured before the corrections: overtreat the correction of the torque on the upper incisor up to +17 degrees and upright the lower incisor up to -1 degree. The goal of this overcorrection is to provide positive overjet to correct the class II
- If the anterior overjet is less than the distance necessary to correct the class II in the molars, it will not be possible to achieve a final class I relationship, for that purpose before starting to use class II elastic, enough positive anterior overjet should be provided
- In the class II division 2, the upper incisors torque is essential for the correction. The more retroclined the upper incisors are, the more posterior anchorage will be needed. This is the reason why, in some severe class II division 2, a posterior microscrew is needed to provide enough posterior anchorage for the correction
- Sequential upper distalization can be requested, together with the expansion and rotation corrections
- Distalization and protrusion of the incisors should be sequenced to prevent losing posterior anchorage during the distalization; alternatively, distalization can be done simultaneously with proclination movement of the incisors (labial crown torque) and correction of rotation movements of the incisors (aesthetic start)
- Before correcting a class II, the staging of movement on the incisors should be considered:
  - *Class II division 2*: remove first the root of upper incisor from the cortical bone. First procline and then apply retrusion, intrusion and lingual root torque

- Procline crown (which is eqivalent to taking the root out of the cortical bone)
- Intrusion
- Retrusion + lingual root torque

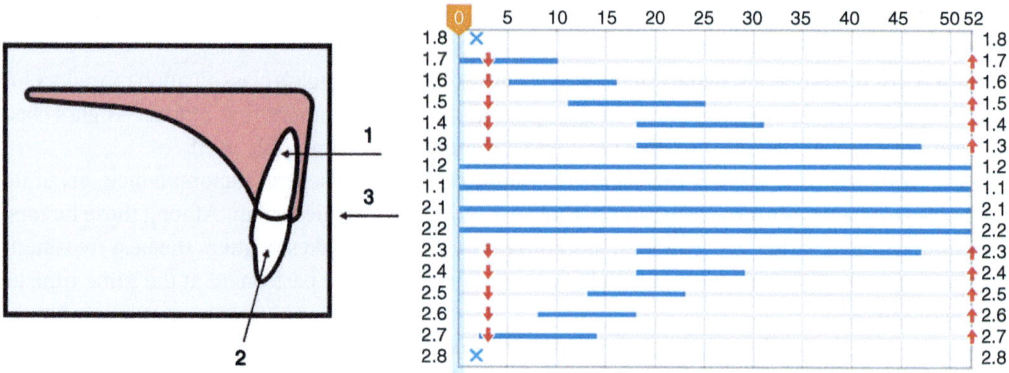

Fig. 20.21 Class II division 2 incisors need treatment sequence like this: procline crown, intrude, retrude. This makes the 'V' pattern change, owing to anterior incisor movement.

- *Class II division 1*: First ensure the four upper incisors, torque is the same and then apply retrusion, intrusion and lingual root torque. Note that the more lingually torqued the four upper incisors are, the more posterior anchorage we will need:
  - The same torque for the four incisors
  - Simultaneous movement: Intrusion + retrusion + lingual root torque

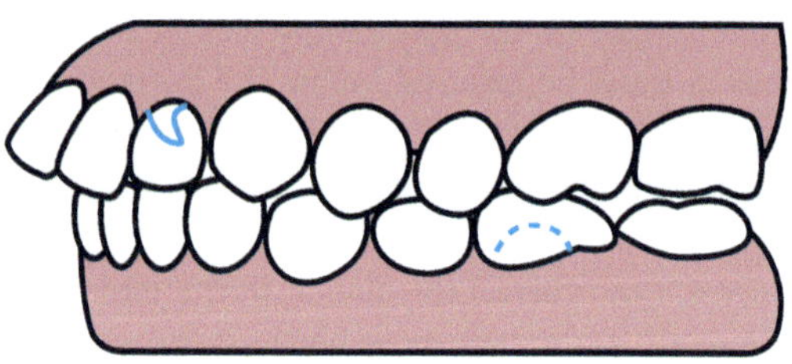

Fig. 20.22 Class II division 2 incisors need a treatment sequence such as: procline crown, intrude, retrude.

Treatment Options for Class II Patients

Our protocol to correct class II cases is outlined here:

- **Mandibular advancement** (mandibular hypoplasia in growing patients)
- **Expansion + virtual jump** (teenage patients with narrow arches and incomplete class II)
- **Upper sequential distalization** (adults with incomplete class II and teenagers with full class II and without many possibilities of transversal compensation)
- **Upper simultaneous distalization** assisted with TAD (adults with full class II or class II division 2)
- **Lower simultaneous mesialization** assisted with TAD or Locatelli (adults with mandibular hypoplasia and retruded profile). These will be shown in the multidisciplinary treatments in Chapters 22 and 24

Extra Resources for Class II Patients

As with brackets and wires, patient condition might make it more favourable to solve the class II situation than just upper distalization or lower mesialization. This is summarized in Table 20.1.

Expansion

As upper arch expansion is higher on upper arch, arch depth reduction is also greater than in the lower arch, leading to an overjet reduction as a result of the 'pearl necklace effect', with an estimated 0.5 mm class II reduction.

Table 20.1 Extra resources for class II patients

Resource	Maximum effect
Expansion	0.5 mm
Molar rotation	1 mm
IPR	2 mm
Upper distalization	4 mm
Upper distalization + TAD	8 mm
Lower mesialization	2 mm
Extractions	8 mm

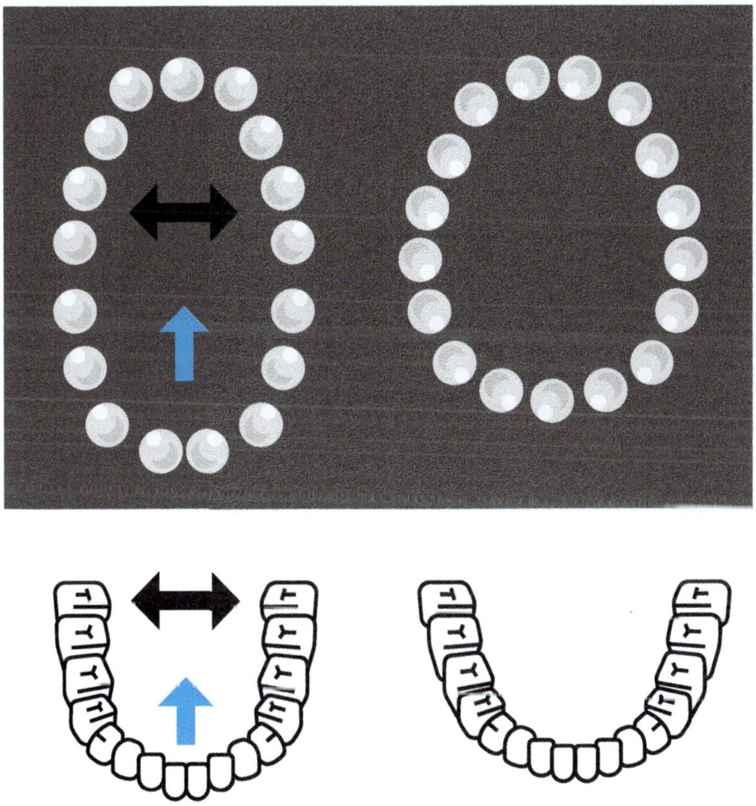

Fig. 20.23 Upper expansion leads to higher arch depth reduction and resolving of class II.

Molar Derotation

Severe upper first molars rotation can result in these teeth using more space in the upper arch than predicted, leading to an increased class II anterior–posterior relationship. This therefore is a simple way of reducing the amount of class II.

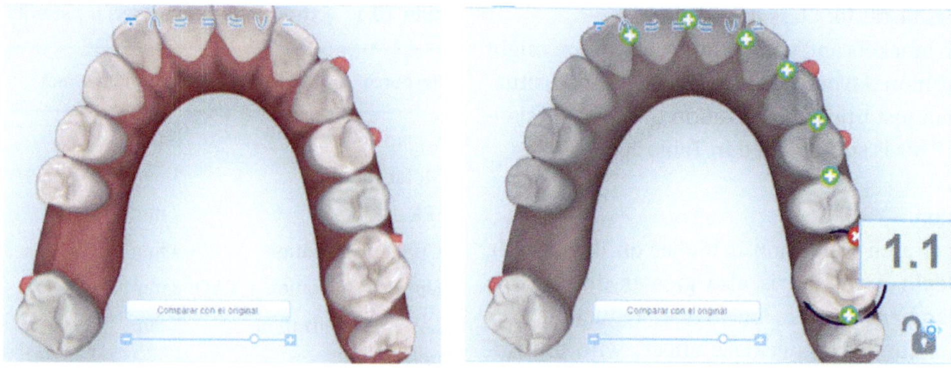

Fig. 20.24 ClinChecks: a 45 degree upper molar derotation solves up to 1 mm class II. For this, a vertical bevelled to mesial attachment or an optimized rotation attachment on affected molars is suggested.

Upper Distalization

This might happen predictably up to 4 mm on upper arch, and can be managed for a full class II patient with skeletal anchorage with TADs as an auxiliary technique. Once again, it is important to understand that without TADs there is always a proclination effect on anterior incisors whenever posterior sectors are distalized.

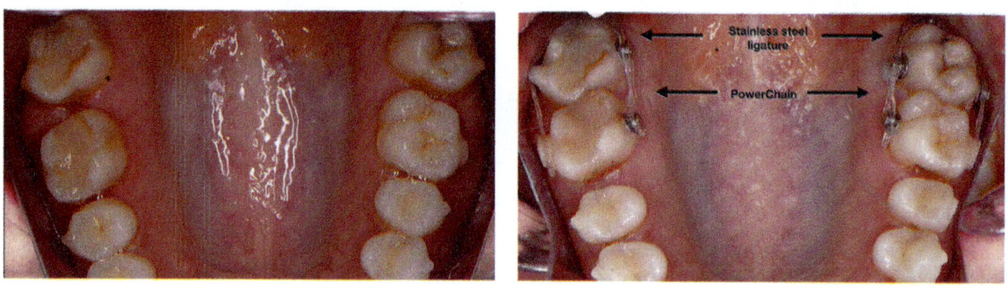

Fig. 20.25 Intraoral views: a 45 degree upper molar derotation solves up to 1 mm class II. For this, a vertical bevelled to mesial attachment or an optimized rotation attachment on affected molars is suggested.

Lower Mesialization

This is an effect of the use of elastics to lower molars, which make the same mesialization as previously achieved with brackets and wires. For this reason, the use of elastics will have to be based on lower incisor proclination with regard to mandibular bone and cephalometric values, as will be shown in the clinical case later in this chapter.

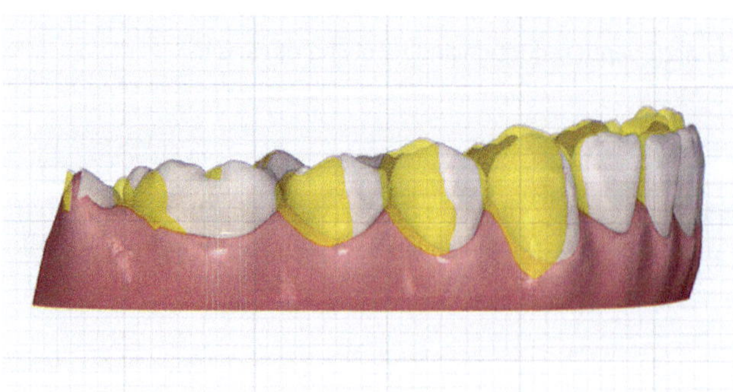

Fig. 20.26 Lower mesialization is represented in yellow, and results from the use of intermaxillary elastics.

Extractions

Again, classic resources for patients with braces can be used with aligners, while considering different biomechanical approaches because of the differences between techniques.

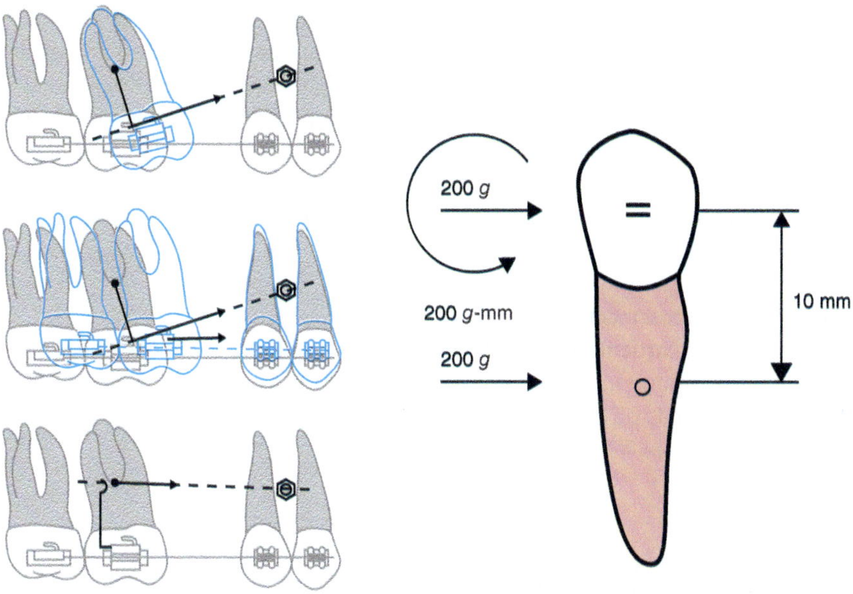

Fig. 20.27 Biomechanics is the basis of an orthodontic treatment, regardless of which technique is used, there may be similar results, such as a bowing effect after posterior mesialization, resulting from a lack of force from the centre of resistance of the tooth (on the root, not the crown, where the aligners deliver their force).

Extraction of Wisdom Tooth

It is possible to take advantage of the rapid acceleratory phenomenon (RAP) if extracting upper wisdom teeth before starting distalization, which leads to a natural accelerated osteoblastic procedure.

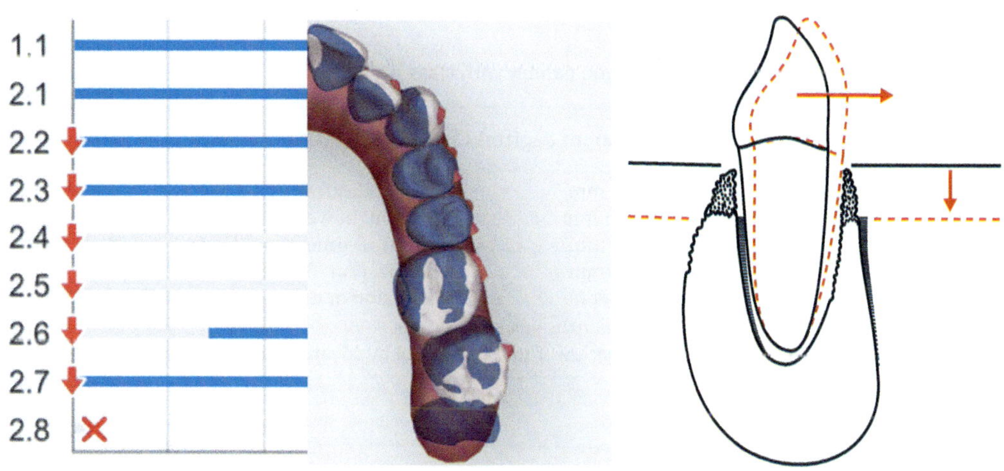

Fig. 20.28 Distalization should start just after wisdom tooth extraction so as to optimize treatment length.

20.2.2 Mandibular Advancement

Mandibular advancement through the use of functional appliances is considered a popular treatment approach in growing individuals, which makes Invisalign Mandibular Advancement a unique tool for practitioners when facing class II growing patients.

While some researchers have found favourable outcomes based on mandibular growth, attributed to either mandibular length augmentation or effective condyle growth, others distrust the magnitude of these effects. Moreover, evidence indicates that the dentoalveolar changes produced by functional treatment outweigh the skeletal changes attained.

That said, as it is not the objective of this book to cover these aspects, the focus will be on Invisalign Mandibular Advancement device characteristics for these patients, which might benefit from a deep knowledge of its protocols.

Ideal Moment for Mandibular Advancement

When treating growing patients, particularly when the objective is to achieve not only orthodontic, but also orthopaedic changes, timing may be more significant than the appliance chosen for the treatment. Optimal timing depends on the skeletal maturation of each individual, which can be accurately determined by using the CVM method of Baccetti.[2]

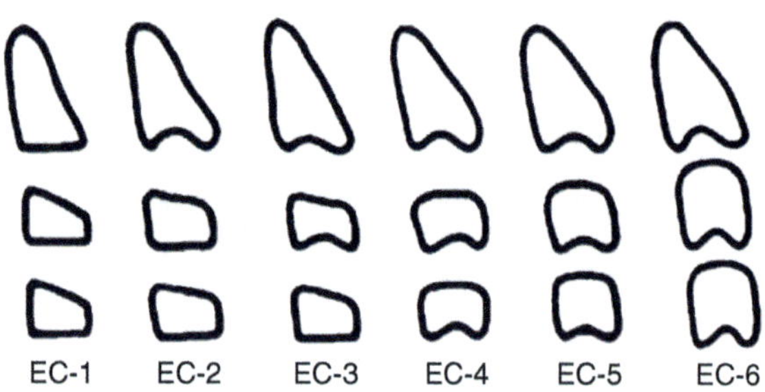

Fig. 20.29 Growth has to be carefully checked before a mandibular advancement.

Baccetti stated that the ideal time to make an orthopaedic treatment was when the patient was in CS3 and CS4 of the maturation in the vertebrae. The protocol we apply when we treat a growing patient with class II is provided in Table 20.2.

Table 20.2 Protocol when treating a growing patient with class II

CS1	**No Permanent Sagittal Correction**	
CS2		
CS3/4	Overjet <3 mm	Class II elastics
	Overjet 3–6 mm	MA + night wear elastics
	Overjet >7 mm	MA + full-time wear elastics
CS5	Overjet <3 mm	Distalization
	Overjet >4 mm	Extraction or distalization with TADs
Second phase	At least 6 months wearing elastics	
Mandibular advancement	Offers better lower incisor control by covering labial surface	

Features of MA

- Aligner features: compensation for eruption and mandibular advancement plus the normal features of treatment of teenage patients
- Aligners and power wings are made of the same proprietary SmartTrack material as Invisalign aligners
- The most characteristic features are the Precision Wings, which are positioned between first molars and premolars
- It is important to consider that in order for the technician to make the precision wing, they need all the premolar erupted or a stable late-mixed dentition

How Does it Work?

- In exactly the same way as a twin-block, the precision wings force the patient to occlude in a forward position, advancing and holding the mandible in a forward position. However, during the night, the only way to hold the mandible in position is by placing class II elastics (our method of using the class II elastic is from lingual to the upper first premolar to labial of the lower second molars). In this way, the elastic does not interfere with the precision wings.
- At the same time that we advance the mandible, the teeth can be levelled and aligned.
- We can ask to show the mandibular advancement with only one jump or gradually.

MA Protocol

Pre-MA Phase (Light Blue Colour)

Purpose:

- Level Spee curve, create >2 mm overjet to allow mandibular advancement
- Other minimal tooth movements to facilitate precision wings placement

Clinical treatment:

- Incisors proclination in division 2
- Anterior intrusion in deep bites
- Molar rotations
- Crossbite corrections

Aligners:

- Standard aligners
- Attachments
- No precision wings

MA Phase (Dark Blue Colour)

Purpose:

- Advance mandible (2mm every 8 aligners)
- Simultaneous tooth movement (limited in teeth covered by precision wings)
- Attachments in molars will be removed
- >26 aligners phase

Clinical treatment:

- Class II correction
- Arch coordination

- Overjet reduction
- Teeth alignment and levelling

Aligners:

- Aligners with precision wings
- Limited features under PW

Transitional Phase (Dark Blue Colour)

Purpose:

- Hold the mandible in advanced position while waiting for additional aligners
- No additional tooth movement
- 4 aligners phase

Clinical treatment:

- Hold the mandible in advanced position

Aligners:

- Aligners with precision wings

Features of Treatment in Teenage Patient

Compensation of Eruption for Canines or Second Premolars

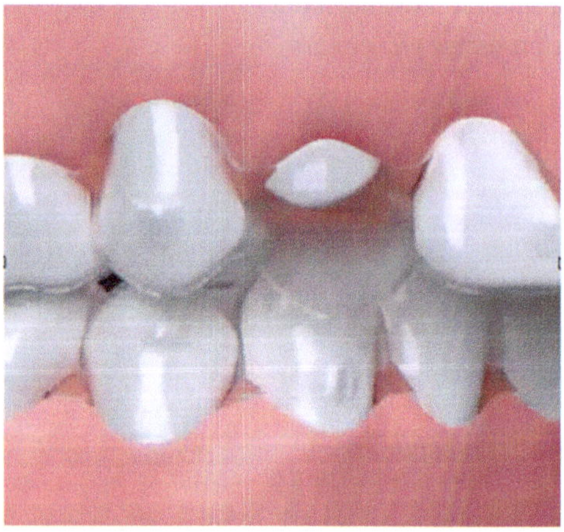

Fig. 20.30 Eruption compensator in a canine.

These are designed to accommodate the natural eruption of canines and second premolars while the patient is wearing aligners, allowing the necessary room for erupting teeth. These are really important as a light force applied to an erupting tooth might interfere in the process, stopping it and altering patient's natural exfoliation process. In the past this used to occur with conventional devices such as the Schwartz removable appliance but, thanks to an algorithm that calculates tooth movement, it no longer happens.

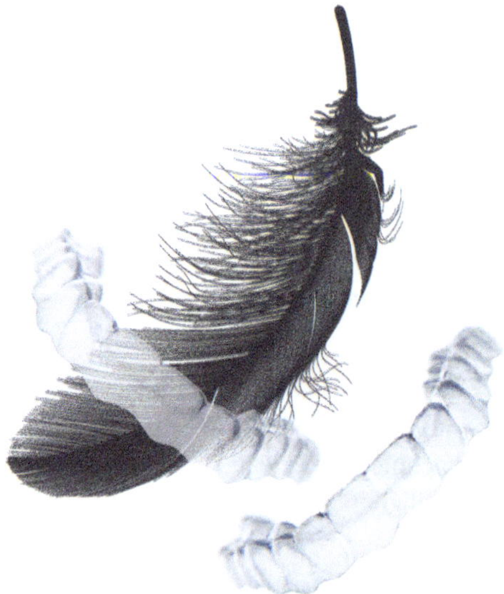

Fig. 20.31 Any contact over 12 g will interrupt the tooth eruption.

Terminal Molar Tabs for Second/Third Molars

The eruption tab extends over the mesial cusp of the terminal molar and helps prevent supra-eruption of the terminal molars.

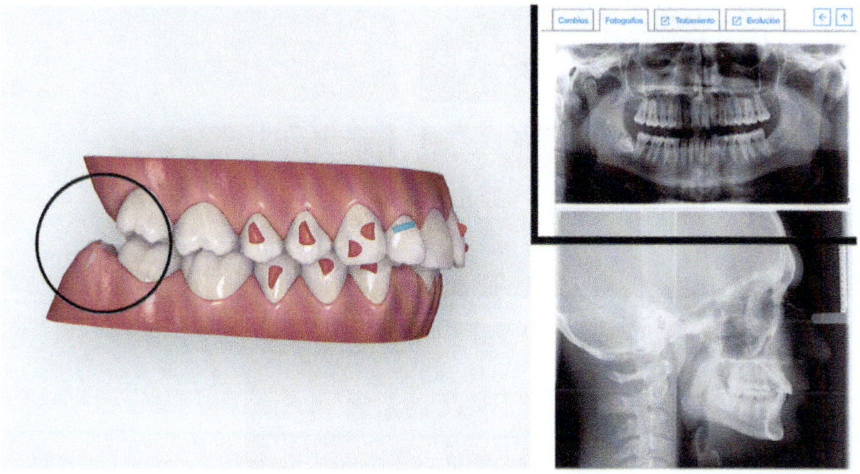

Fig. 20.32 Terminal molar tabs prevent molars supra-eruption creating posterior interference that may lead to an anterior open bite, as used to happen with brackets and wires when wisdom teeth erupted.

20.2.3 Conventional Mandibular Advancement + Aligners

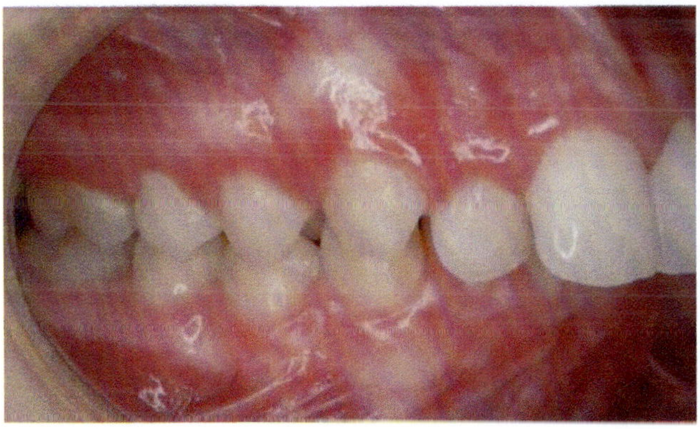

Fig. 20.33 Initial intraoral view.

Diagnosis

A 12-year-old patient presented with a normodivergent skeletal class II with mandibular hypoplasia. They had narrow arches, upper incisor proclination, a deep bite, 10 mm of overjet, labial incompetence and a retruded chin.

Treatment Plan

- This case occurred before the launch of Invisalign MA, so there was a first phase with Herbst appliance and D-Gainer (started on Jan 2014, finished on Nov 2015)
- After the orthopaedic treatment an Invisalign Lite case was made
- Using two devices can now be avoided because the first and second phase can be made with the appliance of MA

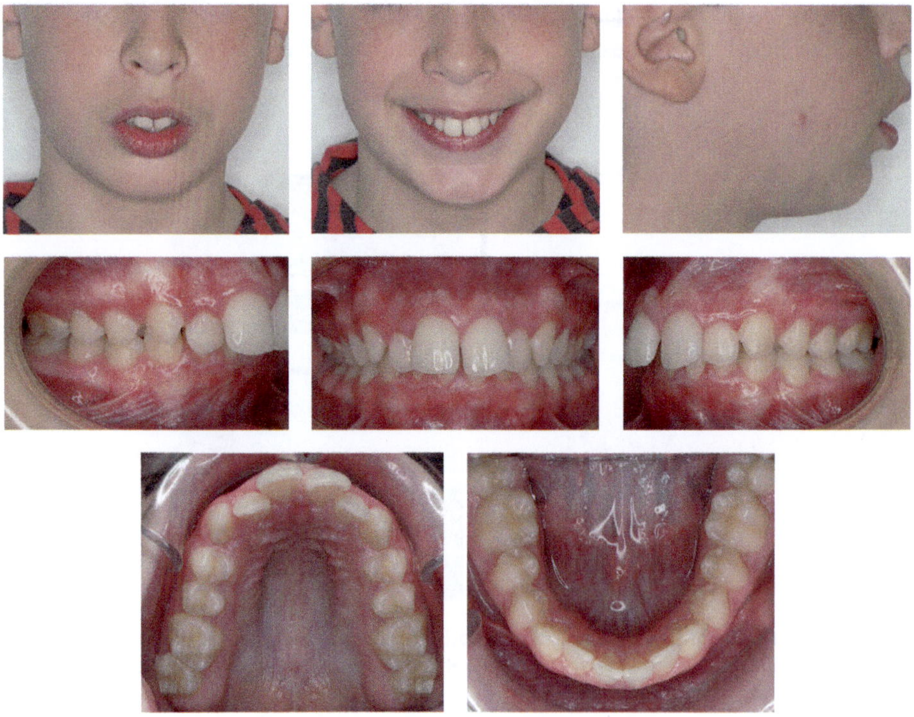

Fig. 20.34 Pretreatment extraoral and intraoral views.

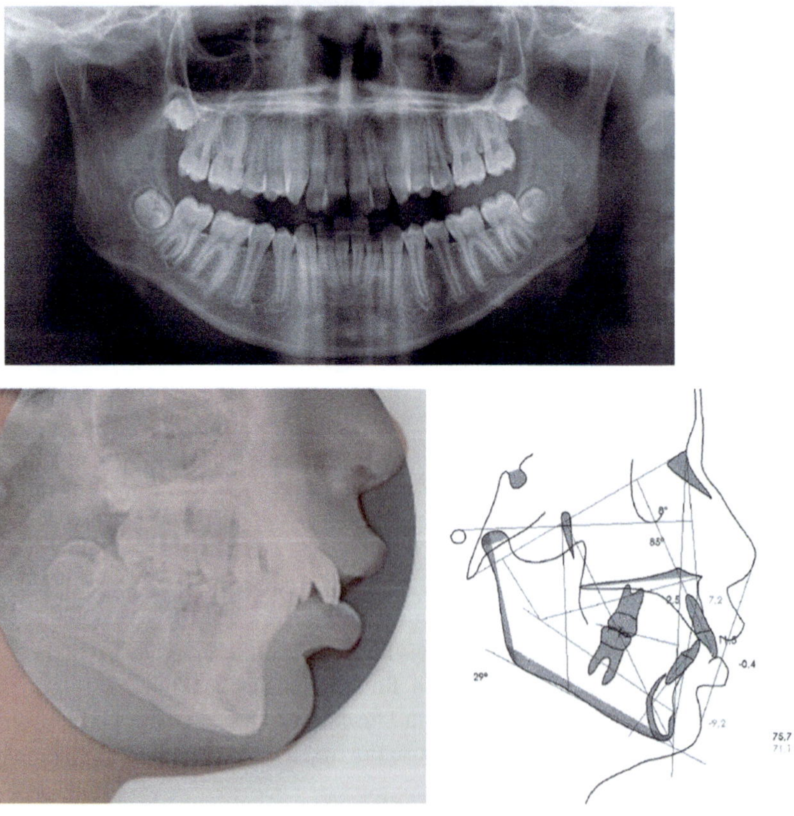

Fig. 20.35 Initial panoramic X-ray, teleradiograph and cephalometry.

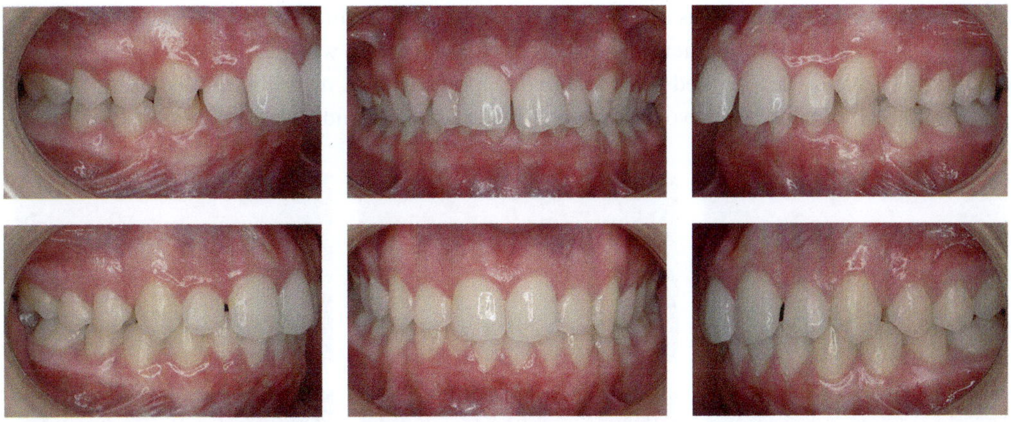

Fig. 20.36 Intraoral situation after Herbst appliance. After the first phase with Herbst appliance, the mandible had advanced into a class I position. Upper diastemas needed to be closed in the second phase.

Requirements for the Technician

- *Maxilla*: As it was necessary to close the upper diastemas without losing torque of upper incisors maximum anchorage in the posterior zone was needed; for that purpose molars were not moved and retrusion, intrusion and lingual root torque were applied to the upper incisors simultaneously.
- *Mandible*: A positive overjet was needed to close upper diastemas, so in order to have adequate anchorage to retrude the lower incisors the lateral zone was not moved; the technician was asked to make IPR on contact points between 33 to 43 and to retrude the lower incisor, applying lingual root torque simultaneously.

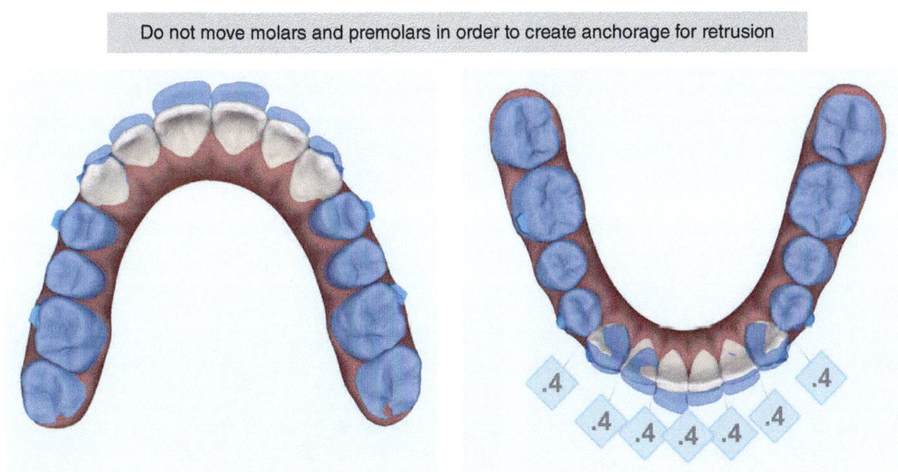

Fig. 20.37 Upper and lower ClinCheck views.

Treatment Summary

- After the first orthopaedic phase a dental class I molar and canine was achieved.
- Time of treatment 1 year and 5 months.
- During Lite treatment the upper diastemas were corrected and both midlines centred.

- The patient needed 14 months of Invisalign treatment: 14 aligners, changed every 14 days and another 14 aligners of refinement. Normal overjet and overbite were achieved.
- 12 and 22 had to be proclined with a D-gainer previously to mandibular advancement with Herbst appliance in order to avoid the interferences for the mandibular protraction.

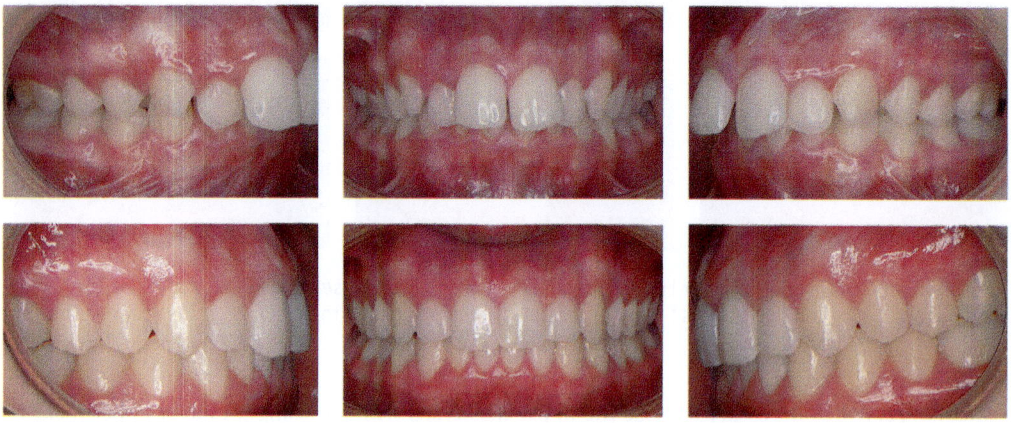

Fig. 20.38 Comparison of initial (upper row) with final result (lower row).

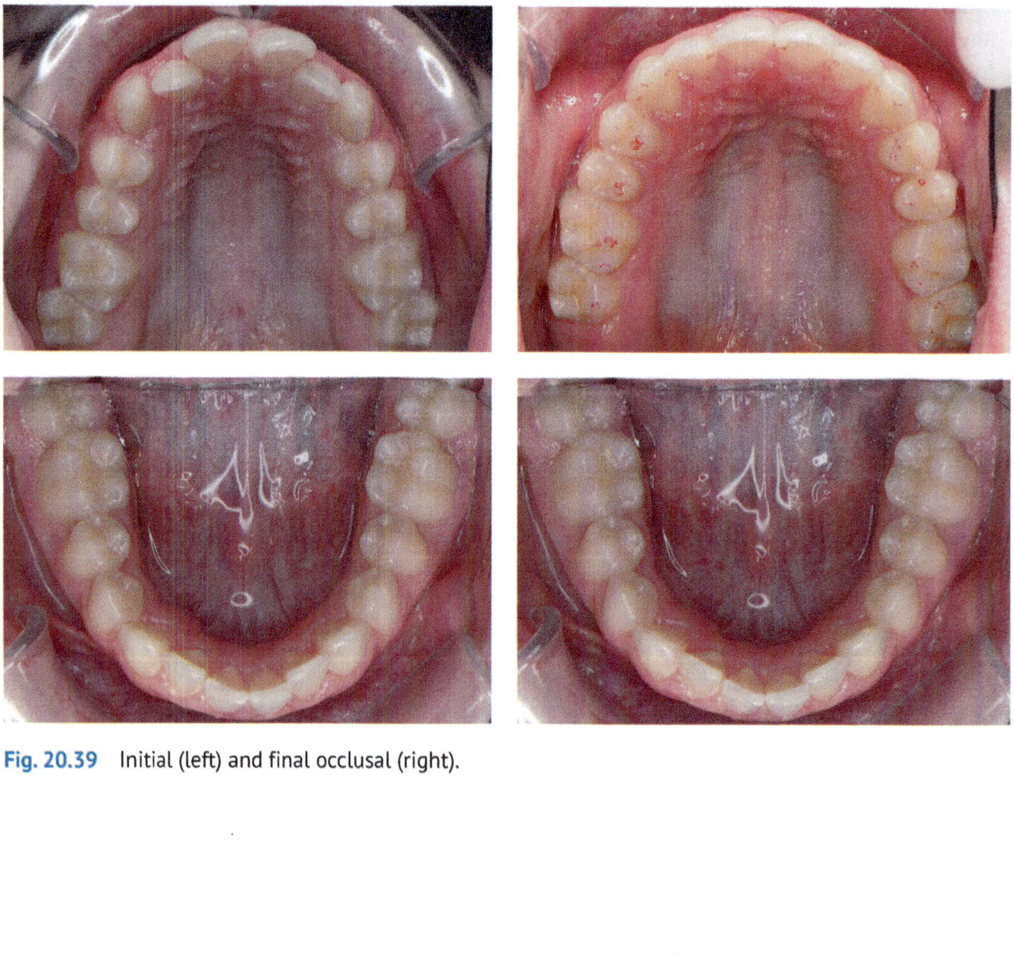

Fig. 20.39 Initial (left) and final occlusal (right).

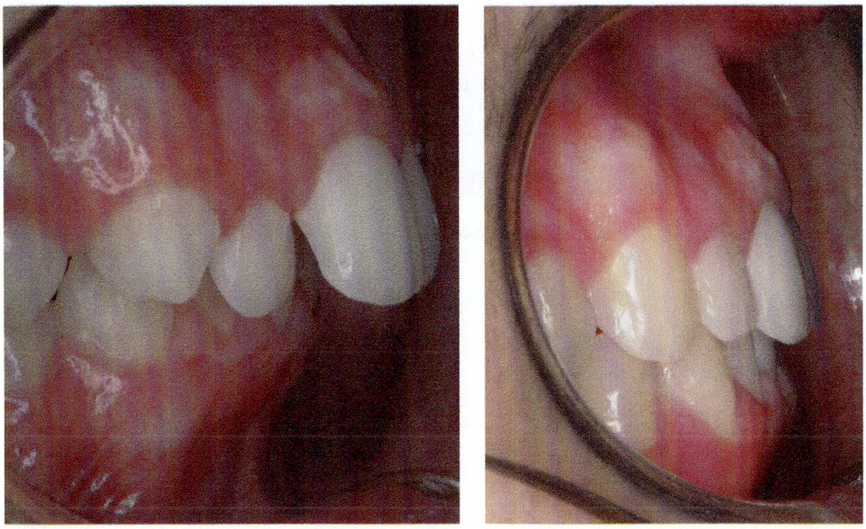

Fig. 20.40 Initial (left) and final overjet (right).

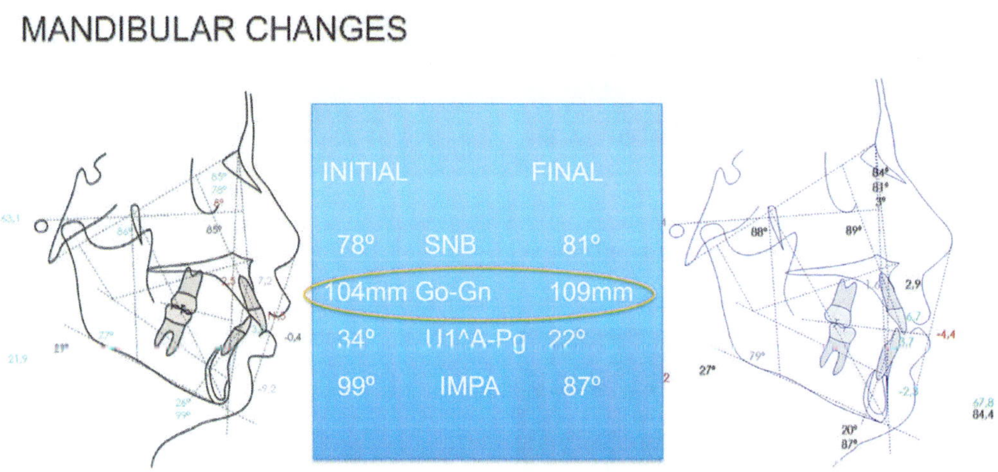

Fig. 20.41 Mandibular changes.

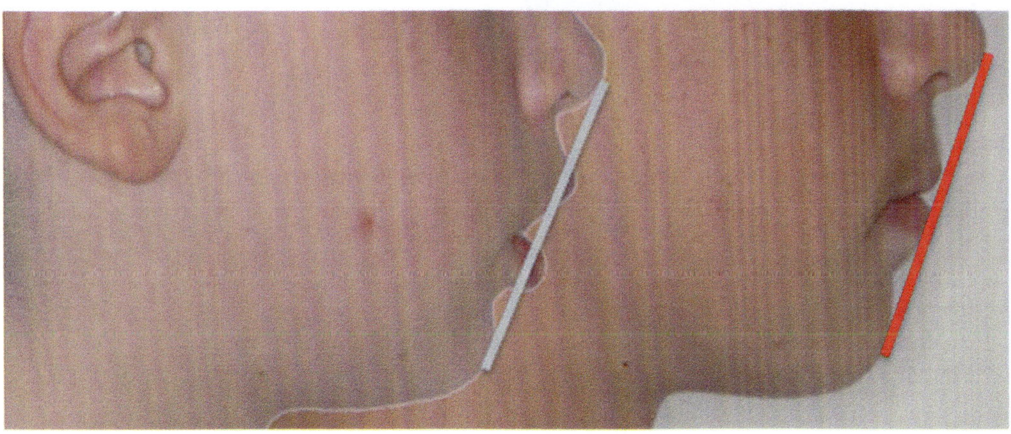

Fig. 20.42 Changes in profile.

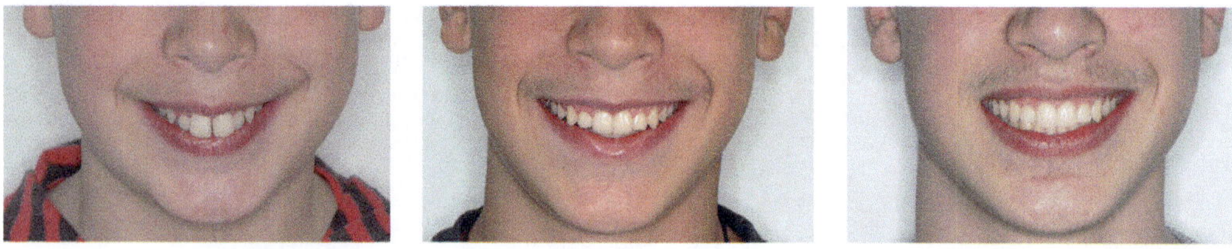

Fig. 20.43 Initial smile (left), smile at the end of first phase (middle) and final smile (right).

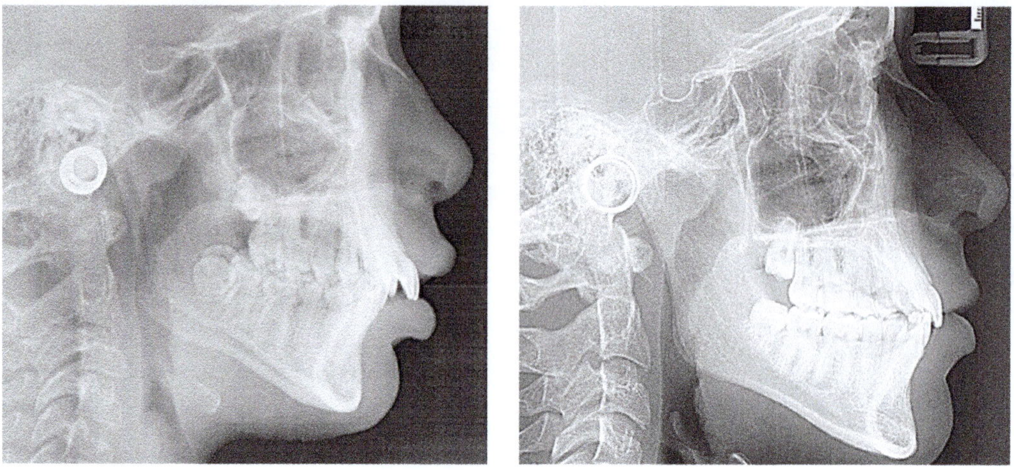

Fig. 20.44 Initial and final lateral X-rays.

20.2.4 Invisalign Mandibular Advancement

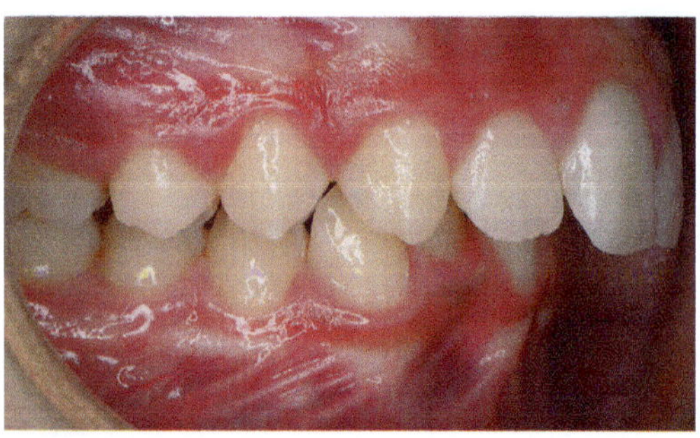

Fig. 20.45 Intraoral initial picture.

Diagnosis

A 14-year-old patient had class II division 1 with mandibular hypoplasia and a bilateral scissor bite. The had a class II profile with labial competence, centred upper midline, 90% deep bite and a 9 mm overjet.

Treatment Plan

- First orthopaedic phase of mandibular advancement with MA to help the mandible grow
- Second Invisalign comprehensive phase once the mandible was in a class I relationship

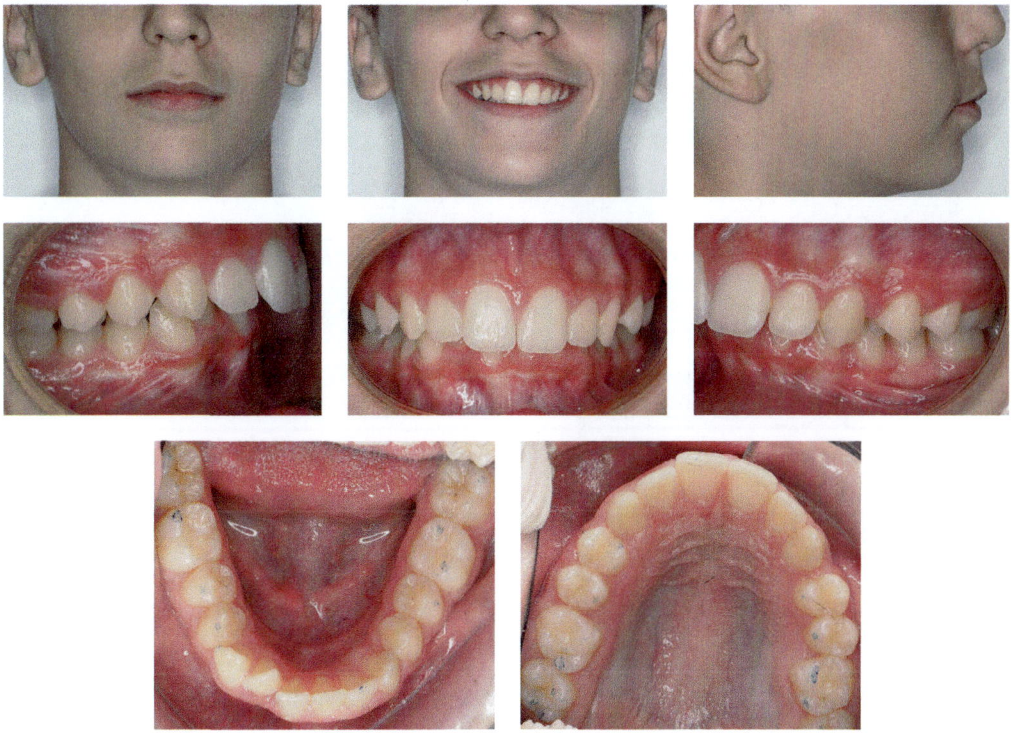

Fig. 20.46 Initial extraoral and intraoral views.

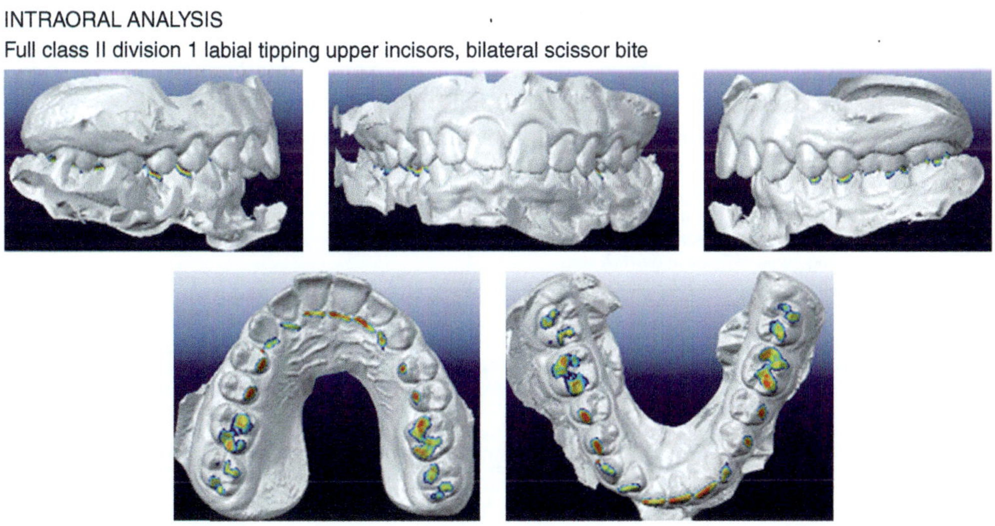

Fig. 20.47 Occlusal contact at the beginning of the treatment.

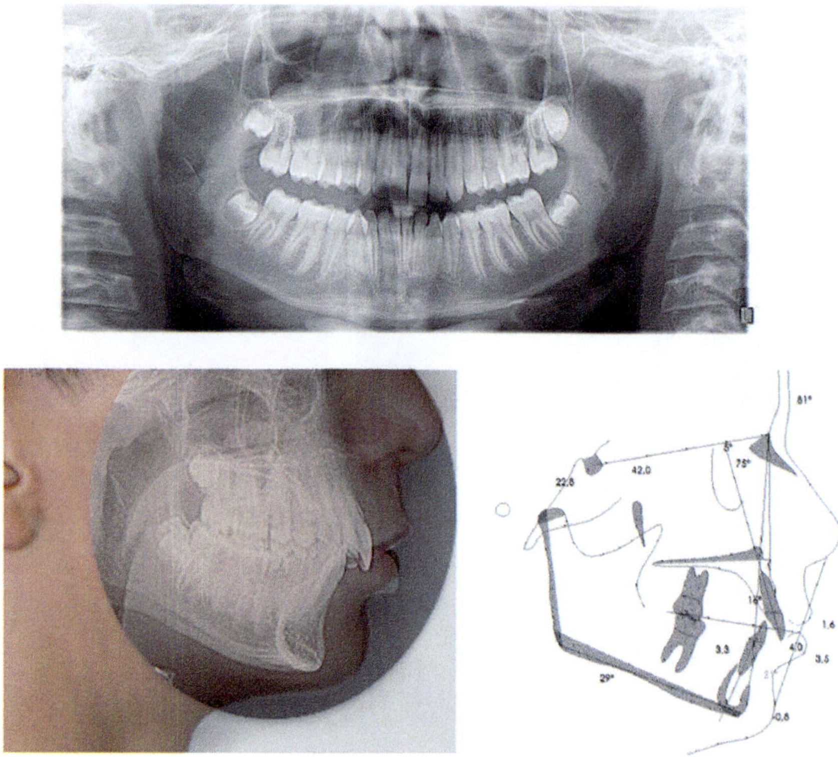

Fig. 20.48 Initial panoramic X-ray, teleradiograph and cephalometry.

Requirements for the Technician

- As there was enough overjet, the MA phase was started straight away without a pre-advancement phase. (As we learned later, this was a mistake, as a pre-advance phase to level the curve of Spee before starting the advance phase is mandatory to avoid future interference when the mandible acquires an advance position and subsequent distortion in the precision wings.)
- Arches to be coordinated in shape, size and torque during the mandibular advancement.

- Coordinate arches (parabolic arches, symmetric in shape, torque and size)
- Intrusion + upper incisors lingual torque
- Levelling curve of Spee in pre-MA stage
- Mandibular advancement + class II elastics night use

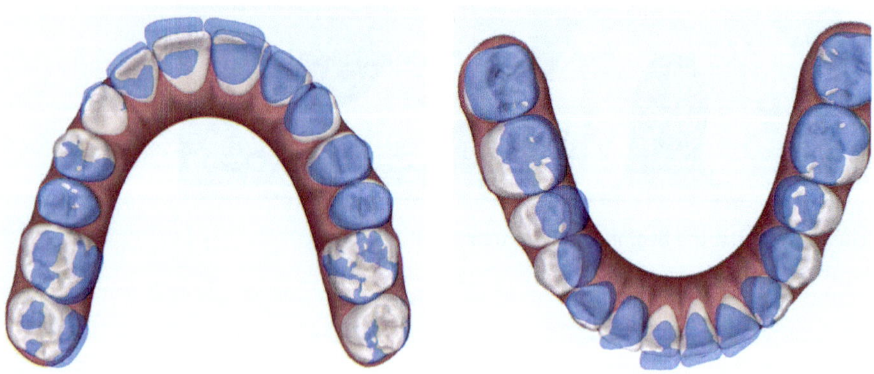

Fig. 20.49 Initial upper and lower ClinCheck views.

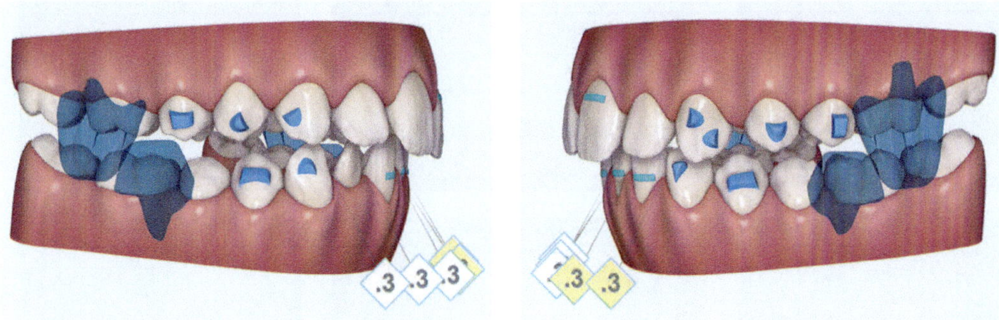

Fig. 20.50 Initial right and left ClinCheck views.

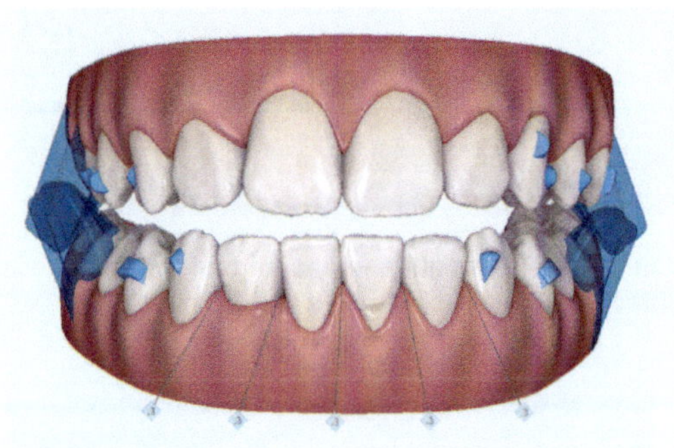

Fig. 20.51 Initial frontal ClinCheck view.

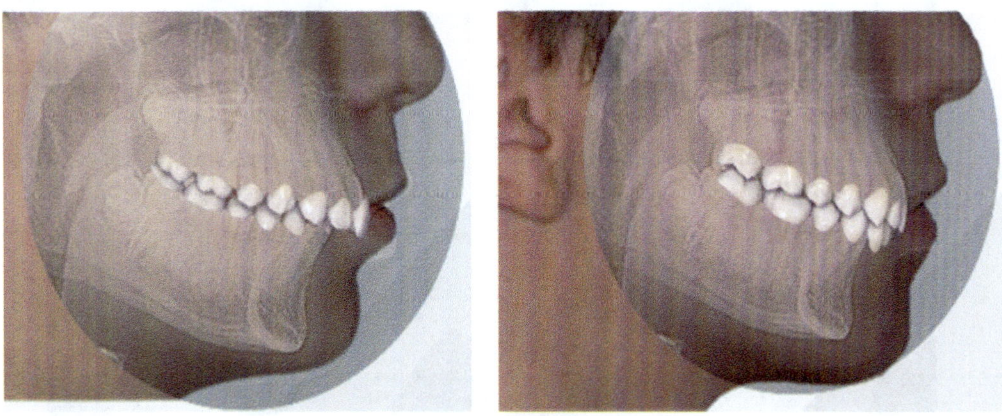

Fig. 20.52 Goal of treatment: mandibular advancement into a bilateral class I.

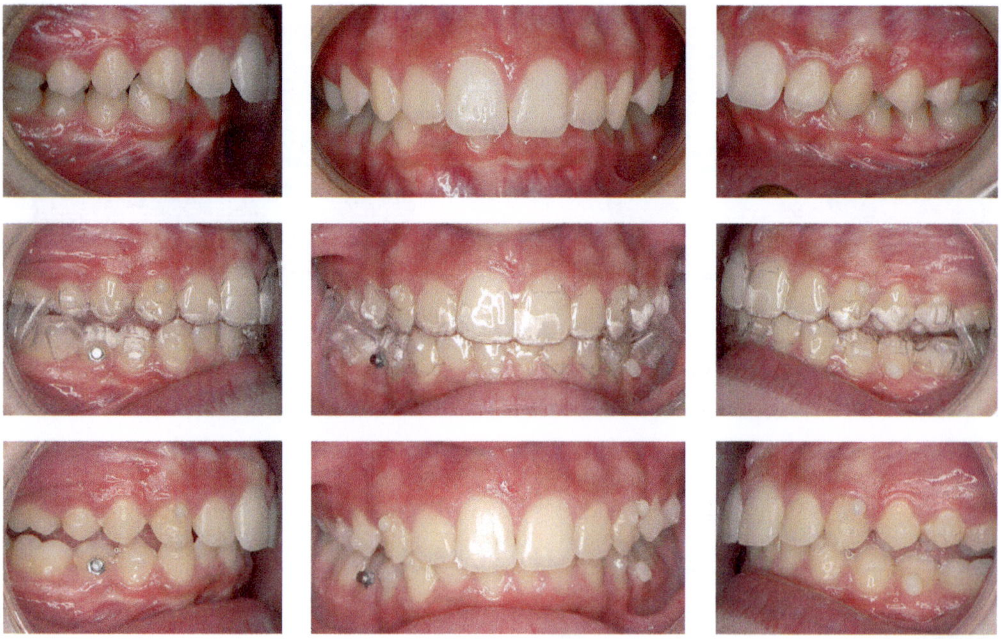

Fig. 20.53 Initial occlusion (upper), month 6 of evolution (middle), with aligners/month 6 of treatment without aligners (lower) showing anterior premature contact.

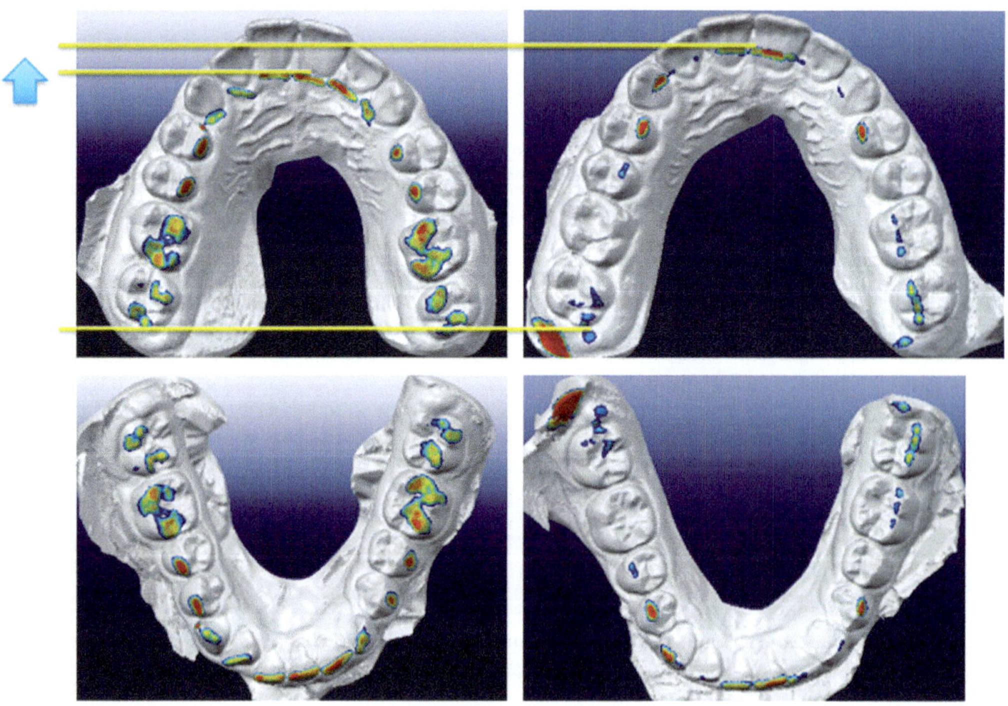

Fig. 20.54 Mandibular advancement in the first six months of treatment.

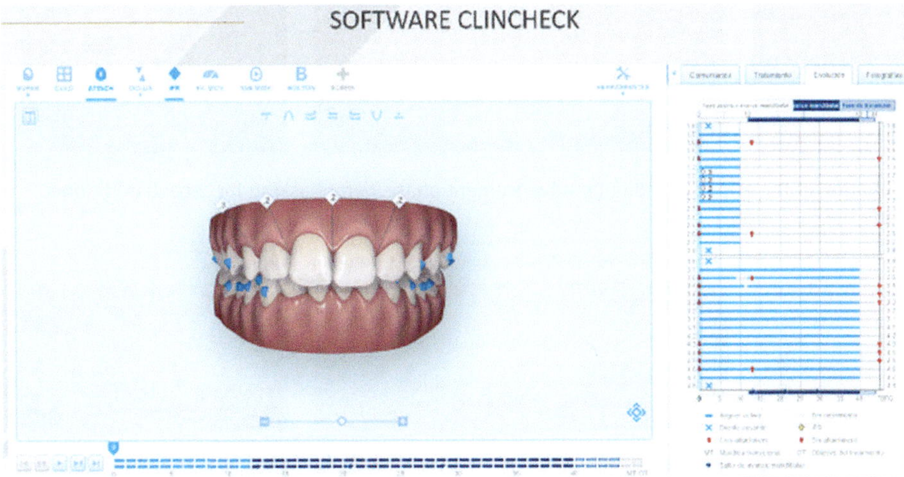

Fig. 20.55 New ClinCheck, asking to level the curve of Spee before continuing advancement of the mandible. A pre-mandibular advancement phase is used to intrude lower incisors and provide positive torque to upper incisors. During pre-MA phase ensure you over-correct the labial root torque of molars that are going to support the PW.

Treatment Summary

- Total treatment time was 18 months
- Arches were transversally coordinated by the lower expansion after 6 months of treatment
- After the six months, as no pre-MA phase was performed and the curve of Spee was not levelled, premature contacts were found on incisors and the precision wings had distortion problems that forced the taking of a new scan and additional aligners being required after only 6 months of treatment
- In the time the patient starts the MA phase, it is convenient to indicate class II elastics for night wear, in order to hold the mandible in place during the night in an advance position and prevent the distortion of the precision wings (class II elastics were used from aesthetic buttons attached on upper canines to the second lower premolars)
- Scissor bite was corrected and a bilateral class I was achieved, with normal overjet and overbite and an appropriated anterior guidance at the end of the treatment; the patient also had a better chin projection

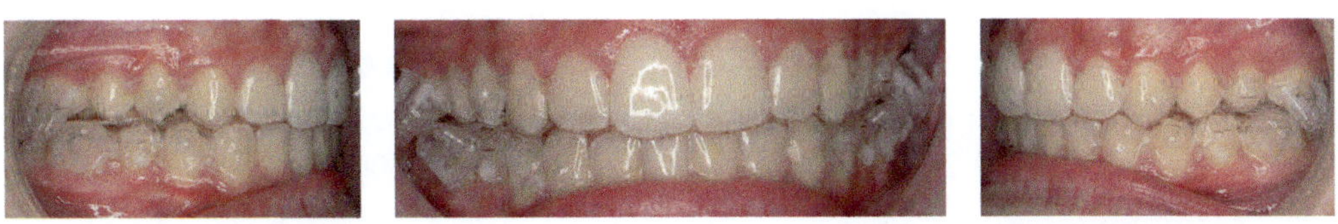

Fig. 20.56 Aligner 17 of additional aligners using class II elastics.

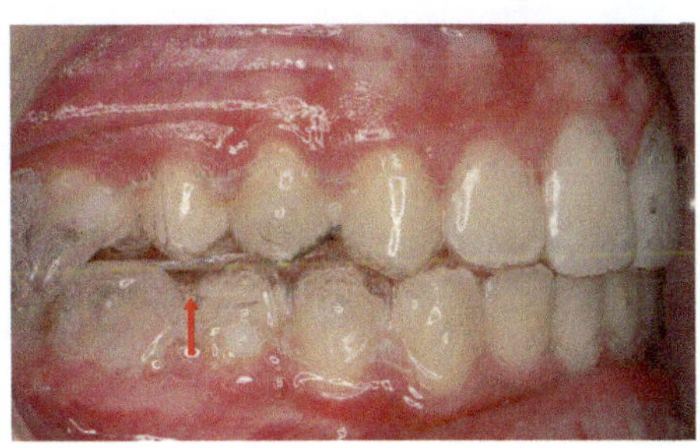

Fig. 20.57 Position of class II elastics (from lingual of upper first premolar to labial of lower second molar) to avoid interference with precision wings.

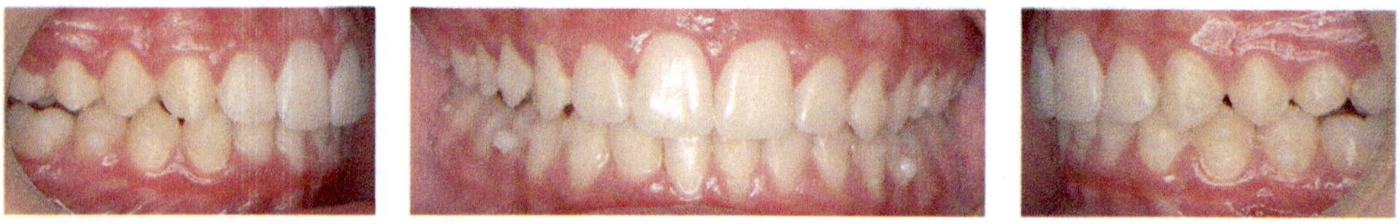

Fig. 20.58 Situation at the end of mandibular advancement phase, before asking for second additional aligners to settle the occlusion.

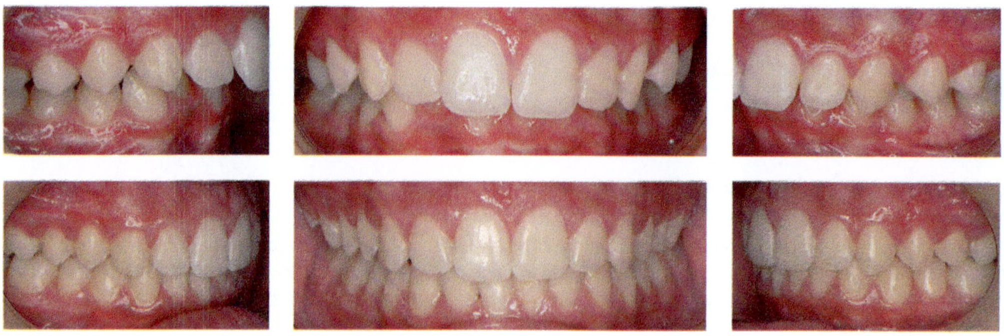

Fig. 20.59 Comparison between initial (upper) and final occlusion (lower).

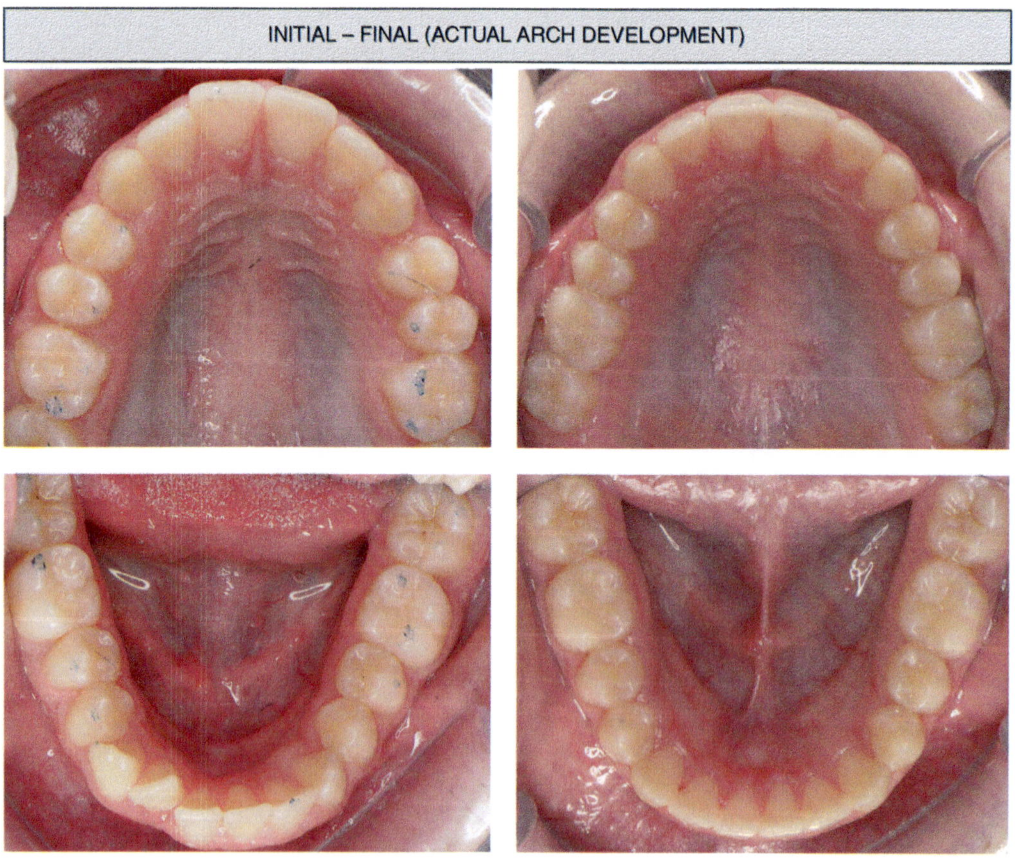

Fig. 20.60 Final arch development.

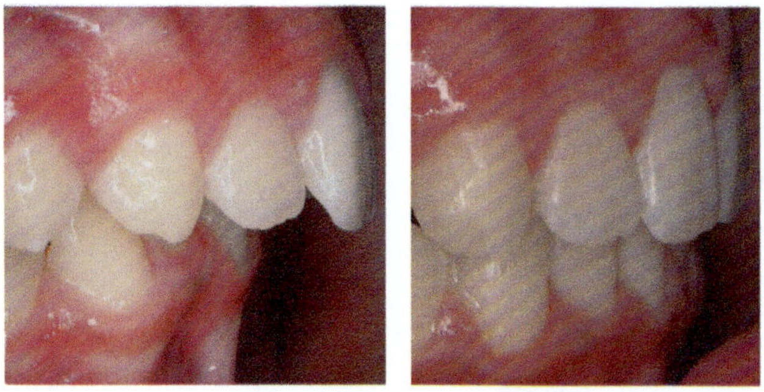

Fig. 20.61 Comparison of initial and final overjet.

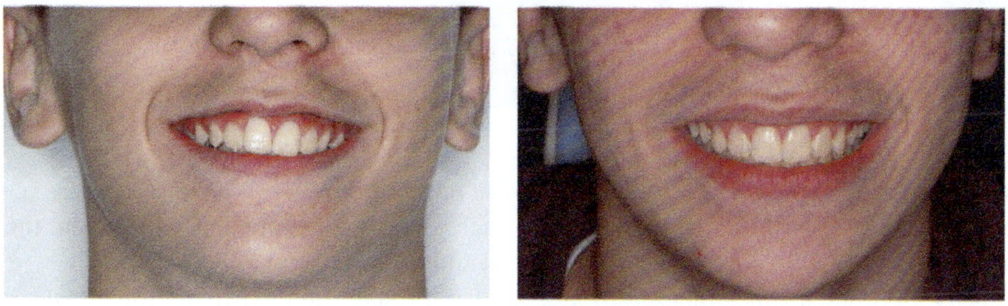

Fig. 20.62 Comparison of initial and final smile.

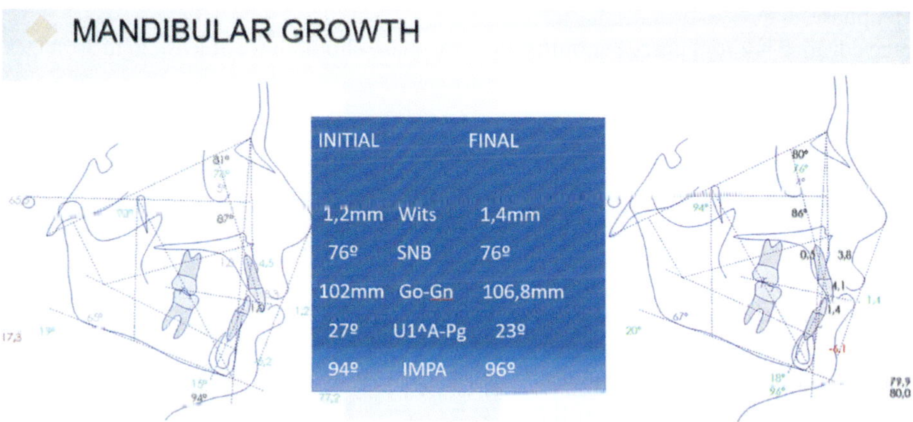

Fig. 20.63 Mandibular changes after 18 months of treatment.

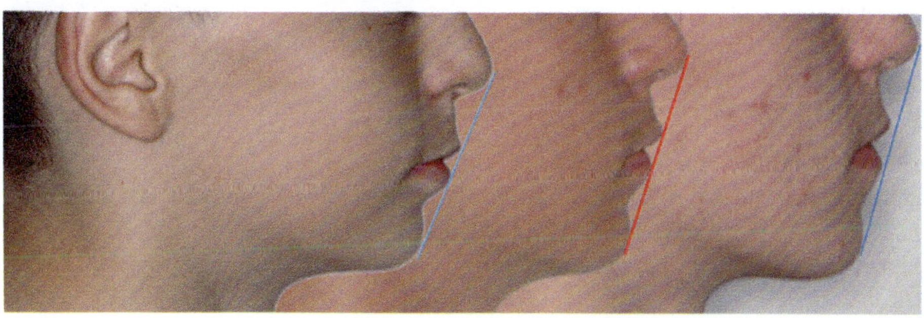

Fig. 20.64 Comparison in chin projection between initial, before additional aligners and at the end of the treatment.

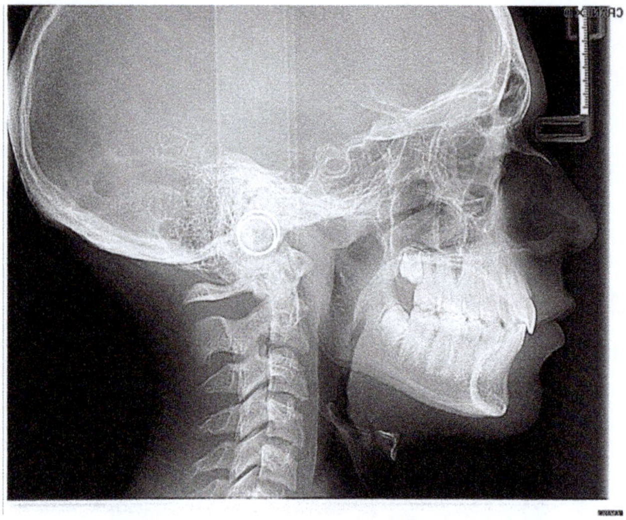

Fig. 20.65 Final lateral X-ray.

Tips for Class II Patients Treated with Invisalign Mandibular Advancement

- In the same way that other functional appliances, such as the Herbst appliance, function, the correction of class II by MA requires growth potential and patient compliance
- It is necessary for a pre-advance phase to level the curve of Spee, and to expand the arches in order to avoid interferences during mandible protraction
- In class II division 2, the upper incisors need to be procline into a class II division 1 before starting the MA phase
- The average advance is 2 mm every 8 months, the MA phase should have at least 26 to 30 stages to allow the mandible to grow

20.2.5 Class II Corrected by Transverse Arch Development and Intermaxillary Elastics

Diagnosis

A 17-year-old patient presented with mandibular asymmetry, a normodivergent class II profile and retruded chin. The upper midline was centred and the mandible was shifted to the right. They had dental full class II subdivision on the right, and class I on the left, with narrow arches and negative torque of upper canines.

Teleradiograph analysis: Normodivergent skeletal class II with labial tipping of lower incisors.

Right-side unilateral chewing.

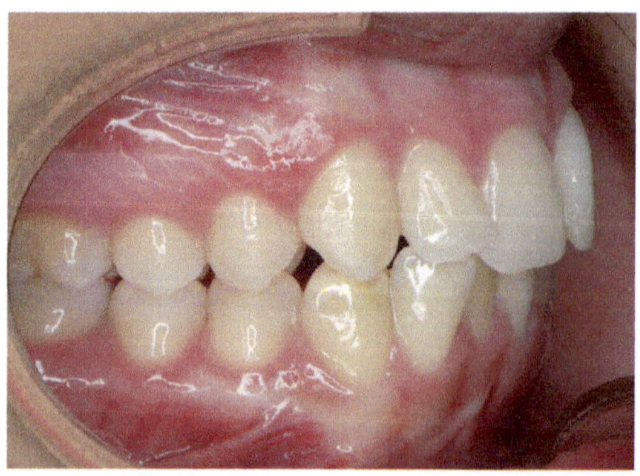

Fig. 20.66 Initial intraoral view.

For the Asymmetric Mandibular Growth

- TMJ examination: irreducible dislocation on the right side with no pain and no movement limitations.
- The functional disability of the right joint was probably one of the cofactors responsible for the asymmetric mandibular growth.

Treatment Plan

- Correction of the mandible asymmetry and the unilateral class II without extraction of upper right premolar to avoid impairing the profile
- Re-centre the mandible and achieve a more prominent chin projection

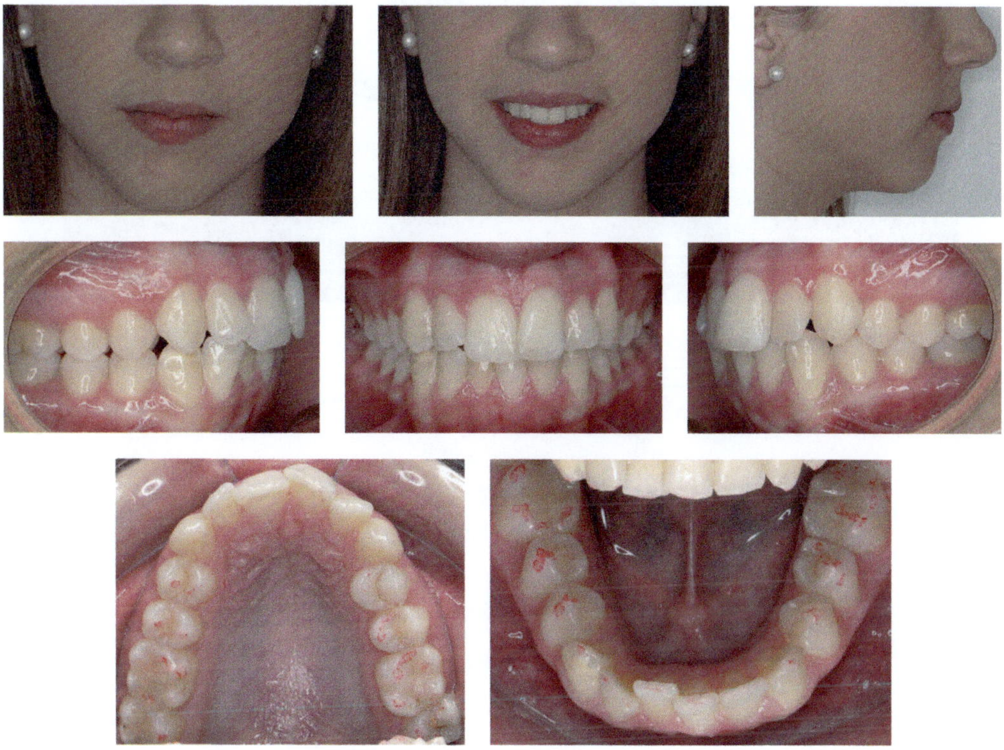

Fig. 20.67 Pretreatment extraoral and intraoral views.

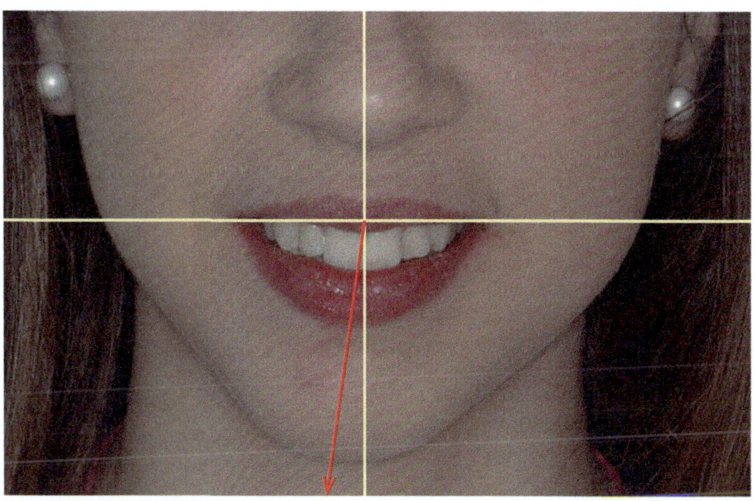

Fig. 20.68 Lower skeletal asymmetry. Normal upper incisors exposure at rest and no gum exposure when smiling. Upper midline centred. No frontal canting occlusal plane. There is lower skeletal asymmetry with a 4 mm right-side deviation and a narrow smile.

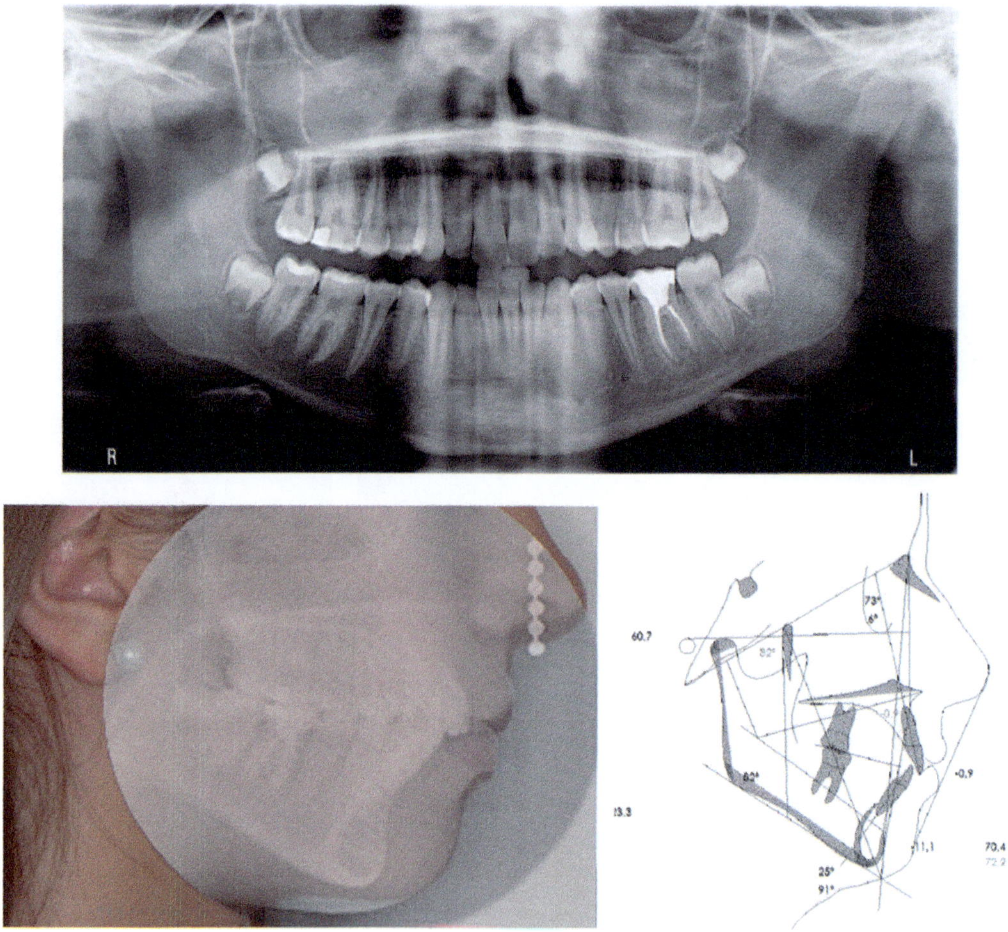

Fig. 20.69 Initial panoramic X-ray, teleradiograph and cephalometry. The aim was to correct the mandibular asymmetry and the unilateral class II malocclusion without recourse to premolar extractions in order to avoid impairing the profile (forestall excessive flattening of the upper lip and opening of nasolabial angle) by seeking to re-centre the right TM and to achieve more prominent chin projection.

Requirements for the Technician

- Arch expansion
- Upright lower incisor to create positive overjet
- Make a virtual jump to coordinate arches

Maxilla:

- Mesial-out rotation of the molars at the same time as expansion.
- AT HBG bevelled attachments to gingival 4 mm in U4 and U6 to control the posterior torque during expansion.

Mandible:

- Expansion and simultaneous retraction of lower incisors to create positive overjet for the virtual jump (elastic simulation)

Maxillary staging:
- No sequential distalization. Expansion, molar derotation and virtual jump.

Mandibular staging
- Correct crowding by expansion and IPR. No Proclination of lower incisors. We need overjet for the virtual jump

- Anchorage Attachment: HBG U4 + U6 and optimized attachments in canines.
- Class II elastic on right side 24 hours and night use on left side

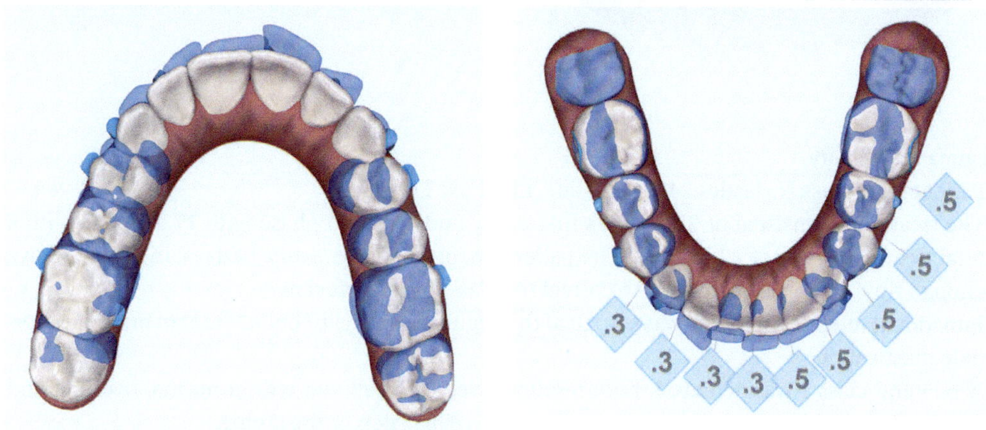

Fig. 20.70 Initial upper and lower ClinCheck views.

- Re-centre the lower jaw by upper and lower expansion and upright lower incisors to allow the virtual jump using class II elastics.
- Functional re-education: Initiate it at the beginning of treatment in order to promote alternate mastication.

- **Anchorage attachment:** HBG bevelled attachment to gingival U4 + U6 and optimized attachments in canines.

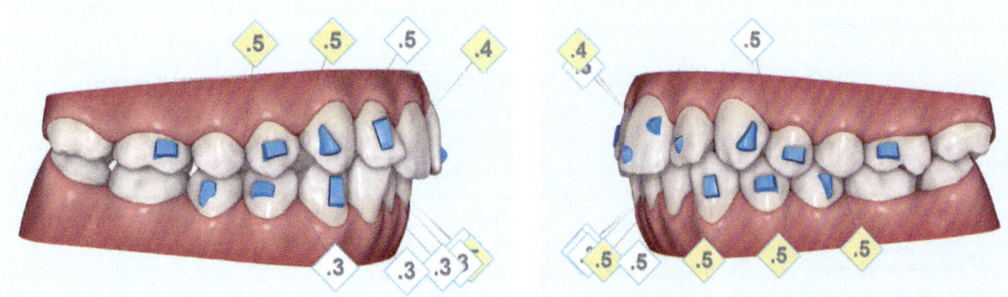

Fig. 20.71 Lateral ClinCheck views.

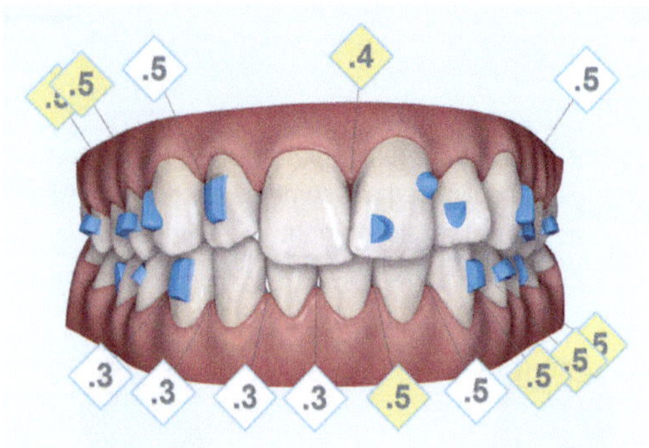

Fig. 20.72 Initial frontal ClinCheck view.

Treatment Summary

- Patient wore class II elastics 24 h right-side, night use left-side
- The treatment consisted of 27 aligners first phase and a second phase with 17 aligners, with a total treatment time of 22 months. The patient changed aligner every 14 days, in order to have enough time using class II elastic to correct the class II malocclusion
- Functional re-education: this was started at the beginning of treatment in order to promote alternate mastication
- A bilateral class I was achieved, both midlines were centred and with a normal overbite and overjet. The smile improved considerably owing to expansion of the arches

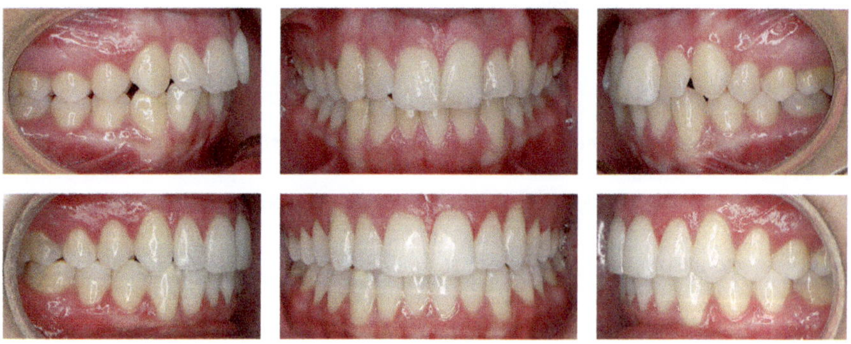

Fig. 20.73 Comparison between initial (upper) and final occlusion (lower).

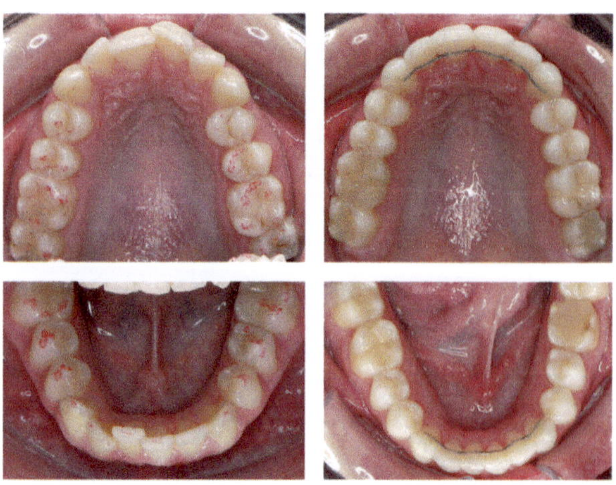

Fig. 20.74 Initial (left) and final occlusal (right).

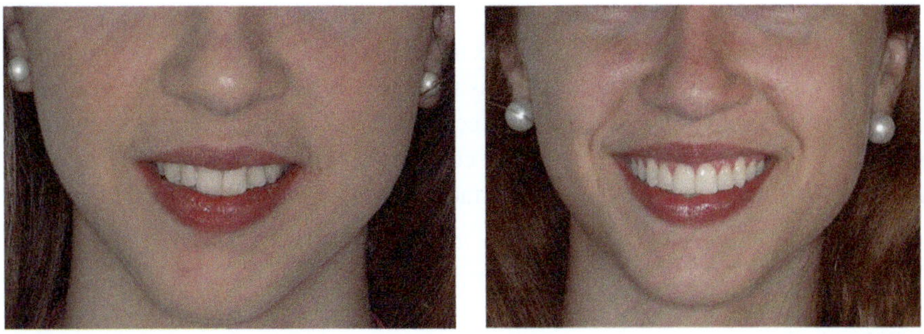

Fig. 20.75 Initial and final smile.

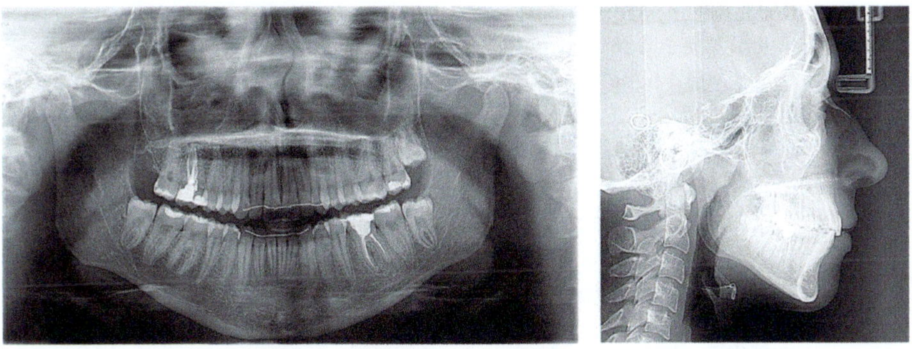

Fig. 20.76 Panoramic and lateral X-rays.

Tips for Class II Correction with Intermaxillary Elastics

- The key to correct class II is the transversal development of the upper arch. Narrow arches in young patients will be able to be corrected by expansion and elastic virtual simulation.
- Class II elastics should be in full-time wear to achieve the correction.
- Provide a positive overjet, uprighting lower incisors to counteract the side-effects of the class II elastic.
- In case of lower crowding, ask the technician to correct by expansion and IPR, with no proclination, to create a positive overjet to correct the class II.
- Change aligners every 14 days, instead of every week, to ensure enough time for the use of elastic.

20.2.6 Sequential Upper Distalization and Lower Mesialization

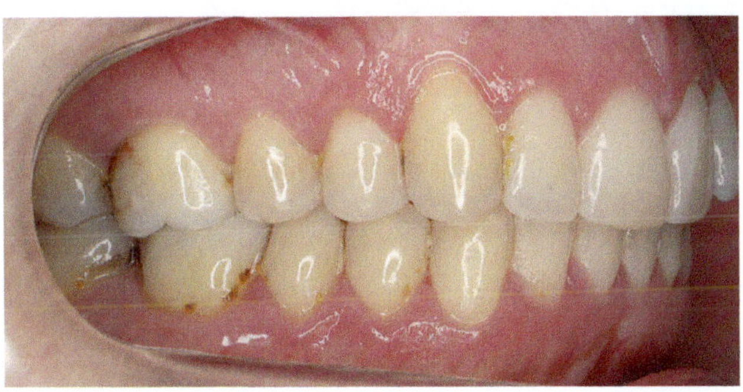

Fig. 20.77 Initial intraoral view.

Diagnosis

A 37-year-old patient treated with braces when she was a child demanded orthodontic treatment with aligners to improve her smile. A chief concern was the narrow smile and 22 misalignments. She had normodivergent skeletal class I, wide buccal corridors and incomplete class II in both sides, with lingual torque of upper incisors. Instead of contact points between the teeth she had been treated with a lot of IPR and presented contact surfaces instead of contact points. Her overjet was reduced.

Treatment Plan

- Symmetrical expansion of the upper arch.
- Maxillary: sequential upper distalization simultaneous to expansion and labial torque to the upper incisors during posterior distalization.
- Mandibular: sequential lower mesialization using the labial position of lower incisors as anchorage for the mesialization. The lower incisors were slightly proclined, so the root of the lower incisor anchored to the cortical bone would create the necessary anchorage for the sequential lower mesialization.

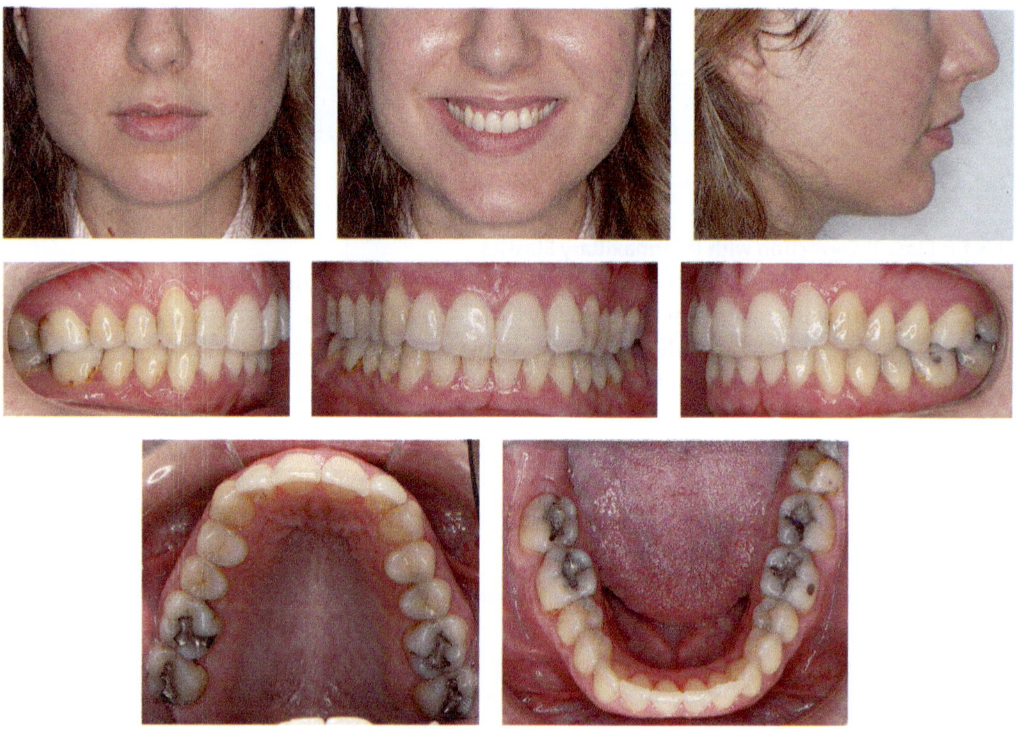

Fig. 20.78 Pretreatment extraoral and intraoral views.

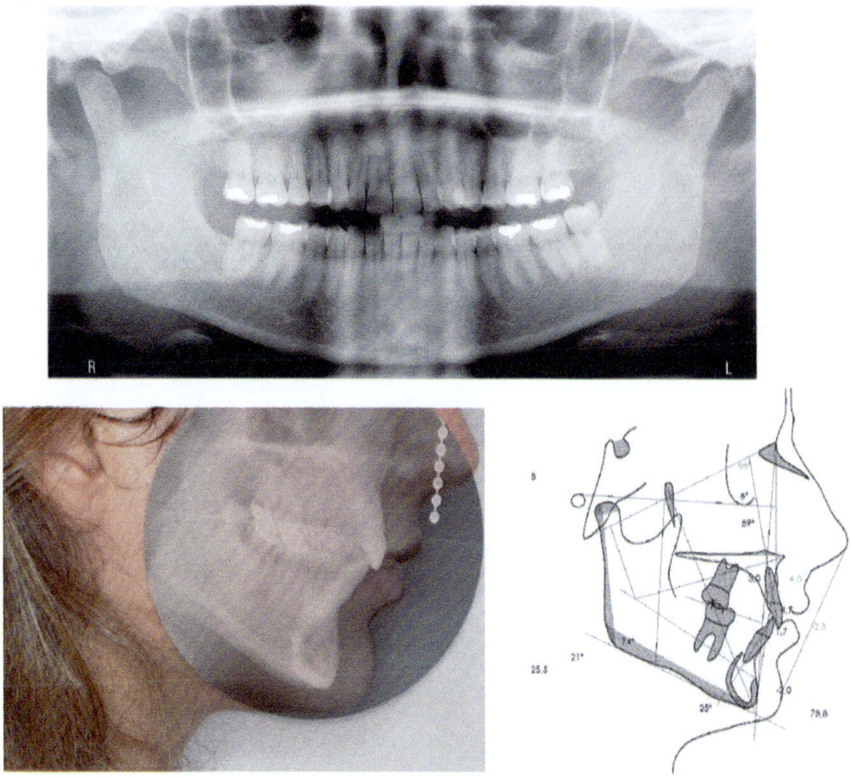

Fig. 20.79 Initial panoramic X-ray, teleradiograph and cephalometry.

Requirements for the Technician

- Maxilla: start applying labial torque to the upper incisors straight away. Class II elastics could not be started without providing a positive overjet.
- Expand the upper arch during the sequential distalization and coordinate arches with a parabolic shape.

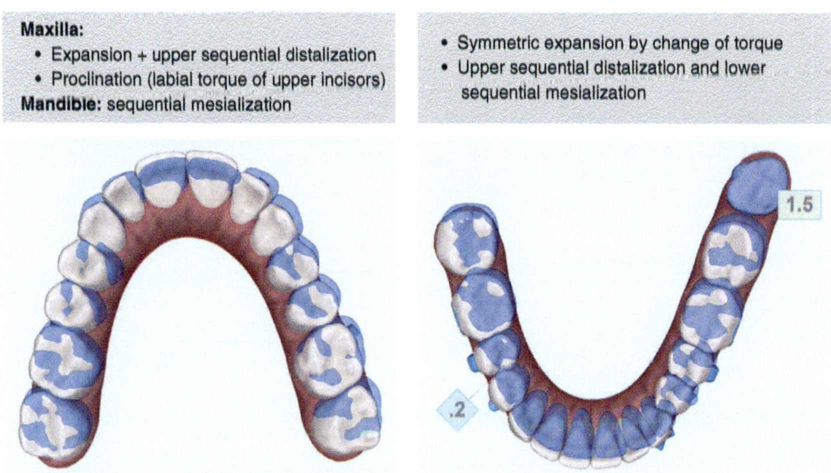

Fig. 20.80 Initial upper and lower ClinCheck views

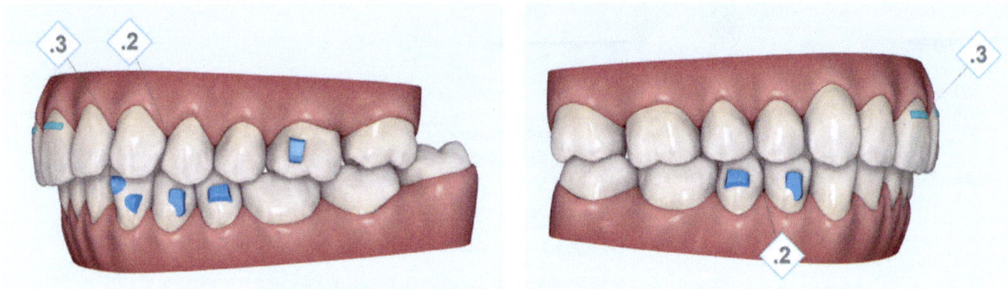

Fig. 20.81 Initial right and left ClinCheck views.

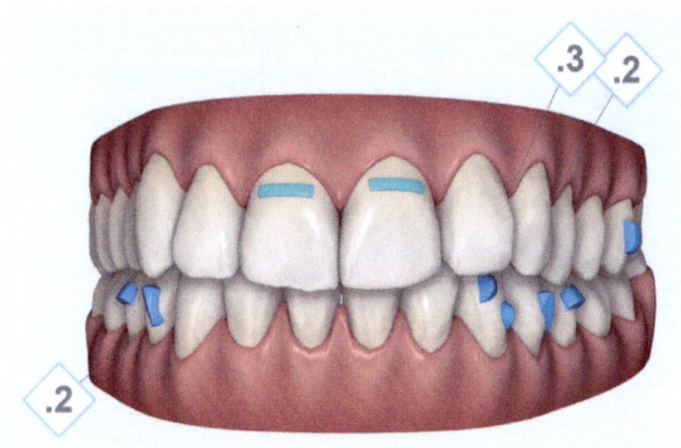

Fig. 20.82 Initial front ClinCheck view.

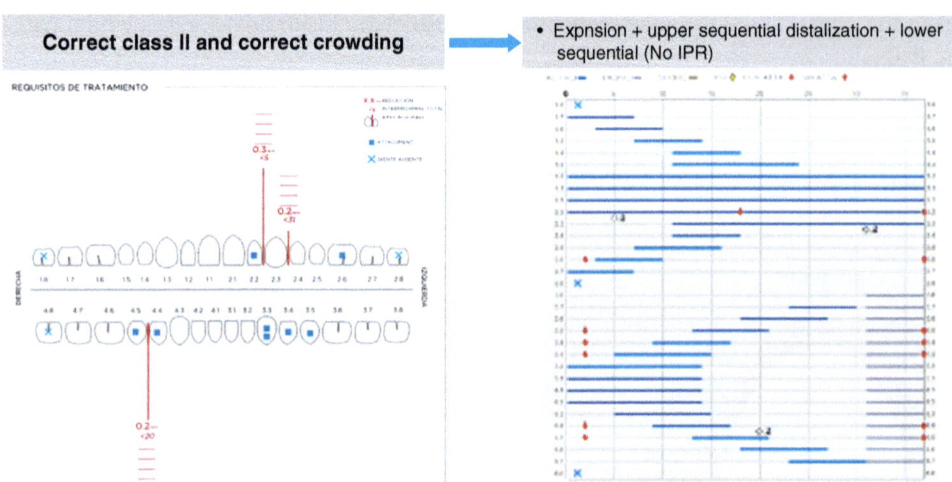

Fig. 20.83 Upper sequential distalization and lower sequential mesialization.

Treatment Summary

- Total treatment time was 18 months
- The patient wore 36 aligners with changes every 10 days followed by a set of additional aligners.
- The patient got a wide smile at the end of the treatment with a bilateral class I and almost no IPR performed on her teeth
- The midlines at the end of the treatment were centred to obtain the correct overbite and overjet

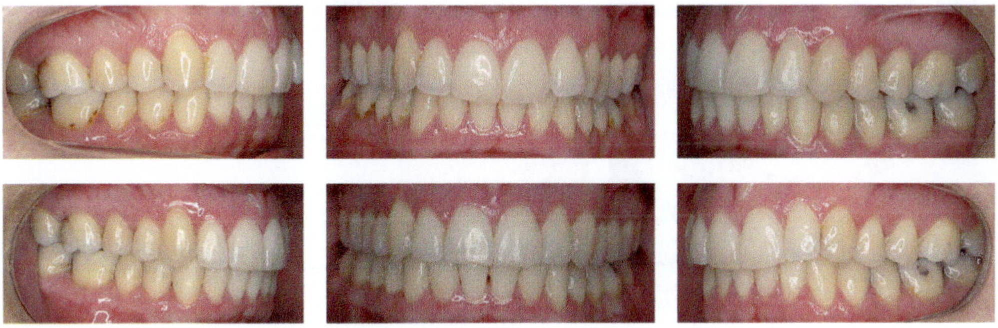

Fig. 20.84 Comparison between initial (upper) and final (lower) occlusion.

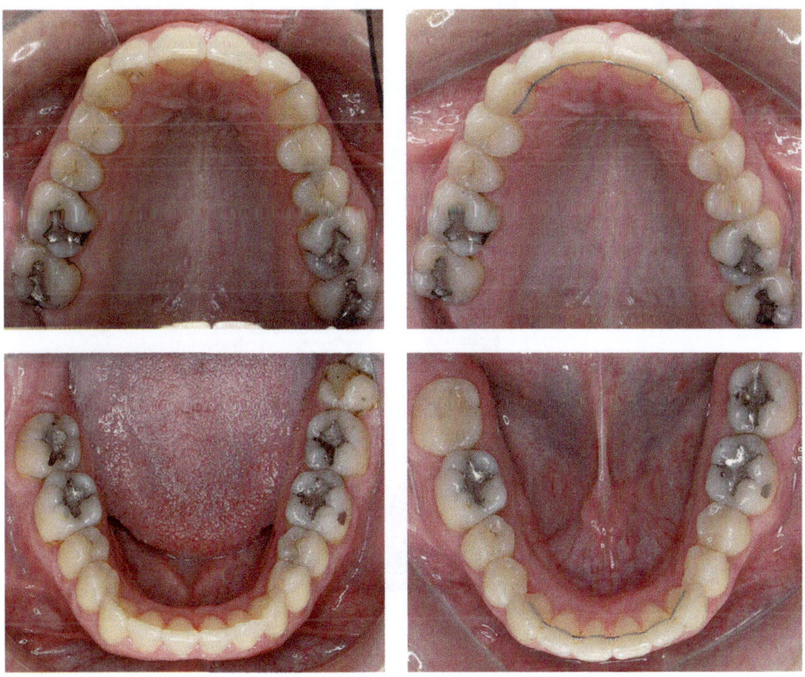

Fig. 20.85 Before (left) and after (right) lower occlusal views.

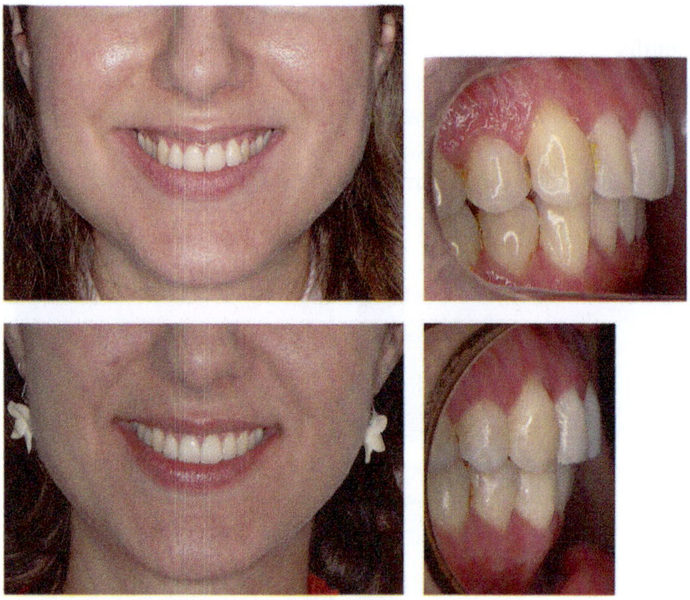

Fig. 20.86 Initial and final smile and overjet.

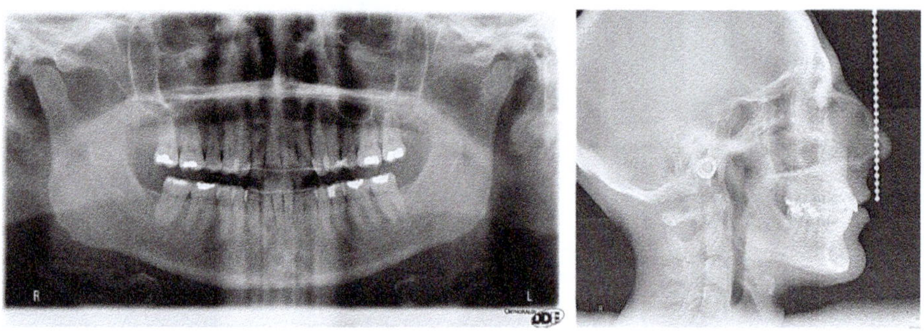

Fig. 20.87 Final panoramic and lateral X-rays.

20.2.7 Sequential Distalization

Diagnosis

A 26-year-old normodivergent patient presented with class II division 2, no anterior guidance and painful TMJ symptoms. The patient had received orthodontic treatment before. The patient's chief concern was the TMJ pain, and there was limitation of movement. The upper incisor had a lingual crown tipping and the third upper molars were impacted on bone.

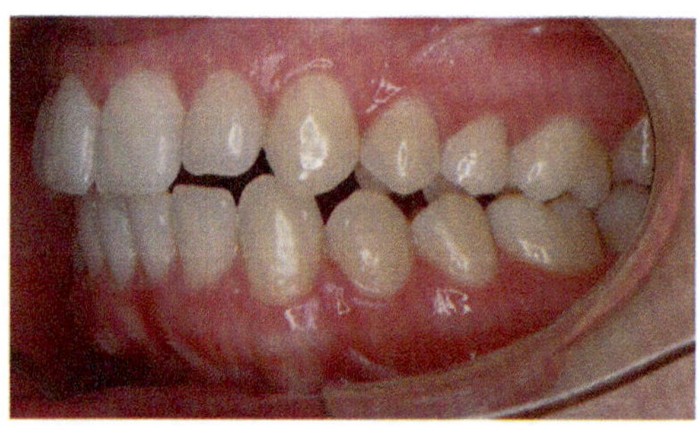

Fig. 20.88 Initial intraoral view.

Treatment Plan

- Extract upper third molars
- Apply a sequential upper distalization
- During the molar distalization, labial crown torque will be applied to upper incisors
- In order to provide the case with positive overjet, there would be IPR on the anterior incisors and retrusion of lower incisors

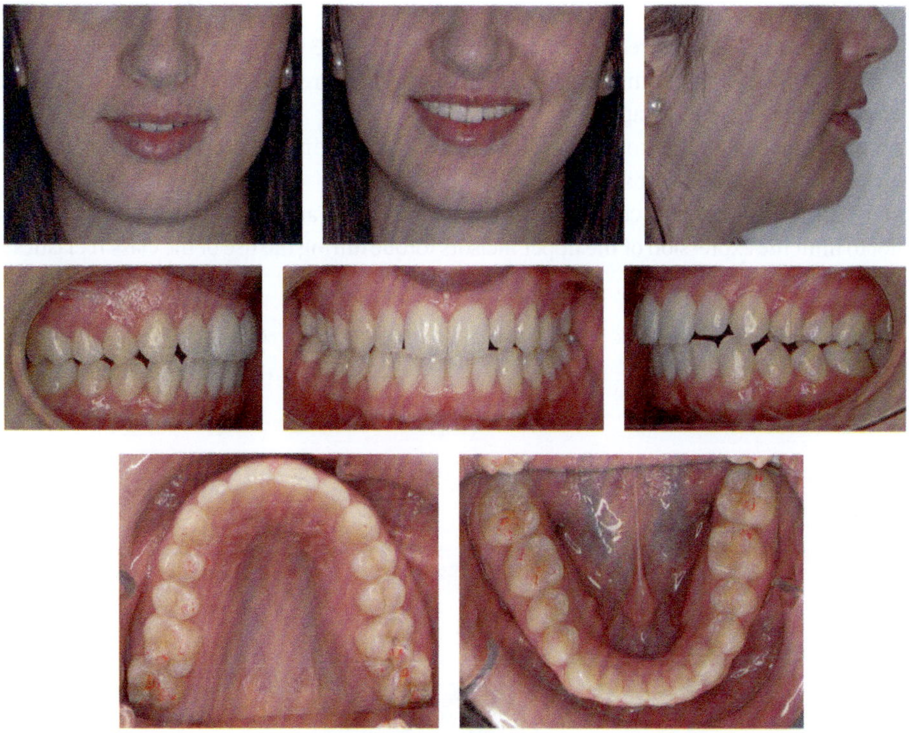

Fig. 20.89 Pretreatment extraoral and intraoral views.

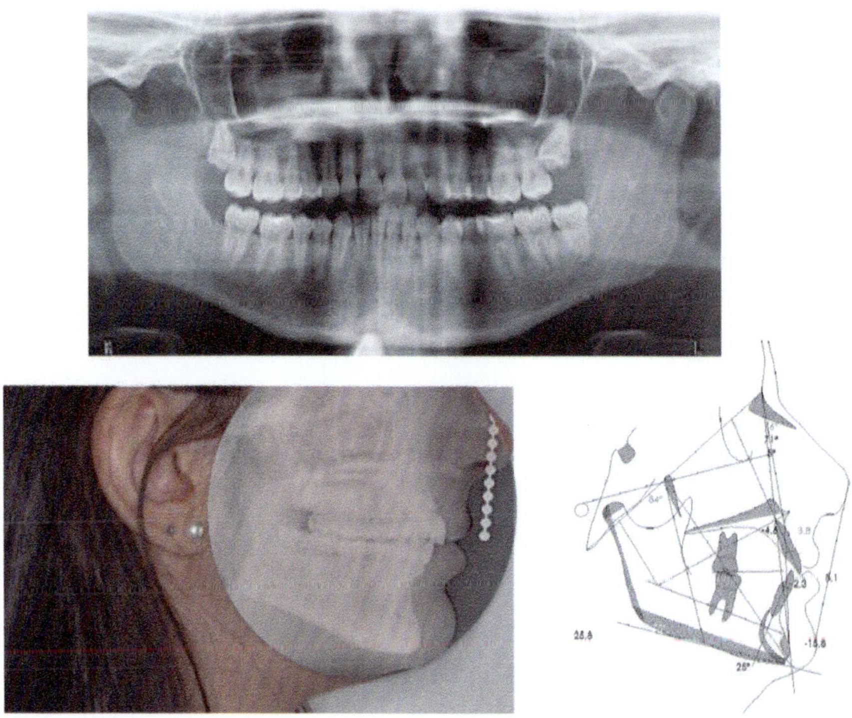

Fig. 20.90 Initial panoramic X-ray, teleradiograph and cephalometry.

Requirements for the Technician

- A positive overjet would be required, by making a lower IPR 3 to 3 and by applying labial crown and lingual root torque to upper incisors from the beginning of treatment. All upper and lower incisors would be moving from stage 1.
- At the end of the treatment, overcorrection aligners of the upper incisors torque and uprighting of the lower incisors in order to ensure the overjet correction.
- Button cutouts instead of precision cuts on the upper first premolars and in the second lower molars, in order not to limit the expression of the upper incisors torque during the use of the class II elastics.

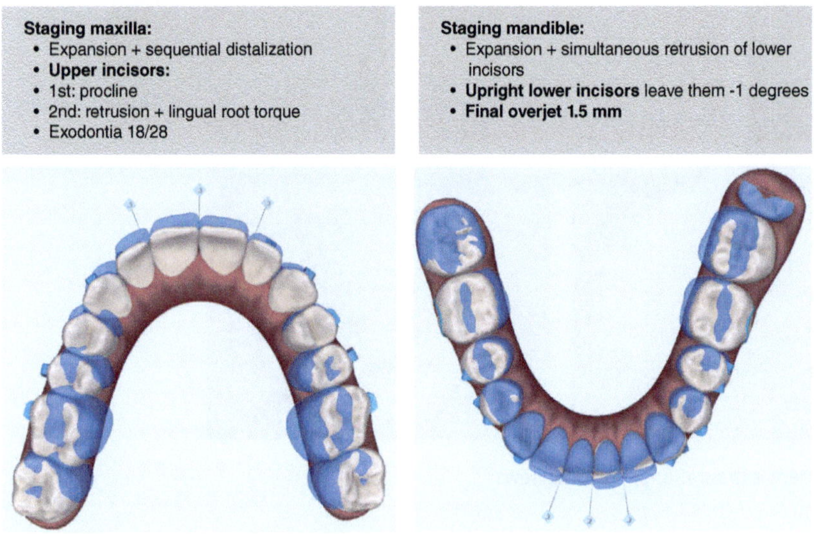

Fig. 20.91 Upper and lower occlusal ClinCheck views.

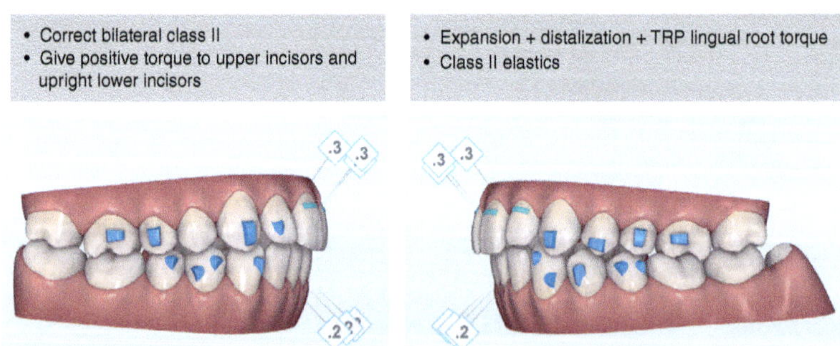

Fig. 20.92 Right and left ClinCheck views.

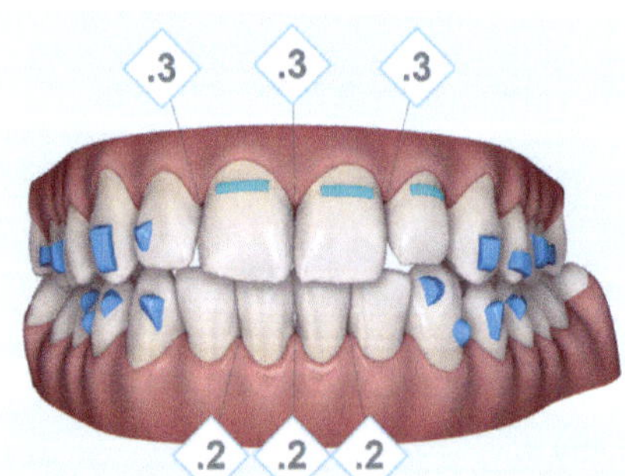

Fig. 20.93 Front ClinCheck view.

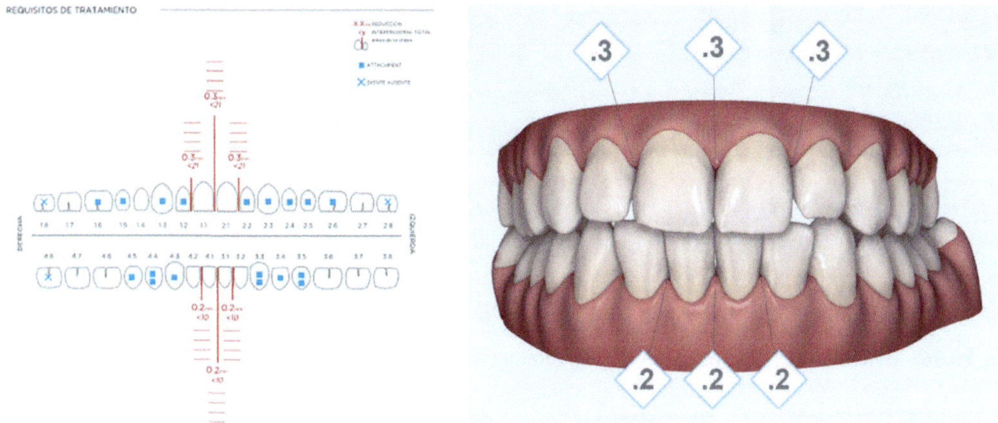

Fig. 20.94 Treatment for interproximal reduction.

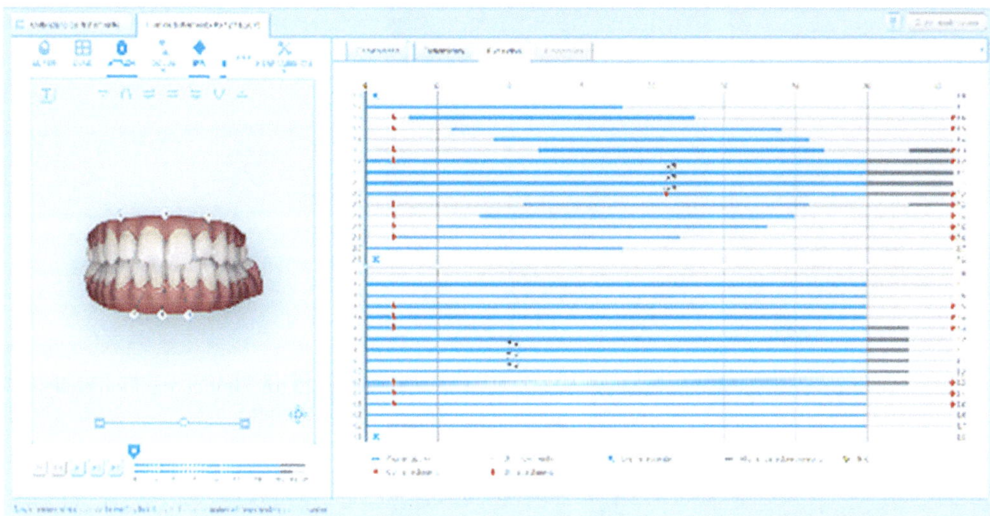

Fig. 20.95 Sequential upper distalization pattern.

Treatment Summary

- Treatment time was 19 months
- Total treatment required 35 active aligners, the final aligners of overcorrection were not used as a set of additional aligners were used
- The aligners were changed every 10 days
- Class II elastics were used full-time until the second upper premolar started distalization. A bilateral class I was achieved, with normal overjet and overbite and appropriated anterior guidance at the end of the treatment

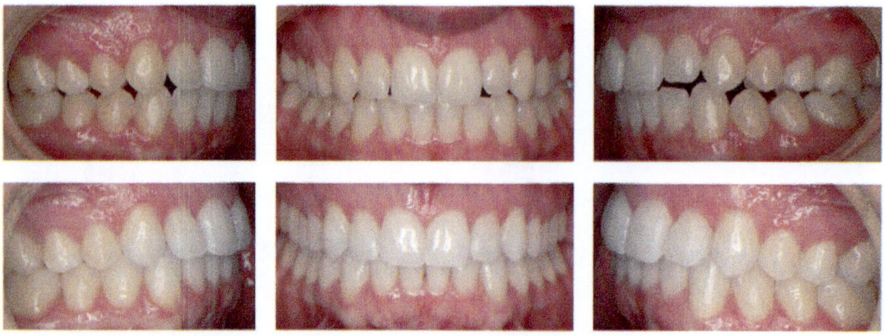

Fig. 20.96 Before (upper) and after (lower) intraoral views.

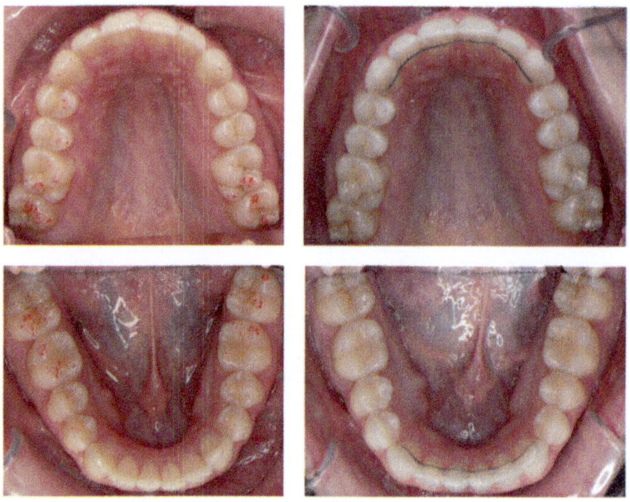

Fig. 20.97 Initial (left) and final (right) occlusal.

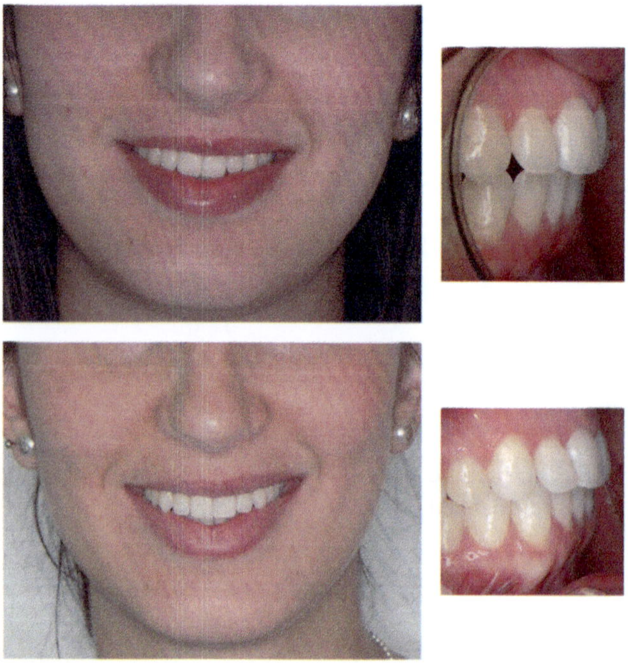

Fig. 20.98 Initial and final smile and overjet.

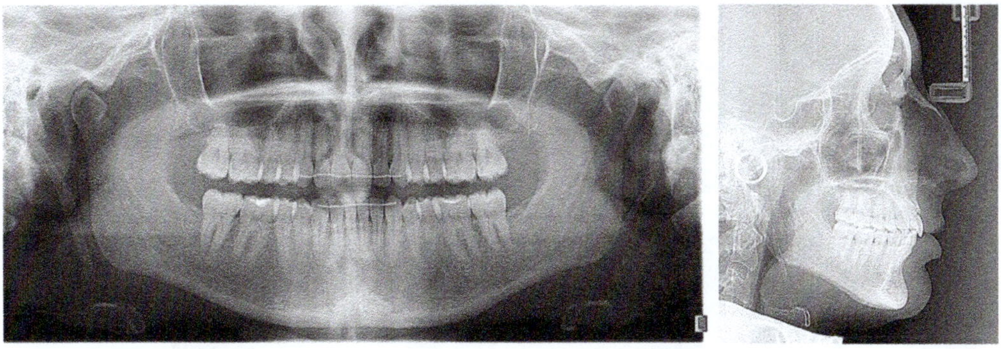

Fig. 20.99 Final panoramic and lateral X-rays.

Tips for Sequential Distalization

- Indicated to correct class II in adult patients, or in growing patients whose arches do not allow much transversal compensation.
- The third molars need to be extracted before starting the upper distalization. If the third molars are germs in growing patients, they do not need to be extracted.
- If upper incisors have a lingual torque, start providing labial crown torque to the upper incisors during the posterior distalization.
- Class II elastics are necessary until the second upper premolars start the distalization.
- Where there is lower crowding, do not procline the lower incisors; correct by expansion and IPR in order to provide positive overjet to correct the class II.
- In severe class II, attachments bevelled to gingival of 3 mm in the lingual surface of upper incisors can be used to provide extra anterior anchorage during the sequential distalization.

20.2.8 Simultaneous Distalization

Diagnosis

A 30-year-old patient with hyperdivergent skeletal class II presented with full class II on right side, incomplete class II on the left, proclination of upper incisors and narrow arches. They had a canted occlusal plane, more descended on right side, and mottled enamel (dental fluorosis).

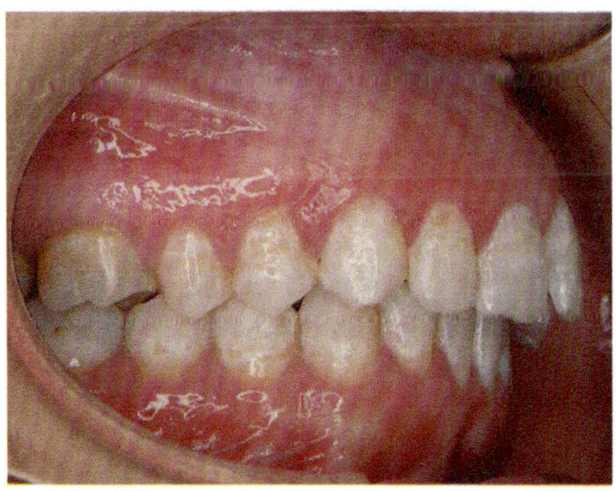

Fig. 20.100 Initial intraoral view.

Treatment Plan

- Sequential distalization of upper molars and, once achieved, using TADs as anchorage, simultaneous retraction 5 to 5.
- Intra-arch elastics would be used from upper canines to the microscrew.
- Intermaxillary elastics would be used in full-time wear from the moment the first molars got into their final position.
- On the lower arch, expansion and simultaneous retraction of lower incisors was planned, in order to create positive overjet to correct the class II.

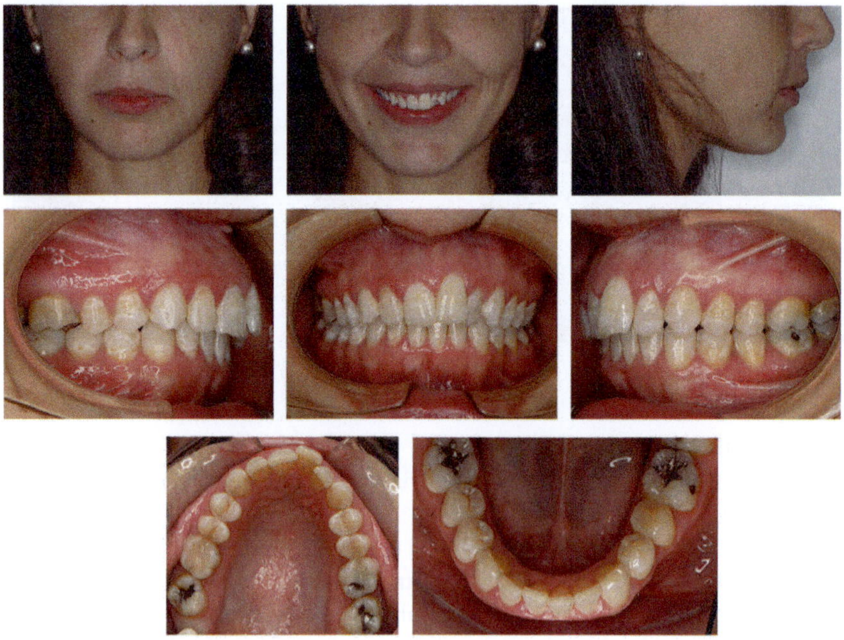

Fig. 20.101 Pretreatment extraoral and intraoral views.

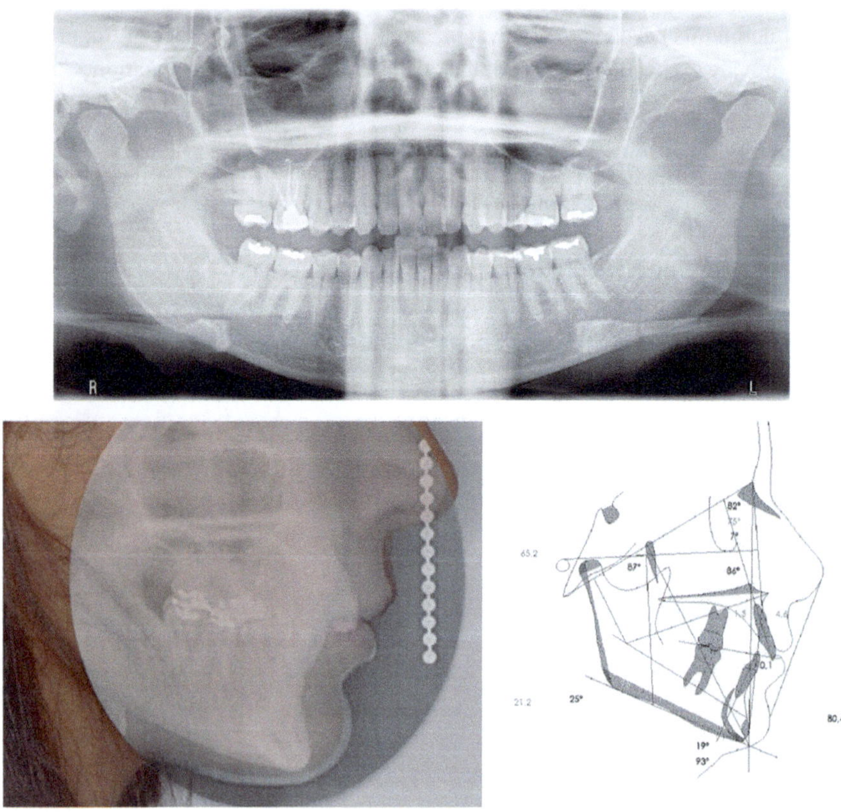

Fig. 20.102 Initial panoramic X-ray, teleradiograph and cephalometry.

Requirements for the Technician

- Distalize sequentially the second and first upper molars, while at the same applying lingual root torque to the upper incisors
- Afterwards, every tooth on the upper arch (except the molars) to move simultaneously together with lingual root torque to the upper incisors during the retraction

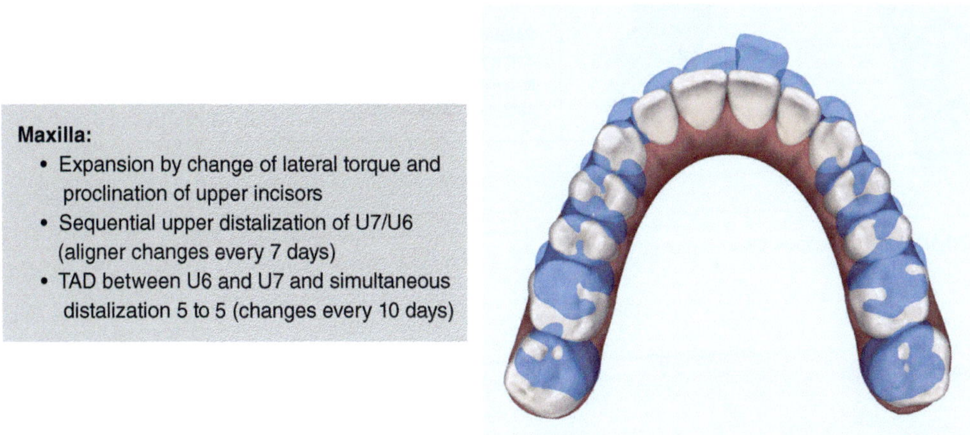

Fig. 20.103 Superimposition, upper occlusal ClinCheck view.

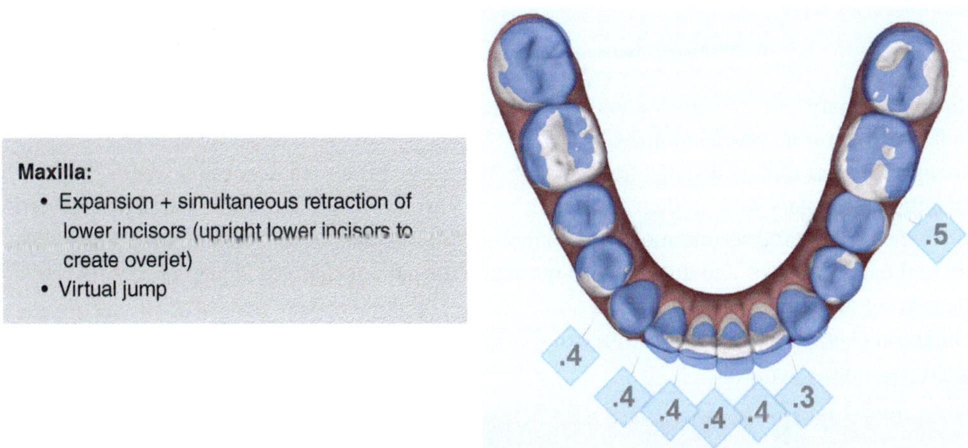

Fig. 20.104 Superimposition, lower occlusal ClinCheck view.

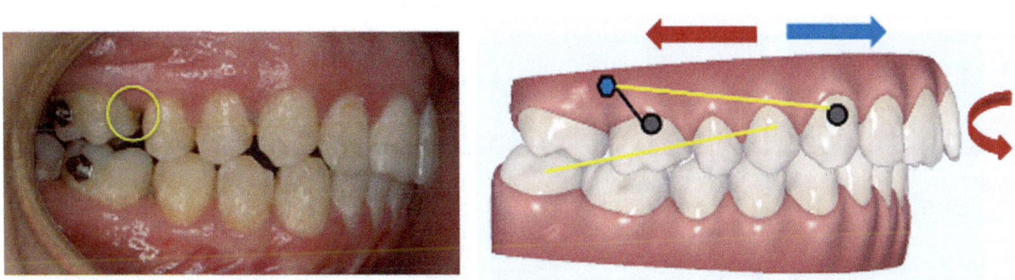

Fig. 20.105 Biomechanics for simultaneous distalization.

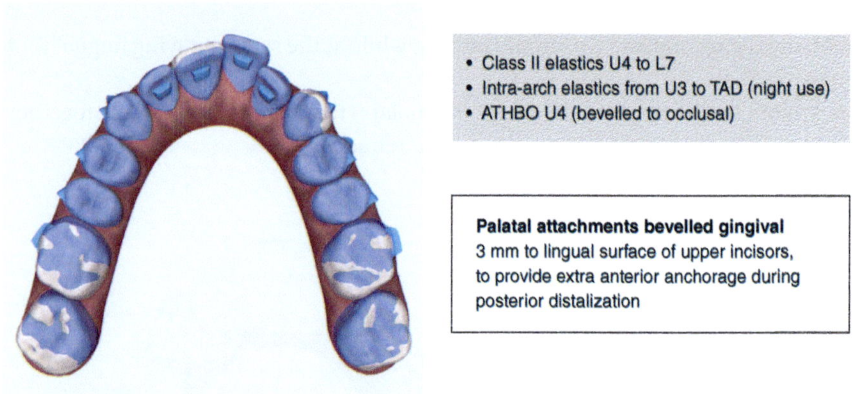

Fig. 20.106 ClinCheck view.

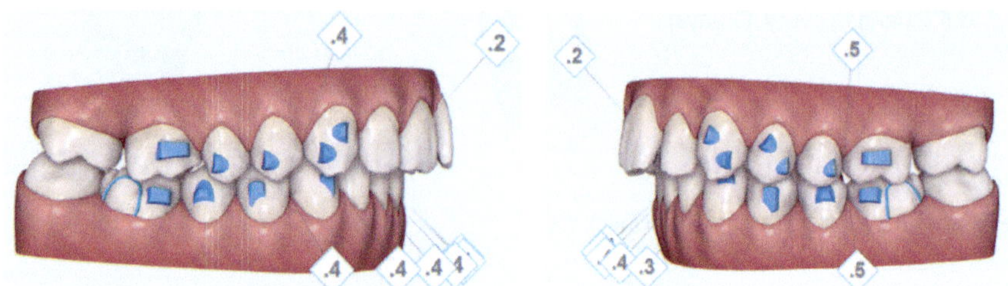

Fig. 20.107 Right and left ClinCheck views.

Treatment Summary

- Total treatment time was 23 months.
- During the upper molars distalization, the patient changed their aligners every week.
- Once the first molars were in their final position, a yuxtacigomatic microscrew was placed vertically between first and second molars of 10 mm, the first molars were attached using a steel ligature to the microscrews, and during 5 to 5 retraction the patient changed aligners every 10 days.
- The first set of aligners were 54 and an additional set of aligners were needed.
- A bilateral class I relationship with normal overjet and overbite as well as occlusal plane corrected was finally achieved.

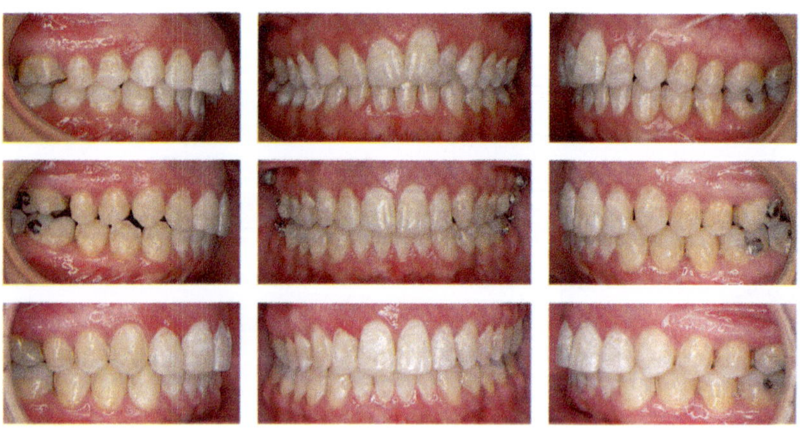

Fig. 20.108 Initial views (upper), before additional aligners (middle) and final views (lower). The incisal edge of 11 was repaired with composite at the end of the treatment.

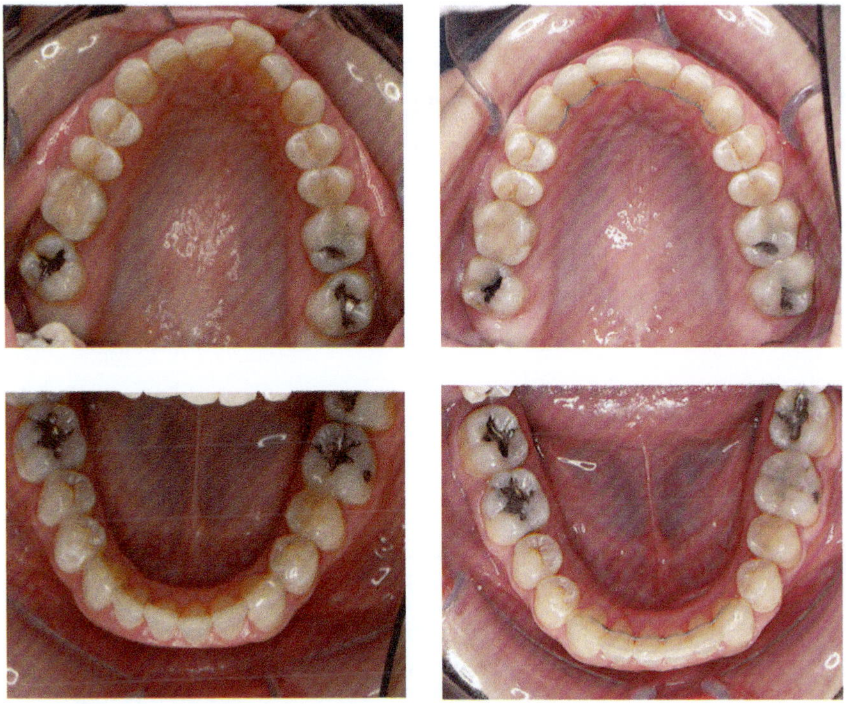

Fig. 20.109 Before (left) and after (right) occlusal views.

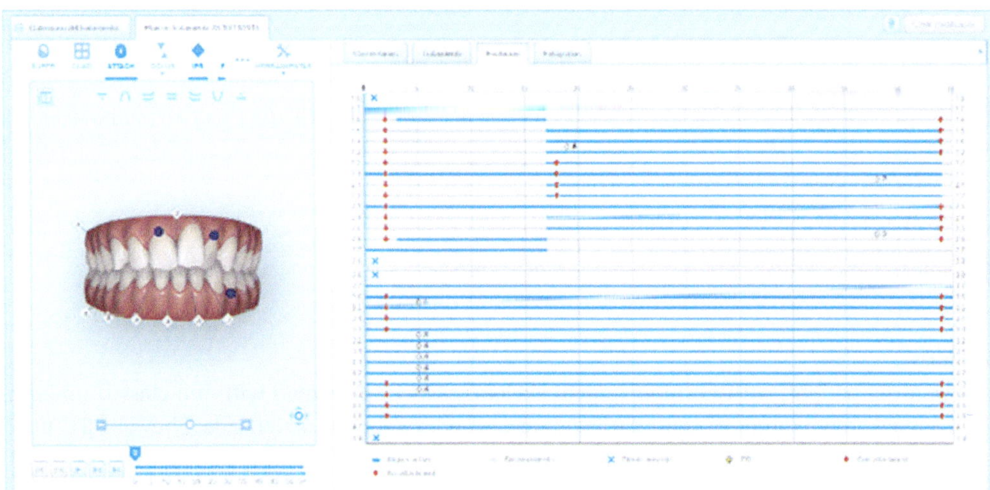

Fig. 20.110 Simultaneous distalization pattern.

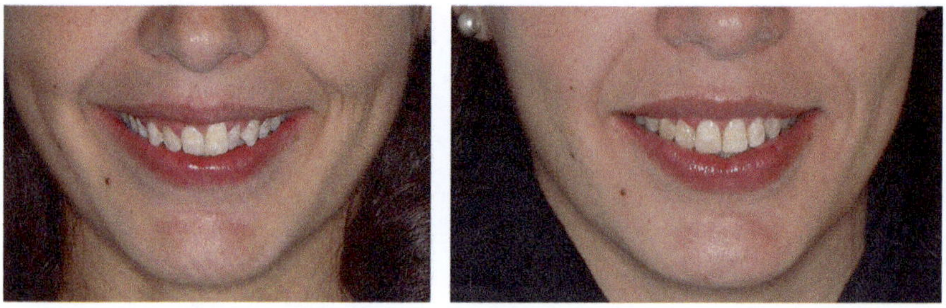

Fig. 20.111 Before and after treatment smile.

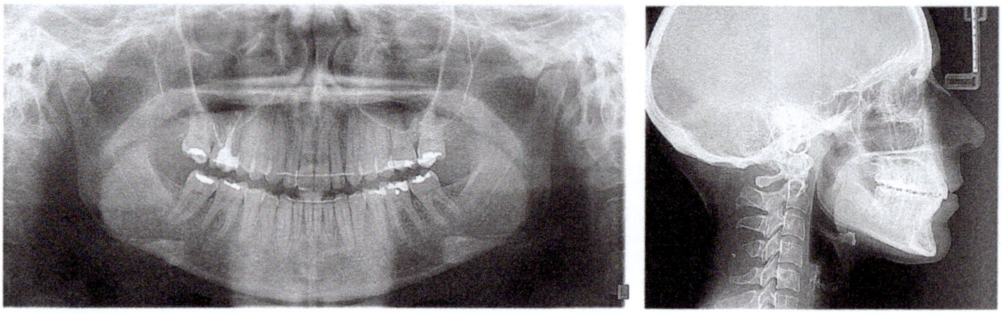

Fig. 20.112 Final panoramic and lateral X-rays.

20.2.9 Simultaneous Distalization with TADs in Tuberosity

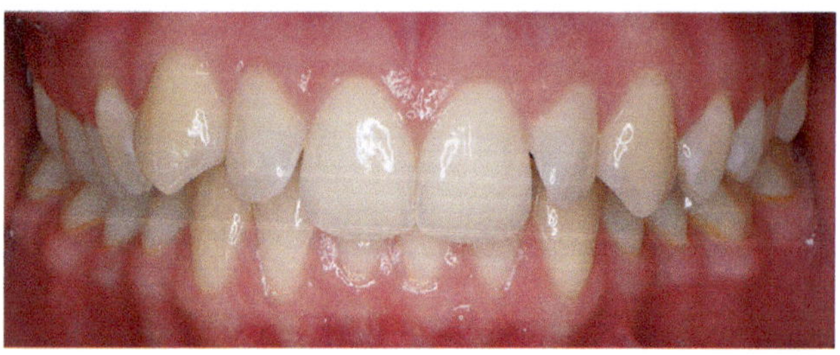

Fig. 20.113 Distalization from 3 to 7 in a row pattern.

Diagnosis

A 24-year-old patient, with normodivergent skeletal class II, presented with full class II on both sides, lingual crown torque of central upper incisors and scissor bite on left side. They had a canted occlusal plane, more descended on left side, mandibular asymmetry with right-side deviation of the mandible and TMJ disorder.

Treatment Plan

- Simultaneous distalization from 3 to 7 on both sides, using TADs in tuberosity as anchorage
- Intermaxillary elastics would be used with full-time wear from the beginning of the treatment
- On the lower arch, expansion and simultaneous retraction of lower incisors was planned to create a positive overjet to correct the class II

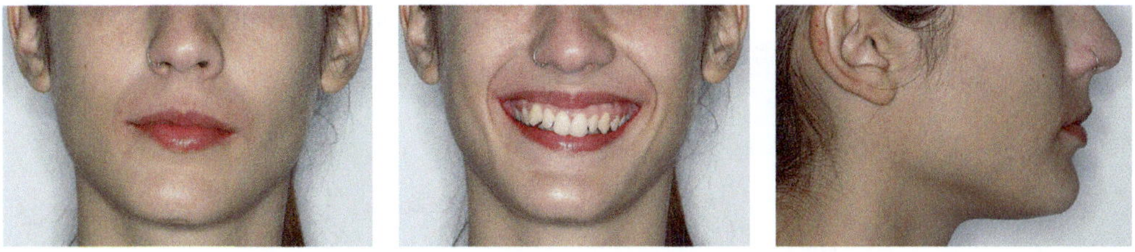

Fig. 20.114 Extraoral analysis: mandibular asymmetry.

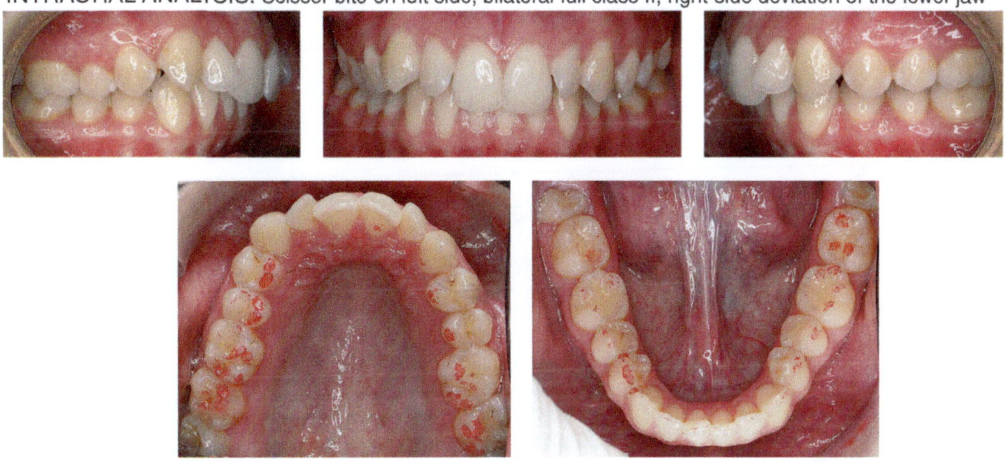

Fig. 20.115 Initial intraoral views.

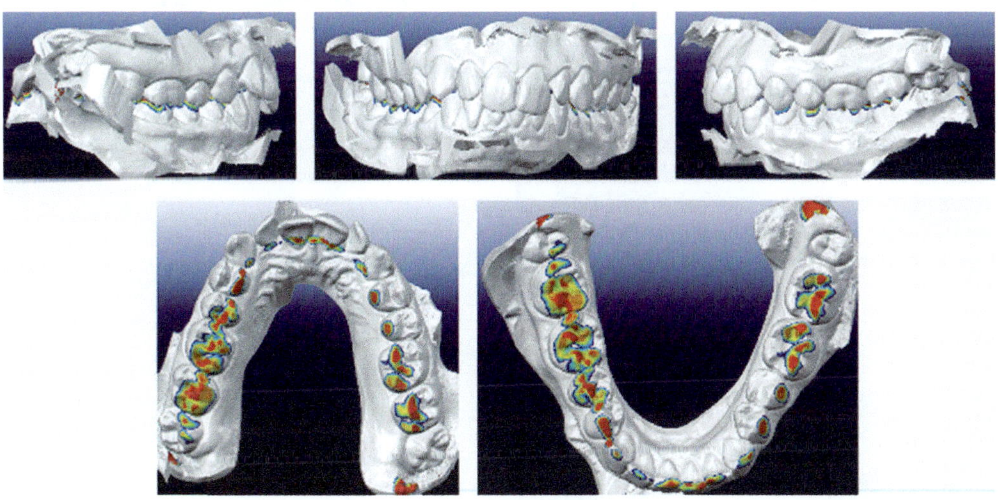

Fig. 20.116 Scissor bite on left side.

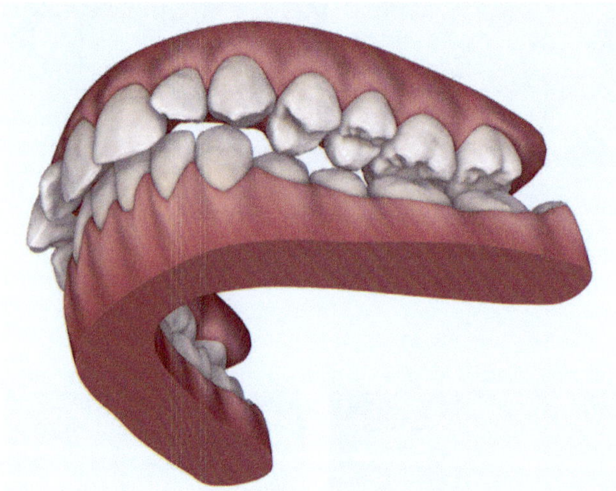

Fig. 20.117 Scissor bite on left side.

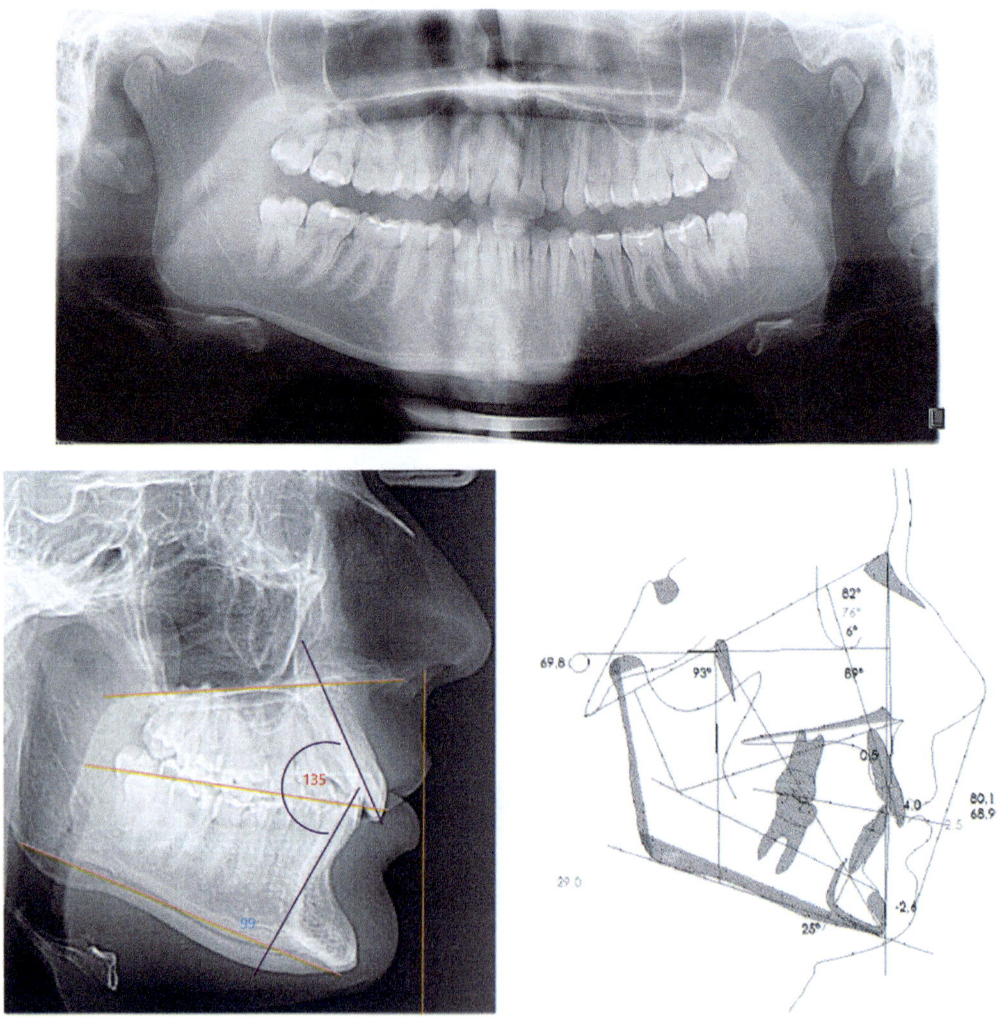

Fig. 20.118 Initial panoramic X-ray, teleradiograph and cephalometry.

Requirements for the Technician

- Distalize simultaneously from canine to second molar applying, at the same time, labial crown torque of upper incisors
- Once the molar achieves its final position, start retruding upper incisors at the same time that lingual root torque is applied to the root

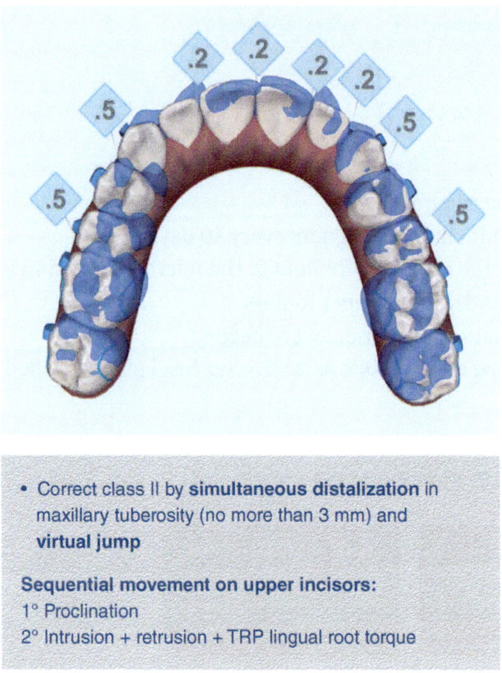

Fig. 20.119 ClinCheck upper occlusal view. Correct class II by simultaneous distalization in maxillary tuberosity (less than 3mm) and a virtual jump. Sequential movement on upper incisors: first proclination, second intrusion + retrusion + palatal root torque.

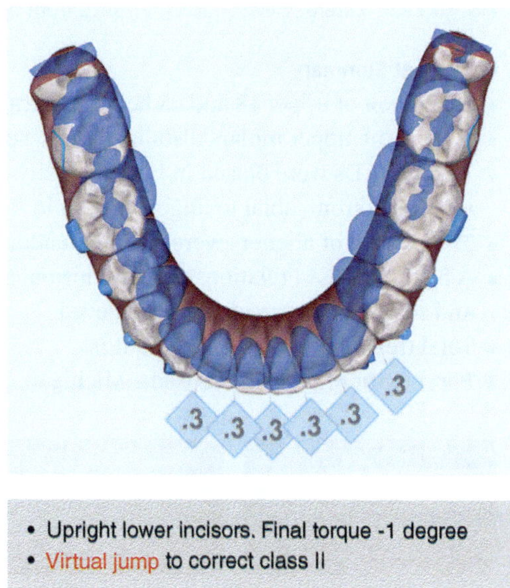

Fig. 20.120 ClinCheck lower occlusal view.

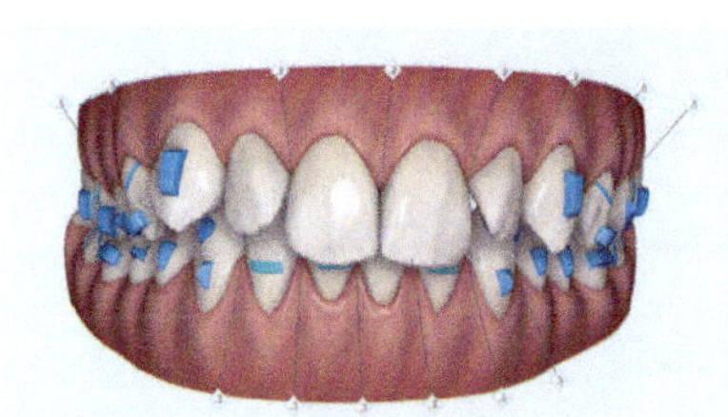

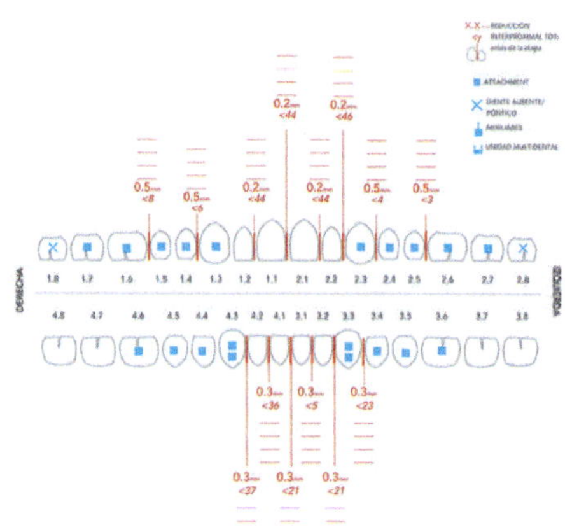

Fig. 20.121 Interproximal reduction.

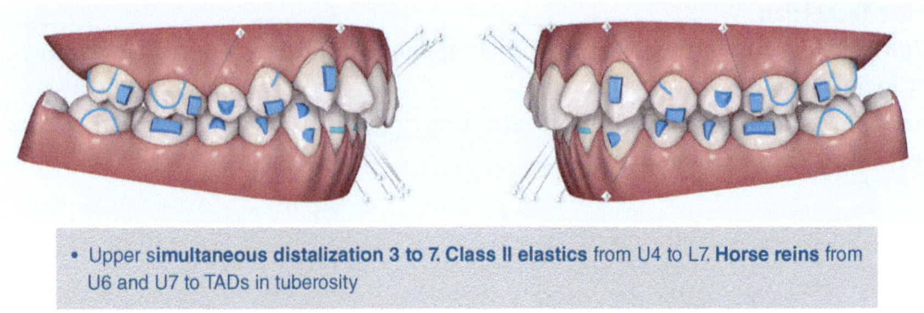

Fig. 20.122 Lateral views: Class II elastics from upper 4 to lower 7.

Treatment Summary

- Extraction of upper 18 and 28 before starting the treatment.
- During the upper molars distalization, the patient changed aligners every 10 days.
- 12 mm TADs were placed in the tuberosity and the molars were held to the microscrew using a rein horse from labial to lingual button in first and second upper molars.
- The first set of aligners were 48 and an additional set of aligners were needed.
- A bilateral class I relationship with normal overjet and overbite as well as occlusal plane levelled and scissor bite corrected was achieved.
- Total treatment time was 23 months.
- For retention, the patient used a Michigan splint.

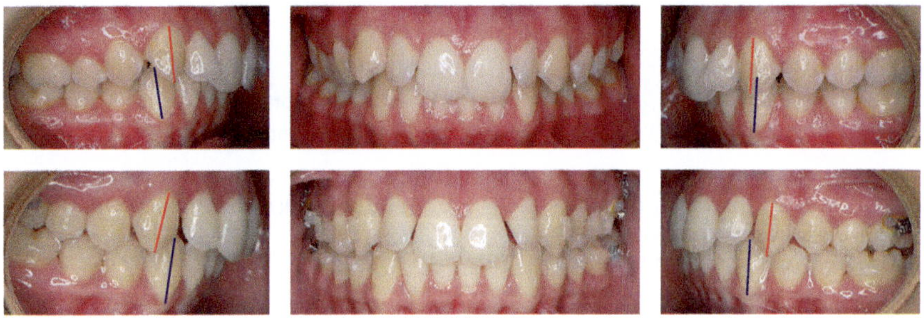

Fig. 20.123 Evolution after 13 months.

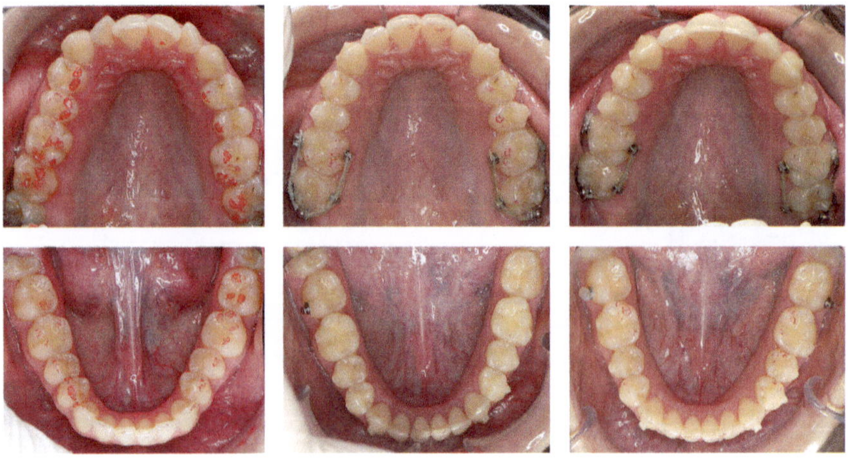

Fig. 20.124 Rein horse to distalize upper molars from TADs in the tuberosity.

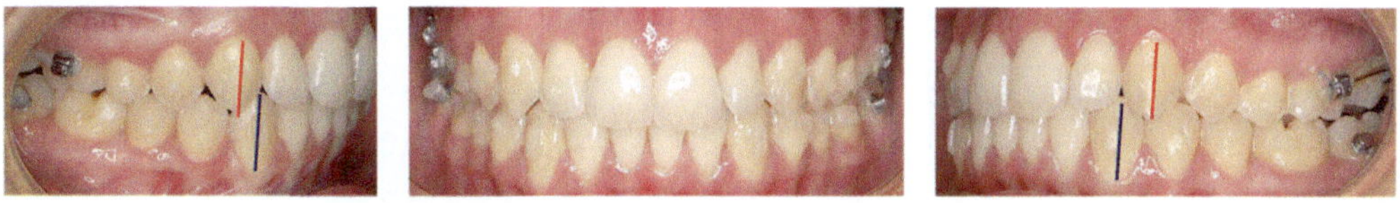

Fig. 20.125 Evolution after 17 months.

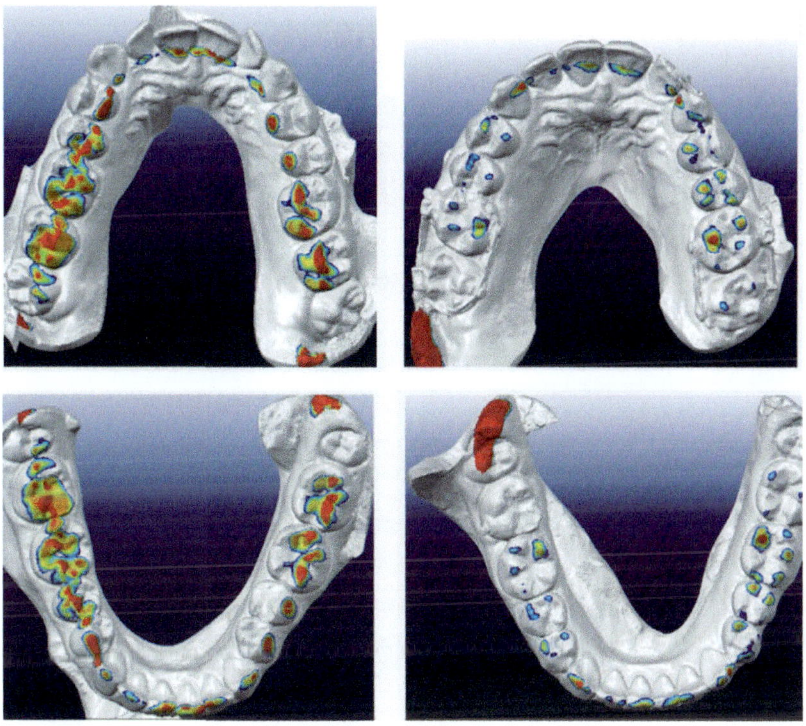

Fig. 20.126 Correction of scissor bite.

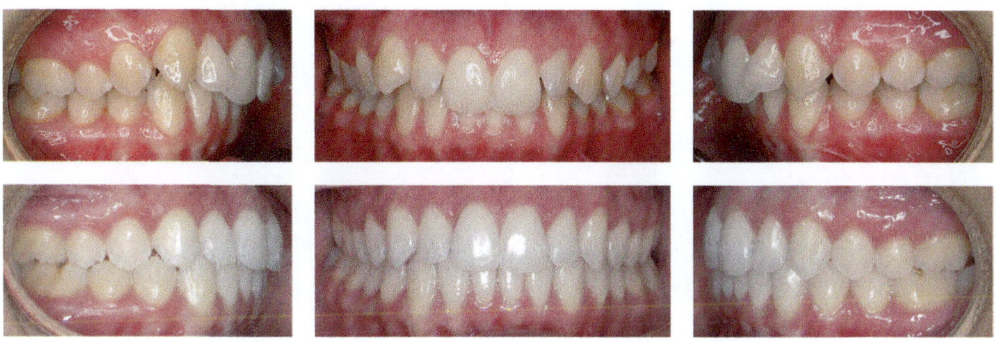

Fig. 20.127 Initial (upper) and final occlusion (lower).

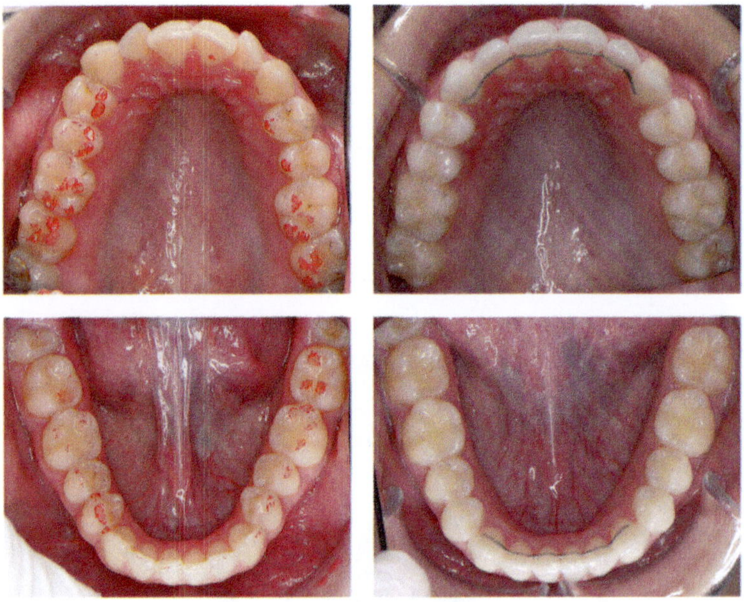

Fig. 20.128 Before (left) and after (right) occlusal.

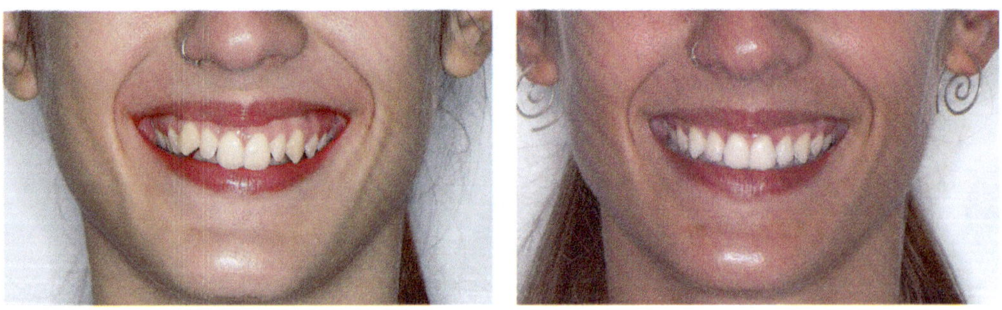

Fig. 20.129 Comparison of before (left) and after smile (right).

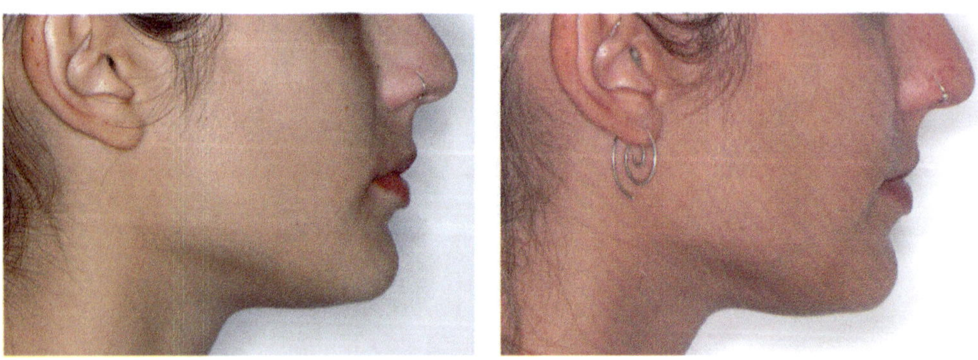

Fig. 20.130 Before (left) and after (right) profile.

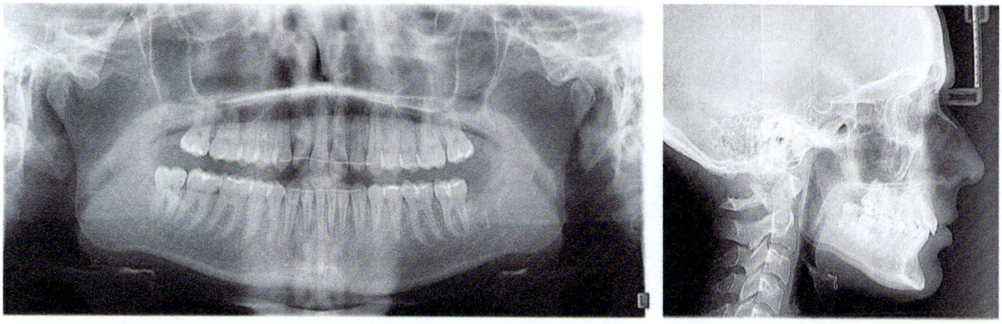

Fig. 20.131 Final panoramic and lateral X-rays.

20.2.10 Simultaneous Distalization with TADs in Tuberosity

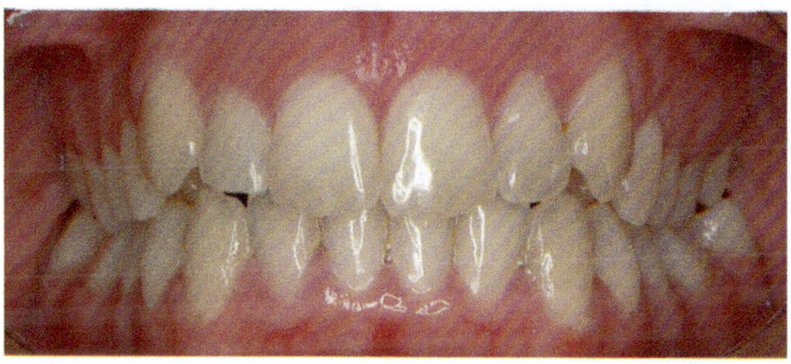

Fig. 20.132 Simultaneous distalization from 5 to 5 pattern.

Diagnosis

A 27-year-old patient with hyperdivergent skeletal class II presented with incomplete class II on both sides, class II division 2 malocclusion, lingual crown torque of upper incisors, lingual torque of upper premolars and canines. She had symmetric arches, lip competence, a retrognathic mandible and opened nasolabial angle.

Treatment Plan

- Simultaneous distalization of molars on both sides, using TADs in tuberosity as anchorage and rein horse from the beginning of treatment
- Intermaxillary elastics would not be needed as the upper anchorage to correct class II will be provided by upper TADs
- On the lower arch, in order to create positive overjet to be able to correct the class II, expansion and simultaneous retraction of lower incisors was planned using IPR between lower incisors

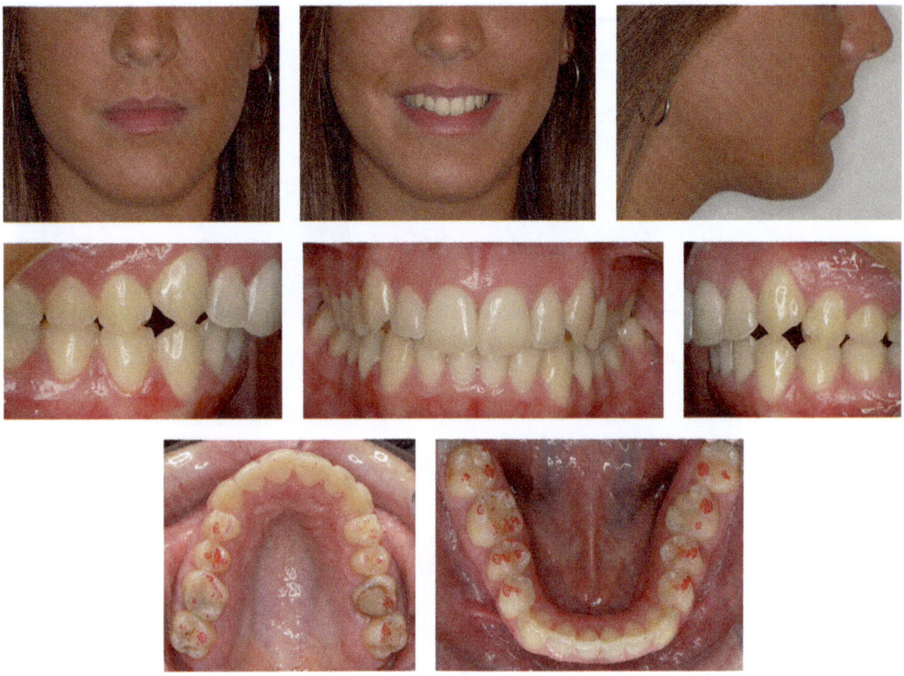

Fig. 20.133 Pretreatment extraoral and intraoral views.

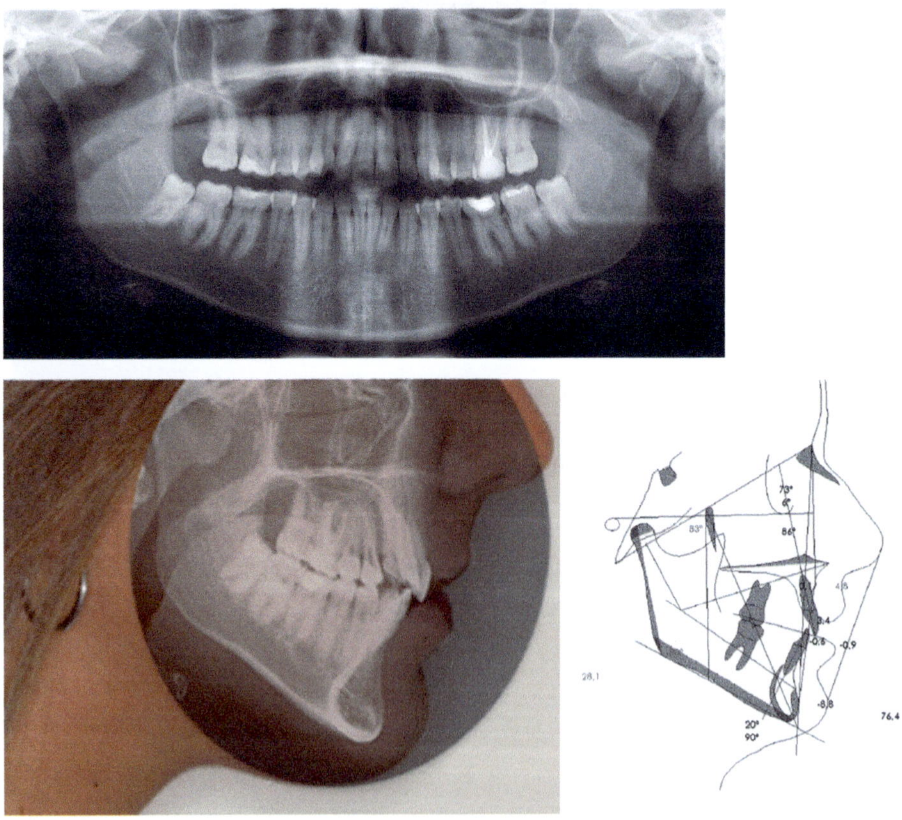

Fig. 20.134 Initial panoramic X-ray, teleradiograph and cephalometry.

Requirements for the Technician

- Distalize simultaneously upper 6 and upper 7, applying labial crown torque to the upper incisors at the same time
- Once the molar achieves its final position, start retruding 5 to 5 together at the same time that lingual root torque is applied to the upper incisors

Maxilla:

- Sequential distalization of upper molars and simultaneous distalization 5 to 5
- Lingual root torque of upper incisors
- **TADs in tuberosity**

Mandible:

- Expansion + IPR to solve crowding
- **Upright lower incisors to create overjet**
- **Class II elastics**

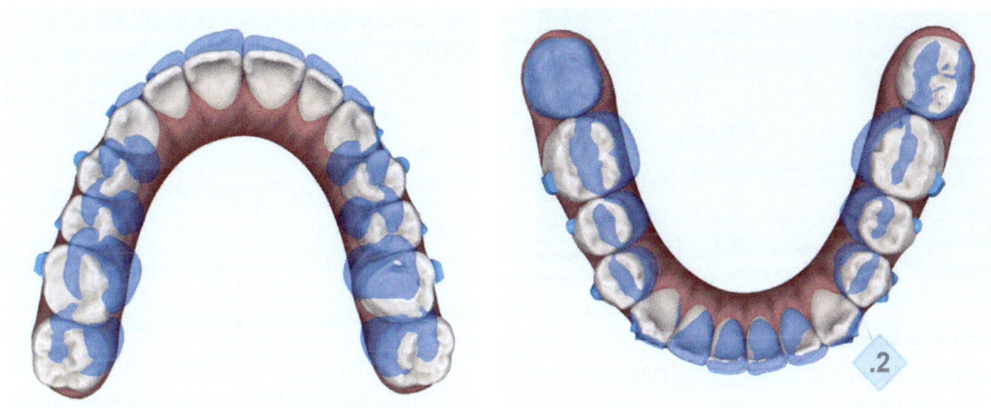

Fig. 20.135 Initial upper and lower ClinCheck views.

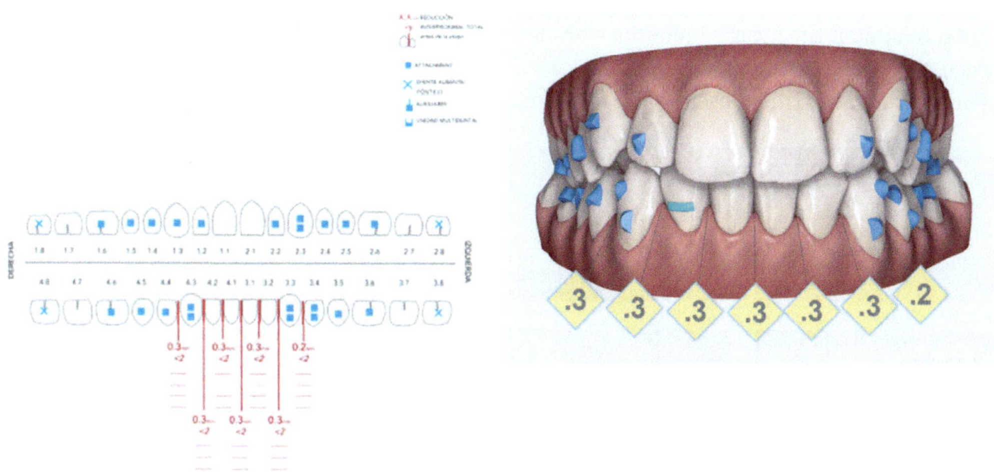

Fig. 20.136 Interproximal reduction from 33 to 43 to upright lower incisors.

- TADs in the tuberosity + direct anchorage to second and first molars for simultaneous distalization 5 to 5 + class II elastics

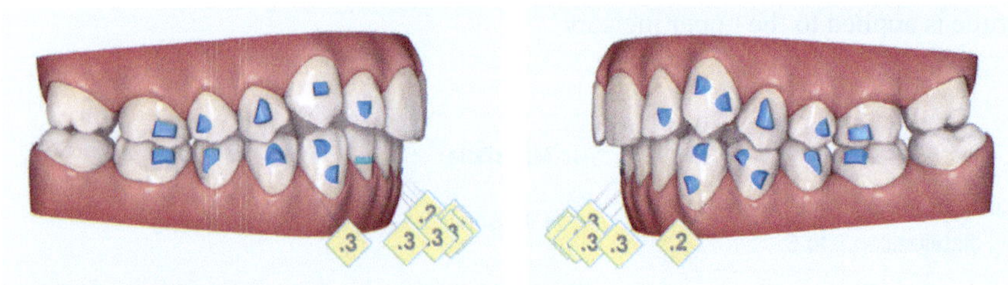

Fig. 20.137 Right and left ClinCheck views.

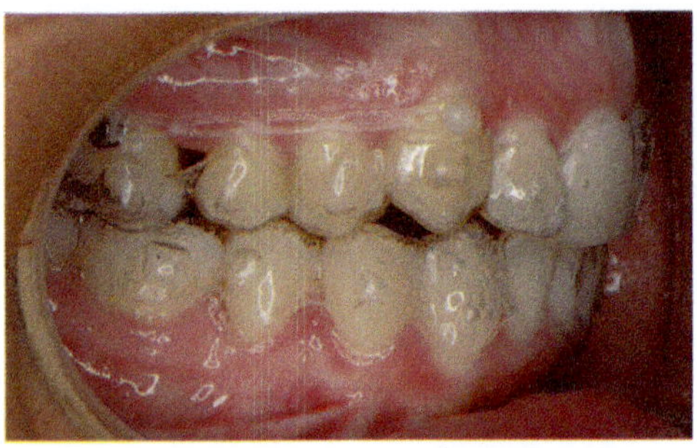

Fig. 20.138 Intra-arch Powerchain from upper canine to first molar to guide 5 to 5 simultaneous distalization.

Treatment Summary

- During the upper molars distalization, the patient changed aligners every 7 days.
- 12 mm TADs were placed in the tuberosity and the molars were held to the microscrew using rein horse from labial to lingual button in first and second upper molars.
- The first set of aligners were 35 and an additional set of aligners was needed.
- A bilateral class I relationship with normal overjet and overbite with both midlines centred and an adequate final torque of upper incisors was achieved.
- Total treatment time was 15 months with no intermaxillary elastics needed except to settle the occlusion at the end of the treatment.
- For retention the patient used vivera retainers.

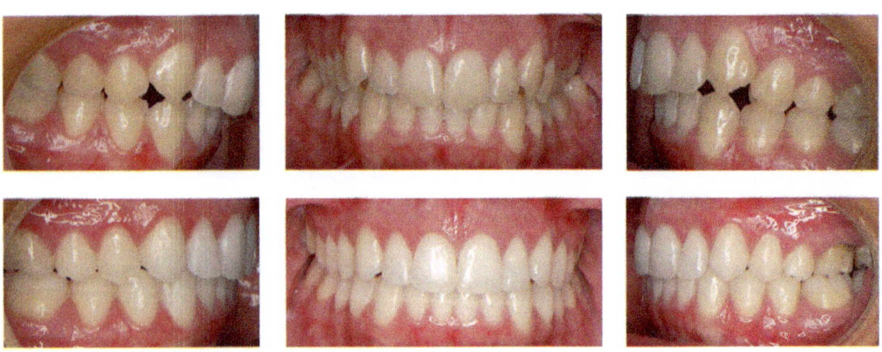

Fig. 20.139 Initial (upper) and final (lowe) intraoral views.

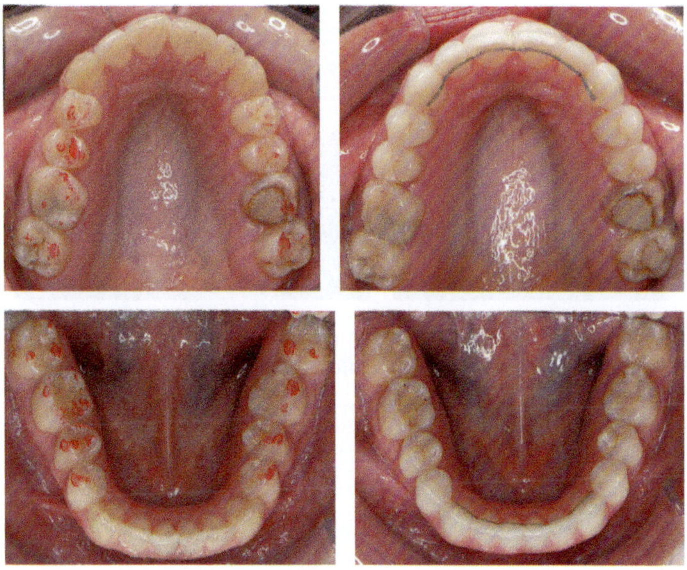

Fig. 20.140 Occlusal before (left) and after (right) treatment.

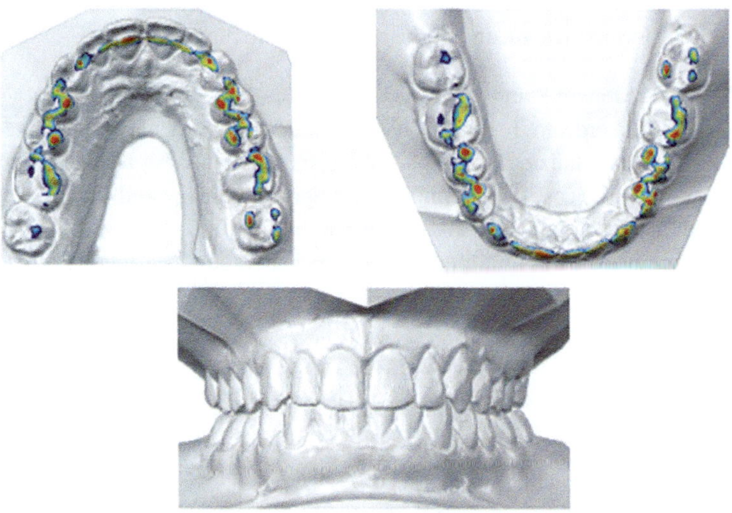

Fig. 20.141 Final occlusal contact.

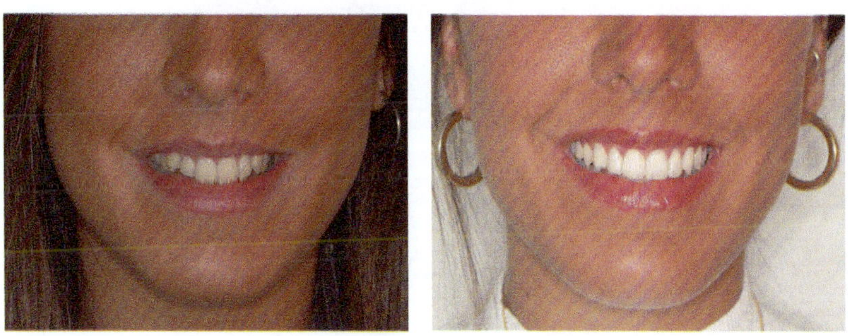

Fig. 20.142 Initial (left) and final smile (right).

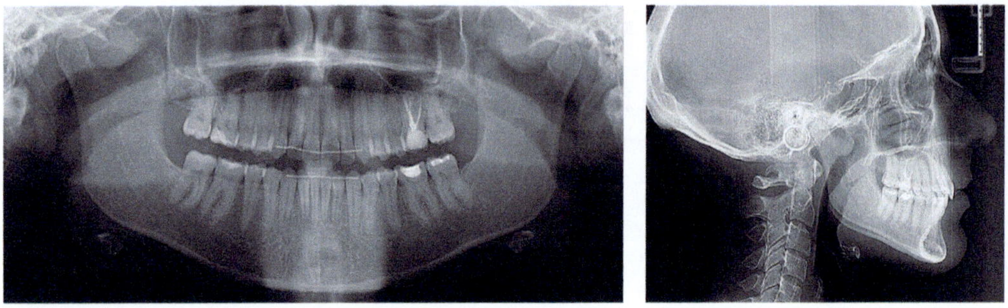

Fig. 20.143 Final panoramic and lateral X-rays: maintenance of lower incisor torque during treatment through not using class II elastics and using TADs instead to distalize upper arch.

20.2.11 Top Jet

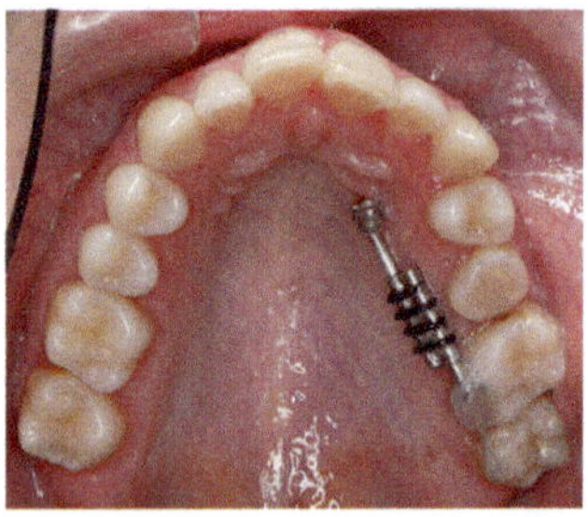

Fig. 20.144 Top jet appliance.

Diagnosis

A 38-year-old brachyfacial patient with a skeletal class I pattern and dental class II malocclusion presented with full class II on the left and an incomplete class II on the right, minor crowding, upper incisor proclination and an upper right midline deviation from facial midline. They had an asymmetric smile as a result of asymmetric raising of the corners of the mouth.

Treatment Plan

- In order to shorten the treatment time, the treatment plan consisted of distalizing both upper left molars simultaneously using a top jet
- After the molars achieved a class I, the case was submitted to Align Technology and the malocclusion correction completed by sequential upper distalization in both arches
- The distalization of the molars would be maintained by using a clear vacuum-formed retainer full-time until the first aligner was delivered

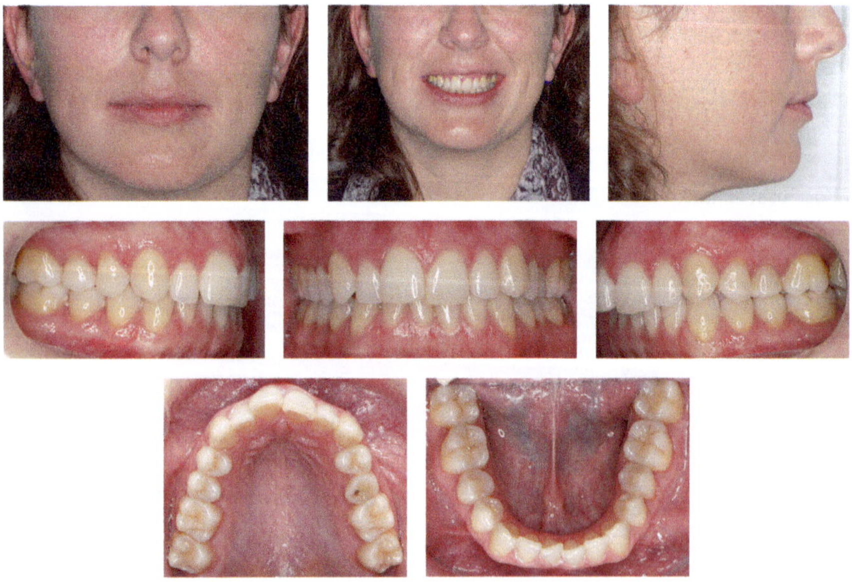

Fig. 20.145 Pretreatment extraoral and intraoral views.

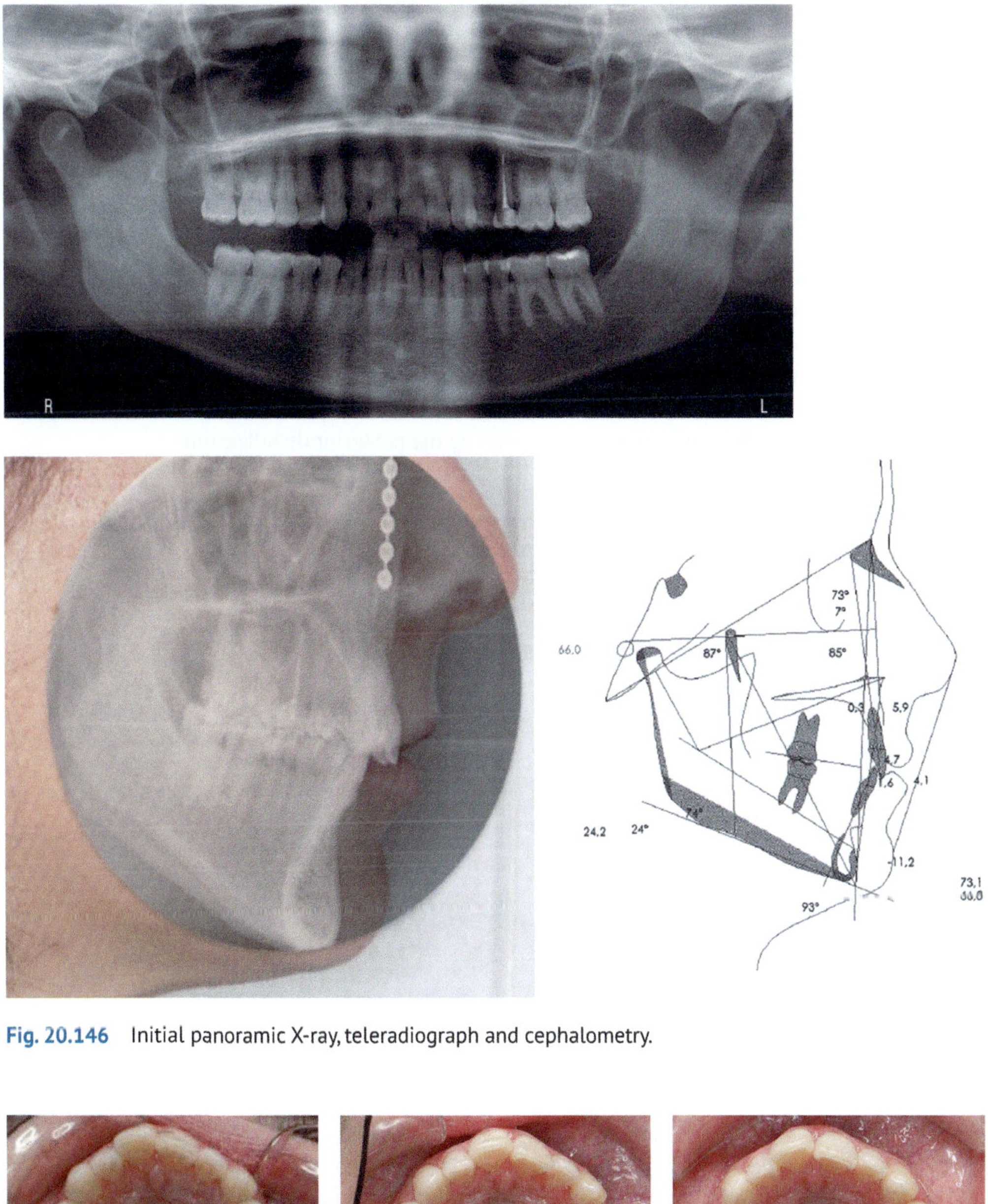

Fig. 20.146 Initial panoramic X-ray, teleradiograph and cephalometry.

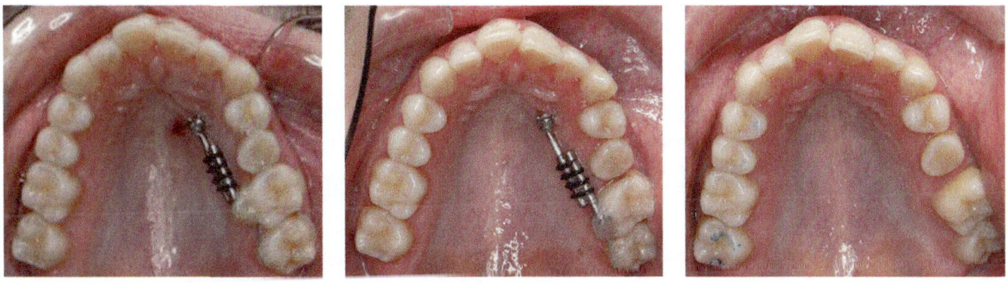

Fig. 20.147 Distalization with top jet before Invisalign treatment.

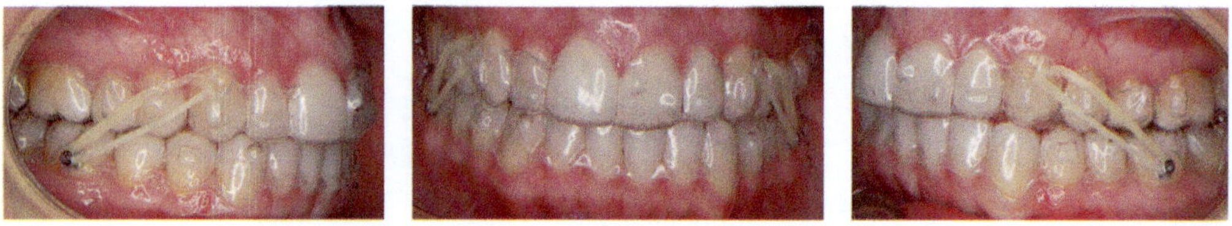

Fig. 20.148 Sequential distalization with class II elastics.

Requirements for the Technician

- When the records were sent to Align Technology, molars on the left side were already in class I, so the technician was required to start from the first aligner with a bilateral sequential distalization using the standard staging.
- Bevelled attachments were required on incisal edges of upper lateral incisor and lingual ellipsoidal attachment for better anterior anchorage during the posterior distalization.

Maxilla:

- Upper sequential distalization
- Correct upper midline

Mandible:

- Expansion + IPR to upright lower incisors

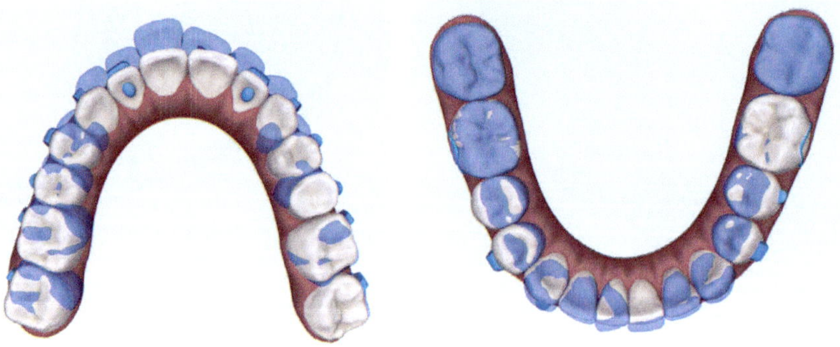

Fig. 20.149 Upper and lower ClinCheck views.

Bilateral sequential distalization (previous distalization of 26 and 27 with top jet)

- Anchorage attachments: Horizontals U4 and U6 and vertical attachment on canines.
- Class II elastics

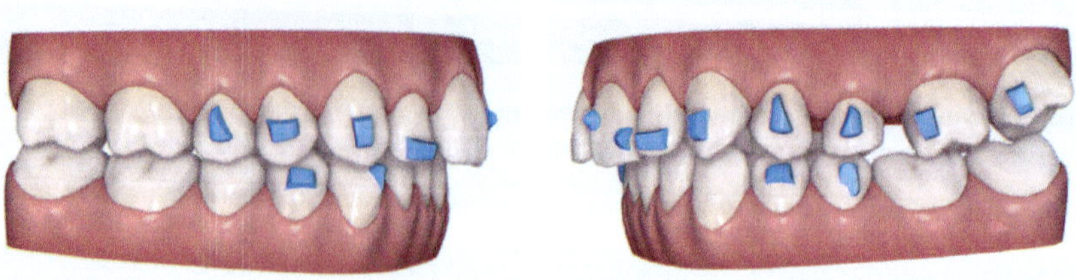

Fig. 20.150 Lateral ClinCheck views.

Treatment Summary

- The patient had 3.5 months of treatment with the top jet before Invisalign treatment. The top jet was activated every 2 weeks.
- After 3.5 months, the case was submitted to Align Technology; the patient had 43 aligners with class II elastic with full-time wear and the aligner was changed every 10 days.
- After the 43 aligners, a new set of additional aligners was requested.
- Total treatment time was 18 months.
- Class I was achieved in both sides. Both midlines were centred and the improvement in incisor inclination and interincisal angle is shown in the cephalometric radiograph (Fig. 20.155).

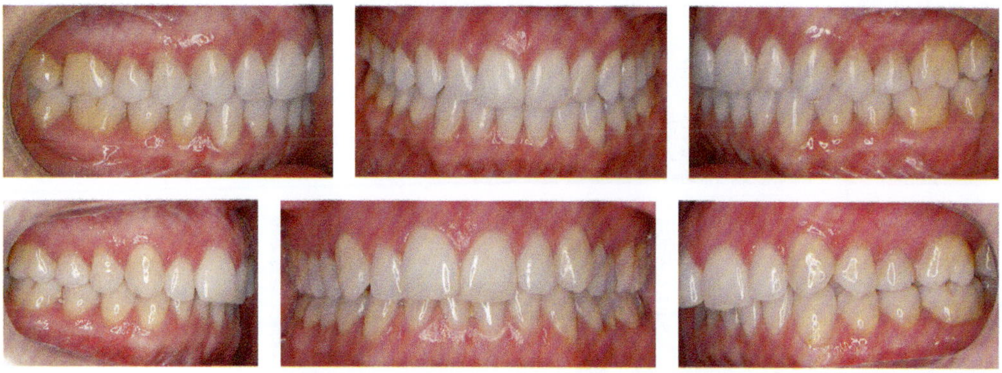

Fig. 20.151 Comparison of initial (upper) and final (lower) intraoral views. Both midlines centred and bilateral class I.

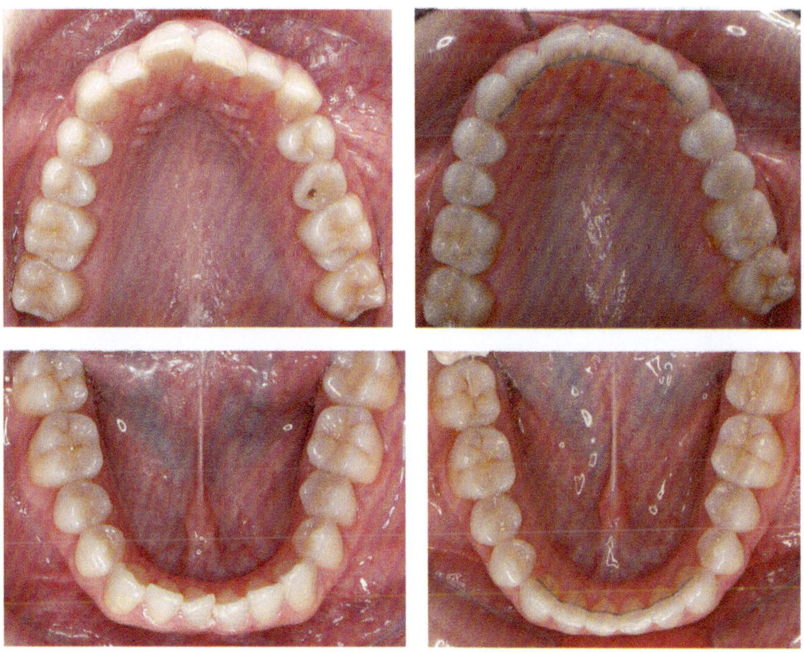

Fig. 20.152 Initial (left) and final (right) occlusal.

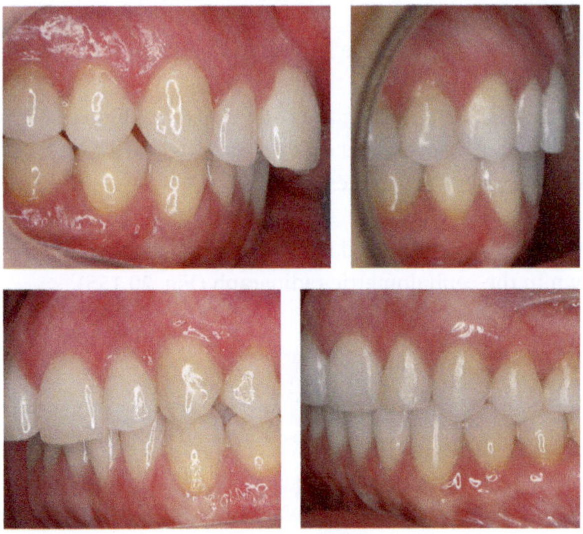

Fig. 20.153 Initial (right) and final overjet (left).

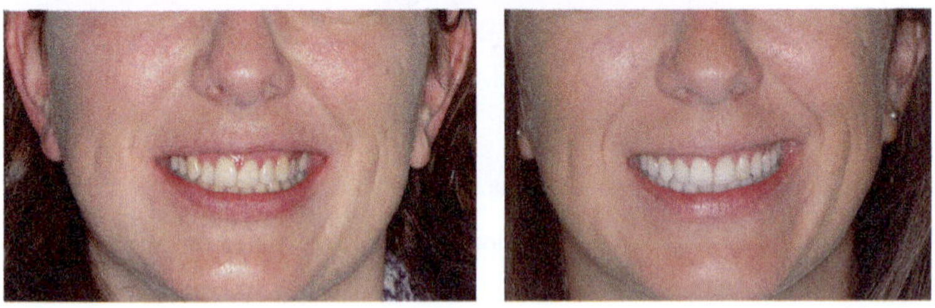

Fig. 20.154 Initial and final smile.

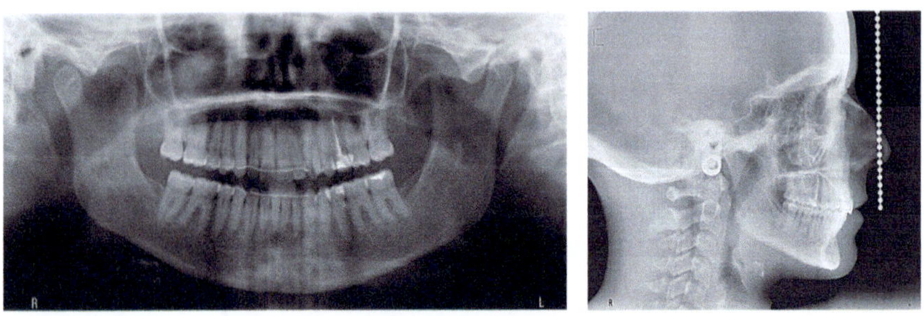

Fig. 20.155 Final panoramic and lateral X-rays.

20.2.12 Class II with Proclined Lower Incisors

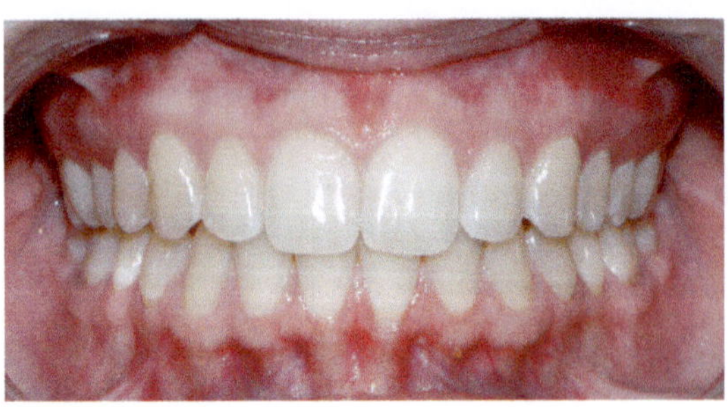

Fig 20.156 Initial intraoral view.

Diagnosis

A 29-year-old brachyfacial patient with a skeletal class I pattern and dental class II malocclusion presented with half cusp class II on the right and mild class II on the left, lower incisor proclination and a relapse from previous treatment with intensive use of class II elastics.

Treatment Plan

- Treatment consisted of upper sequential distalization with reduced use of elastics thereby avoiding mesialization on the lower arch
- IPR on lower arch, as well as extra lingual root torque from 32 to 42 helped improve their position in relation to bone

ClinCheck 1: Requirement for the Technician

Upper:

- Use second quadrant as anchorage until molars finish their movement, after that proceed with slight expansion
- Deferred sequential half distalization on the upper arch, combined with expansion to reduce arch depth

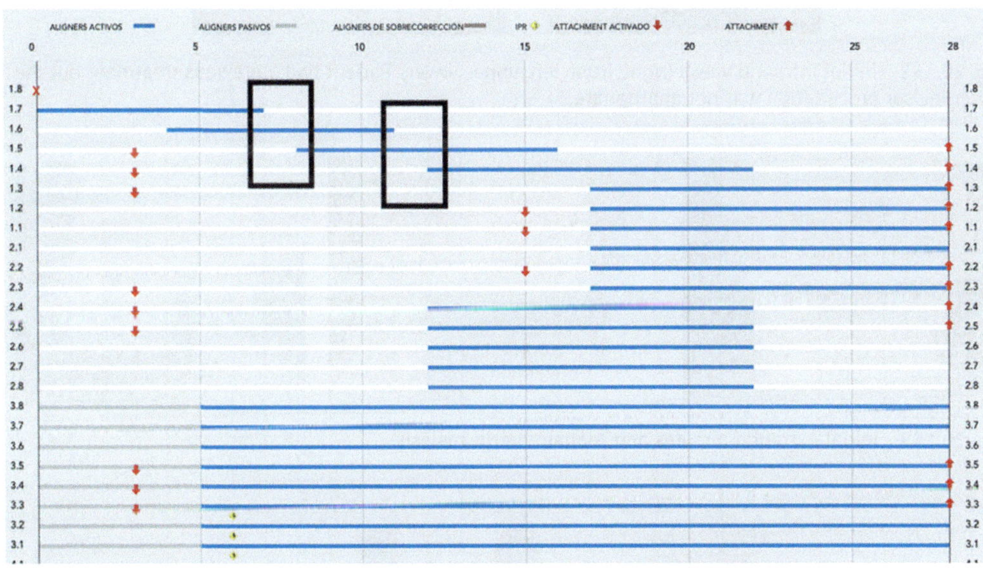

Fig 20.157 Deferred sequential distalization, in which some teeth move 'alone' in order to maximize anchorage because of the lack of intermaxillary elastics use.

Lower:

- Expansion and lower IPR to reduce intercanine distance
- Extra lingual root torque 32-42 to improve their position inside the bone, using buccal power ridges

Treatment Summary

- Patient had 20 months of treatment with aligner change every 2 weeks, and night use elastics on the second stage.
- After the 28 aligners, a new set of 20 additional aligners was requested.
- Class I was achieved in both sides. The improvement in lower incisor inclination in relation to the bone is shown in the cone beam computed tomography (CTCB) radiograph (see Fig. 20.164).

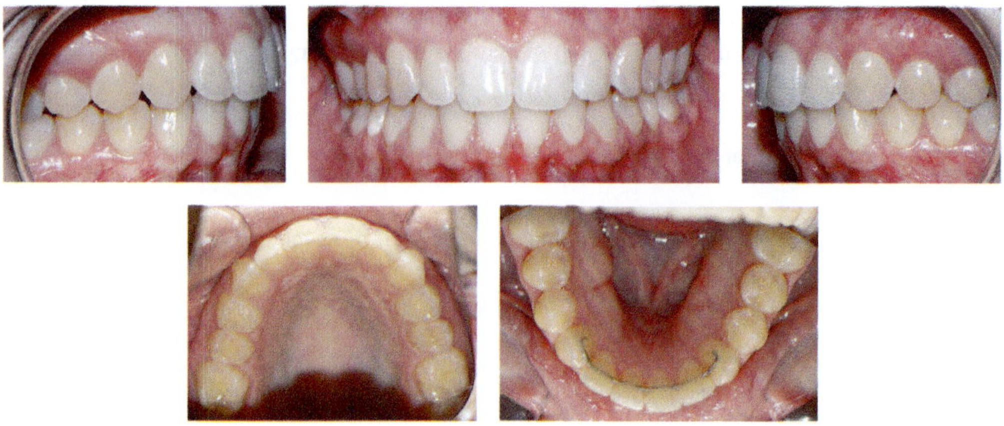

Fig. 20.158 Initial intraoral views (right, front, left, upper, lower). Patient had a previous treatment but the lower incisor proclination was not appropriate.

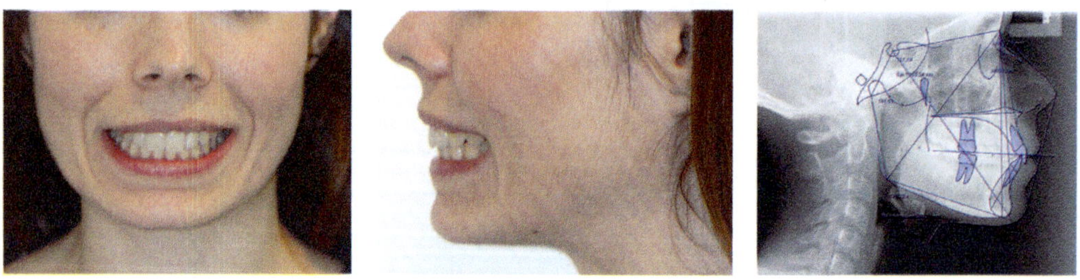

Fig. 20.159 Initial extraoral pictures and cephalometric analysis.

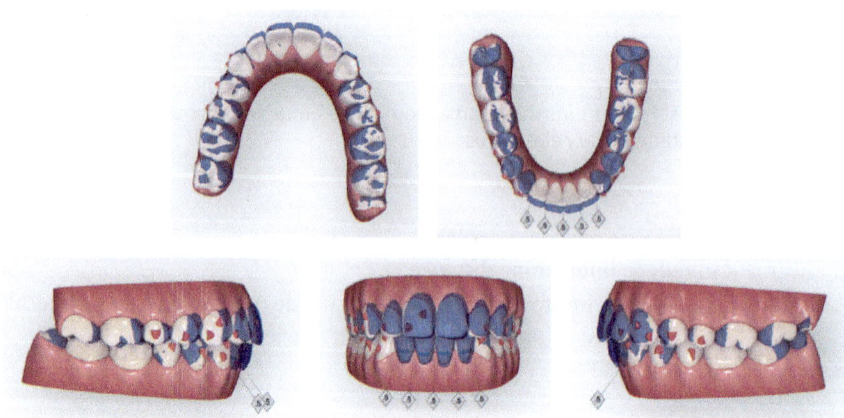

Fig. 20.160 Initial ClinChecks.

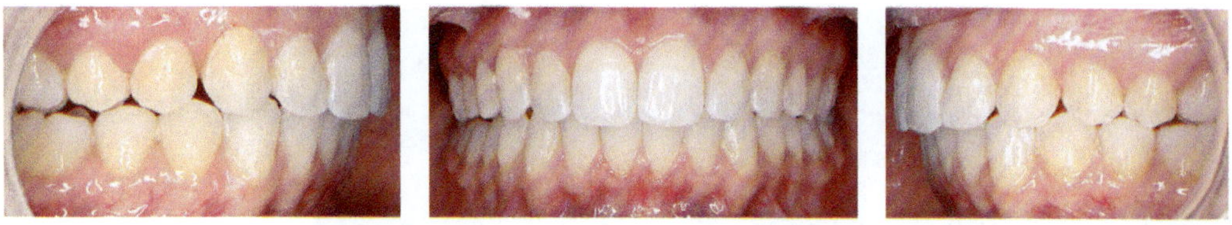

Fig. 20.161 Intraoral pictures at refinement.

ClinCheck 2: Requirement for the Technician

- Sequential distalization on upper arch, together with night class II elastics for a sagittal and vertical component
- Expansion to help with retrusion
- Anterior intrusion combined with posterior extrusion so as to hypercorrect anterior deep bite and posterior deep bite

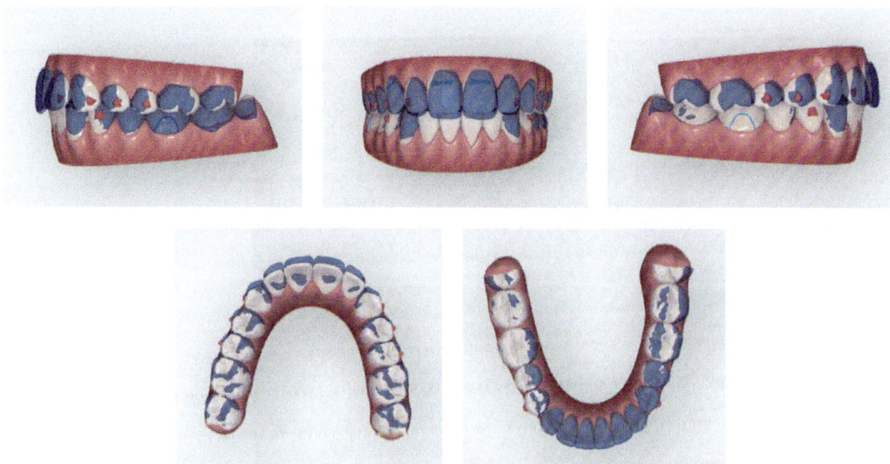

Fig. 20.162 Refinement ClinChecks.

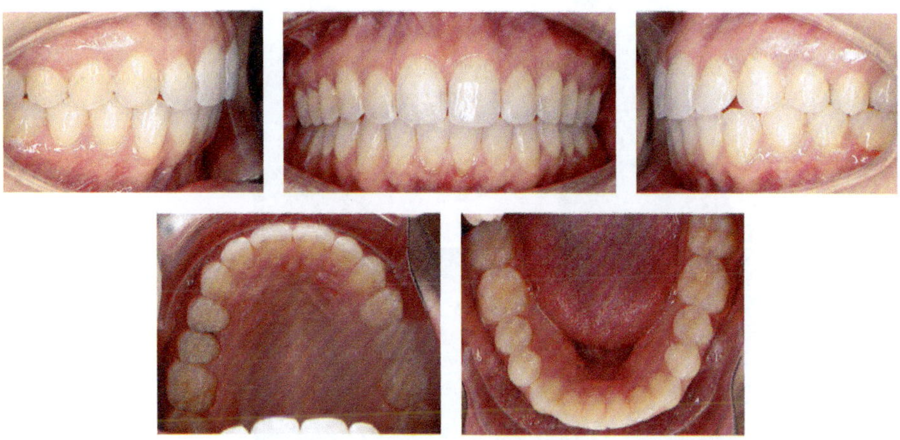

Fig. 20.163 Final: intraoral pictures showing improvement of the lower incisor position as well as a stable class II occlusion.

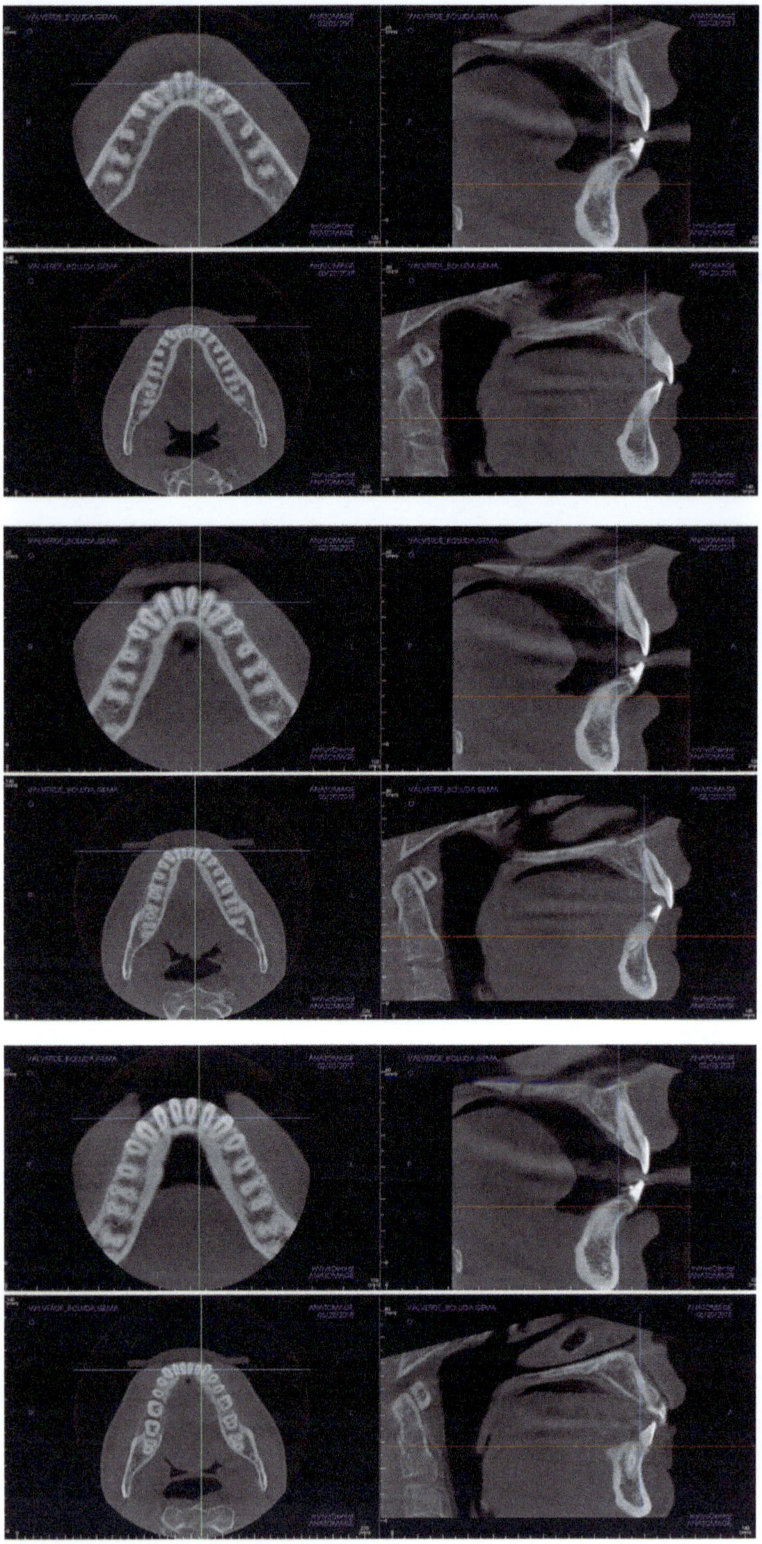

Fig. 20.164 The cone beam computed tomography comparisons show how the lower incisor position was improved in relation to the bone.

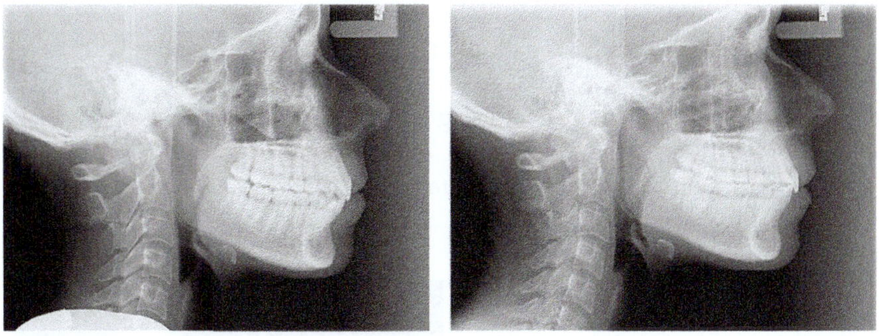

Fig. 20.165 Final comparison of lateral X-rays.

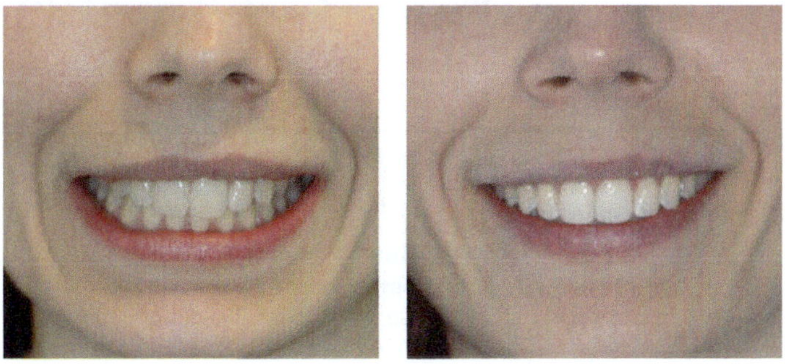

Fig. 20.166 Comparison of before and after smile.

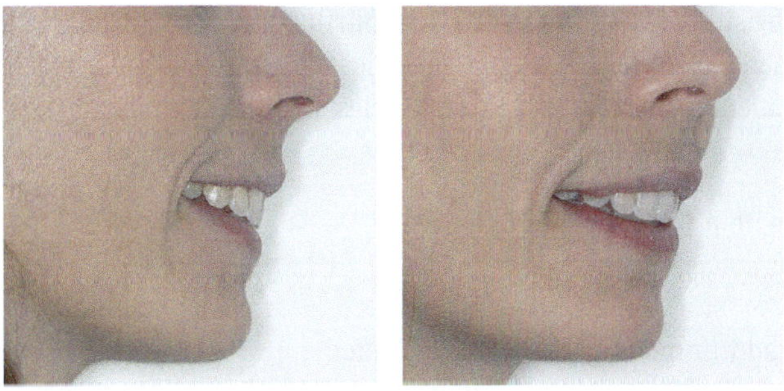

Fig. 20.167 Extraoral profile views.

20.2.13 Full Class II with Posterior Crossbite

Diagnosis

A 34-year-old brachyfacial patient with a skeletal class II pattern and dental class II malocclusion presented with full cusp class II on the right and class I on the left, posterior crossbite on the right side and a deep bite.

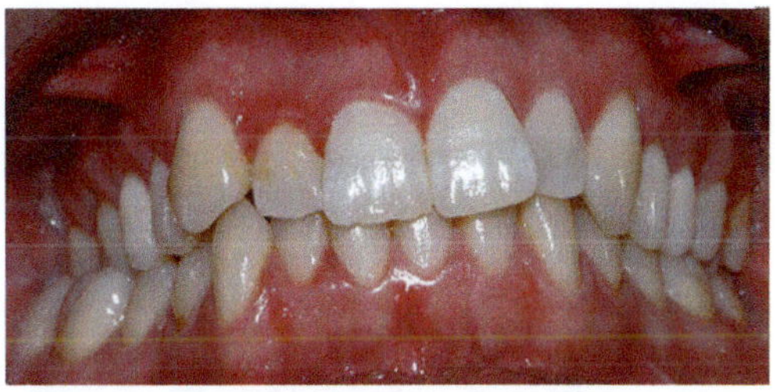

Fig. 20.168 Initial intraoral view.

Treatment Plan

- Treatment consisted of upper sequential distalization on first quadrant together with lower mesialization on that arch
- Crossbite protocol was applied, with the patient using criss-cross elastics during upper molars expansion
- Contralateral sides were used on both sets of aligners to create anchorage allowing movement

ClinCheck 1: Requirement for the Technician

Upper:

- Use second quadrant as anchorage until premolars finish their movement, after that proceed with slight expansion on left side
- Place precision cuts for criss-cross on posterior sector (palatal upper molars, buccal lower molars)
- Manual precision cuts added on 13 to help with class II elastics when crossbite was solved
- Start sequential distalization at the same time as anterior torque correction, applying biomechanical concepts seen before in the book
- Combine both distalization and expansion (for this instruct the patient to wear elastic from upper 6 to lower 7, creating a class II vector + expansion force)

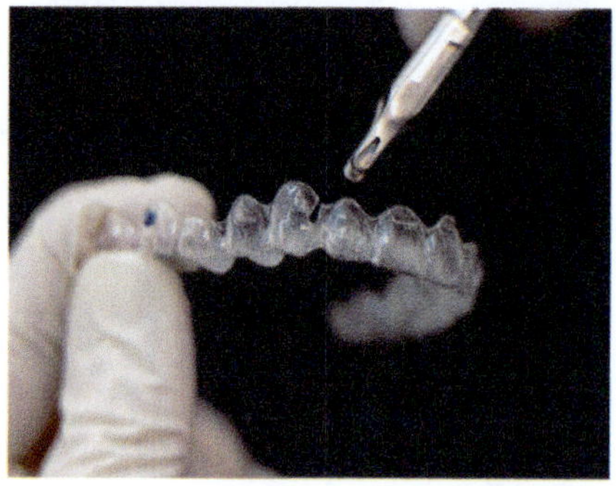

Fig. 20.169 Manual precision cut on 13 allows optimized attachment on this tooth, otherwise it would be changed to a different one with less root control.

Lower:

- Expansion on third quadrant and protrusion of lower incisors using fourth quadrant as anchorage
- Start fourth quadrant mesialization when lower incisors are proclined, leaving a space distal to them by arch expansion. At the same time patient would start using class II elastics as crossbite is solved

Treatment Summary

- Patient had 20 months of treatment with a 1 week aligner change
- Criss-cross elastics until crossbite was solved
- After that, class II elastics
- After the 61 aligners, a new set of 22 additional aligners were requested
- Class I was achieved in both sides, solving the deep bite and expanding both arches to create a more pleasing smile

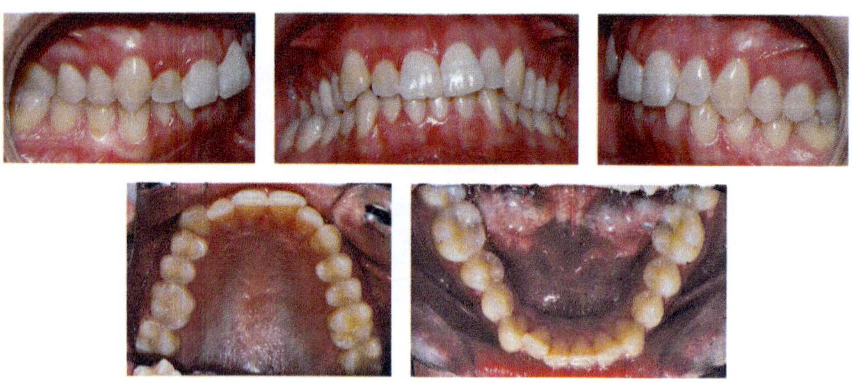

Fig. 20.170 Initial intraoral views (right, front, left, upper, lower).

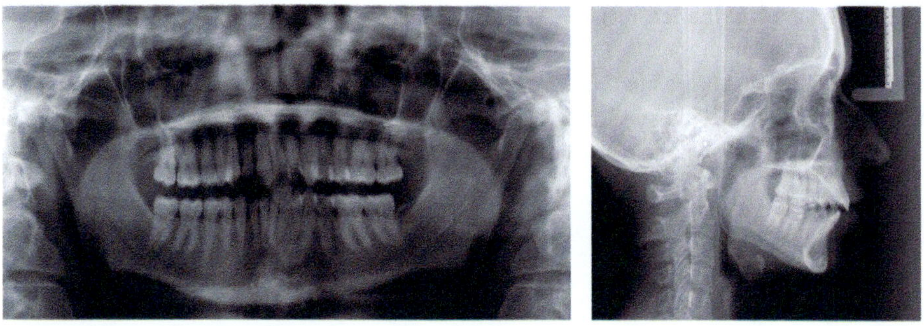

Fig. 20.171 Initial panoramic and lateral X-rays.

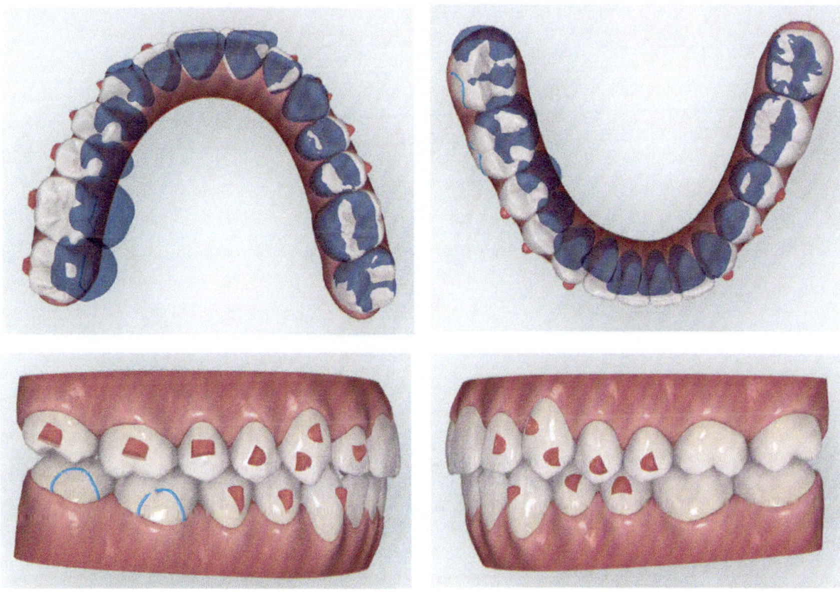

Fig. 20.172 Initial ClinChecks.

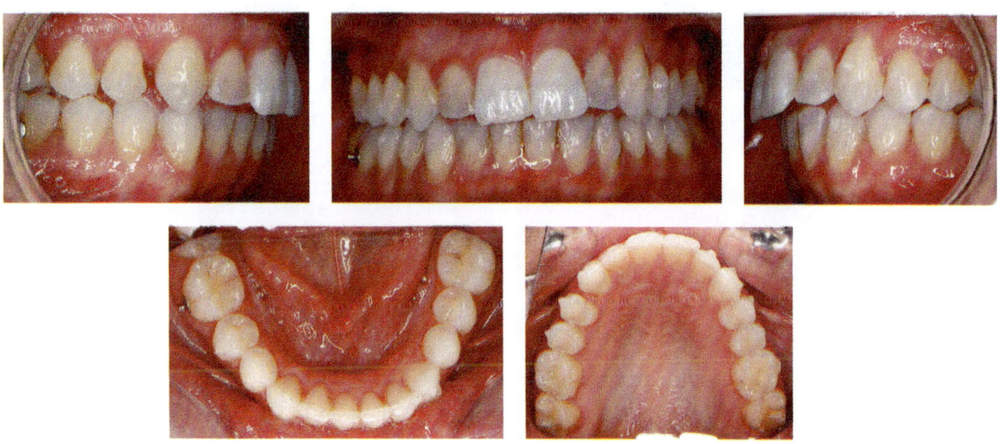

Fig. 20.173 Refinement: initial intraoral views (right, front, left, upper, lower).

ClinCheck 2: Requirements for the Technician

- Use second quadrant as anchorage
- Posterior precision button cutouts for vertical elastics, day wear
- Precision hook on 13, class II elastics for night use

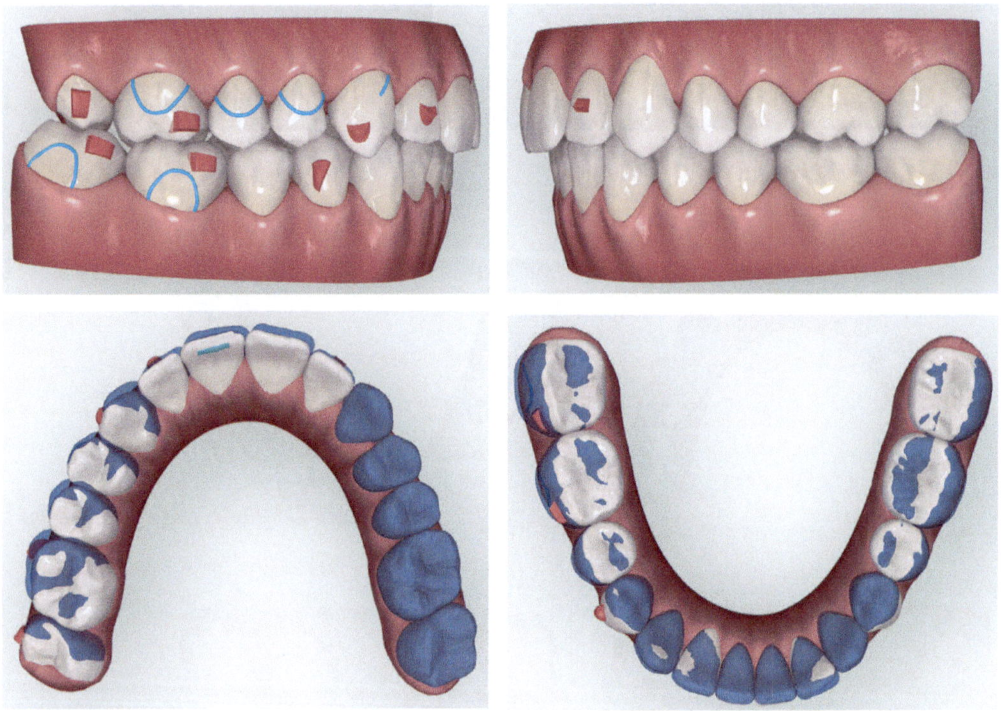

Fig. 20.174 Refinement ClinChecks.

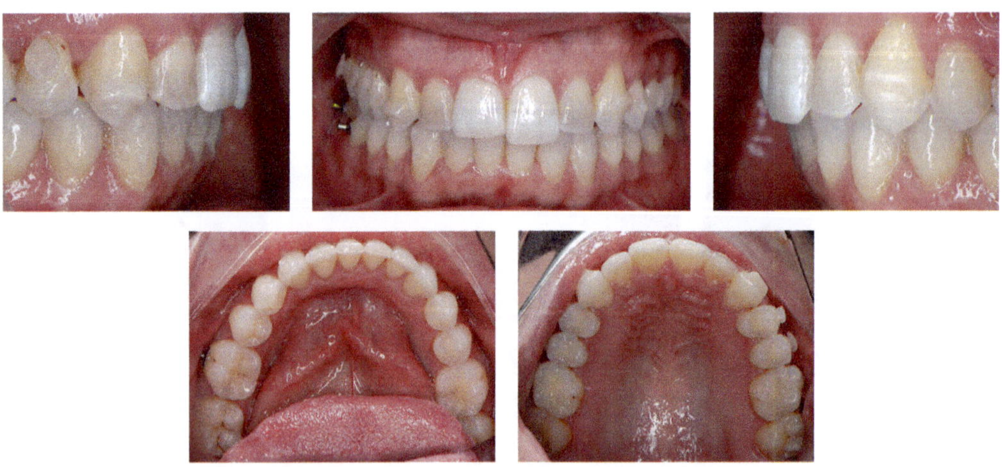

Fig. 20.175 Final intraoral views (right, front, left, lower, upper).

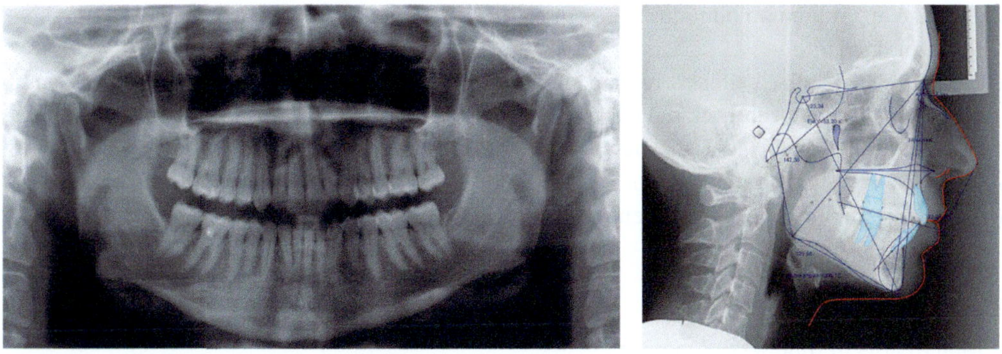

Fig. 20.176 Final panoramic and lateral X-rays.

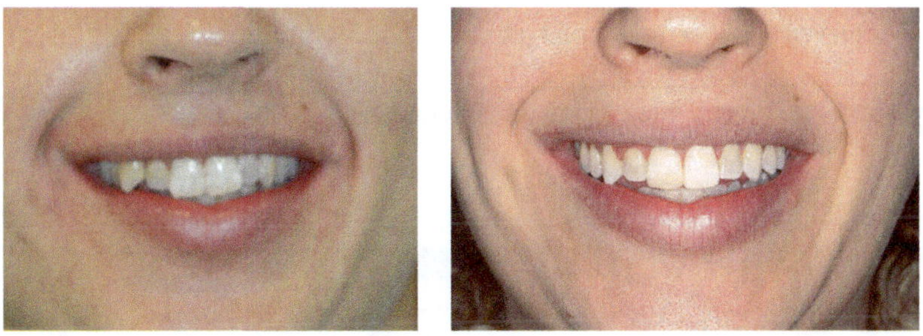

Fig. 20.177 Before and after smiles, before aesthetic anterior restoration.

20.2.14 Class II Patient with Anterior Open Bite and Crossbite

Diagnosis

A 20-year-old man with a skeletal class II pattern presented with anterior crossbite 22, open bite tendency, posterior compression, short incisor display and half cusp class II on both left and right side

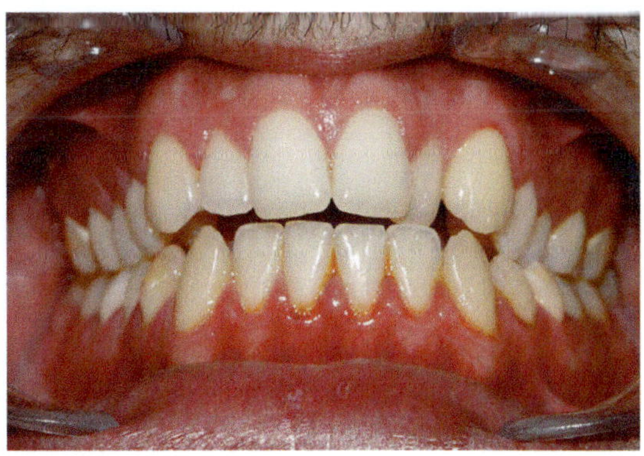

Fig. 20.178 Initial intraoral view.

Treatment Plan

- Upper wisdom teeth were extracted before the orthodontic treatment
- Anterior crossbite to be corrected
- Expand arches to improve smile aesthetics
- Intrude posterior teeth so as to close the anterior bite by mandibular rotation, which would help in solving class II

ClinCheck 1: Requirements for the Technician

- Anterior extrusion attachments protocol to help with posterior intrusion
- Expand at the same time as anterior torque is lost to help with relative extrusion

- Distalize upper arch on both quadrants intruding upper molars at the same time, to end with a posterior open bite
- Lower arch mesialized after correcting lower incisors torque and intruding them, therefore creating space that is usually closed by retrusion but to be used for posterior sector mesialization, thanks to 24/7 use of class II elastics
- Extra BRT to 22 to help take the root to its perfect position with regard to torque
- Place attachments on 13 to 23 when their extrusion movement starts, so as to keep anterior aesthetics free from attachments

Treatment Summary

- Total treatment time was 17 months
- A total of 44 active aligners were used on a 7-day change interval and an additional set of 11 aligners were used
- Class II elastics were worn continuously
- Bilateral class I was achieved with dentoalveolar expansion in both arches resulting in an improved smile
- Retention was provided with Vivera, increasing the thickness on posterior sectors to prevent relapse

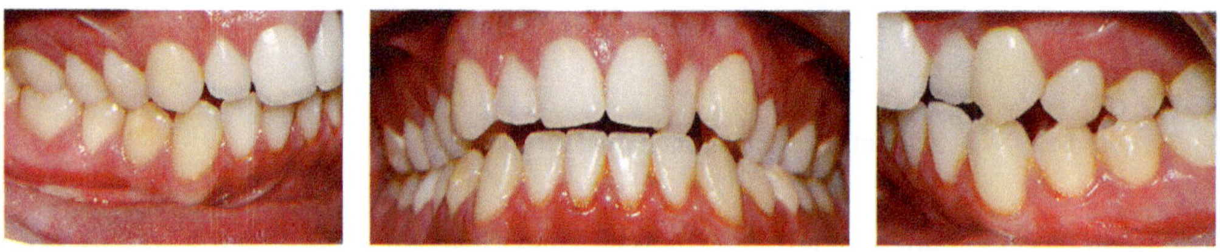

Fig. 20.179 Initial intraoral views (right, front, left, upper).

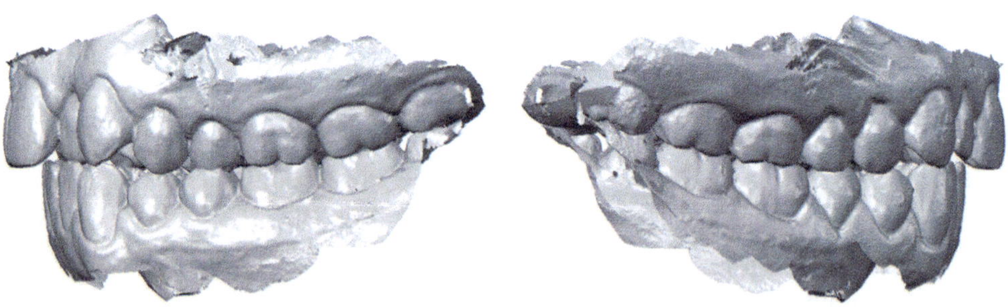

Fig. 20.180 Initial intraoral models to check class II relationship before 18 and 28 were extracted.

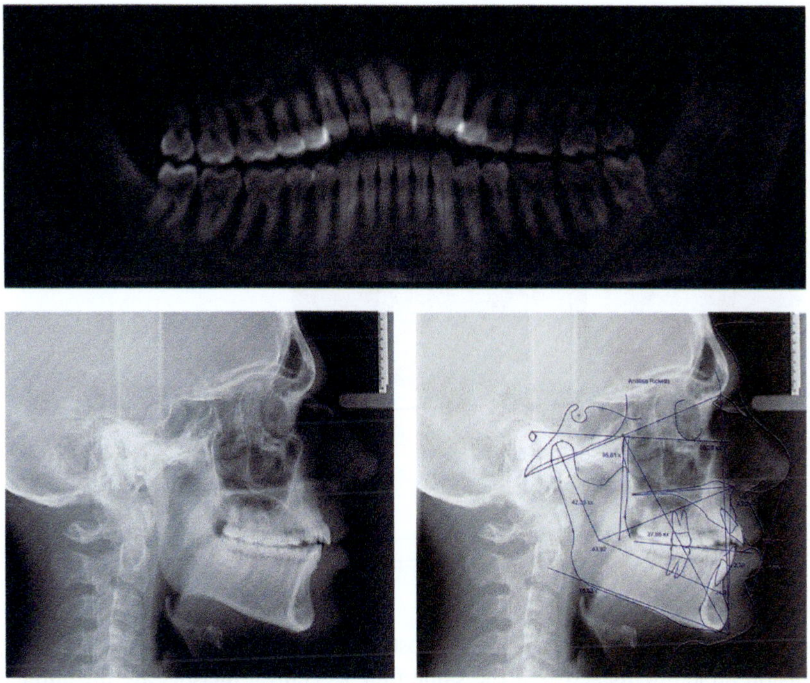

Fig. 20.181 Pretreatment panoramic and lateral X-rays and cephalometry.

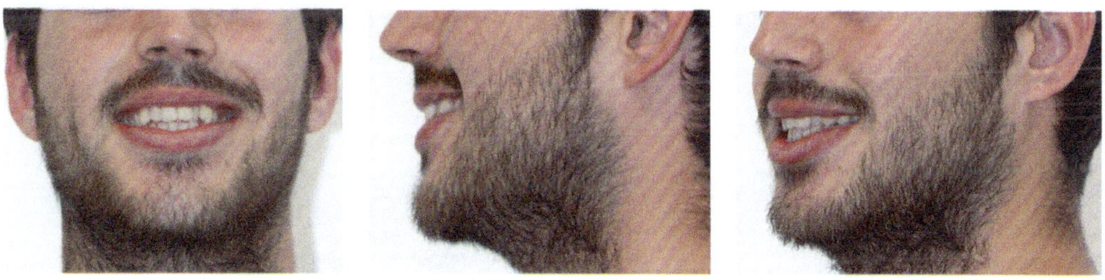

Fig. 20.182 Initial extraoral views.

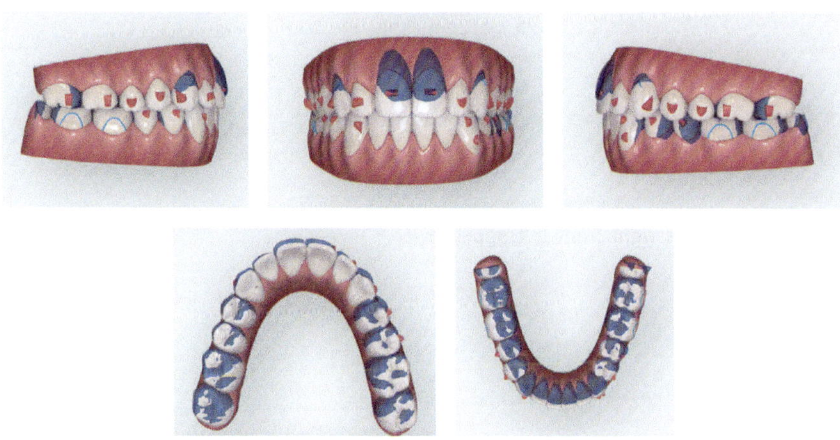

Fig. 20.183 Initial ClinChecks (right, front, left, upper, lower).

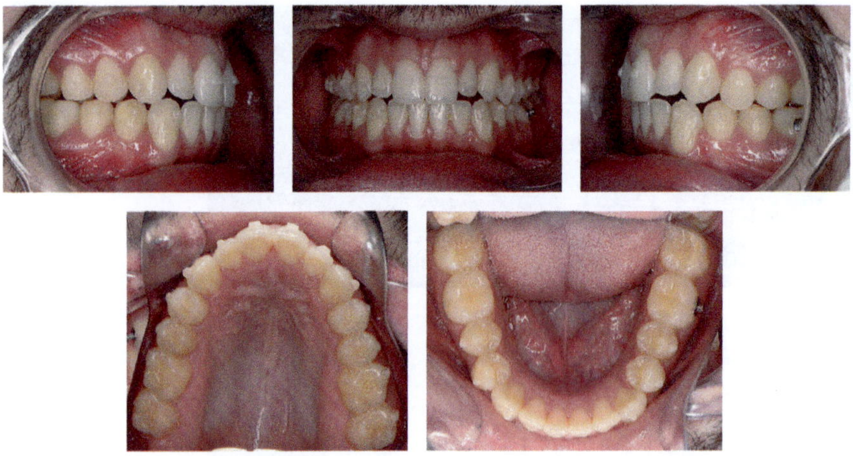

Fig. 20.184 Intraoral refinement (right, front, left, upper, lower).

ClinCheck 2: Requirements for the Technician

- Posterior precision cuts to allow final settlement with posterior extrusion
- Upper lateral extrusion attachments active at the same time as central incisors are intruding, creating a countermovement
- Additional slight expansion and intercuspidation improvement
- Manual precision cuts on lingual surface of 11 and 21 to help solve the tongue thrusting habit and prevent relapse

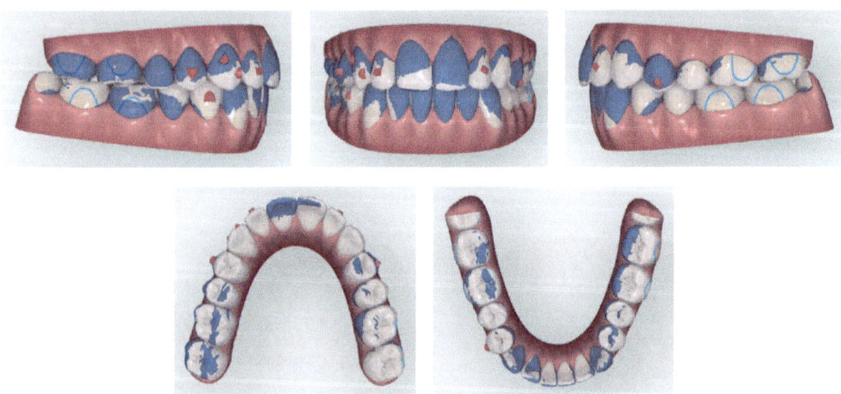

Fig. 20.185 Refinement ClinChecks: right, front, left, upper, lower.

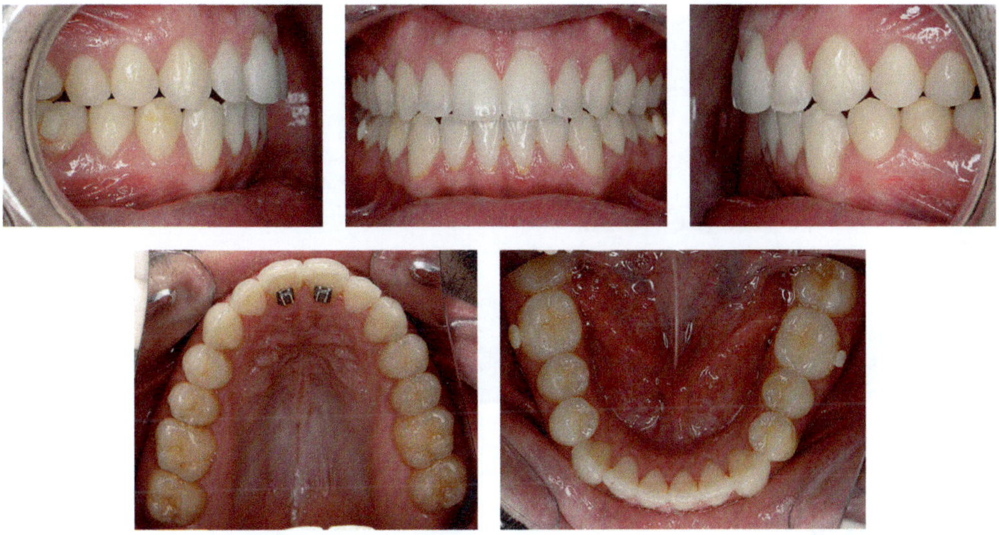

Fig. 20.186 Final intraoral views: right, front, left, upper with tongue tamers lower.

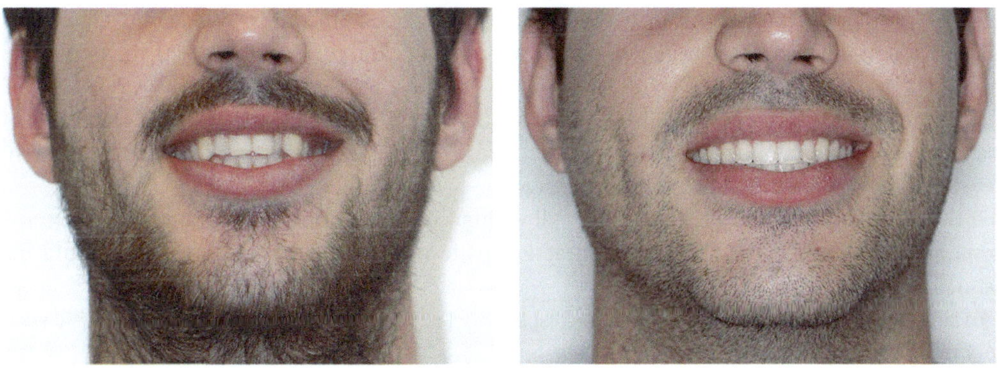

Fig. 20.187 Before and after smile, showing improvement in upper incisor display.

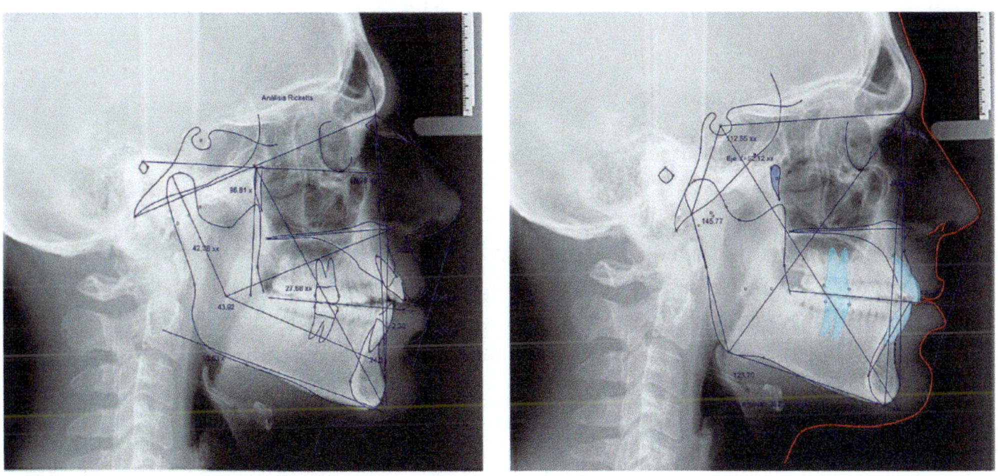

Fig. 20.188 Final cephalometric measurements (before and after).

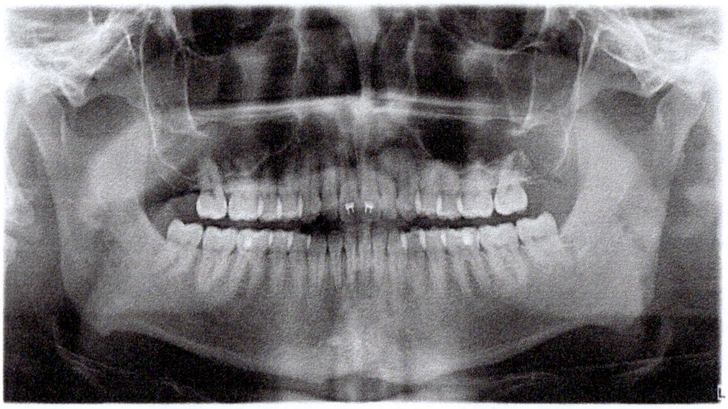

Fig. 20.189 Final panoramic X-ray.

20.3 Class III

A skeletal class III malocclusion in a growing patient will require growth modification with a first orthopaedic phase. This modification of the growth needs a combined treatment with a functional device to open the palatal suture, such as a Hyrax expander, and then proceeds with aligners therapy, as shown in the chapters on growing patients.

In adult/non-growing patients with either a dental class III malocclusion or a mild skeletal discrepancy, non-extraction treatment may be attempted with aligners asking for transversal arch development and lower IPR or lower distalization.

If the skeletal discrepancy is greater but still within the possibility of dental camouflage, extractions may be required. The common extraction patterns for class III malocclusions would be extraction of the first lower premolars.

In severe skeletal class III malocclusions, especially the ones with asymmetry, orthognathic surgery might be required.

Class III Features

The innovations for class III corrections are the same as for class II:

- Precision cuts
- Button cutouts
- Power ridges
- Optimized root control attachments

Precision Cuts and Button Cutouts

- Normally, button cutouts are requested in first upper molars and precision cuts in lower canines (we use button cutouts by lingual of the first upper molars in cases where, at the same time, upper expansion required).
- Elastics from upper 6 to lower 3 will create a mesial force on the entire maxillary arch and a distal force on the mandibular arch.

Power Ridges

These are normally placed on the mandibular incisors to correct the mandibular incisor inclination while retraction is made after distalization or spacing closure.

Optimized Root Control Attachments

These allow bodily translation of teeth when distalizing mandibular premolars and canines to correct a class III malocclusion. If the software does not place these attachments, the technician can be asked to do it or place vertical rectangular attachments to prevent the tipping problems during the lower distalization.

20.3.1 Posterior IPR

This can be used in class III cases to:

- Correct crowding
- Retract lower incisors and solve an anterior crossbite
- To reduce the overall amount of lower distalization needed to solve class III
- To correct an anterior Bolton discrepancy

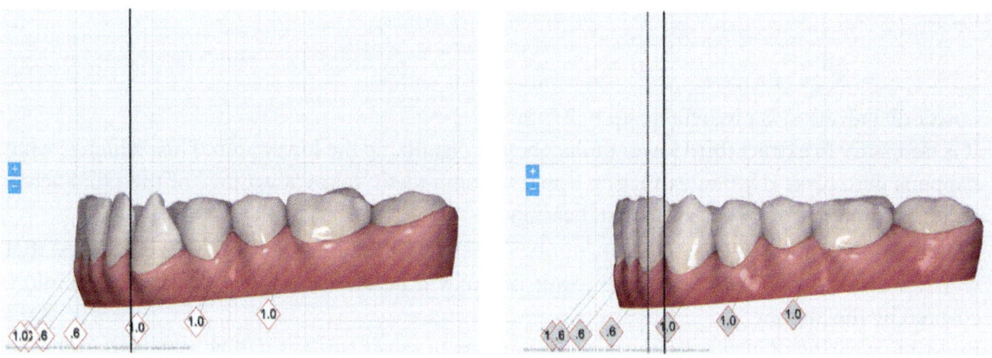

Fig. 20.190 Posterior interproximal reduction will help create space (before and after ClinCheck views)

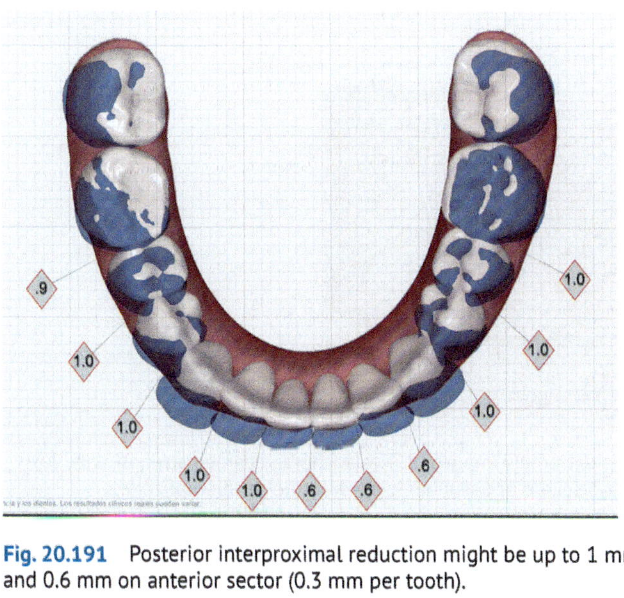

Fig. 20.191 Posterior interproximal reduction might be up to 1 mm per contact point (0.5 mm per tooth) and 0.6 mm on anterior sector (0.3 mm per tooth).

20.3.2 Lower Sequential Distalization

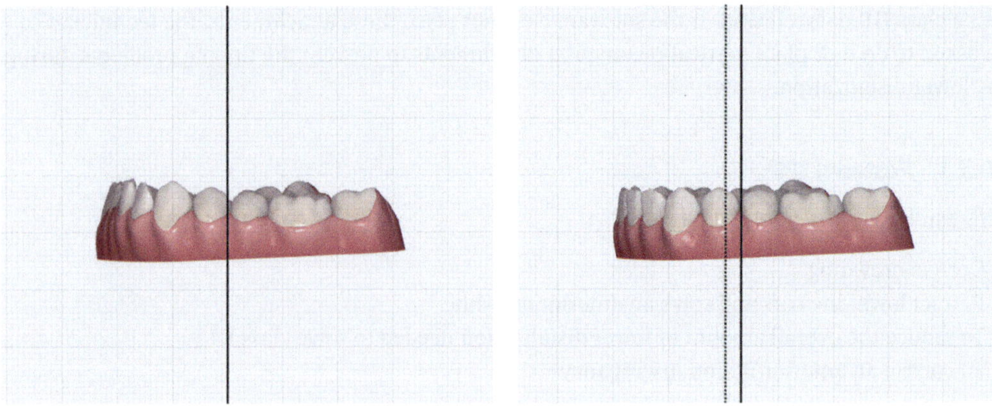

Fig. 20.192 Lower sequential distalization is meant to be predictable up to 2 mm (before and after ClinCheck views).

- Lower distalization is predictable up to 2 mm
- It is necessary to extract third lower molars before distalizing the lower arch. This, which is what happens with class II when extracting upper wisdom teeth, takes advantage of the rapid acceleratory phenomenon to speed up distalization
- The best approach is to take the scan/impressions after extracting the third lower molars: that way the distal surface of the second lower molar will be completely registered and therefore covered by the aligner
- Full-time wearing of elastic from upper first molars to lower canines will be necessary from the beginning of lower distalization
- In cases of lower distalization of 3 mm or more, a microscrew in the retromolar zone will be necessary

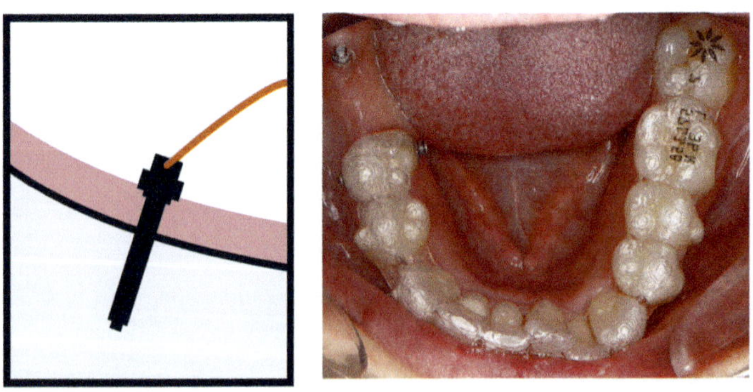

Fig. 20.193 In class III cases, anchorage is extremely important. The anchorage can be strengthened just with class III elastics if the class III is not too severe or use a microscrew in the retromolar zone.

If upper incisors have a labial tip inclination at the beginning, in order to prevent side effects of the class III elastics, which would procline the upper incisors even more, a microscrew distal to the first upper molar and a steel ligature from the upper first molar to the microscrew can be used to avoid mesialization of the upper arch by the class III elastic.

In cases with missing molars and class III, in order to provide the necessary anchorage to correct the class III, implants and provisional crowns would need to be placed before starting the treatment.

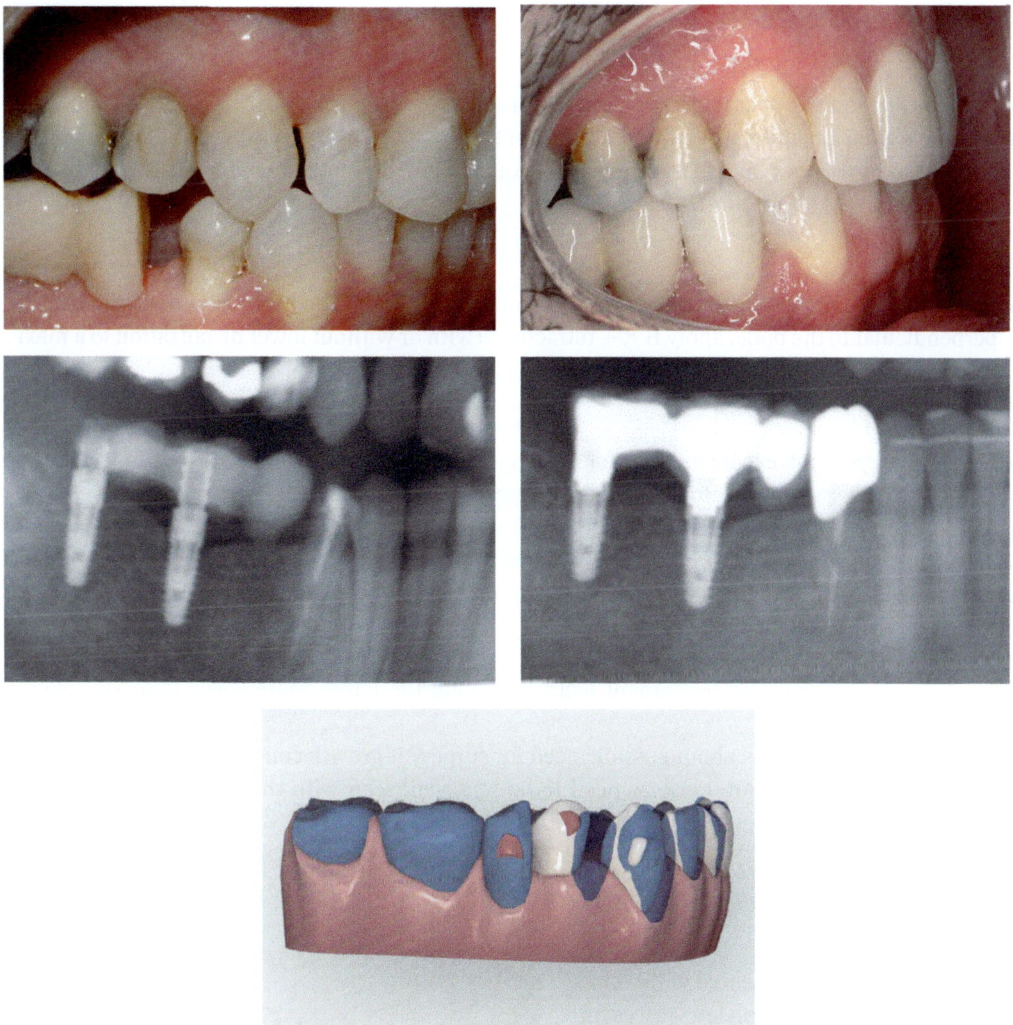

Fig. 20.194 Temporary implant supported crowns help create posterior anchorage, and when final position is achieved they will be substituted for permanent ceramic crowns.

- When the patient presents an **anterior crossbite**, sagittal preference needs to be applied and instead of starting with the expansion it is more effective to make the sagittal correction first
- First: ask for protrusion of upper incisor to anchor root to the cortical bone

- Second: ask for expansion, mesialization and simultaneous retrusion of upper incisors
- In the lower arch, class III elastic cannot be used until we have fully uprighted lower incisors
- Aligners act as a bite plane to disocclude the teeth where they are in crossbite or where there is a CO-CR shift.
- Midline correction is very predictable with aligners in cases with asymmetry
- In class III cases, a gentle, uncorrected curve of Spee in the mandibular arch should be left at the end of the treatment to increase the overbite in the final occlusion

Staging for Anterior Crossbites

Maxillary:

- First: protrusion of upper incisors and anchor the root to the cortical bone
- Second: expansion and use the space expansion to mesialize the posterior zone at the same time that the software does the anterior retrusion. Anchorage horizontal attachments should be bevelled to gingival HBG 4 mm U4/U6

Mandible:

- If incisors are torqued to lingual, start treatment by applying labial torque and when they are perpendicular to the bone, apply IPR + retraction. (with or without lower distalization to a maximum of 3 mm)

Tips for Class III

- Overtreat upper arch expansion (ask for 50% more expansion than you need)
- Class III elastics: as soon as lower incisors are perpendicular to occlusal plane
- Ask for a final overjet 1.5 mm on incisors and 1 mm on canines
- Maximum lower distalization is 3 mm (by distal tipping of the crown without moving roots)
- A 4 mm attachment in molars for anchorage in lower sequential distalization

Mixed Dentition

- Create space for erupting permanent teeth by asking for 1 mm more space than you would expect to need
- Communicate effectively about possible need for surgery if growth continues post-treatment
- For primary teeth that are loose or need to be removed, scan with them in and then remove before first aligner delivery

20.3.3 Class III with Anterior Crossbite

Diagnosis

A 44-year-old woman presented with a class III malocclusion subdivision left with asymmetry, anterior crossbite and bilateral posterior crossbite. She had periodontal disease and anterior occlusal trauma, and asymmetric mandibular prognathism with midfacial hypoplasia. The upper midline was centred and there was right-side deviation of the mandible.

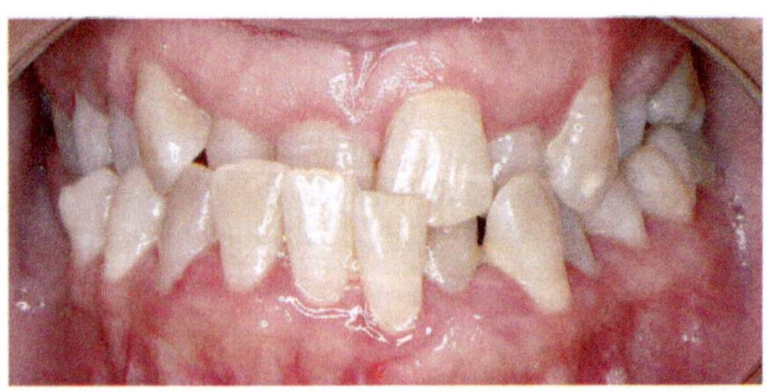

Fig. 20.195 Initial intraoral view.

Treatment Plan

- First, the surgeon was to place an implant on the lower right and a TAD on the lower left. Posterior anchorage was critical to correct the anterior crossbite successfully
- Solve the anterior crossbite and the posterior crossbite to establish an adequate anterior guidance and correction of the class III with mandibular sequential distalization

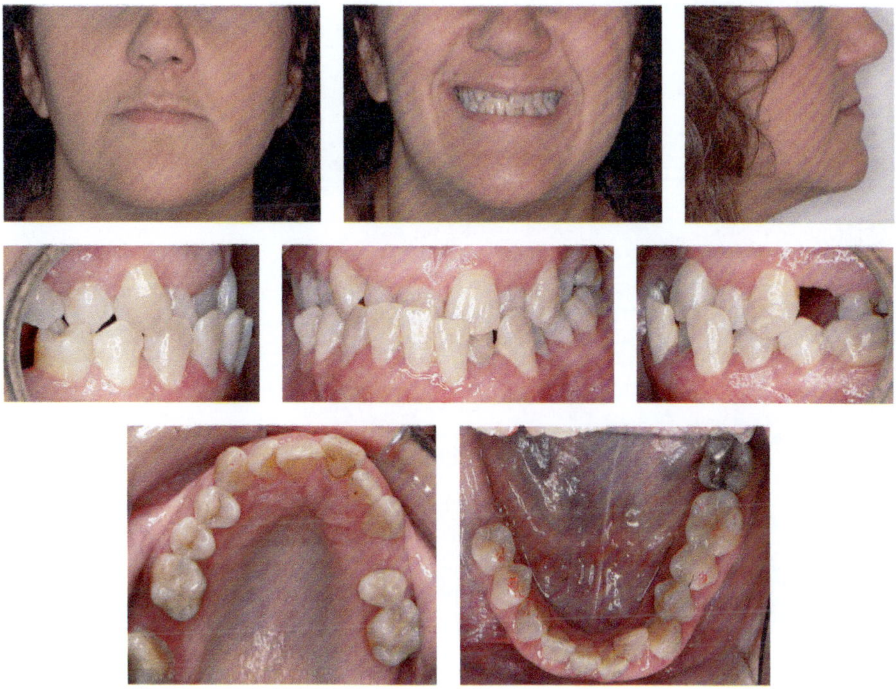

Fig. 20.196 Pretreatment extraoral and intraoral views.

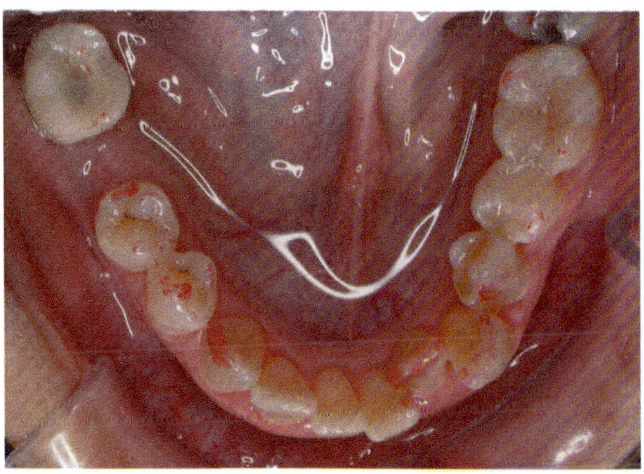

Fig. 20.197 Implant placement on 47 before starting Invisalign treatment.

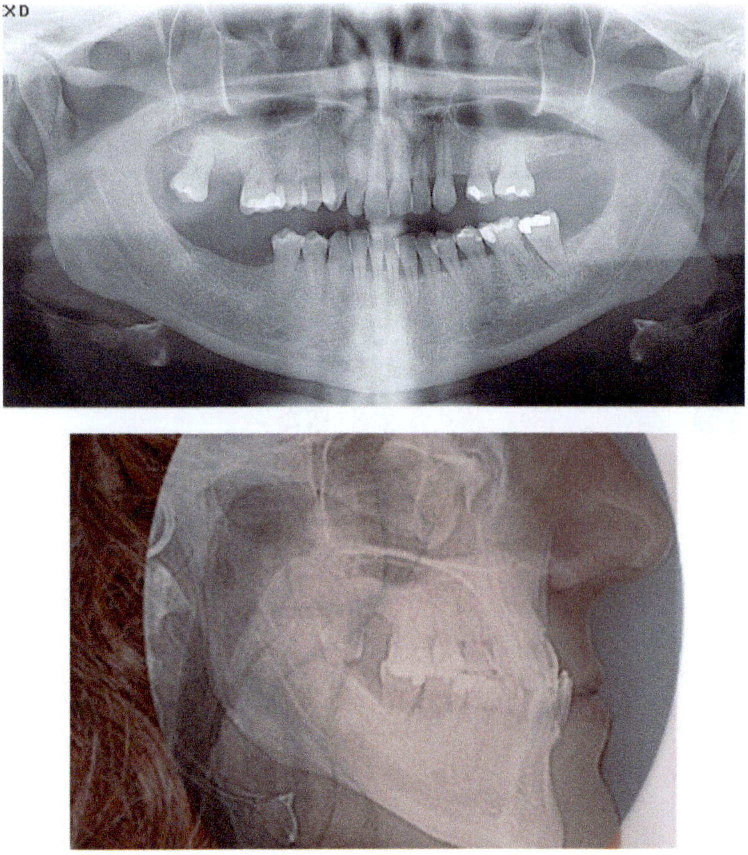

Fig. 20.198 Initial panoramic X-ray, teleradiograph and cephalometry.

Requirements for the Technician

First, provide upper sagittal arch development.

Maxilla:

- Do not move posterior zone and procline upper incisors to anchor the incisor's root to the cortical bone
- Then, using anterior zone as an anchorage, perform a simultaneous movement of expansion and mesialization of the posterior zone
- Use bite ramps in upper canines to assist with the anterior jump

Mandible:

- Distalization and centre the lower midline at the same time
- IPR in the lower arch to help with lower incisor retrusion

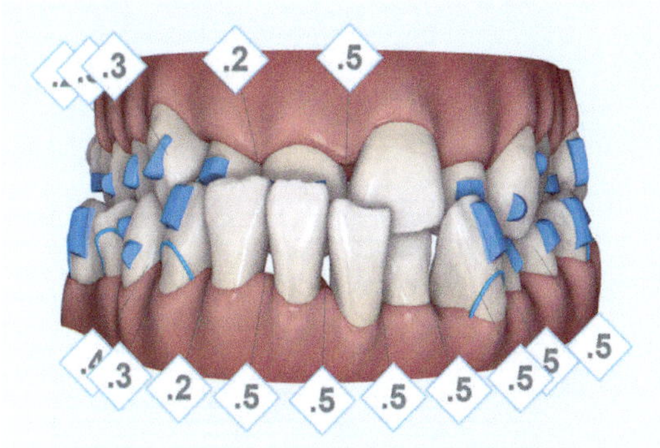

Fig. 20.199 Initial front view.

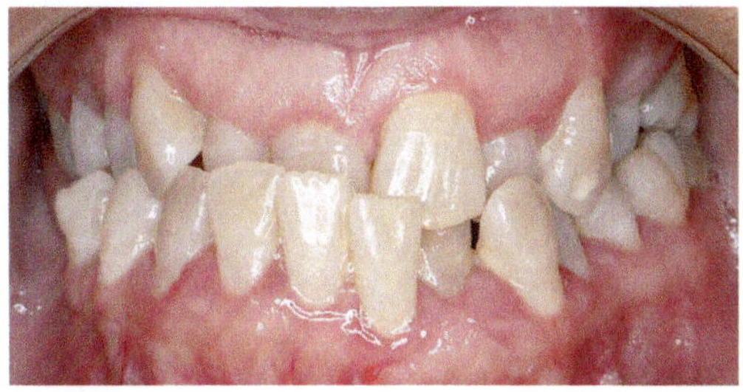

Fig. 20.200 Initial ClinCheck front view.

Treatment goals:
- Correct anterior crossbite by proclination and intrusion of upper and lower incisors
- Posterior anchorage and temporary crowns on implants
- Class III elastics to assist lower distalization and upper protrusion

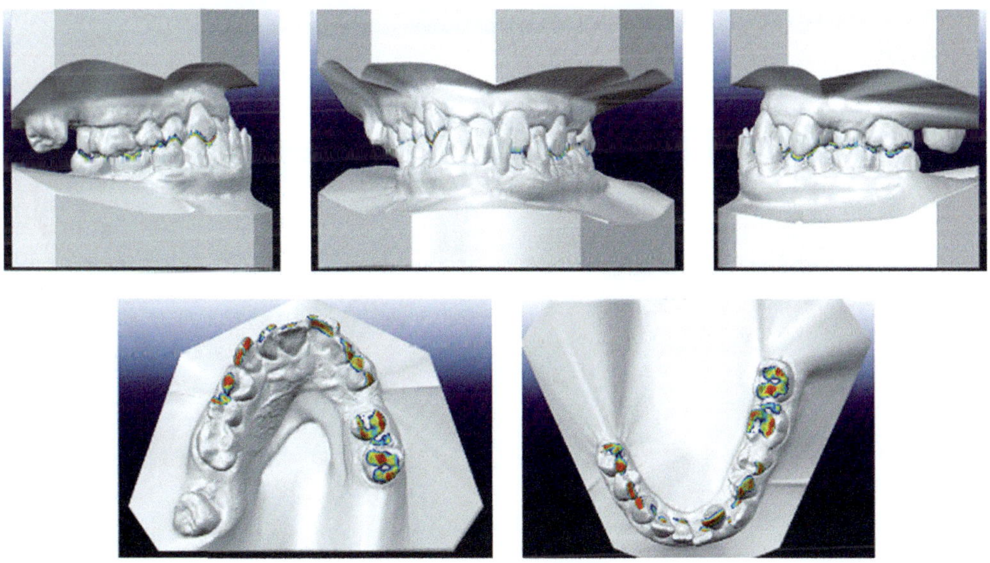

Fig. 20.201 Initial occlusal contact.

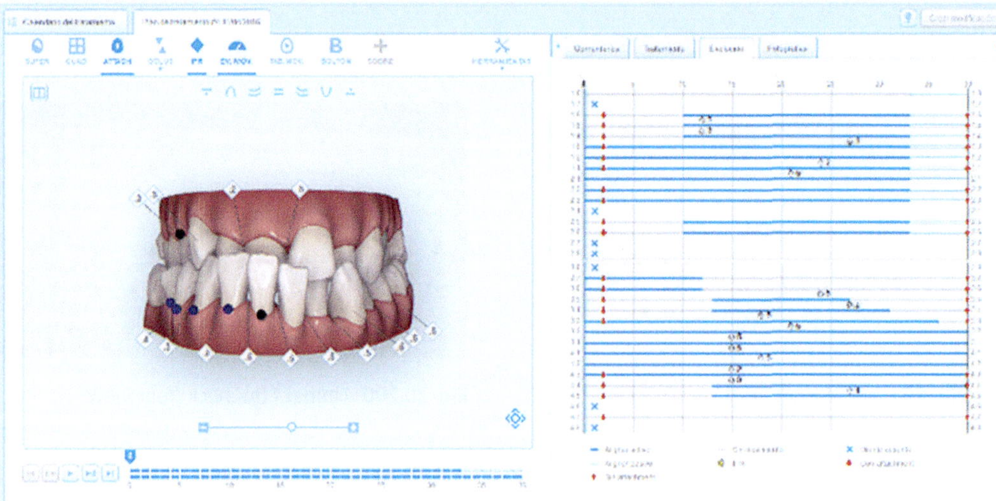

Fig. 20.202 Sagittal priority of movements to solve the anterior crossbite. Periodontal patients benefit from interproximal reduction to make the root become closer and reduce black triangles.

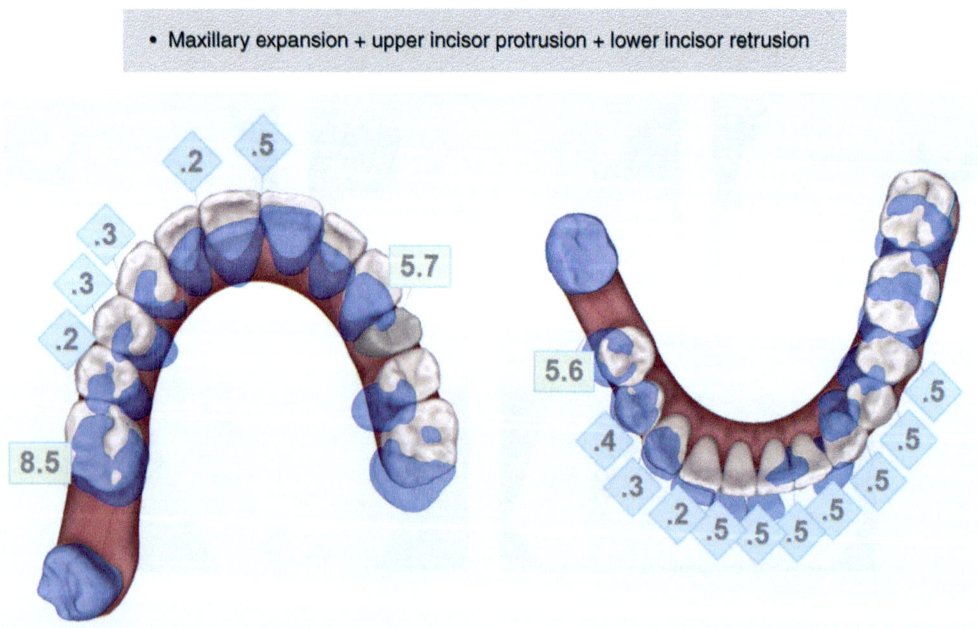

Fig. 20.203 Upper and lower ClinCheck views.

Treatment Summary

- Before starting orthodontic treatment, the surgeon placed an implant for 46 with a provisional crown and placed a microscrew in the retromolar left zone.
- The total number of aligners was 39, with a 10-day aligner change interval; the patient is currently in her 12 months of treatment and is now ready for additional aligners.
- The patient wore class III elastics full-time from lingual of first upper molar to labial of lower canines from aligner 4.
- The posterior and the anterior crossbite were resolved and both midlines were almost centred.

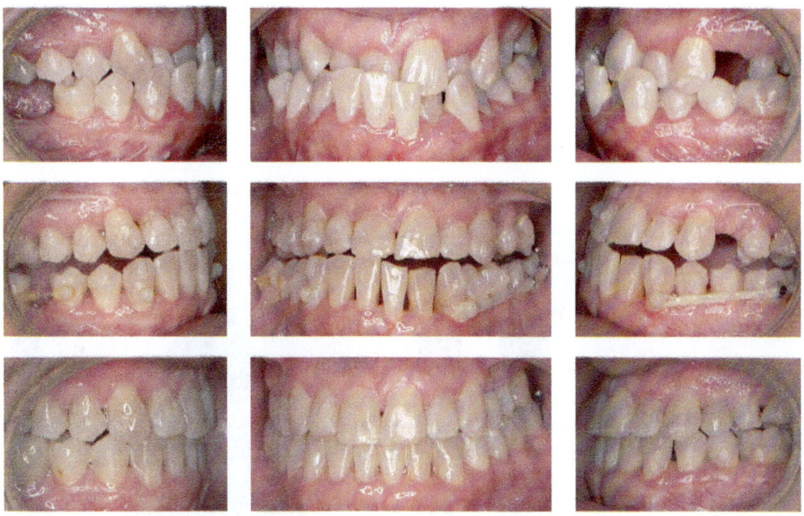

Fig. 20.204 Initial (upper), evolution (middle) and situation after 12 months of treatment (lower).

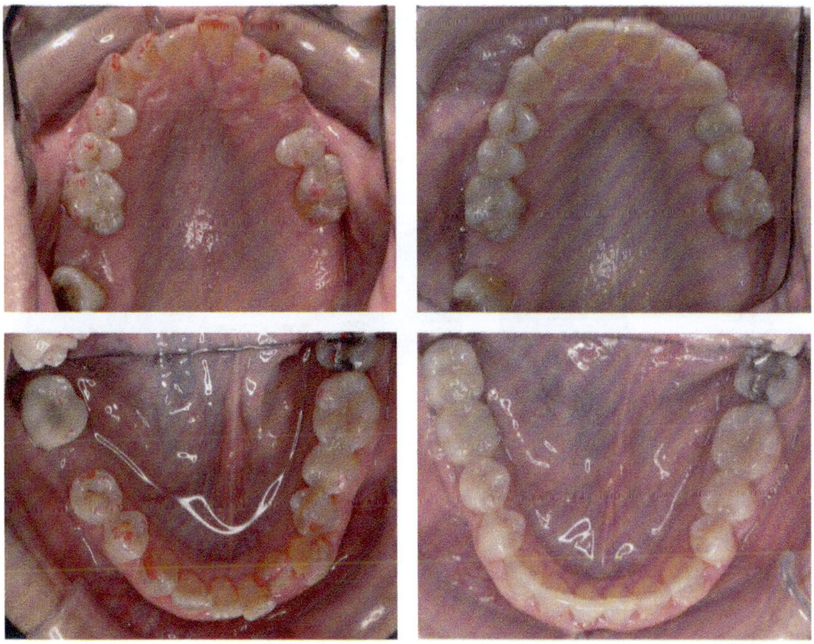

Fig. 20.205 Arch evolution after treatment for 12 months.

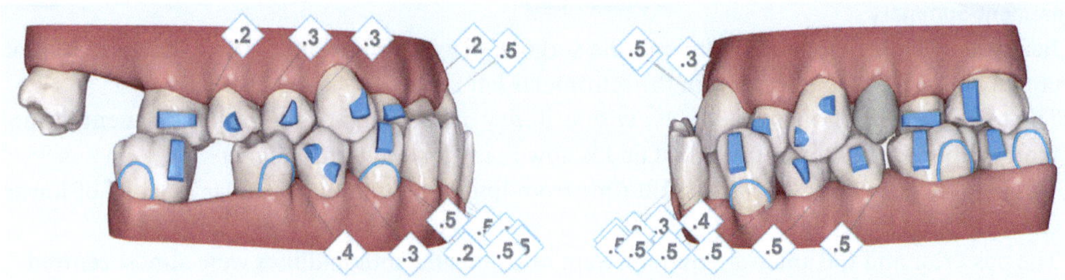

Fig. 20.206 Right and left initial ClinCheck views.

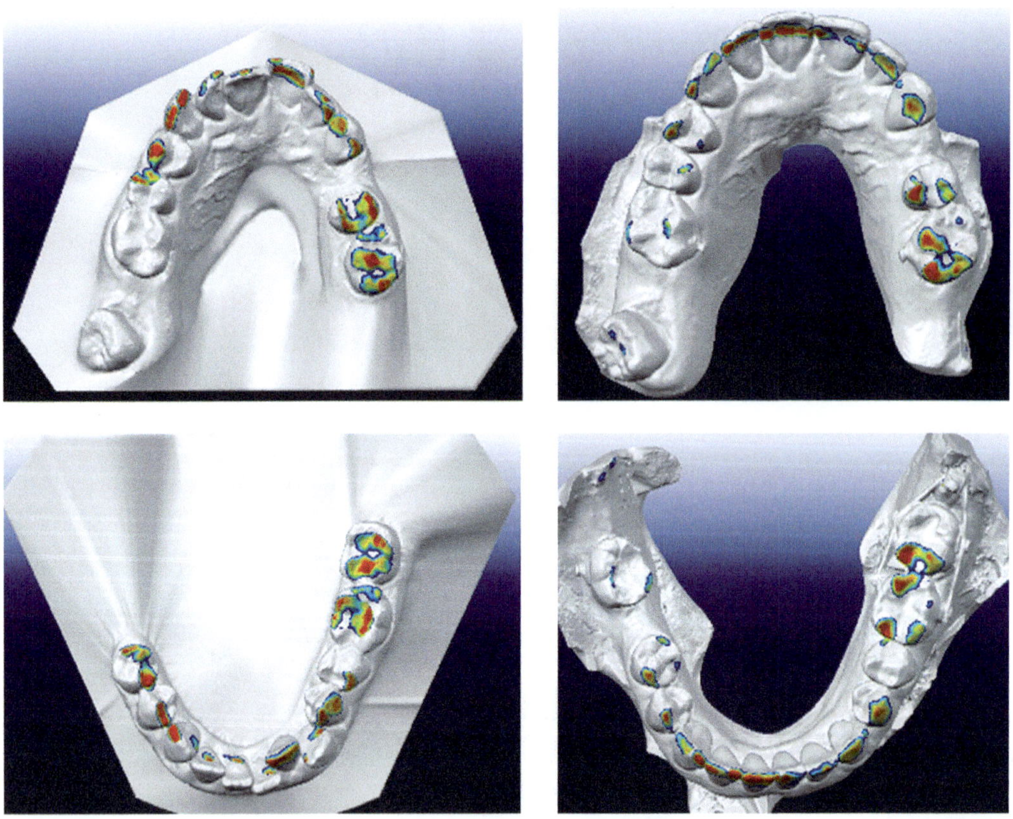

Fig. 20.207 Arch development after 12 months.

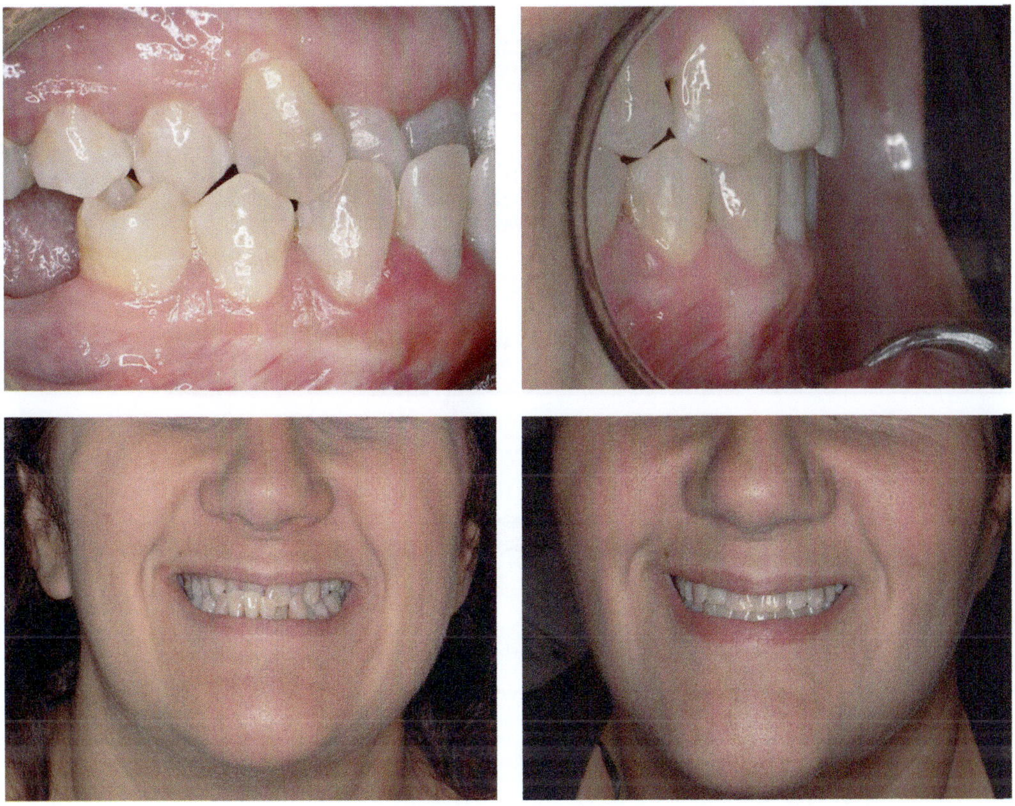

Fig. 20.208 Initial and final overjet and smile.

20.3.4 Dentoalveolar Protrusion, Skeletal Class III

Diagnosis

A 47-year-old woman with a skeletal class III pattern, presented with edge to edge anterior occlusion, open bite tendency, reduced overjet and dento-alveolar protrusion, 27 was extruded. and 47 was missing. In addition she had an anterior crossbite of 12 with right-side deviation of upper midline, and an asymmetric smile as a result of asymmetric raising of the corners of the mouth.

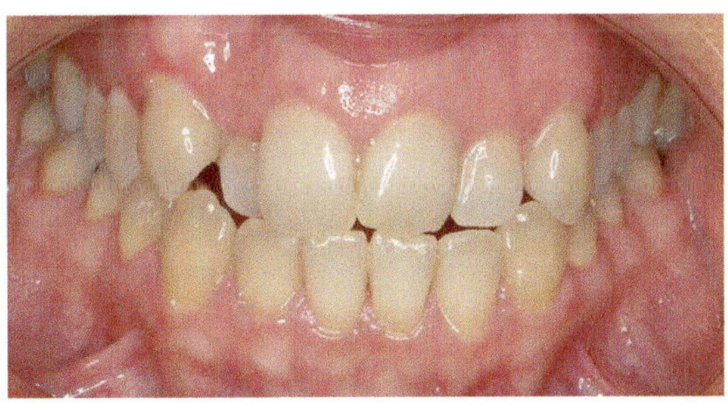

Fig. 20.209 Initial intraoral picture.

Treatment Plan

- Correct anterior crossbite of 12
- Create anterior occlusal clearance
- Increase the overbite
- Intrude 27
- Create space for a restorative treatment for missing 47

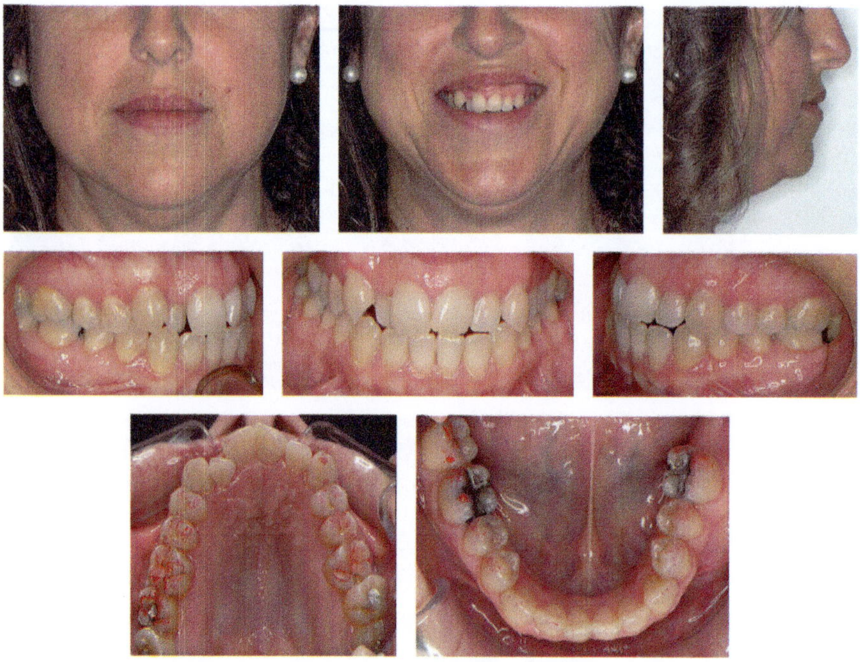

Fig. 20.210 Pretreatment extraoral and intraoral views.

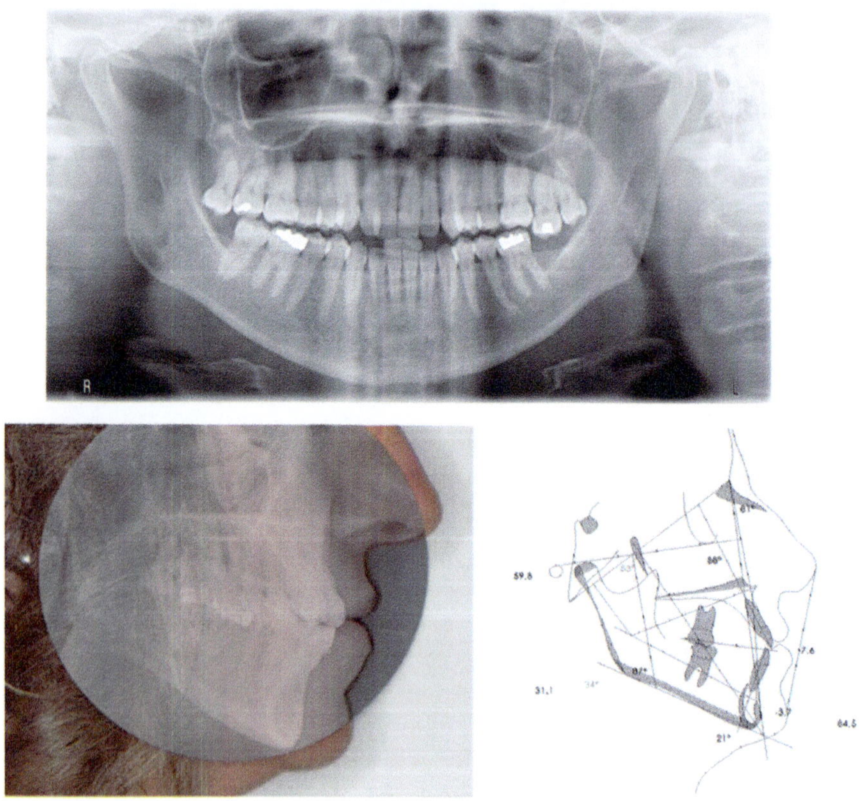

Fig. 20.211 Initial X-ray: panoramic, teleradiograph and cephalometry.

Requirements for the Technician

- IPR 3 to 3 in the lower arch to allow lower incisor retrusion and increase positive overjet.
- Place horizontal attachments in the adjacent teeth to the 27 to assist in intrusion of the molar.
- Precision cuts in lower canines and button cutouts on lingual surface of first upper molar to place class III elastic during the treatment and assist in lower incisor retrusion.
- Horizontal attachment bevelled to gingival in 12 to help with the labial torque of the root requested for this lateral incisor.
- The upper midline is required to be centred with the facial midline during the protrusion movement.
- Aligners of overcorrection of the labial root torque for 12, intrusion of 27 and extrusion of lower incisors are required at the end of the treatment.

1. **Upper symmetric expansion**
2. **IPR** + lower retraction
3. **Class III elastics**
4. TAD to intrude 2.6 (in mesial and distal of 2.6) or implant 36 + provisional crown

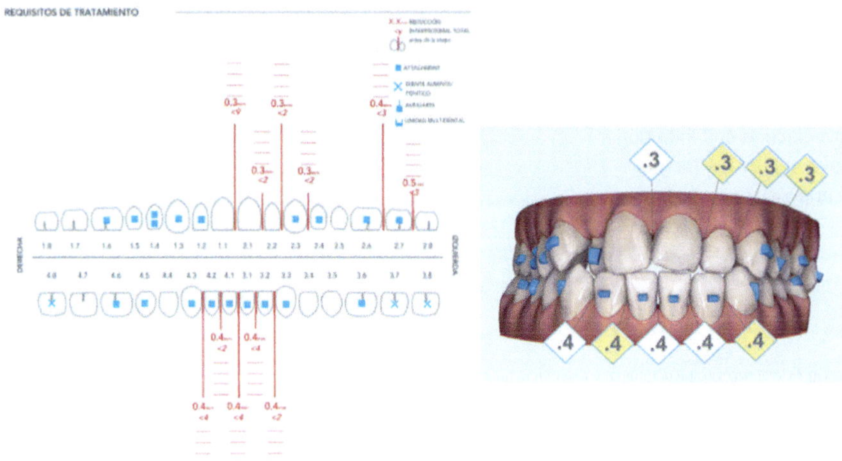

Fig. 20.212 Interproximal reduction.

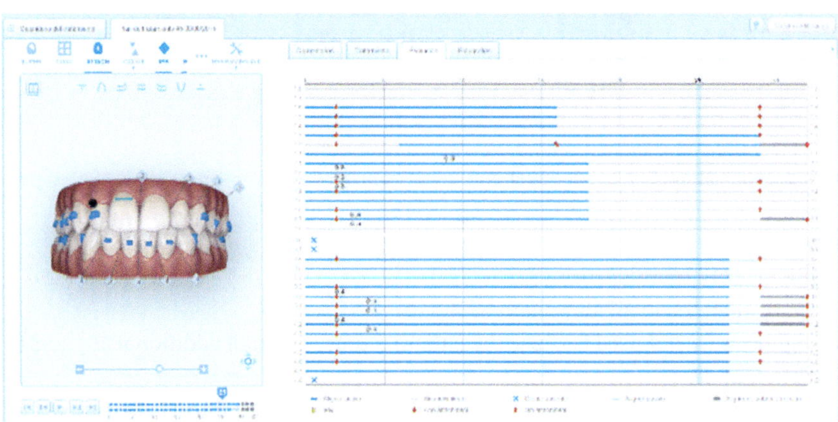

Fig. 20.213 Simultaneous movement pattern.

1. Correct the anterior crossbite of 12, applying labial torque to the root during proclination of the 12.
2. Create positive overjet and increase overbite (by relative extrusion of lower incisors)
3. Intrude 2.6.

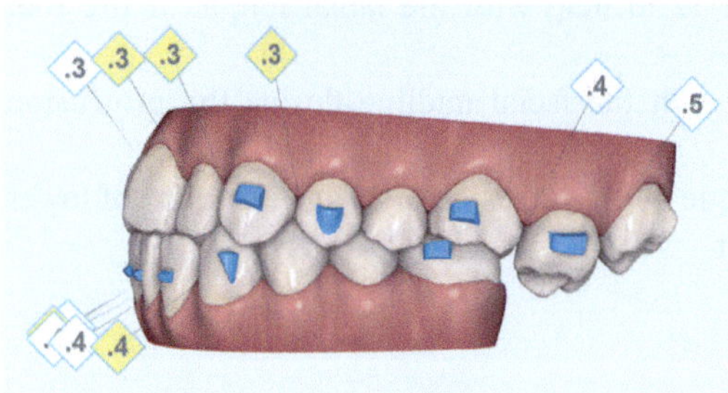

Fig. 20.214 Extrusion of 27 owing to missing 47.

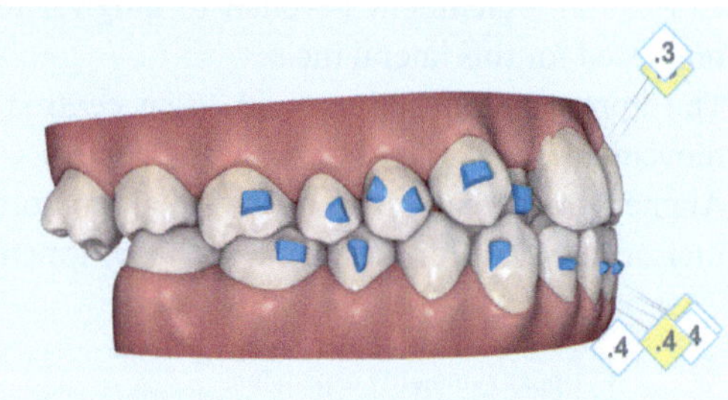

Fig. 20.215 Anterior crossbite of 12.

Maxilla:

- Horizontal attachment bevelled to gingival 4 mm in 12
- Do not move second and third upper molar to have anchorage for the expansion and incisor protrusion

Mandible:

- Lingual root torque to premolars and molars
- IPR + retrusion of lower incisors
- Class III elastics

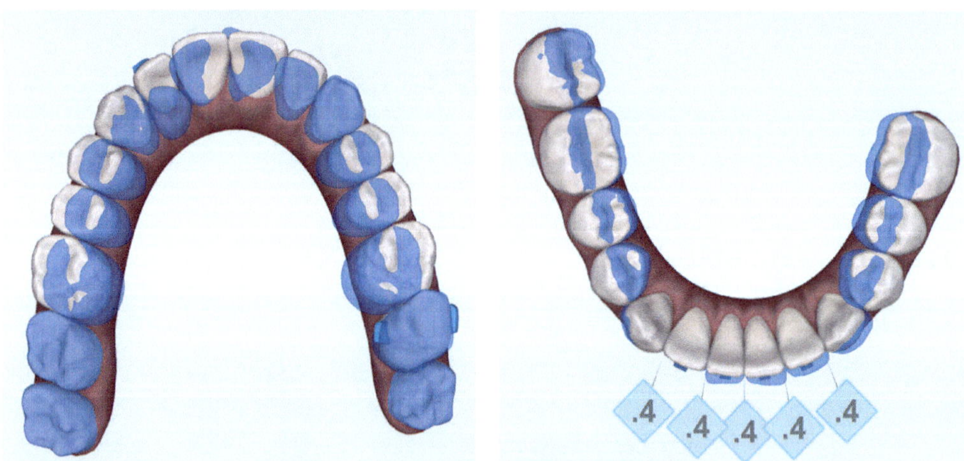

Fig. 20.216 Initial superimposition, ClinCheck upper and lower occlusal views.

Treatment Summary

- Total treatment time was 12 months
- Patient used 29 active aligners on a 7-day change interval
- Overcorrection aligners were not used because the patient required a set of additional aligners to complete the intrusion of 27
- Provisional crown to intrude 27 was not placed until the refinement, as during the first set of aligners the implant for 47 needed to settle

- Correct the anterior crossbite of 12, applying labial torque to the root during proclination of 12.
- Create positive overjet and increase overbite (by relative extrusion of lower incisors)
- Intrude 2.7

- Upper symmetric expansion
- IPR + lower retraction
- Class III elastics
- Implant 37 + provisional crown to assist intrusion of 27

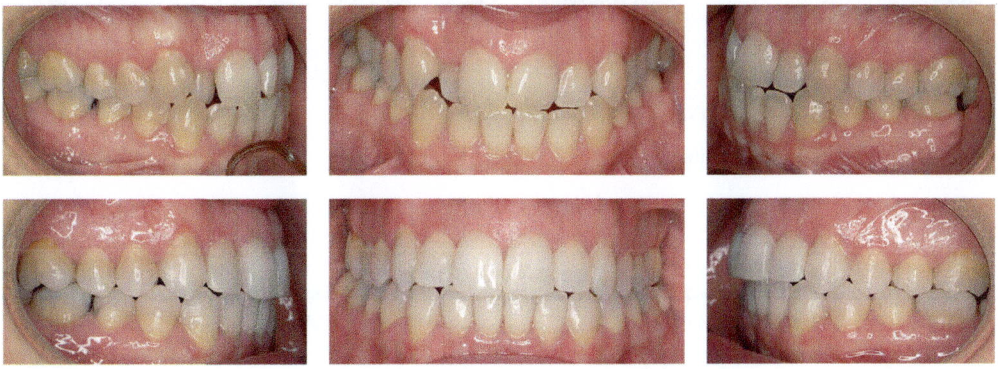

Fig. 20.217 Comparison of initial (upper) and final occlusion (lower).

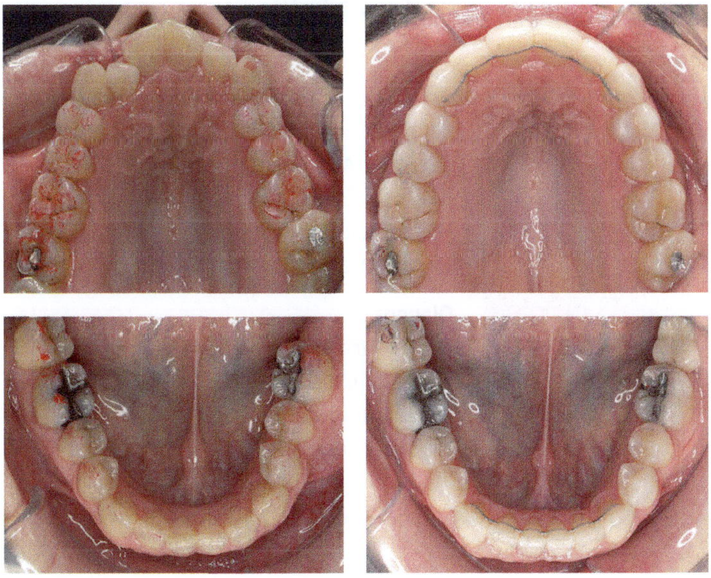

Fig. 20.218 Comparison of initial (left) and final occlusal (right).

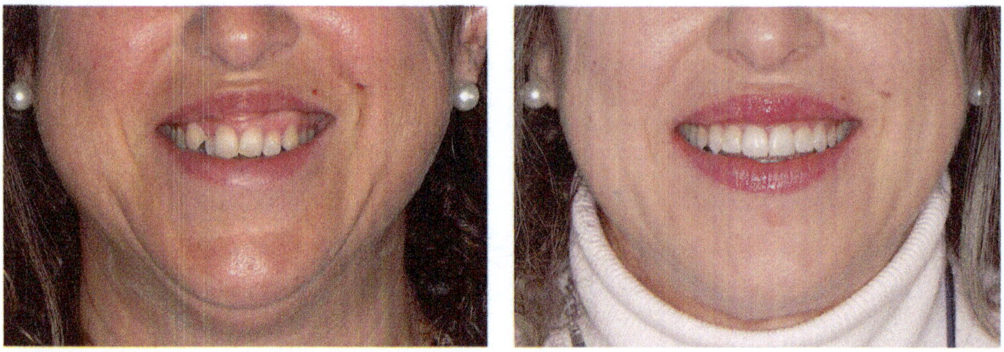

Fig. 20.219 Initial and final smile.

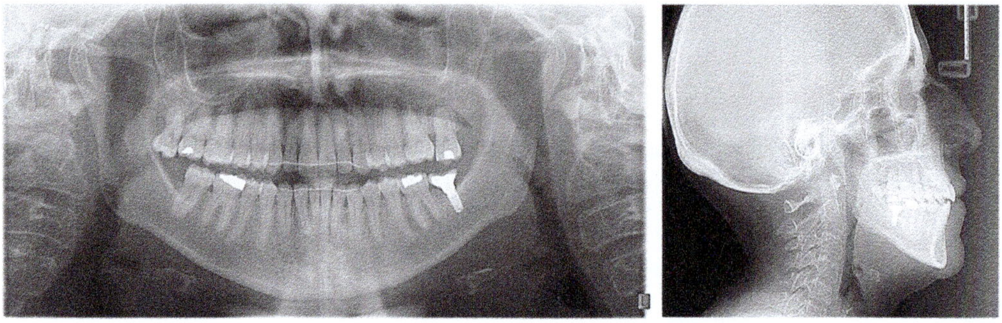

Fig. 20.220 Final panoramic and lateral X-rays.

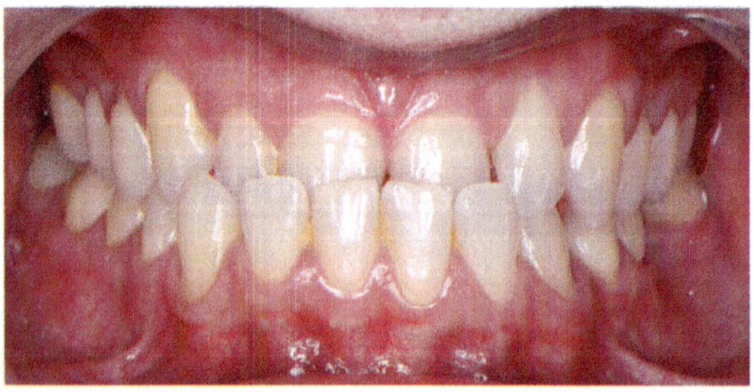

Fig. 20.221 Initial intraoral view.

20.3.5 Anterior Crossbite, Skeletal Class III with Hypoplasic Upper Maxilla, Dentoalveolar Compensation

Diagnosis

A 35-year-old man with a skeletal class III pattern presented with crossbite anterior occlusion, a deep bite tendency, 36 was missing, lower spacing, upper recessions and skeletal hypoplasic maxilla.

Treatment Plan

- Correct anterior crossbite
- Compress upper arch and torque to palatal upper roots
- Compress lower arch and retrude lower incisors to get advantage of lower spacing
- Straightening 37 to have space for an implant on 36

ClinCheck 1: Requirements for the Technician

Upper:

- Dental anchorage on unmovable second molars
- Simultaneous movement: posterior compression combined with anterior lingual root torque
- Anterior power ridges to help with 12–22 torque

Lower:

- Anchorage on 37
- Anterior retrusion with space consumption and additional IPR, combined with extra lingual root torque (LRT) helped by power ridges to help create an 'en masse' movement

Treatment Summary

- Total treatment time was 15 months
- Patient used 36 active aligners on a 7-day change interval and an additional set of 20 aligners
- 24-hour class III elastics were worn on the first set of aligners
- Bilateral class I was achieved with both arches in dentoalveolar compression in order to preserve good tooth position in relation to alveolar bone

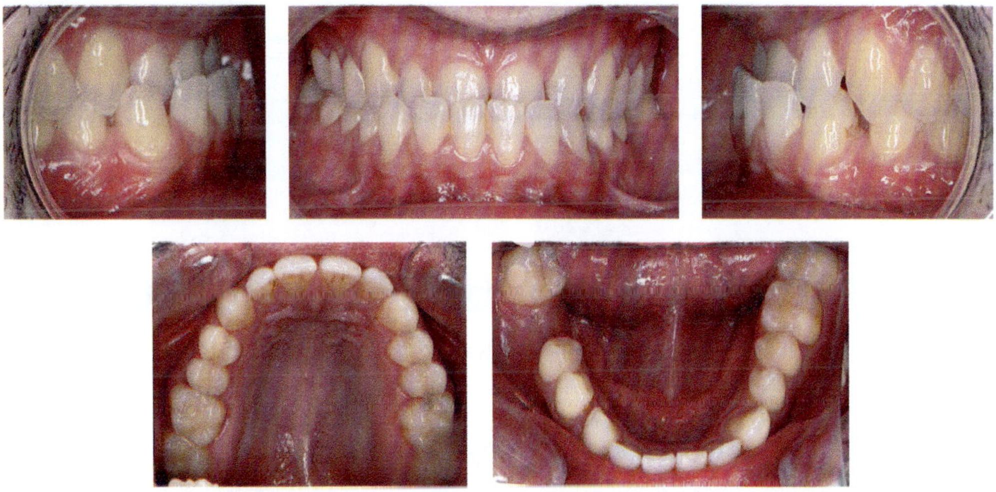

Fig. 20.222 Initial intraoral views.

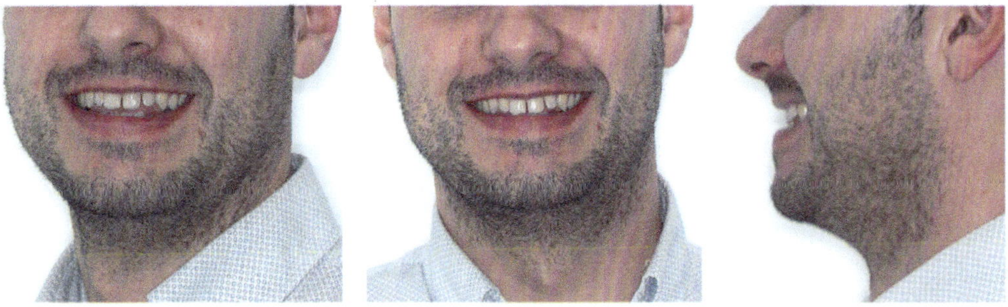

Fig. 20.223 Initial extraoral views.

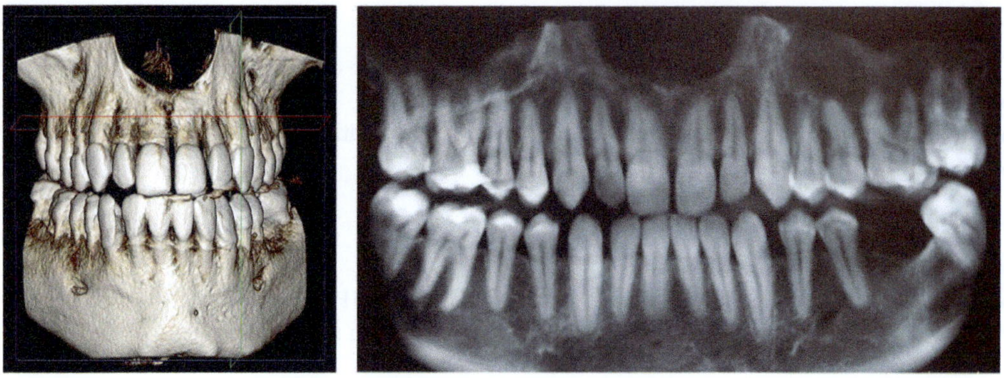

Fig. 20.224 Initial cone beam computed tomography and panoramic X-ray.

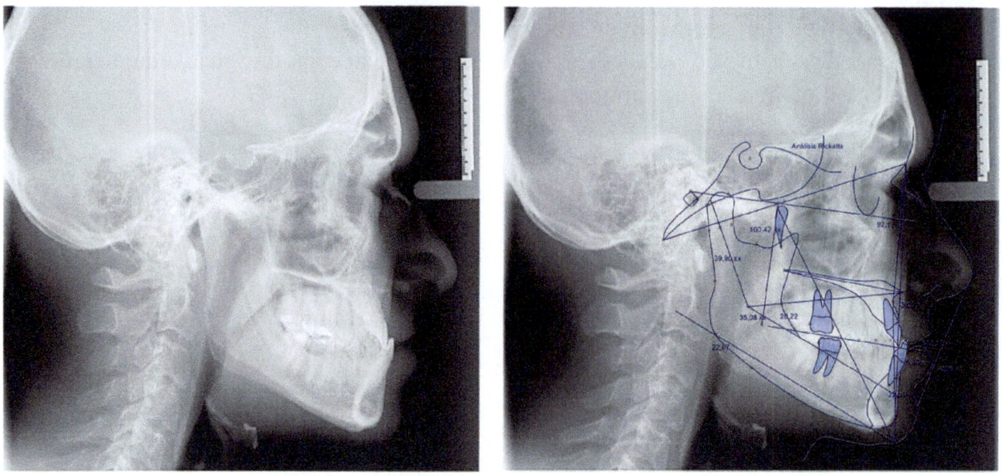

Fig. 20.225 Initial lateral X-ray and cephalometric analysis.

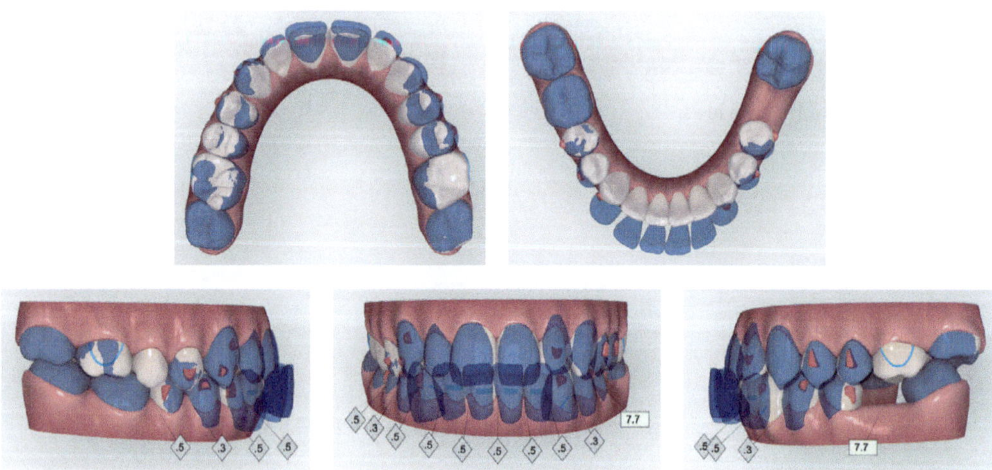

Fig. 20.226 Initial ClinChecks.

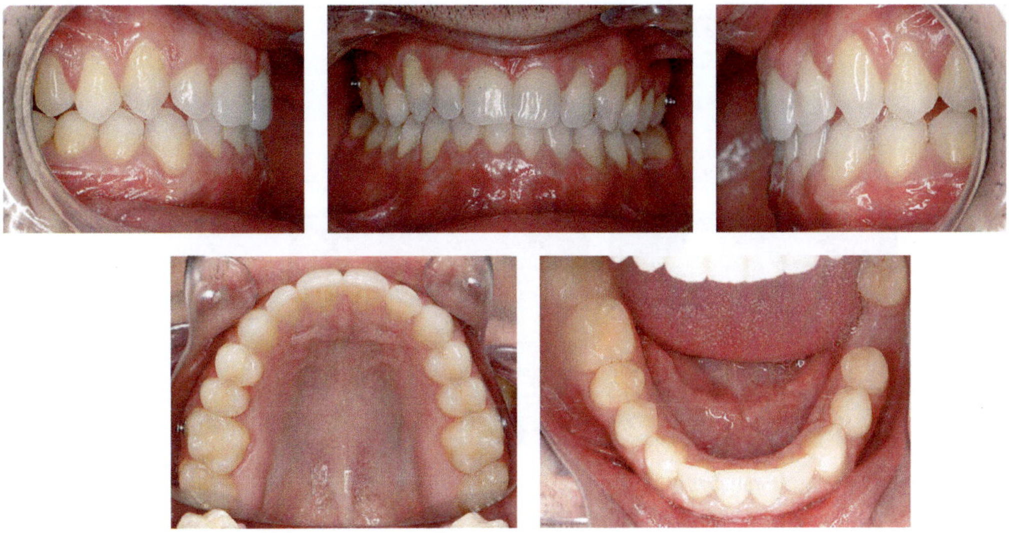

Fig. 20.227 Refinement: intraoral views.

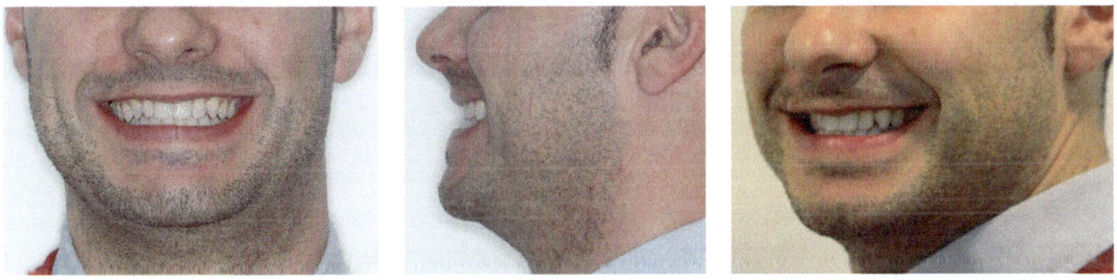

Fig. 20.228 Refinement: extraoral views.

ClinCheck 2: Requirements for the Technician

Upper:

- Anterior power ridges to help with 12–22 torque, solving excessive anterior contact, closing posterior bite and the 'class II' that can be seen after first set of aligners

Lower:

- Straighten 37 by opening space using a virtual 'coil spring', thereby creating more than 12 mm for 36, mesializing third quadrant and leading to a class I occlusion

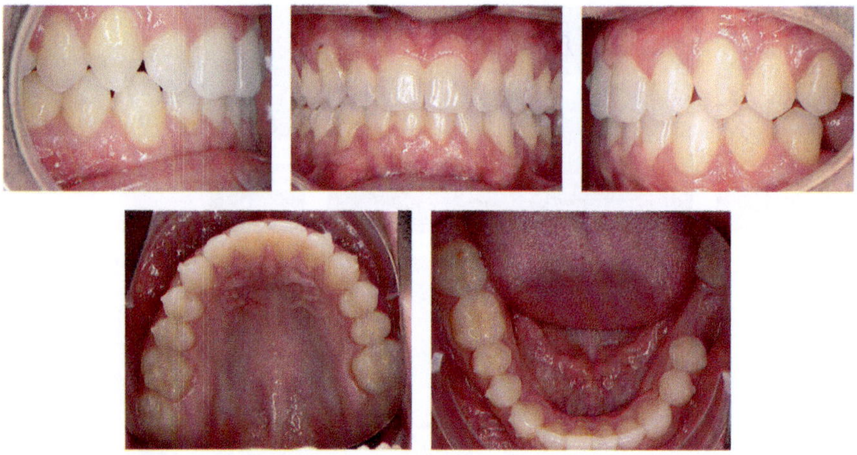

Fig. 20.229 Current intraoral views.

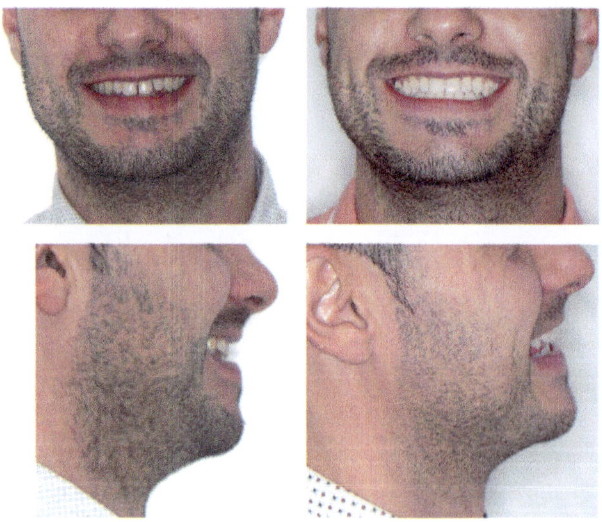

Fig. 20.230 Current smile.

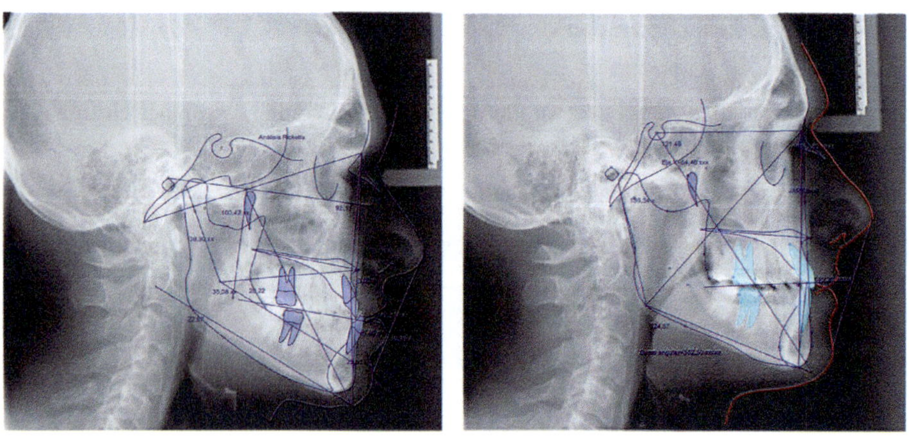

Fig. 20.231 Current cephalometric measurements.

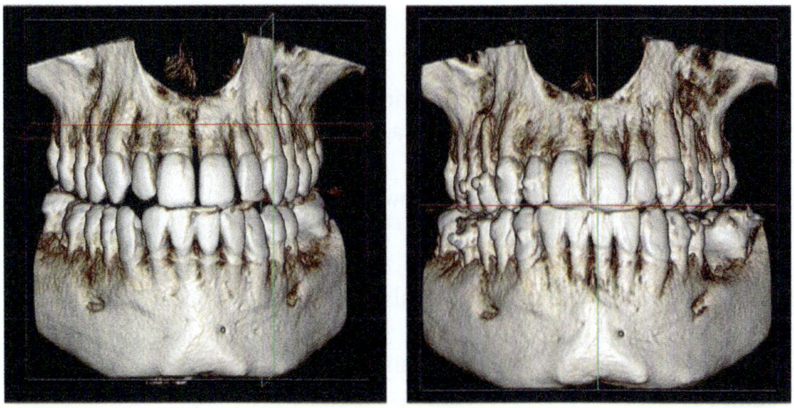

Fig. 20.232 Cone beam computed tomography measurements, before and after treatment.

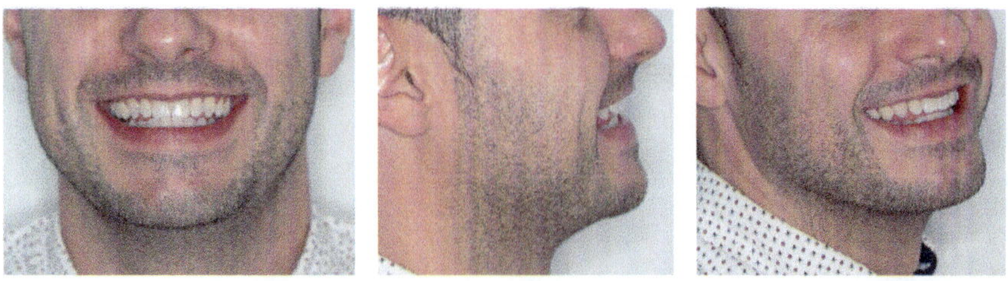

Fig. 20.233 Final smile.

20.3.6 Anterior Crossbite, Skeletal Class III with Hypoplasic Upper Maxilla, Miniscrew-assisted Rapid Palatal Expander (MARPE) Combined with Aligners

Diagnosis

A 34-year-old man presented with a skeletal class III pattern, crossbite anterior occlusion and skeletal hypoplasic maxilla. Both 13 and 23 had been extracted in childhood and 38 was extracted before starting treatment.

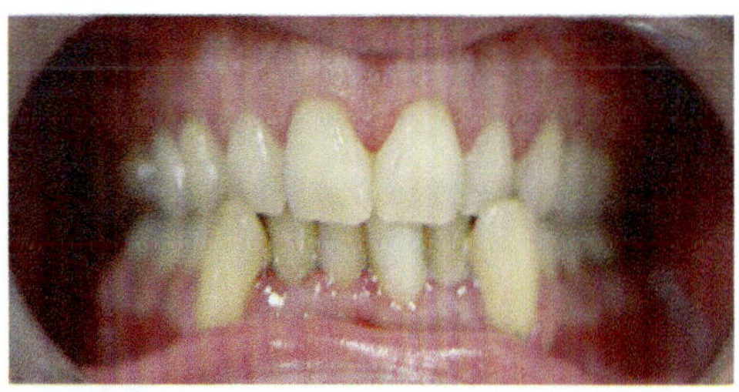

Fig. 20.234 Initial intraoral view.

Treatment Plan

Initial:

- Distalize lower arch with class III mechanics to achieve overjet without considering the sagittal relationship from a class I/II/III classic perspective because of missing canines
- Patient refused surgical approach such as SARPE or MARPE

Changes after 6 months:

- Patient decided to wear a MARPE to obtain a wider arch because he was told it would not be feasible without it
- He also accepted a corticotomy process in palatal suture so as to increase speed of the treatment thanks to rapid acceleratory phenomenon (RAP)
- Therefore plan after this: combine anterior space with MARPE disjunction with class III mechanics

ClinCheck 2: Requirements for the Technician

Upper:

- Open anterior diastema on a 0.25mm rate per aligner during 5 aligners
- Expand using upper wisdom tooth as a hinge and anchorage, creating a better arch form
- Manual precision cuts for class III elastics
- Class III elastics went from upper molar band hooks to lower canines

Lower:

- Half-sequential distalization on both arches, with the goal of not having lower incisors protruding from their initial position
- Lower IPR to avoid black triangles and help avoid proclining lower incisors
- Extra LRT to lower canines because of previous recessions that were to be improved
- Manual button cutouts on lingual surface of lower canines to help with rotation simultaneously with sagittal correction

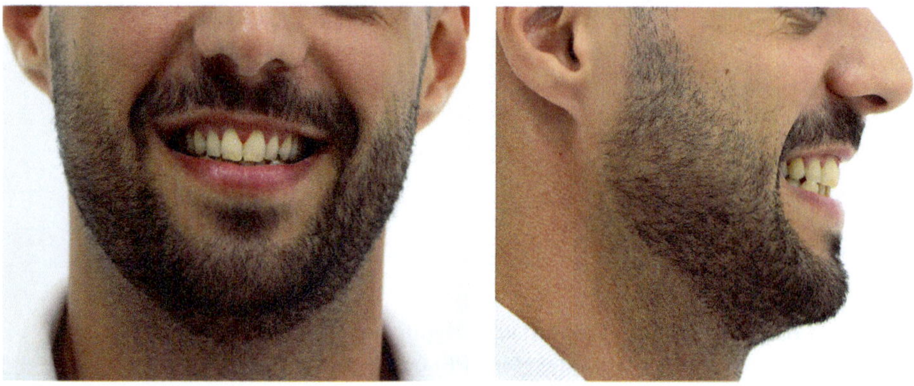

Fig. 20.235 Initial smile.

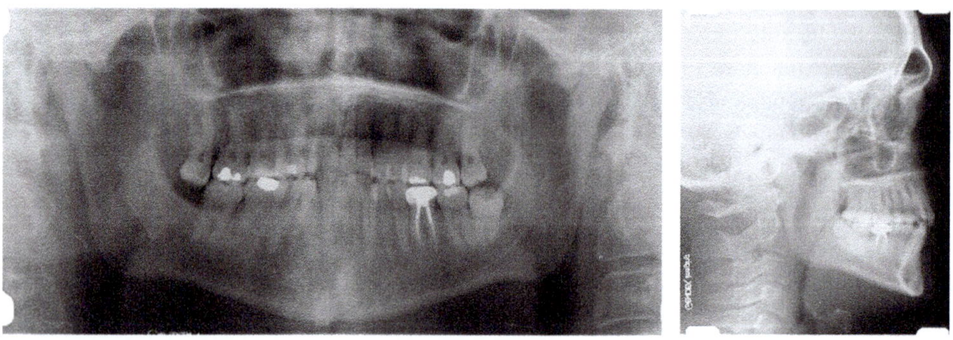

Fig. 20.236 Initial panoramic and lateral X-rays.

Treatment Summary

- Total treatment time was 18 months
- Patient used 36 active aligners on a 7-day change interval and an additional set of 20 aligners
- 24-hour class III elastics were worn
- Proper sagittal, transverse and vertical relationships were achieved thanks to a multidisciplinary approach combining surgery and clear aligners therapy

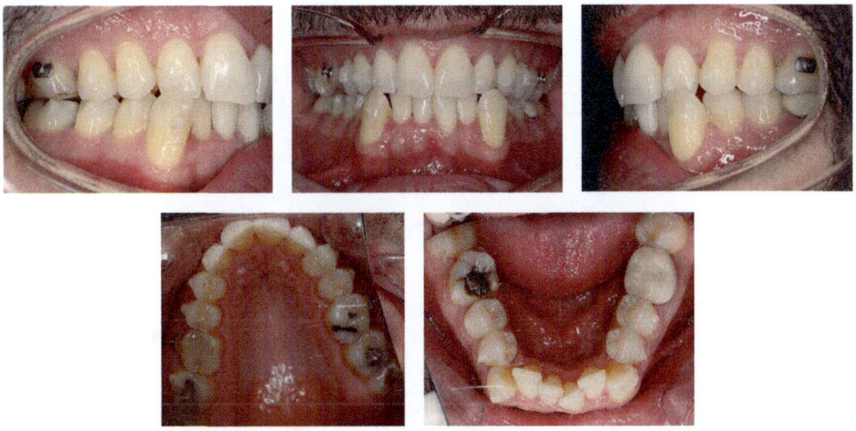

Fig. 20.237 Refinement: initial views after 6 months, when the patient decided to have the miniscrew-assisted rapid palatal expander.

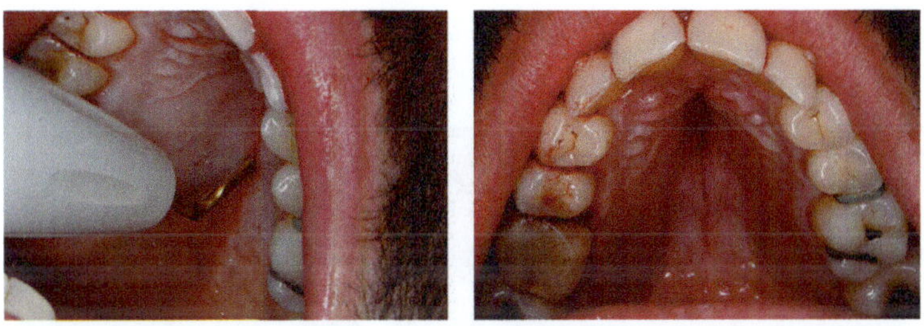

Fig. 20.238 The palatal suture is broken with the same anaesthesia that will used for the miniscrew-assisted rapid palatal expander.

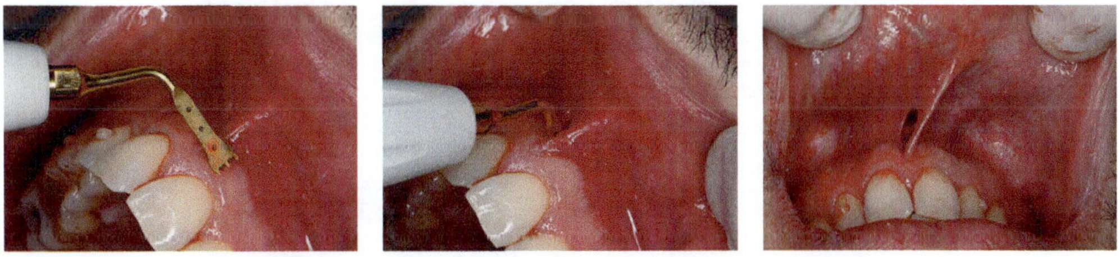

Fig. 20.239 The palatal suture is broken with the same anaesthesia that will be used for the assisted rapid palatal expander miniscrews.

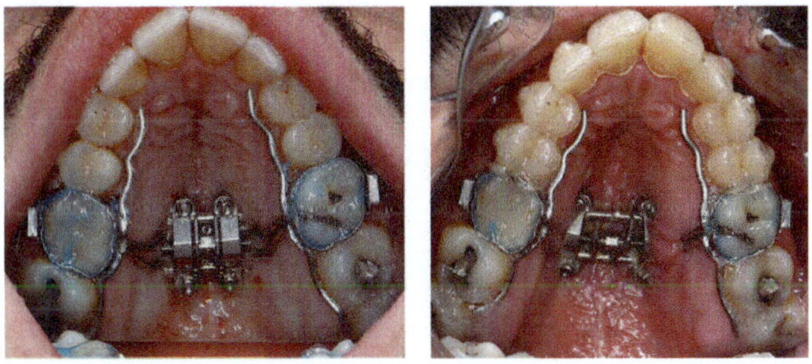

Fig. 20.240 After 2 weeks, the 8 mm screw is fully opened. The palatal surface has healed and the patient is wearing aligners manually trimmed distal to 5s to allow metal bands around molars.

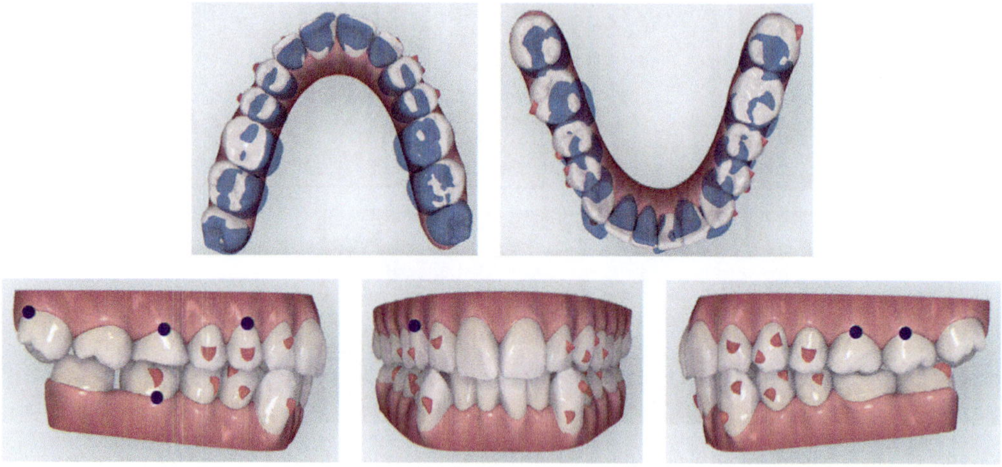

Fig. 20.241 Refinement ClinChecks.

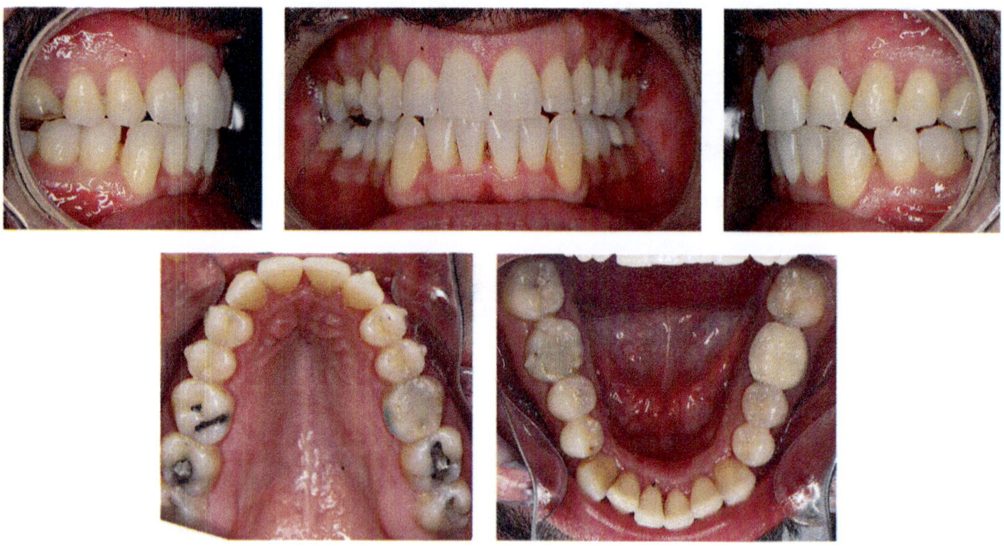

Fig. 20.242 Second refinement: intraoral views.

ClinCheck 2: Requirements for the Technician

- Add slight IPR to final adjustment
- Keep lingual precision cuts on canines to help with its rotation while using class III elastics to upper first molars
- Add extra LRT to lower canines to improve periodontal status

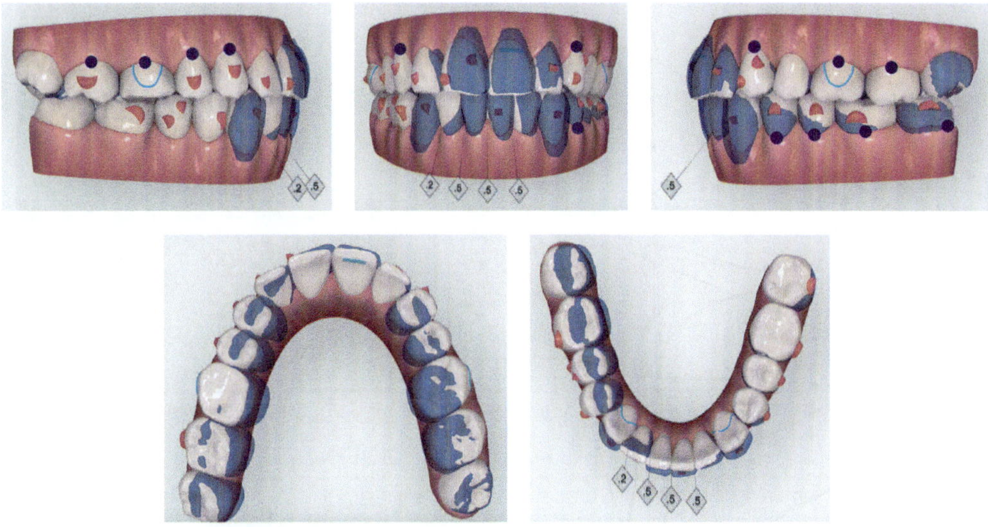

Fig. 20.243 Second refinement ClinChecks.

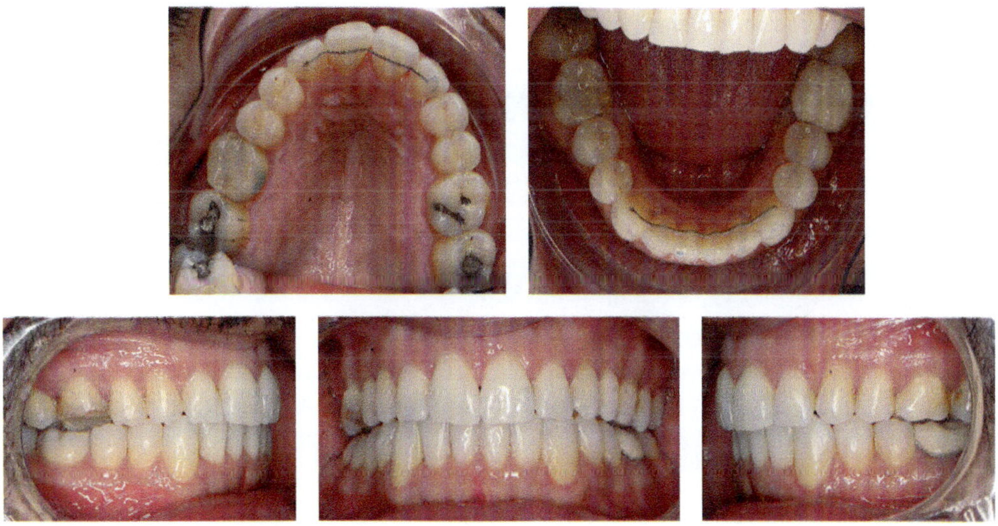

Fig. 20.244 Final intraoral views.

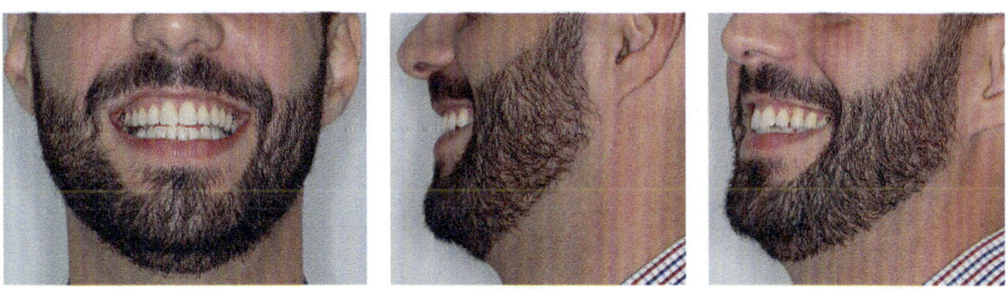

Fig. 20.245 Final smile.

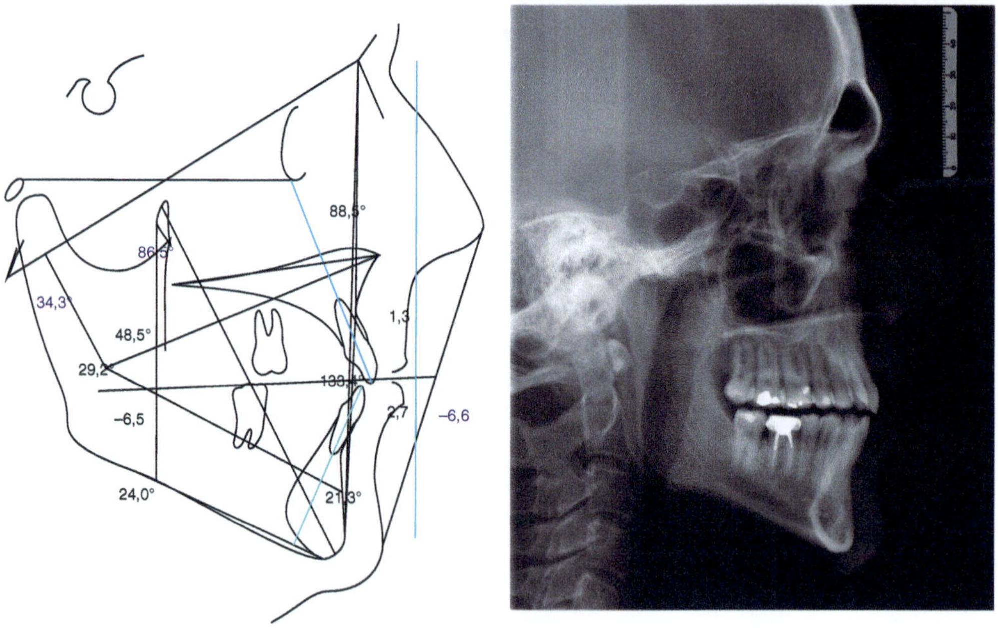

Fig. 20.246 Final cephalometric examination.

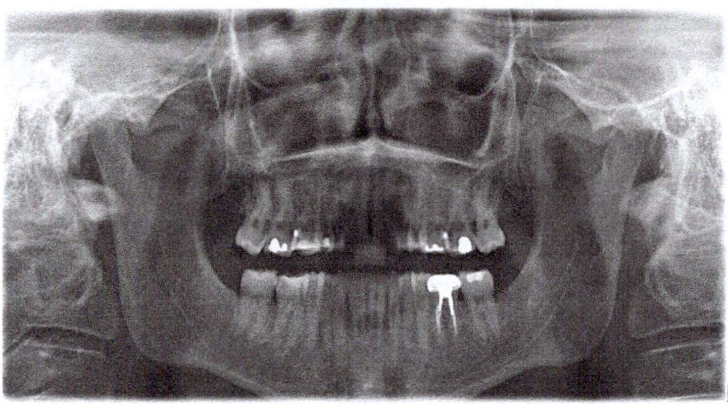

Fig. 20.247 Final panoramic X-ray.

20.3.7 Anterior Crossbite, Skeletal Class III

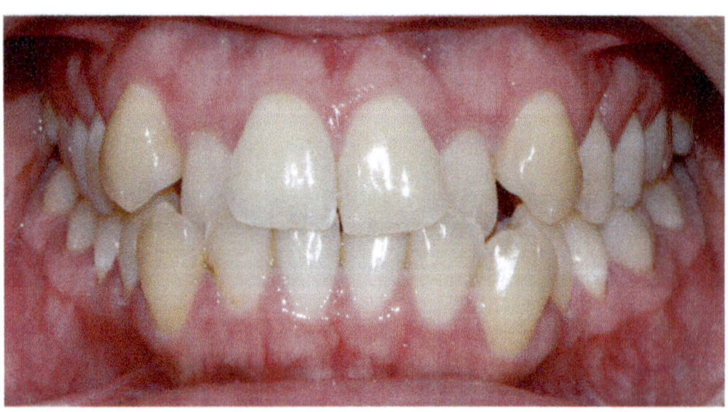

Fig. 20.248 Initial frontal intraoral view.

Diagnosis

A 26-year-old woman presented with a skeletal class III pattern, crossbite anterior occlusion and compressed upper maxilla. She had a hypodivergent profile and an anterior and posterior gummy smile.

Treatment Plan

- Patient refused a four-extraction approach
- A combination of upper arch development by expansion and proclination was planned
- The lower arch was to distalize, to avoid proclining the lower incisors from the initial situation
- Gummy smile was meant to be solved by posterior expansion and anterior proclination

ClinCheck 1: Requirements for the Technician

Upper:

- Expand and procline so as to develop upper arch
- Extra LRT to laterals in order to have a good root torque after solving the crossbite, together with extrusion attachments on these and upper central incisors to control their torque
- Button cutouts on molars to avoid excessive anterior proclination

Lower:

- Half distalization to solve sagittal problem
- Take lower incisors initial position as a reference that cannot be crossed from a sagittal perspective
- Premolar IPR to avoid protrusion
- Lower hooks on canines to maximize effect of class III elastics on lower incisor torque

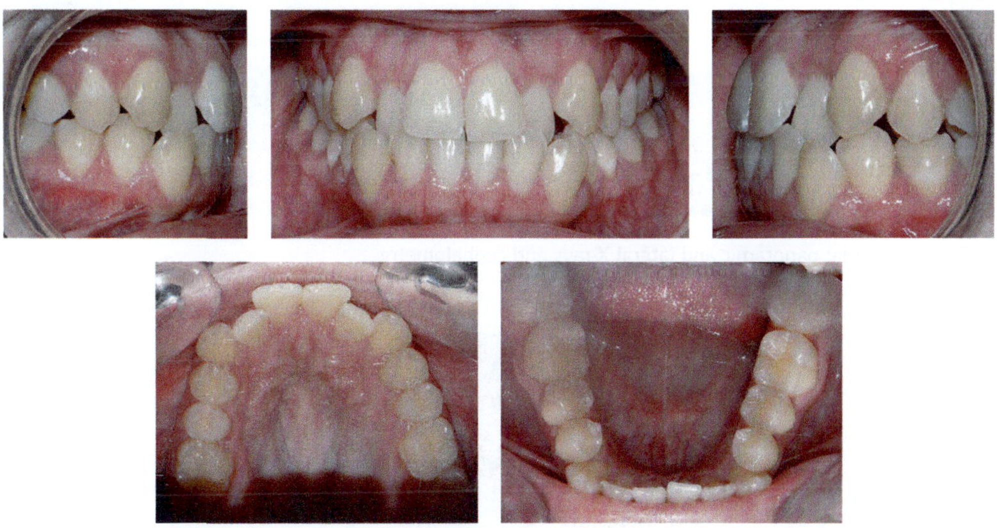

Fig. 20.249 Initial intraoral views.

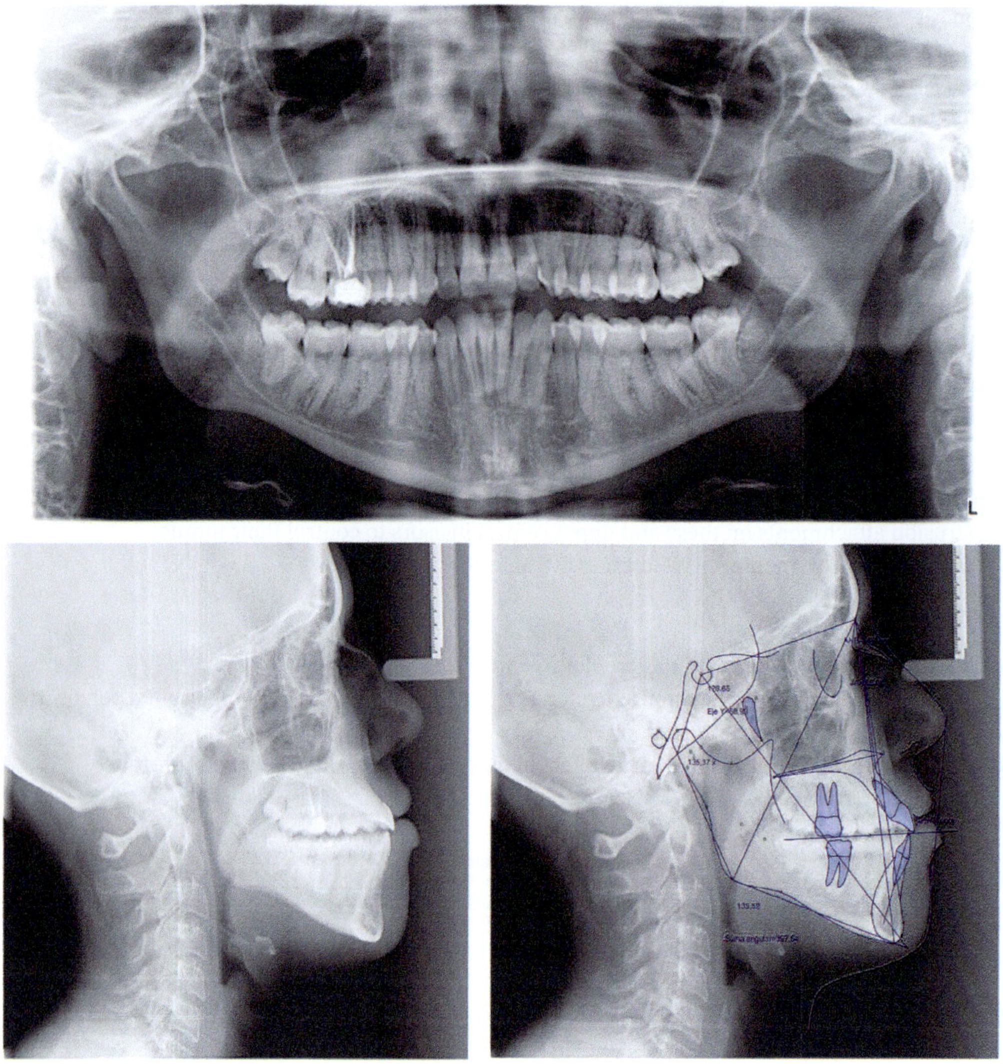

Fig. 20.250 Initial panoramic and lateral X-rays and cephalometry.

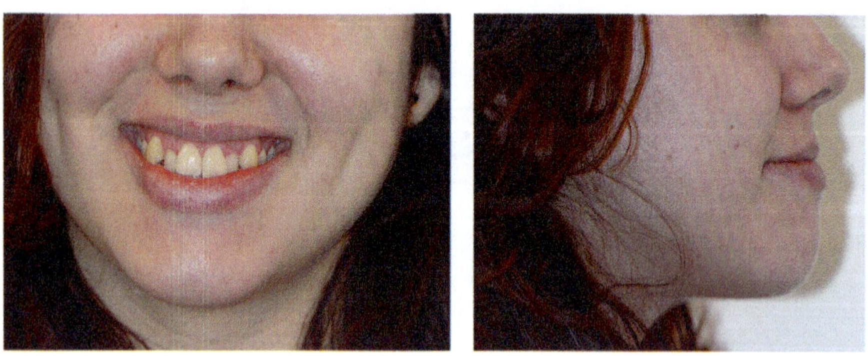

Fig. 20.251 Initial extraoral view.

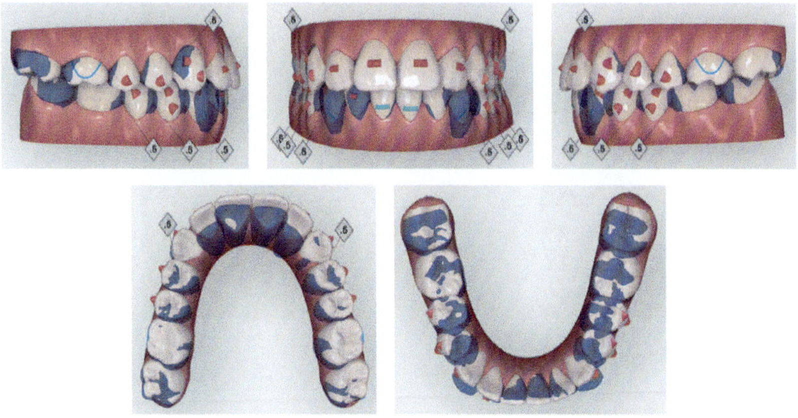

Fig. 20.252 Initial ClinChecks.

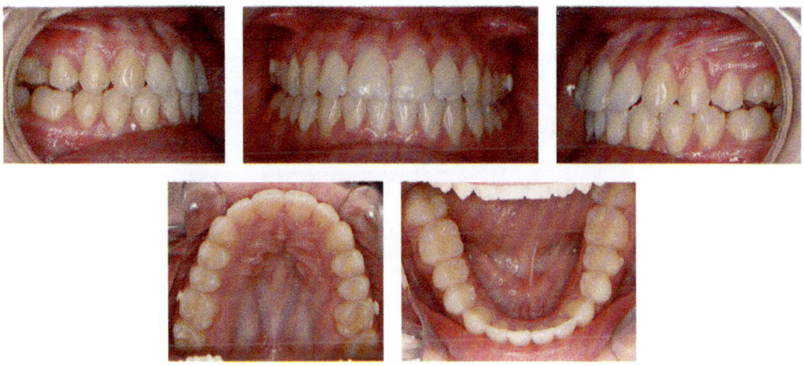

Fig. 20.253 Refinement: intraoral views.

ClinCheck 2: Requirements for the Technician

- Class III elastics button cutouts on right side
- Left button cutouts to close posterior open bite
- Final occlusal adjustments with 3D controls to improve occlusion

Fig. 20.254 Refinement ClinChecks.

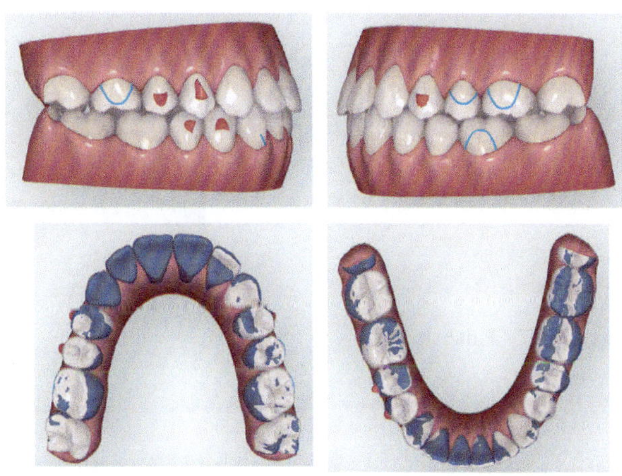

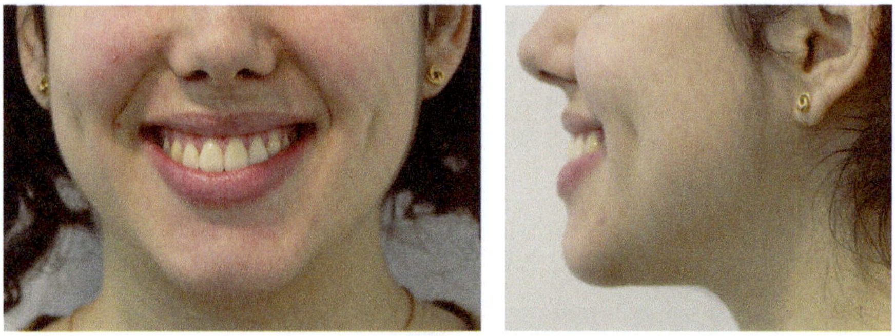

Fig. 20.255 Extraoral view after refinement.

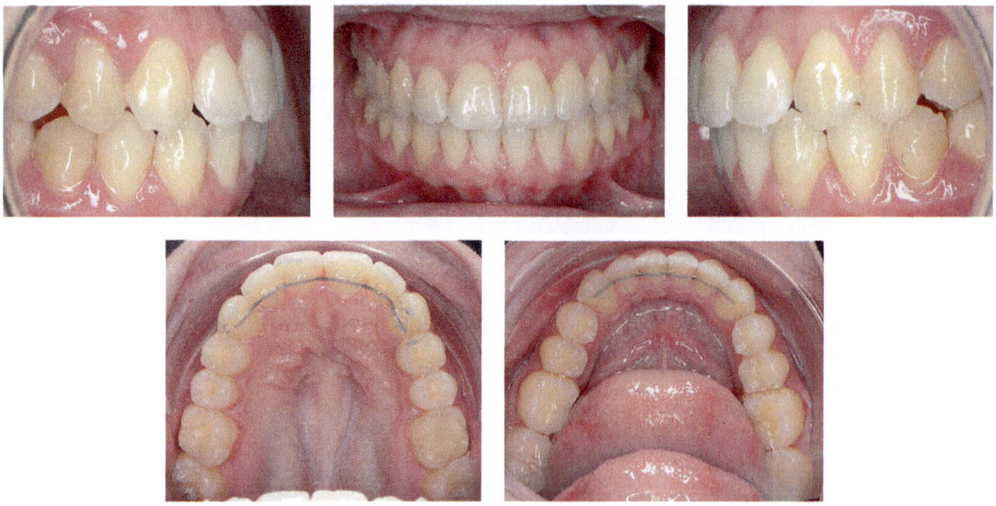

Fig. 20.256 Final intraoral views.

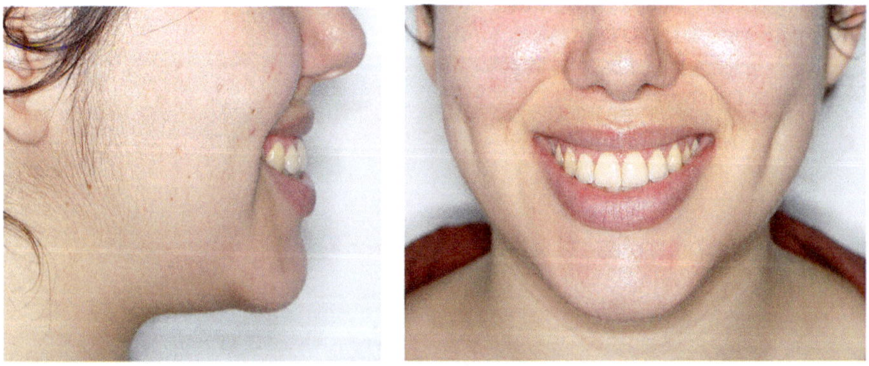

Fig. 20.257 Final smile.

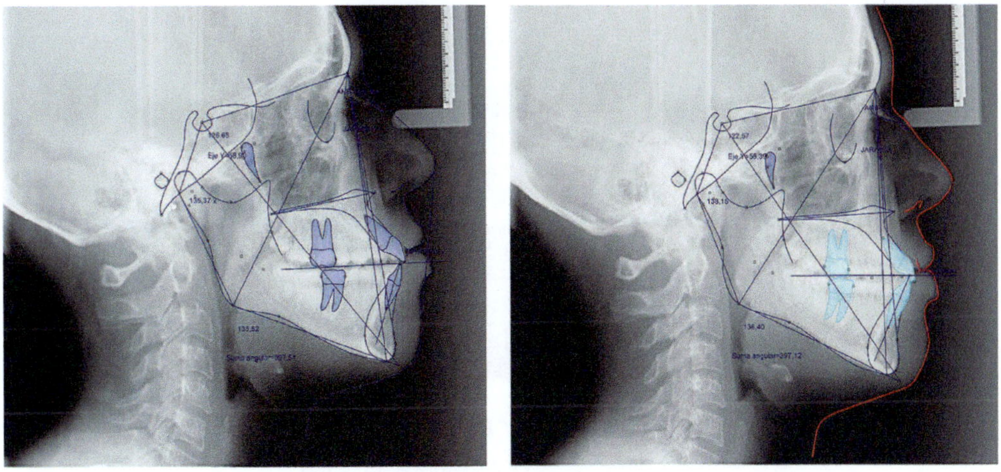

Fig. 20.258 Initial and post-treatment cephalometric analysis.

20.4 Dentoalveolar Protrusion Skeletal Class II

20.4.1 Upper and Lower Simultaneous Distalization Protocol

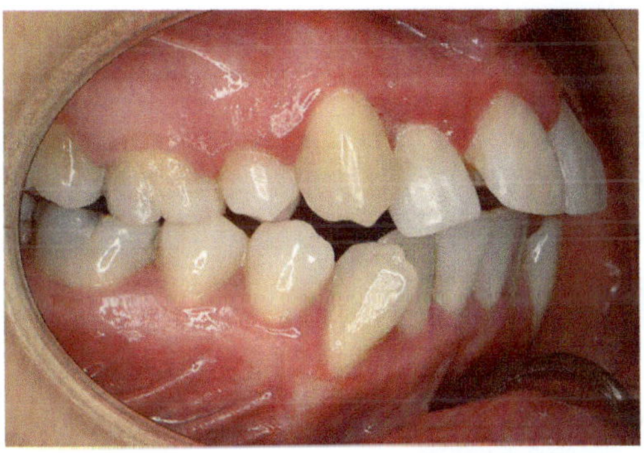

Fig. 20.259 Initial intraoral view.

Diagnosis

A 35-year-old woman presented with a hyperdivergent skeletal class II malocclusion, dentoalveolar protrusion and severe crowding. She was missing 14 and had periodontal disease and a gummy smile. Third molars were present (18/28 and 38 in upper and lower arch), but 48 was missing. She had a 7 mm overjet and open bite tendency with no anterior guidance.

Treatment Plan

- Extraction of 24, 34 and 44 to retrude the incisors and solve the excessive overjet
- Patient refused this, as she was worried about losing more teeth because of her periodontal problem, nevertheless, she accepted an alternative treatment plan extracting the wisdom teeth, which presented periodontal pockets of more than 5 mm, and distalizing upper and lower arches in order to correct the upper and lower proclination without compromising the periodontal situation of the incisors
- After this the patient's periodontal disease was treated by the periodontist
- The wisdom teeth were extracted and the case sent to Align Technology

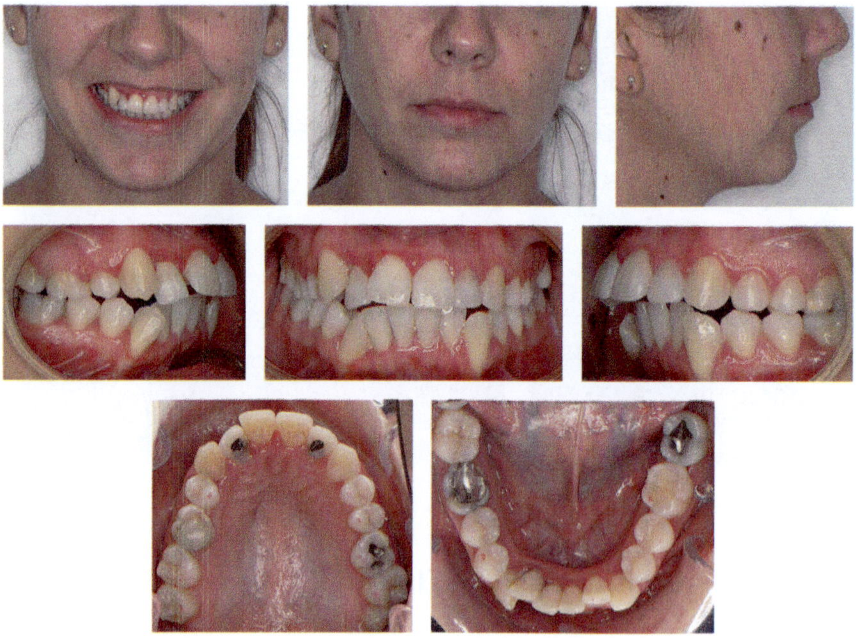

Fig. 20.260 Pretreatment extraoral and intraoral views.

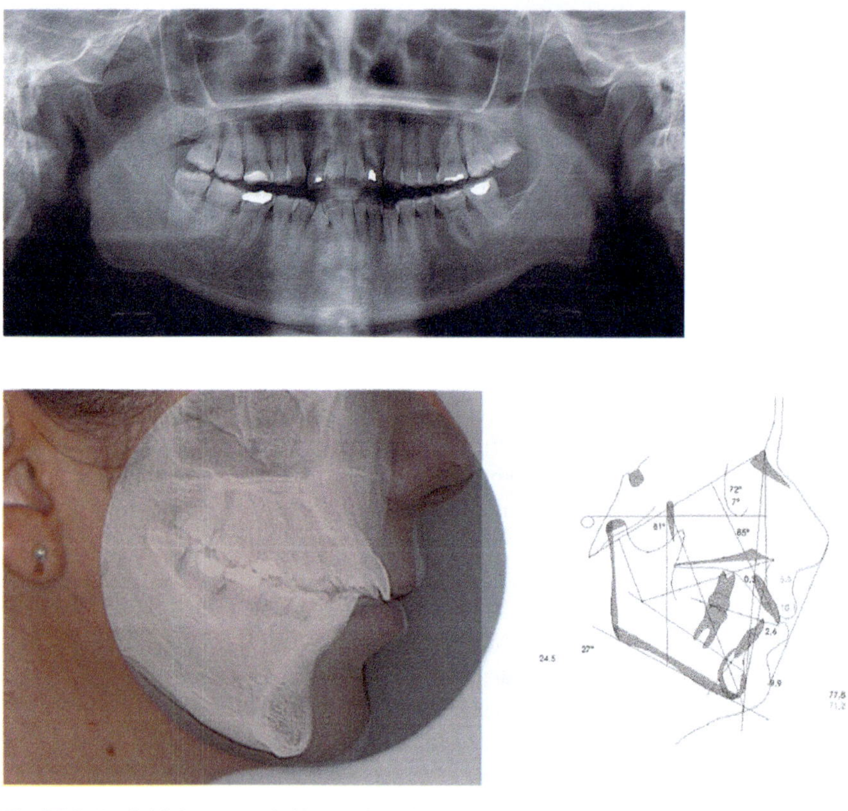

Fig. 20.261 Initial panoramic X-ray, teleradiograph and cephalometry.

Requirements for the Technician

- Simultaneous distalization of the upper and lower molars, once both molars are distalized 2 mm start moving simultaneously to distal 5 to 5 together in the upper and lower arch.
  - Vertical attachments were requested to control the tipping of the canines and premolars during the distalization
  - Maintain the torque of the upper and lower incisor during the retrusion as they would lose torque during the retraction

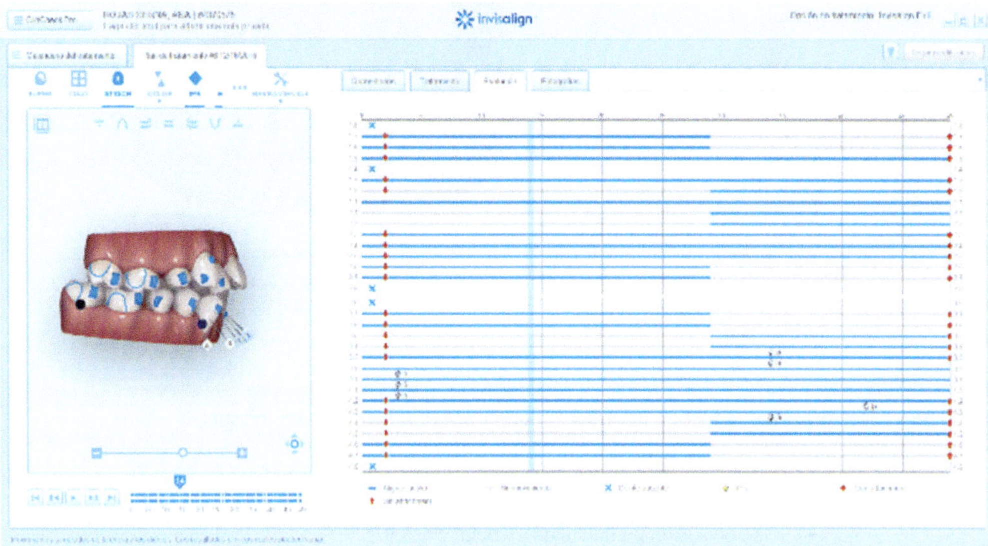

Fig. 20.262 Simultaneous distalization pattern in upper and lower arches.

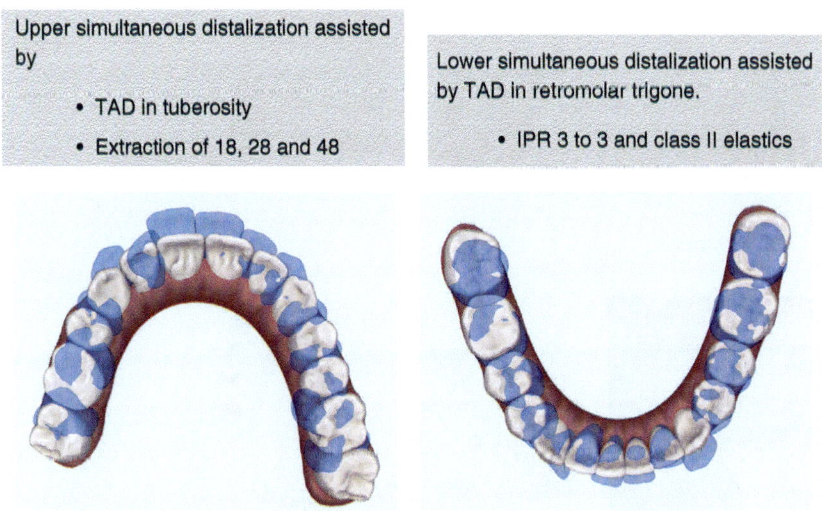

Fig. 20.263 Upper and lower ClinCheck views.

- Expansion + distalization + lower IPR

Correct anterior crowding and overjet

- Finish occlusion in bilateral class I in canine and class II molar on right side and class I molar on left side

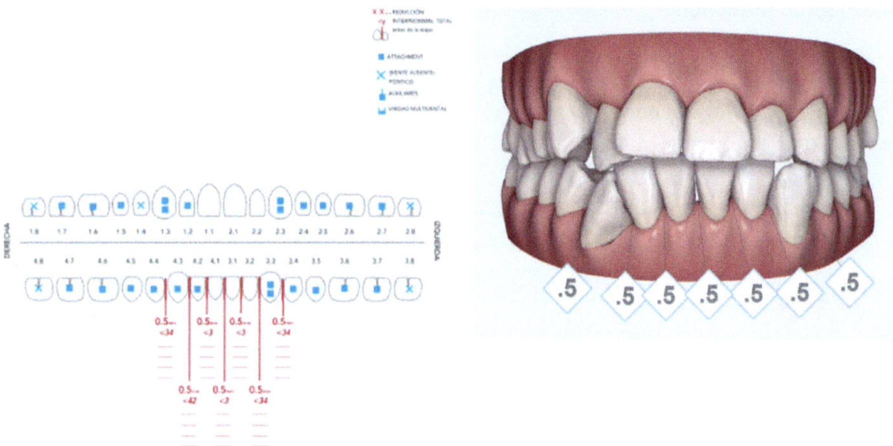

Fig. 20.264 Interproximal reduction necessary in order not to procline lower incisors.

- Achieve bilateral class I
- Finish occlusion on right side in molar class II
- Reduce overjet by incisor retrusion

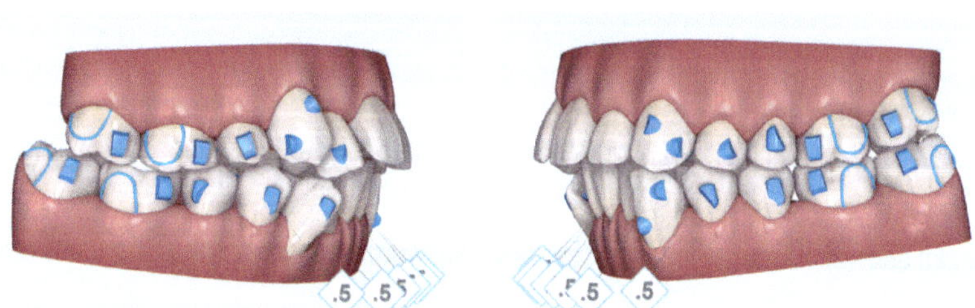

Fig. 20.265 Lateral ClinCheck views.

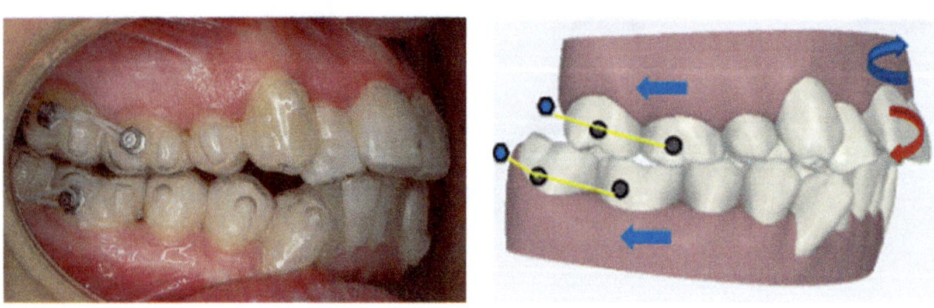

Fig. 20.266 Rein horse with Powerchain to temporary anchorage devices in the tuberosity and retromolar zone.

No proclination:

- Expansion + upper and lower distalization
- Correct open bite by upper and lower incisor retrusion (relative extrusion)
- Correct crowding by expansion, distalization and IPR

- 10 mm TAD in retromolar trigone and tuberosity
- Vertical AT in molars to prevent tipping
- Optimized attachment in canines

- 10mm TAD in maxillary tuberosity
- First the molars are distalized and then 5 to 5 are moved distally together

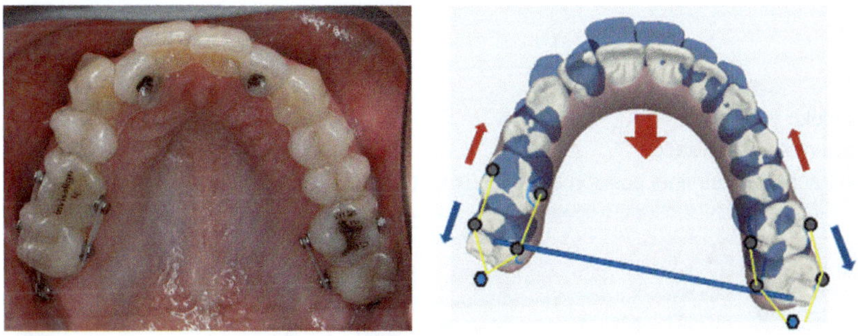

Fig. 20.267 Simultaneous upper distalization using temporary anchorage devices from the tuberosity.

- Correct lower crowding by lower simultaneous distalization + IPR

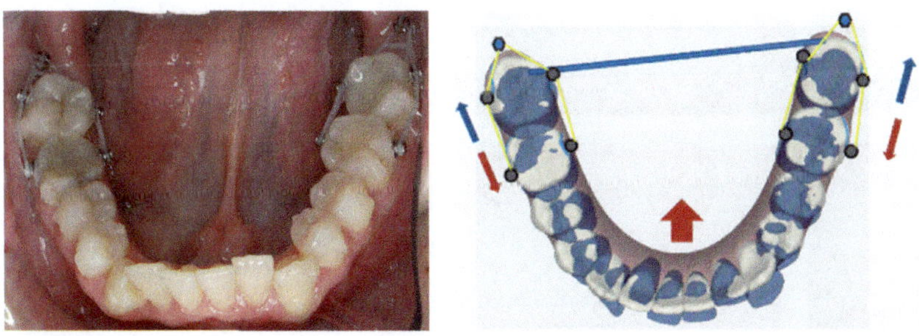

Fig. 20.268 Simultaneous lower distalization using temporary anchorage devices from the retromolar zone.

Treatment Summary

- A microscrew (10 mm) was placed in the upper right and left tuberosity and in the right and left retromolar zone in order to provide anchorage for the simultaneous distalization of both upper and lower molars
- Buttons were placed by labial and by lingual to the four upper and lower molars and a single Powerchain was placed from the labial button to the first molars to the lingual button of the same molar (like a horse rein!)

- This allowed distalization of all the upper and lower arches simultaneously.
- The treatment consisted of 49 aligners, but in aligner 31, because of excessive force activating the Powerchain in the molars, there was a a tipping problem that needed to be addressed with sectional wires in the first and second molars.
- At that time additional aligners were ordered for better adjustment on the molar zone.
- Patient has had 23 months of treatment on 10-day change intervals protocol and she is presently waiting for the second set of additional aligners to complete the closure of the posterior diastemas.
- The open bite was closed without extruding the incisors as the patient had a gummy smile at the beginning of the treatment; the microscrew in the tuberosity and in the retromolar zone allowed not only distalization of the arches but also intrusion of the upper and lower molars, creating an anticlockwise rotation of the mandible and improving the chin projection.
- The periodontal situation of the incisors has improved considerably as a result of the orthodontic treatment as well as the aesthetic of the patient's smile.

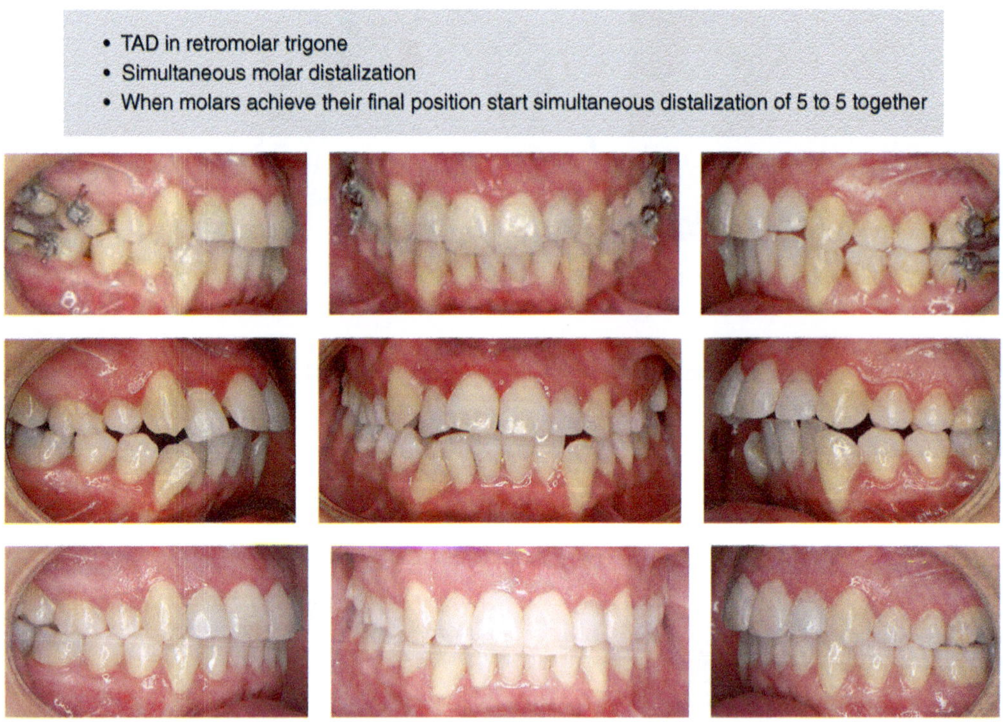

Fig. 20.269 Initial occlusion (upper) and situation at month 17 of treatment (middle) and at the end of treatment (lower).

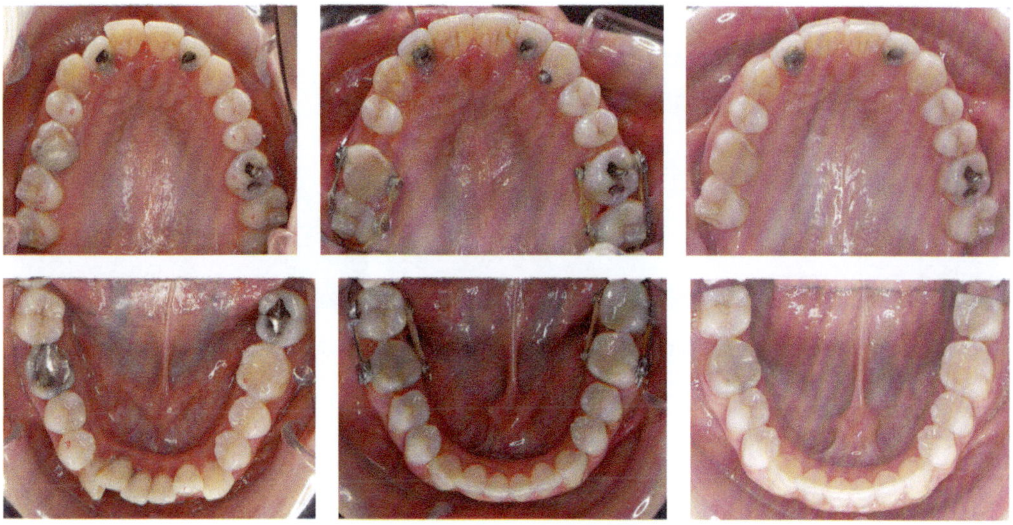

Fig. 20.270 Arch development at 23 months. Powerchain from first upper and lower molars to temporary anchorage devices for simultaneous distalization.

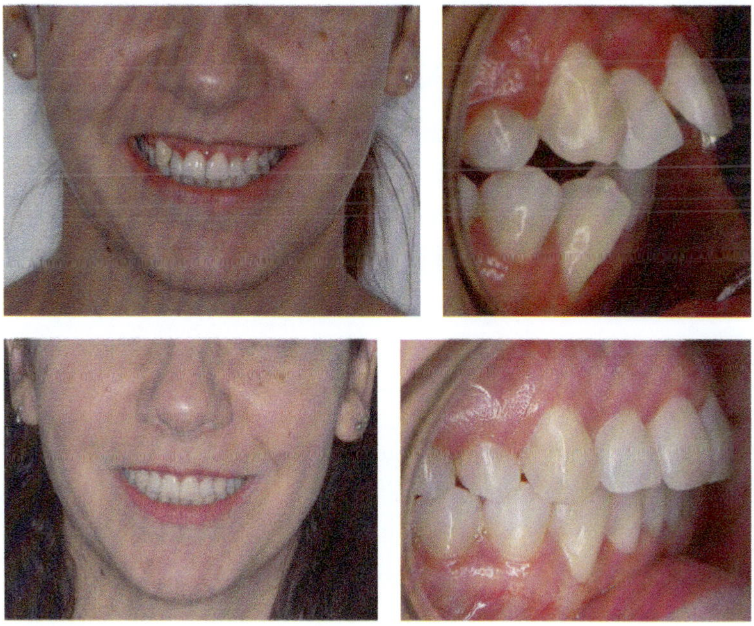

Fig. 20.271 Pretreatment and final smile and overjet.

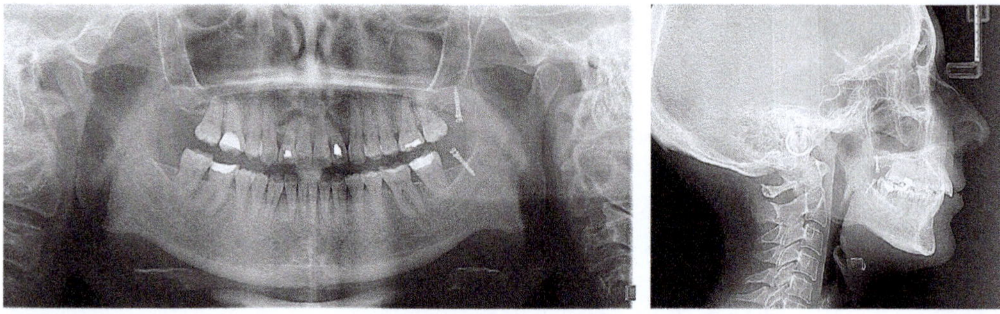

Fig. 20.272 Final panoramic and lateral X-rays.

21

Vertical Problems

21.1 Open Bite

In order to solve an open bite, we need to consider the cause of the open bite, which might be transversal, sagittal or vertical.

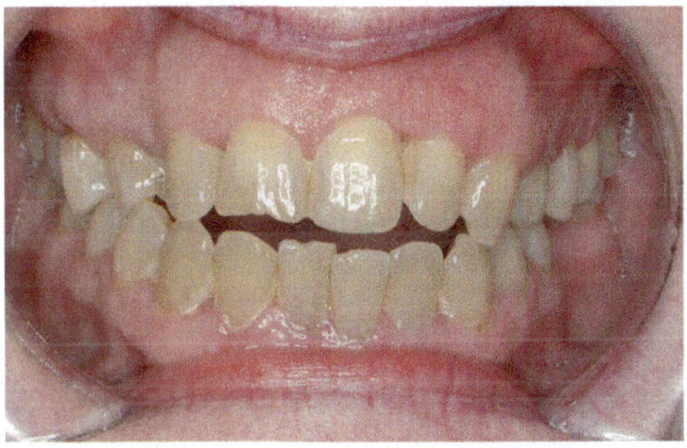

Fig. 21.1 Vertical cause, excess posterior facial height.

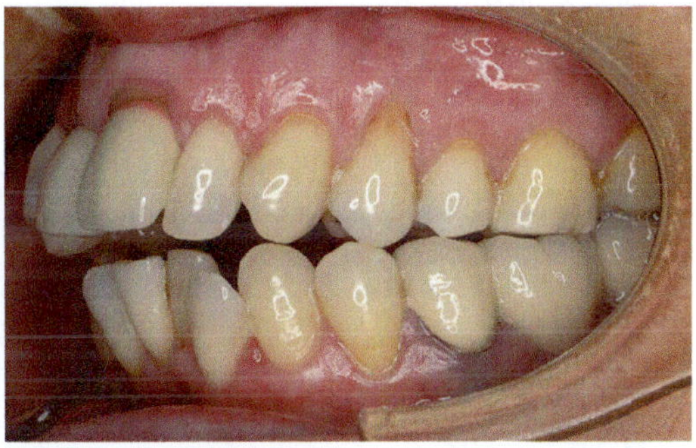

Fig. 21.2 Dentoalveolar cause (protrusion).

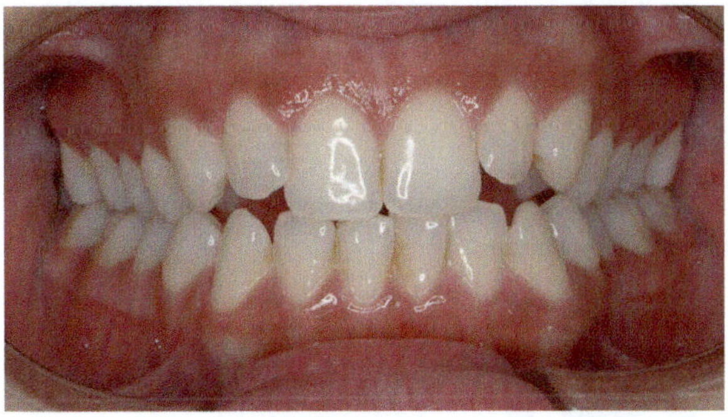

Fig. 21.3 Transversal cause, lingual torque of posterior teeth.

With that in mind, key to correcting an open bite are:

- The amount of posterior expansion which leads to anterior bite closure
- The capacity of tipping to lingual upper and lower incisors, extruding them relatively

Aligner Techniques in Orthodontics, First Edition. Susana Palma Moya and Javier Lozano Zafra.

Companion website: www.wiley.com/go/lozano-zafra/aligner-techniques

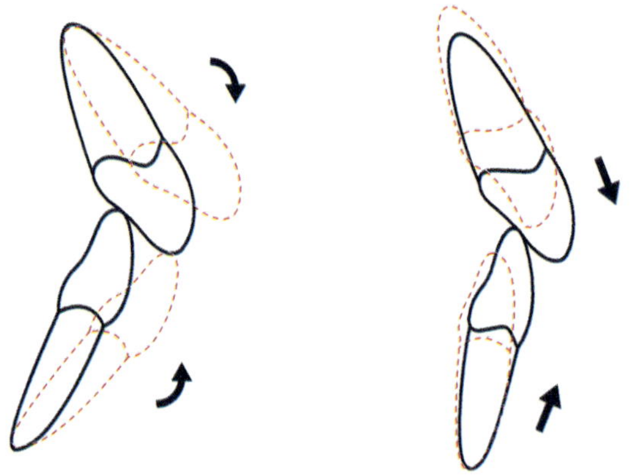

Fig. 21.4 The amount of lingual tipping of upper and lower incisors helps to solve an anterior crossbite by relative extrusion and is a key success factor.

Factors Determining How to Resolve an Open Bite

Smile Analysis If there is a gummy smile, the open bite will need to be corrected by posterior intrusion. However, if there is a low smile, it will be possible to extrude upper incisors to correct the open bite.

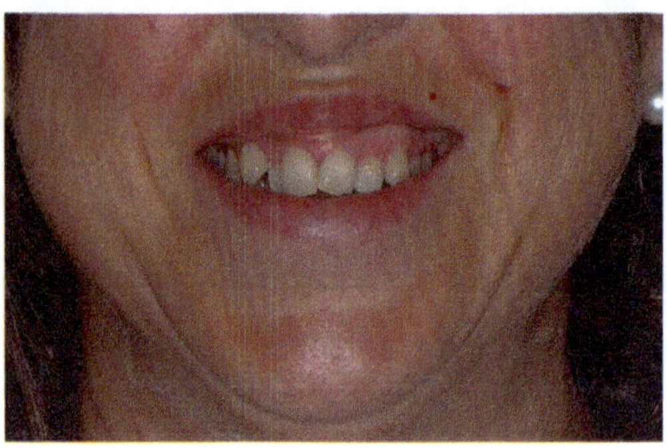

Fig. 21.5 Gummy smile.

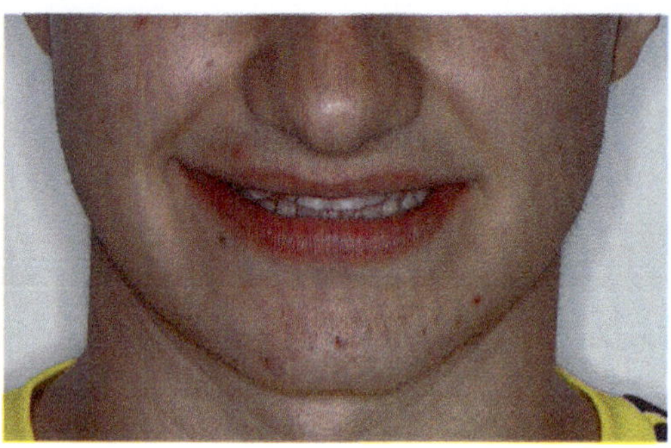

Fig. 21.6 Low smile, short display.

Patient Biotype

Extruding posterior teeth will rotate the mandible and increase anterior facial height, which might be beneficial or not for patient aesthetics.

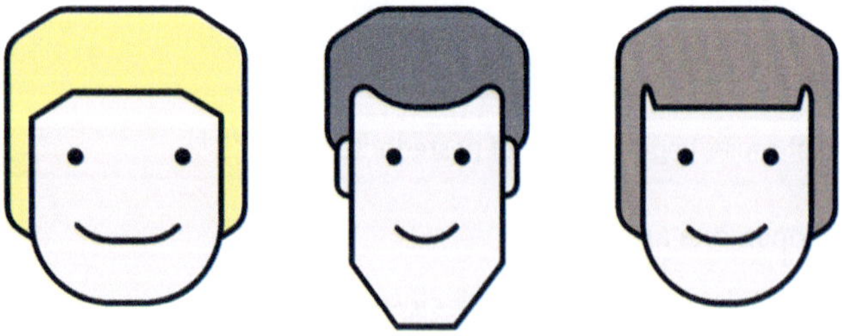

Fig. 21.7 The facial lower third determines whether to intrude or not to intrude posterior teeth.

Posterior Anchorage Analysis

A strong posterior anchorage is needed for effective extrusion of the upper incisors. This anchorage, will be provided by.

- Not moving the posterior lateral zone during the anterior extrusion
- Horizontal 5mm attachments on 4s/6s
- Four lingual attachments on upper incisors during expansion to increase anchorage
- Optimized attachments or conventional vertical in canines

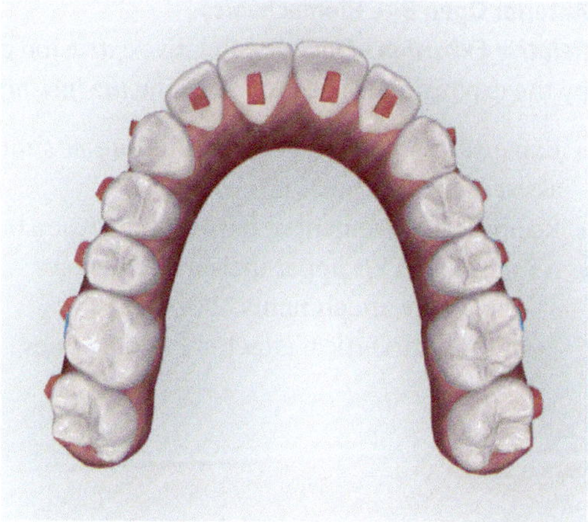

Fig. 21.8 Anchorage attachments.

Anterior Open Bite Anchorage

Although the reciprocal force of the extrusion of the incisor, which in the intrusion of the molars is favourable for the correction of an open bite, attachments are required for the anterior teeth that have to be extruded.

Nevertheless, in the posterior zone, attachments will have the function of controlling the posterior molar torque during the expansion to prevent the labial cuspids of the molar tipping to labial, which could increase the open bite during the correction.

Requirements for the Technician

- Start the correction as soon as possible by transversal development of both upper and lower arches: this will provide space for the retrusion of the incisors (relative extrusion)
- During the expansion, it is advisable to use attachments to the lingual surface of the incisors to increase anterior anchorage
- Postpone absolute extrusion till the end: do not move molars and extrude the upper incisors maintaining torque, remove horizontal bevelled to gingival attachments in lingual and exchange them for optimized extrusion attachments by labial (ask for a reciprocal movement of anterior extrusion and posterior intrusion)
- Minor cases might benefit from 'Chewies'
- Temporary anchorage devices (TADs) should be used to intrude posterior zone (in cases of gummy smile) or when the open bite has a skeletal pattern

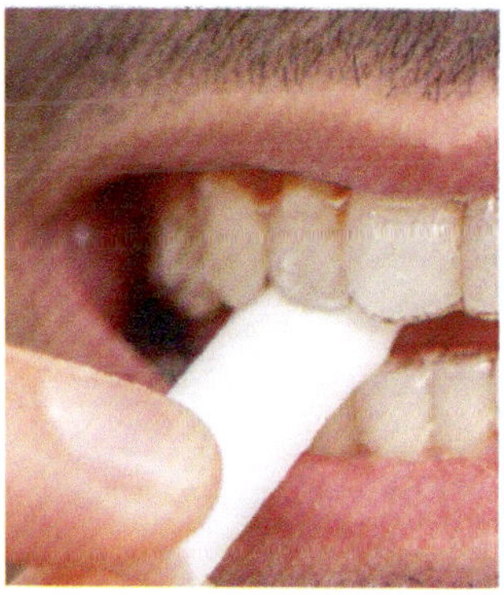

Fig. 21.9 Chewies or fitters are good for minor open bite cases.

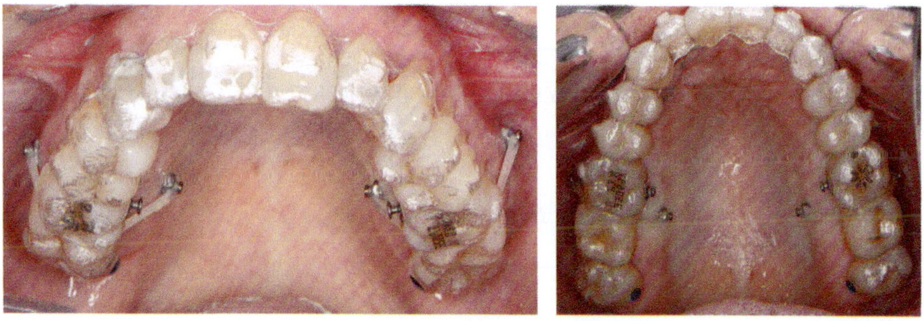

Fig. 21.10 Miniscrews used for absolute posterior intrusion greater than 3 mm, by labial and lingual, and mesial to first molars, enabling the patient to wear an elastic over the aligner.

Anterior Open Bite Biomechanics

Relative Extrusion of Incisors Relative extrusion can be obtained after expansion if the space opened by the expansion is used to retrocline *the incisors:*

- Expansion changing posterior torque + simultaneous incisor retraction + class II elastics to assist incisors retraction
- Reciprocal movement of posterior intrusion 0.5 mm + anterior extrusion at the end of treatment
- AT optimized for upper incisors extrusion
  - Anchorage attachments UA4/5
  - Optimized/vertical attachment in canines

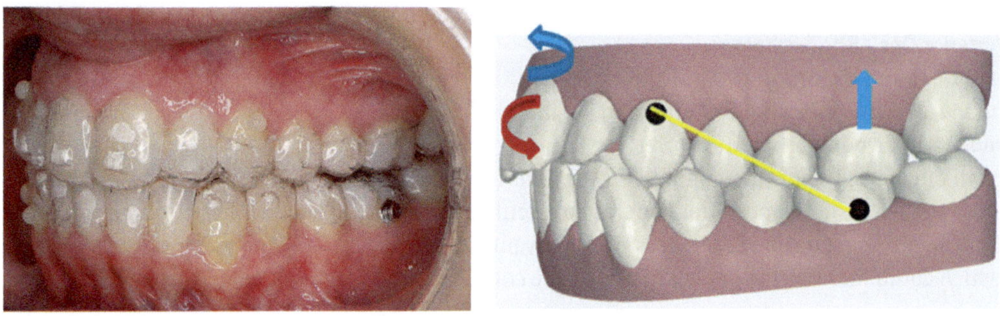

Fig. 21.11 Open bite requires careful biomechanics planning.

Pure Extrusion of Incisors using Multi-tooth Optimized Extrusive Attachments

- The clinician must examine the smile carefully before deciding if upper incisor extrusion is adequate.

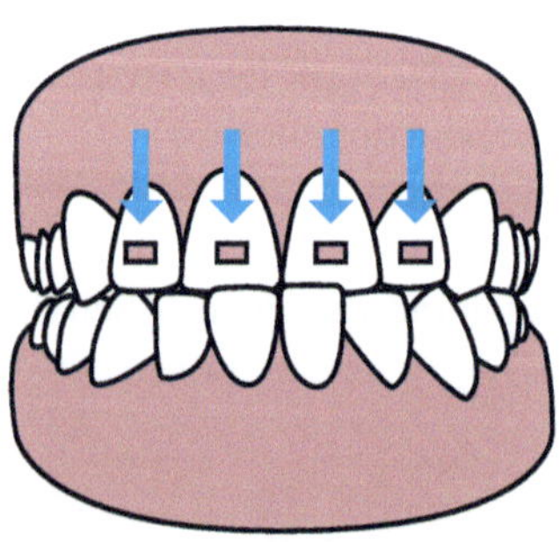

Fig. 21.12 Optimized anterior extrusion is mostly predictable if it is planned at the end of the treatment with posterior sectors unmovable at that time.

- Posterior intrusion of maxillary and mandibular teeth with consequent upward and forward mandibular closure (anticlockwise rotation of the mandible). This is visualized in the ClinCheck as a virtual jump

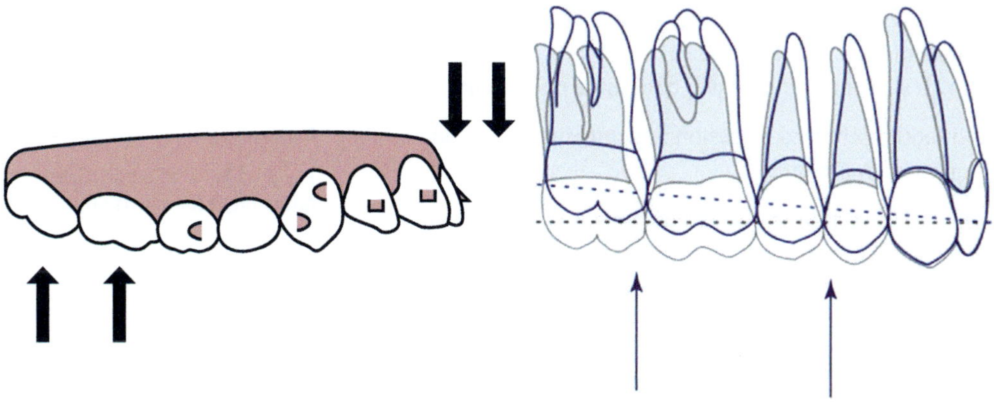

Fig. 21.13 Posterior intrusion will have saggital effects as a result of mandibular rotation.

Open Bite Prescription
- **Easy:** Less than 2.5 mm is very predictable (better if we do not need posterior intrusion)
- **Moderate**: 2.5 mm with less than 1 mm of posterior intrusion
- **Complex:** more than 2.5 mm (auxiliary techniques needed)

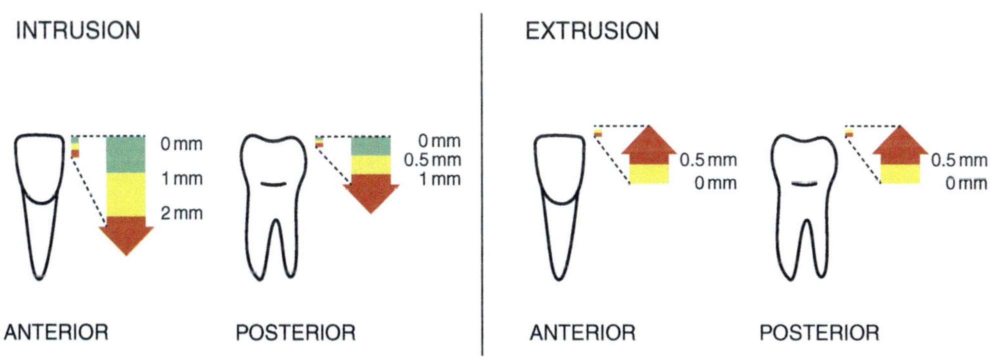

Fig. 21.14 We have to face predictability of vertical movements in order to know whether to plan auxiliary techniques or not.

Question 6 of the Prescription Form How do we want to correct the open bite?

- Only by anterior extrusion?
- By anterior extrusion and posterior intrusion?
- Other like surgery (fill in special instructions)?

Specific Features of an Open Bite

Anterior extrusion:

- Optimized extrusion AT (single tooth more 0.5 mm)
- Automatically placed by the software for extrusion
- Only on upper and lower anterior incisors
- Threshold is 0.5 mm
- Crown size and anatomy will determine placement

Multi tooth optimized extrusion attachments (to extrude all the upper incisors as a unit):

- They will override any other attachment on these teeth
- Placed at the same time
- Automatically placed by the software for extrusion
- Threshold is 0.5 mm

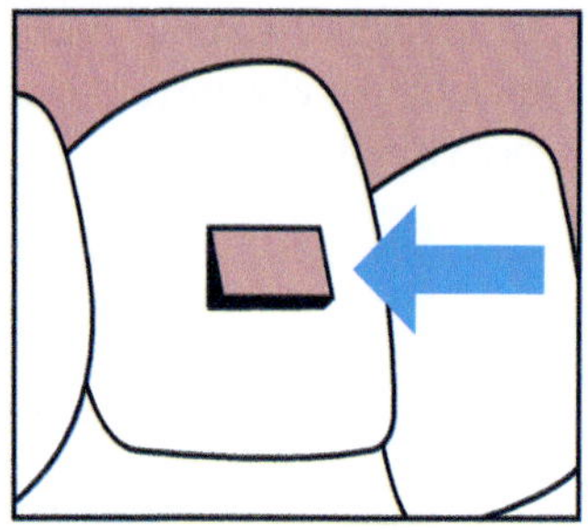

Fig. 21.15 Single optimized attachment for extrusion.

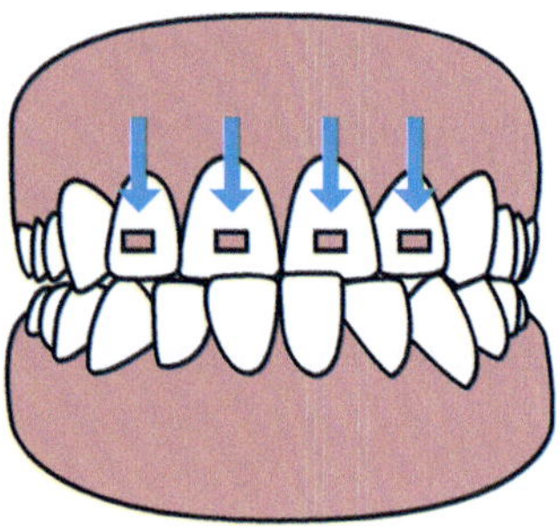

Fig. 21.16 Optimized anterior extrusion is mostly predictable if it is planned at the end of the treatment with posterior sectors unmovable at that time.

Predictability of the Open Bite Treatment

The predictability of treatment will be high when:

- Anterior open bite is dental, not skeletal
- Incisor is proclined at the beginning and can be retroclined, generating a relative extrusion
- The transversal development of arches is possible, as the expansion of narrow arches will provide space to retrocline the incisors
- Open bite can be solved just by anterior extrusion of less than 2.5 mm without the need for intrusion of the posterior molars

Overcorrection

A request for overcorrection could consist of finishing the occlusion with a small gap between the molars or to end up with heavy occlusal contacts, to obtain an overbite of at least 2 mm at the end of treatment.

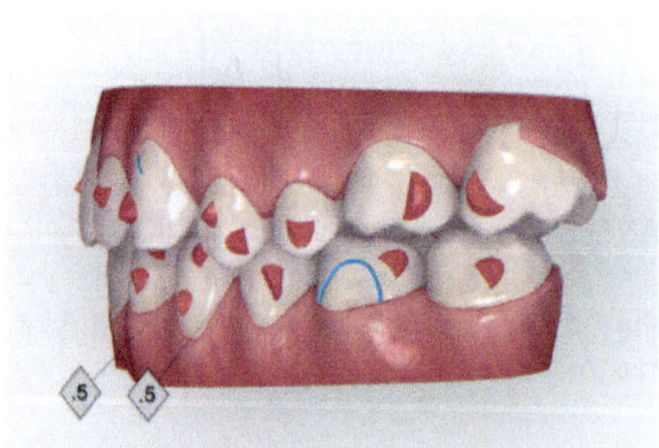

Fig. 21.17 Posterior open bite is a good overcorrection in this case.

Occlusal Attachments

Occlusal attachments might be useful for increasing posterior intrusion forces, as anterior precision bite ramps. They can be filled with composite and then the proper attachments bonded to molar occlusal surfaces or can be left empty, assuming that the plastic will be occluded with more pressure than with a regular aligner.

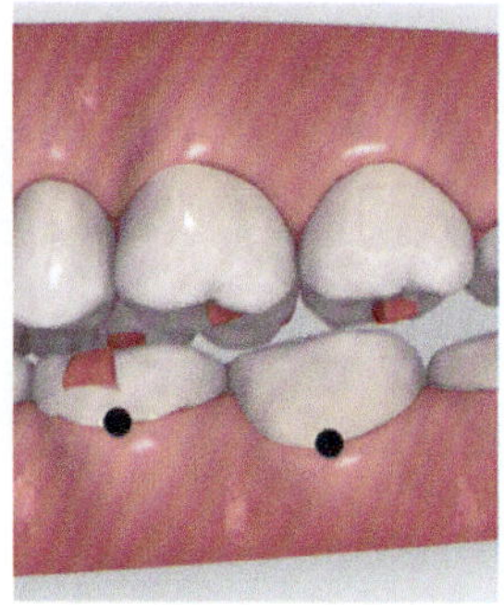

Fig. 21.18 Unpredictable posterior intrusion is assisted by upper and lower occlusal attachments that increase bite forces on posterior sector.

21.1.1 Open Bite: Transversal and Sagittal Cause

Diagnosis

A 31-year-old patient with normodivergent skeletal class I presented with narrow arches with posterior gummy smile and mild crowding.

Treatment Plan

- Correcting the anterior open bite by retroclining the maxillary and mandibular incisors
- Maxillary anterior extrusion and posterior intrusion was also requested at the end of the treatment
- Provide space for retroinclining the incisors, with an expansion that would be performed from the beginning

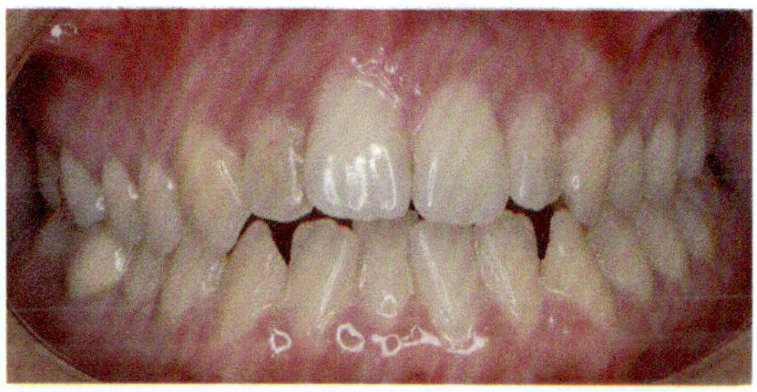

Fig. 21.19 Open bite solved with Lite treatment.

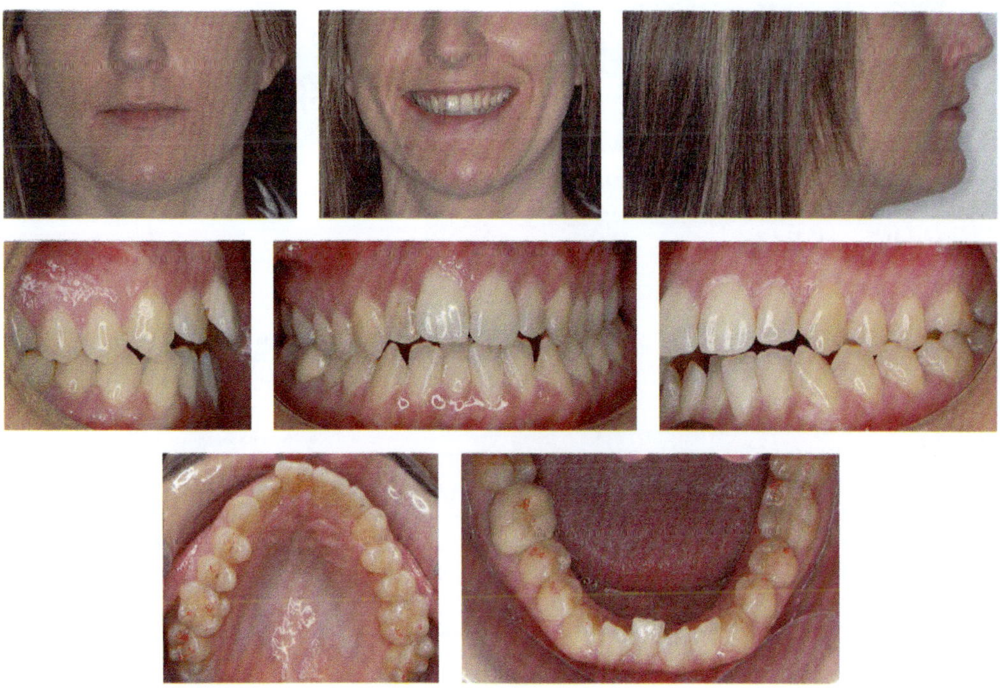

Fig. 21.20 Initial extraoral and intraoral views.

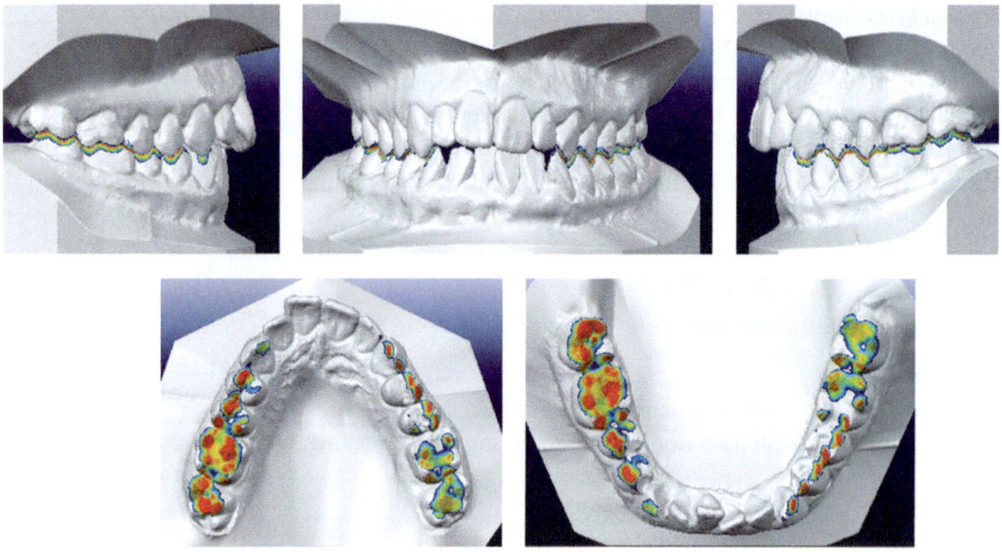

Fig. 21.21 Initial occlusal contact.

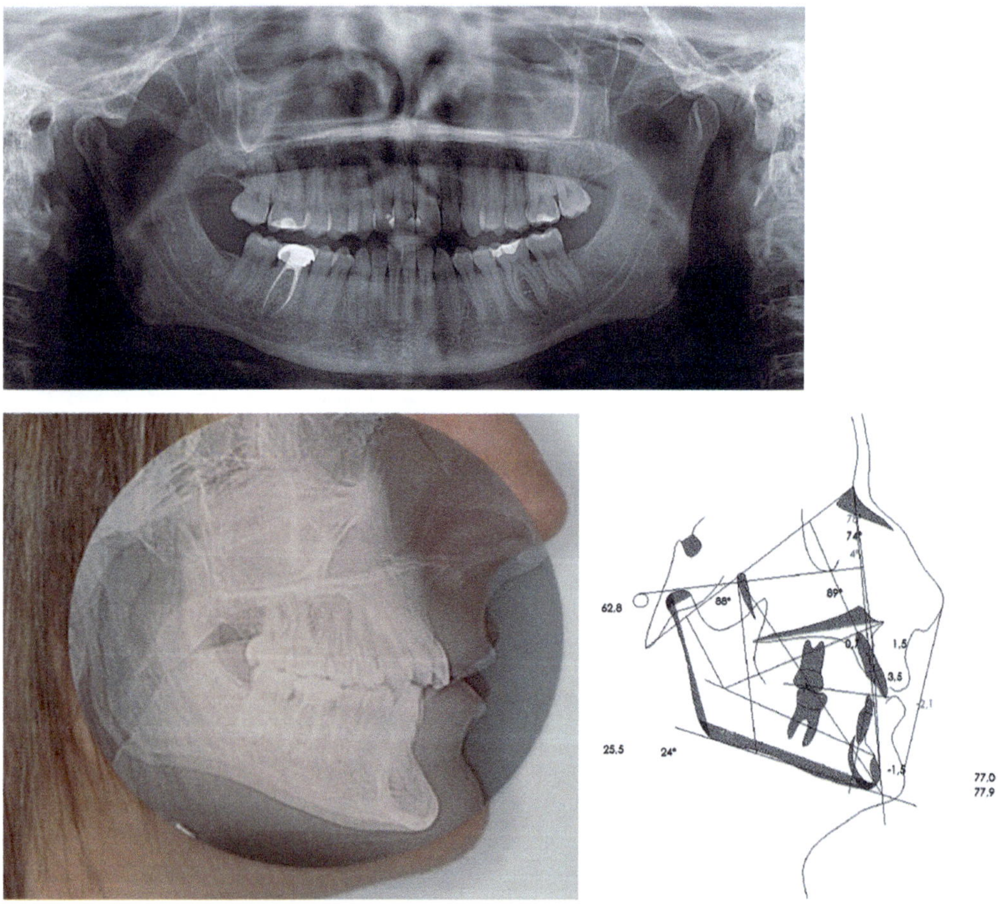

Fig. 21.22 Initial panoramic X-ray, teleradiograph and cephalometry.

Requirements for the Technician

Apply expansion to both arches, perform interproximal reduction (IPR) to correct incisor protrusion and reduce the overjet.

- Do not move molars to use them as anchorage as it is going to be corrected using Lite treatment.
- Multi-tooth anterior extrusive attachments to be placed automatically by the software on the maxillary incisors.
- In the lower arch, IPR to be performed in order to allow for correction of incisor protrusion and alignment without further proclination of the lower incisors.
- A 0.5 mm of posterior intrusion programmed during the incisors extrusion as a reciprocal movement.

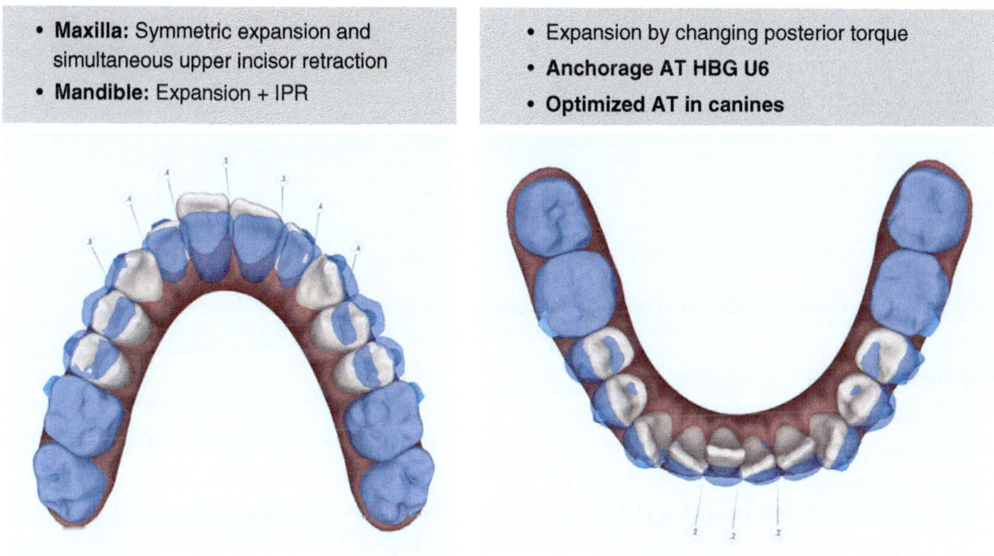

Fig. 21.23 Initial upper and lower ClinCheck views.

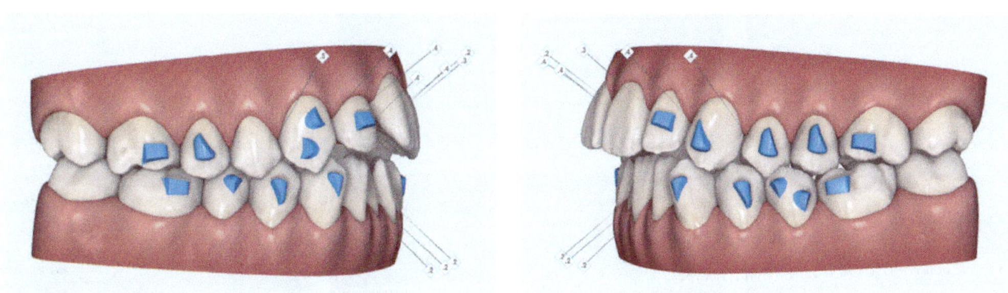

Fig. 21.24 Initial right and left ClinCheck views.

- Postpone upper absolute extrusion until the end
- Do not move molars (during anterior extrusion) to provide posterior anchorage

- Anchorage attachment on posterior teeth
- Class II elastics to assist retraction + relative extrusion of upper incisors

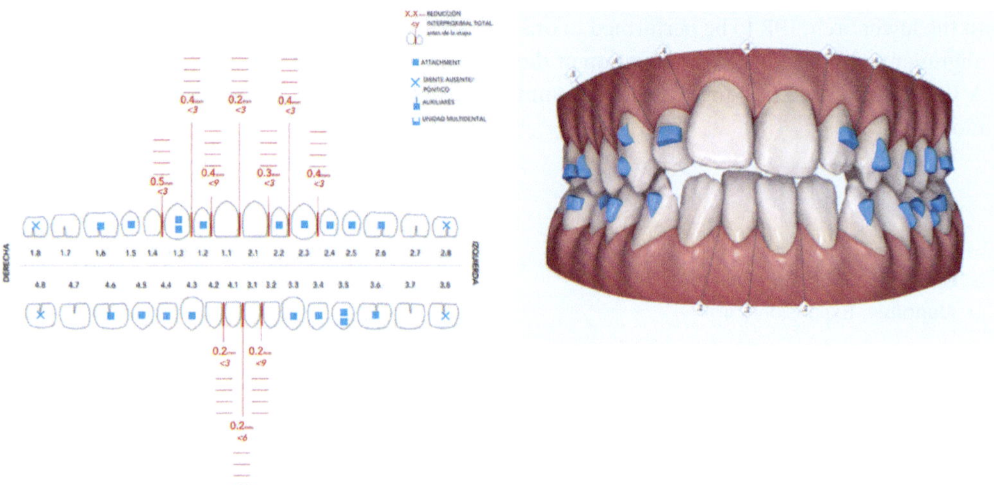

Fig. 21.25 Interproximal reduction necessary for relative extrusion of upper and lower incisors.

Treatment Summary

- The case was completed in 14 months
- The initial case had 14 aligners which were changed on a 2-week interval protocol; after that the patient wore a set of another 14 additional aligners
- The patient used elastics with a class II and vertical pattern for night use during the treatment
- The smile improved considerably as a result of the expansion
- The upper occlusal plane was levelled
- At the end of the treatment the patient had a bleaching and composite veneer in 12

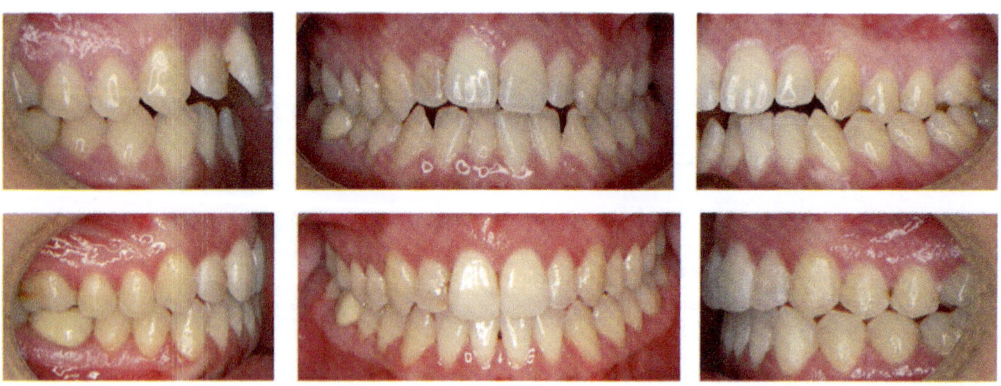

Fig. 21.26 Initial intraoral views (upper) and views before refinement (lower).

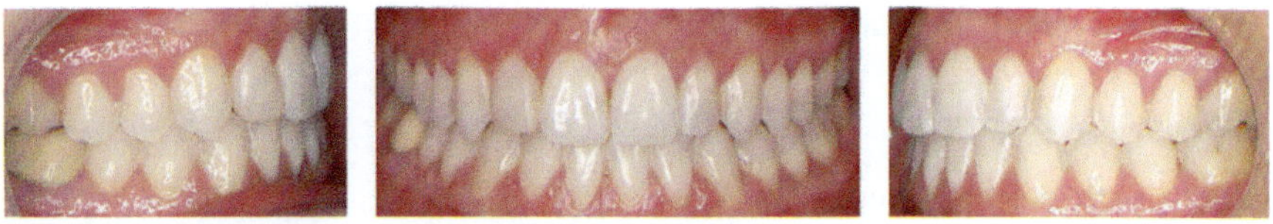

Fig. 21.27 Final intraoral views.

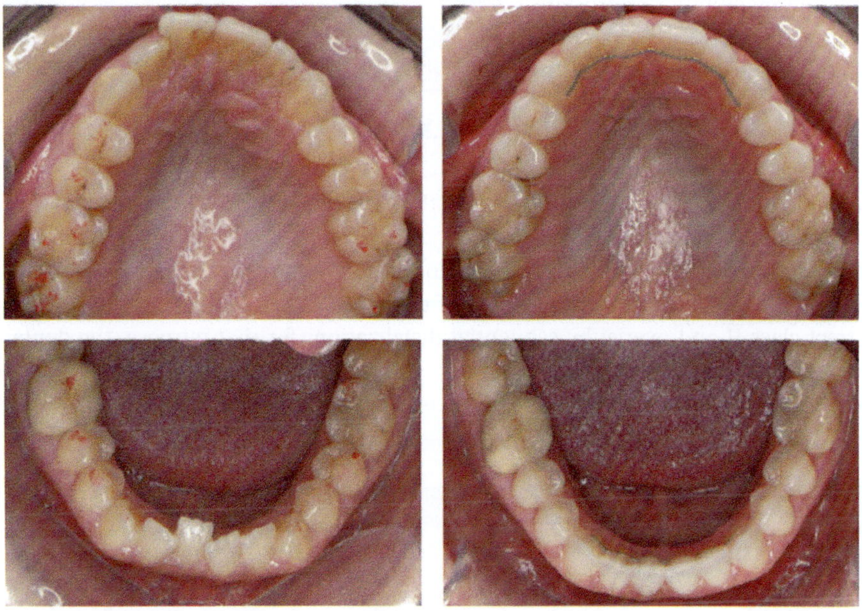

Fig. 21.28 Initial (left) and final occlusal (right).

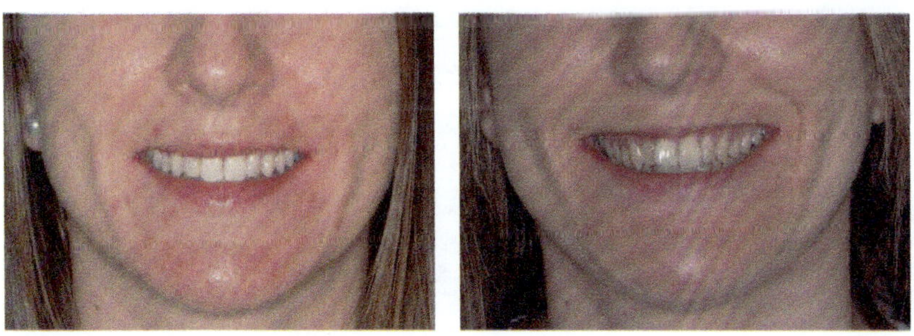

Fig. 21.29 Initial and final smile.

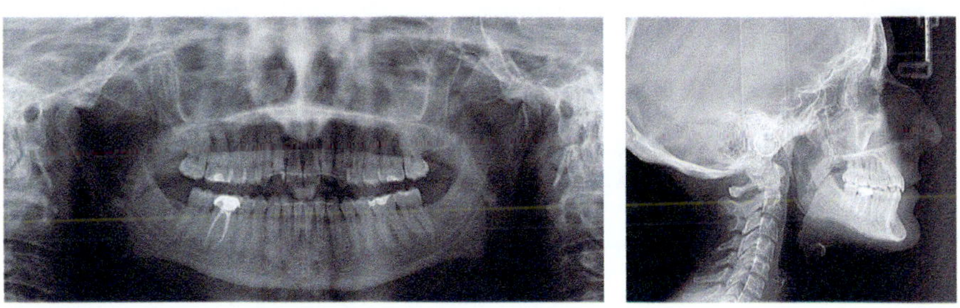

Fig. 21.30 Final panoramic and lateral X-rays.

21.1.2 Open Bite: Transversal, Sagittal and Vertical Cause

Diagnosis

A 62-year-old patient with a hyperdivergent skeletal class II pattern presented with an open bite with transversal, sagittal and vertical problems. She had maxillo-mandibular protrusion, labial incompetence, centred upper midline, constricted arches and dental crowns in 11 and 21.

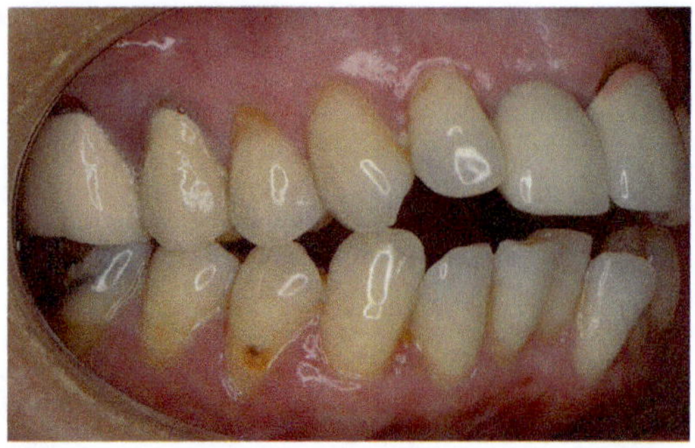

Fig. 21.31 Initial intraoral view.

Treatment Plan

- Expansion, sequential distalization, IPR (to increase the retraction of incisors and the relative extrusion) and simultaneous incisors retrusion
- In order to solve the patient problem, analyse the malocclusion in the different planes of space:
  - transversal: expansion with control of the torque of the premolars and molars
  - sagittal: correct class II and overjet by sequential distalization (for that purpose, the dental bridge needed to be removed in the lower arch)
  - vertical: close open bite by relative and absolute incisor extrusion

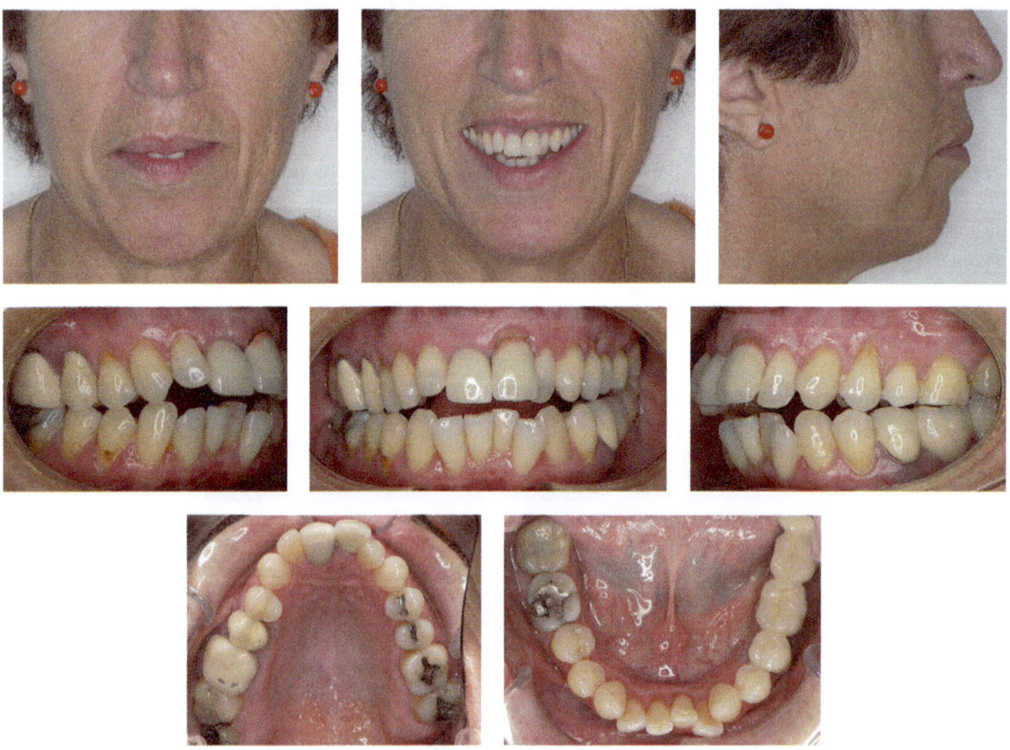

Fig. 21.32 Initial extraoral and intraoral views.

Correction by expansion, distalization and simultaneous upper and lower incisor retraction

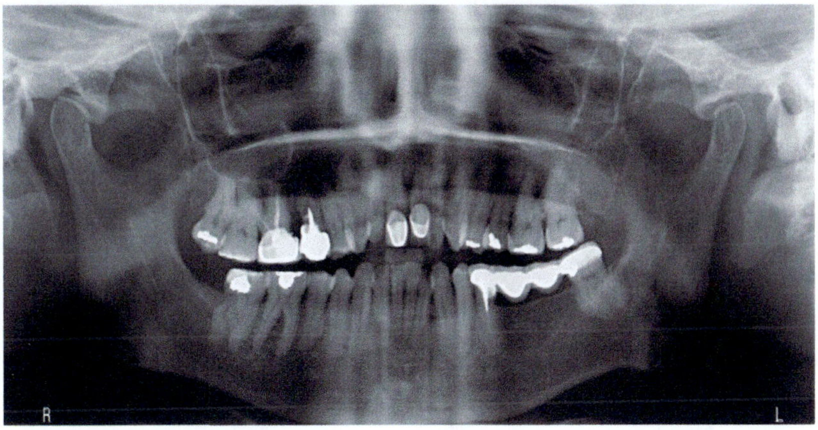

Fig. 21.33 Panoramic X-ray.

The patient has a dental bridge on the lower left quadrant that was cut in order to distalize the lower arch and prevent lower incisors proclination

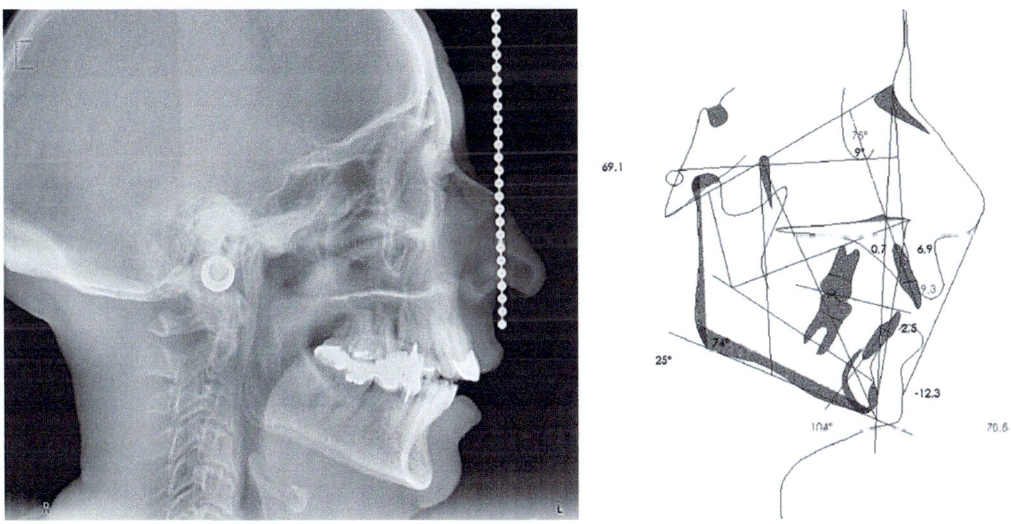

Fig. 21.34 Teleradiograph: proclination of upper and lower incisors, narrow symphysis.

Requirements for the Technician

- Provide expansion to the arches by changing torque and applying labial crown torque to premolars and molars of the upper and lower arches.
- IPR and simultaneous incisors retraction to create relative extrusion of the incisors.
- Lingual attachments bevelled to gingival on the upper incisors (HBG 3 mm), in order to have anterior anchorage during the expansion.
- Simultaneously to the expansion, make sequential distalization of the upper arch to correct the dental class II.

Maxilla:

- First: Expansion, at the same time procline 1.1 and 2.2 to make equal upper incisors torque
- Second: IPR + retrusion upper incisors (relative extrusion of upper incisors)

Mandible:

- Distalization + expansion + IPR + retraction of lower incisors (no proclination)

- Anchorage attachment: AT Horizontal 5 mm U4 and U6
- Optimized AT in canines
- AT palatal attachment HBG 3 mm on upper incisors during expansion, eliminate them when upper retraction starts, and change them by optimizing extrusion AT by labial

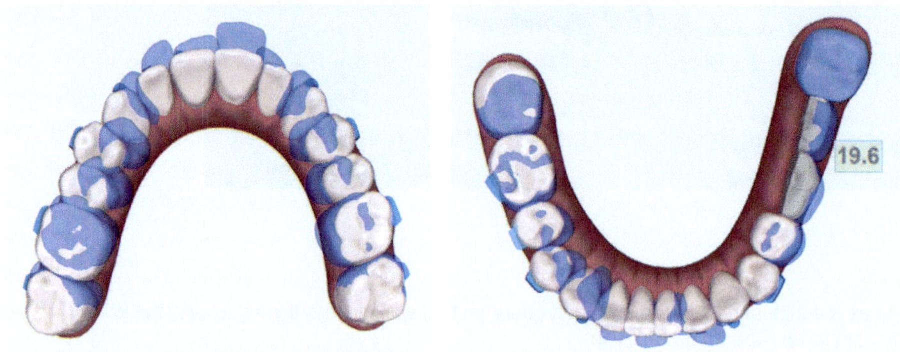

Fig. 21.35 Initial upper and lower ClinCheck views.

Treatment goals:

- Transversal: expansion
- Sagittal: class I
- Vertical: increase overbite

- Expansion by changing lateral torque + IPR + simultaneous loss in arch length
- Dentoalveolar protrusion + open bite = IPR
- Relative extrusion of upper incisors: class II elastics

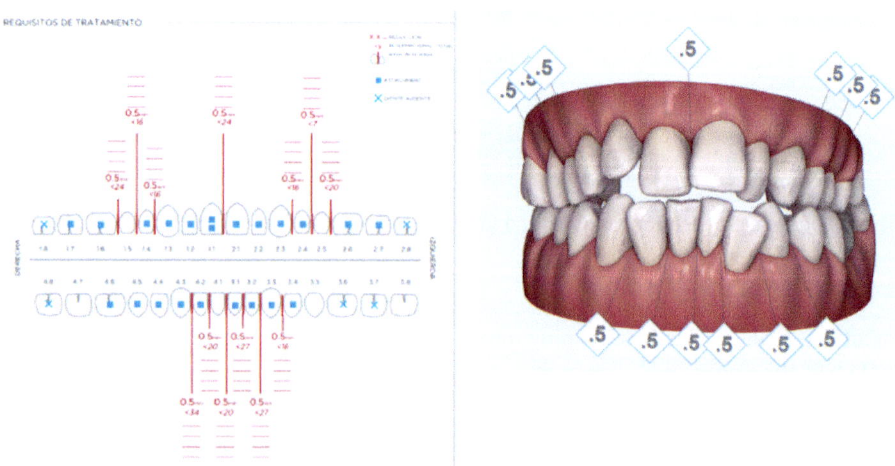

Fig. 21.36 Interproximal reduction to create relative extrusion of incisors.

Resolving the Transversal Problem

Maxilla:

- Expansion by change of lateral torque (tipping teeth to labial without moving the root apex) + simultaneous mesial-out rotation of U6 + IPR
- AT Horizontal 5 mm U4/6
- AT optimized U3
- AT HBG 3 mm palatal of upper incisors (prevent upper incisors intrusion during expansion)

Mandible:

- Expansion + lower sequential distalization + IPR

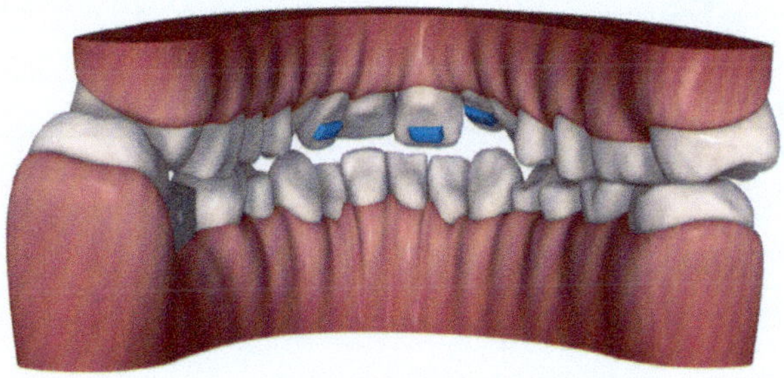

Fig. 21.37 Palatal attachments prevent upper incisors from intrusion during expansion.

Resolving the Sagittal Problem

- IPR + class II elastics (4.5 oz)
- Start with elastics as soon as transverse development is appropriate
- Upright lower incisors (no proclination)
- Lower and upper distalization
- Final overjet on ClinCheck should be 1.5 mm
- Use class II triangular elastics for sagittal and vertical canine movement

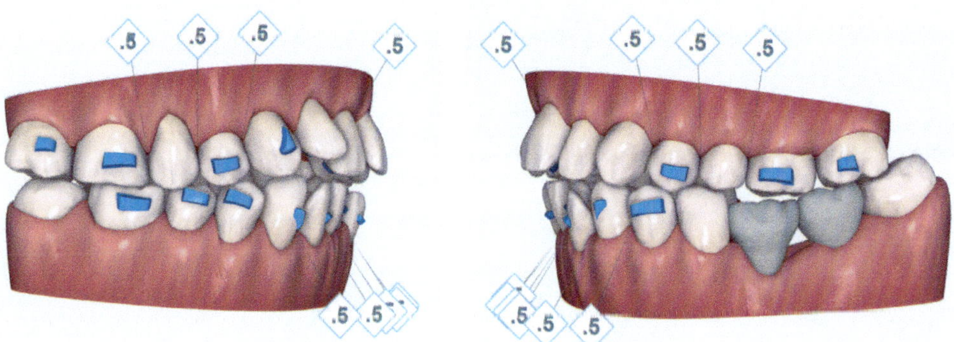

Fig. 21.38 Initial right and left intraoral ClinCheck views.

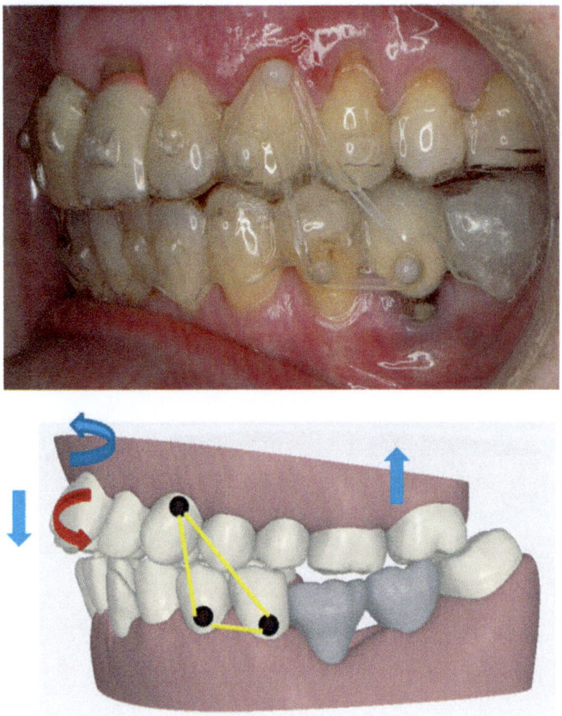

Fig. 21.39 Triangular elastics in class II. The technician was required to extrude upper incisors at the same time as intruding the molar 0.5 mm posterior during the sequential upper distalization.

Resolving the Vertical Problem

Before starting anterior extrusion:

- Eliminate palatal attachments on upper incisors
- Use optimized extrusion attachments on upper incisors
- Plan upper extrusion at the same time as posterior intrusion (0.5 mm)

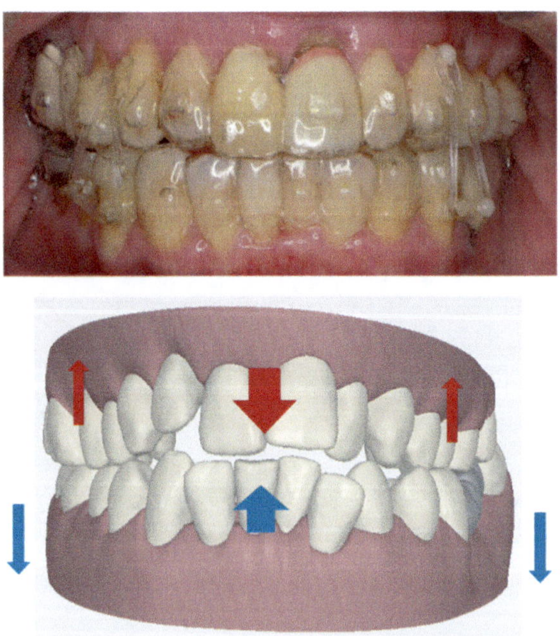

Fig. 21.40 Reciprocal movement of anterior extrusion and posterior intrusion.

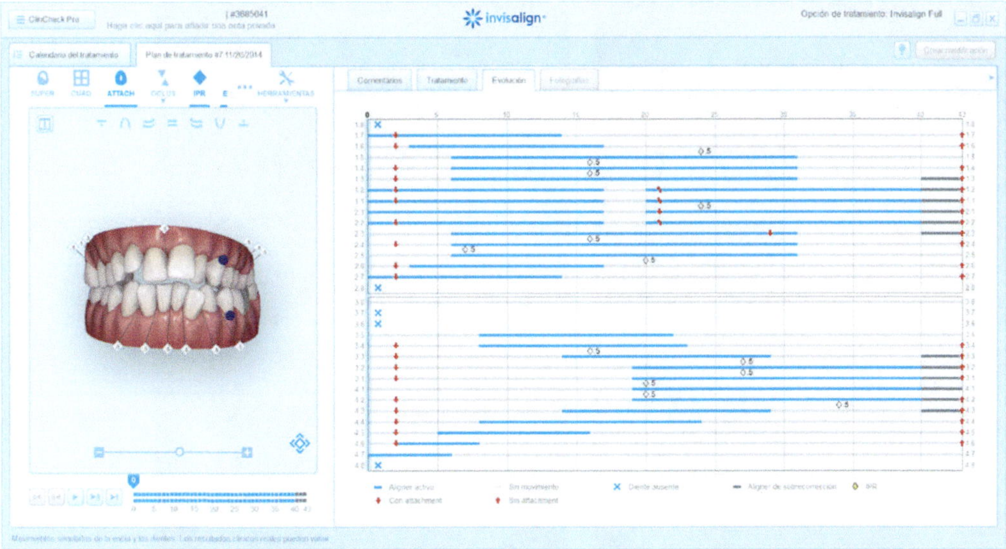

Fig. 21.41 Sequential distalization.

Treatment Summary

- The treatment was completed in 23 months
- For the first set of aligners the initial case had 40 aligners which were changed on a 2-week protocol, and a set of additional aligners which were changed on a 10-day protocol
- The patient used class II elastics and vertical pattern for night use during the treatment to guide the canines to a final class I relationship
- The open bite was closed without increasing the gummy smile of the patient
- The patient is now wearing her aesthetic veneers on the anterior incisors for further improvement of her smile

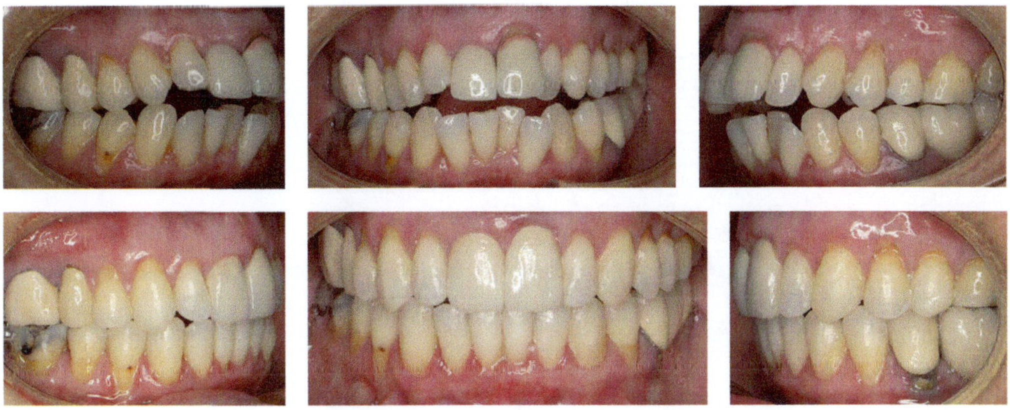

Fig. 21.42 Initial (upper) and final (lower) views.

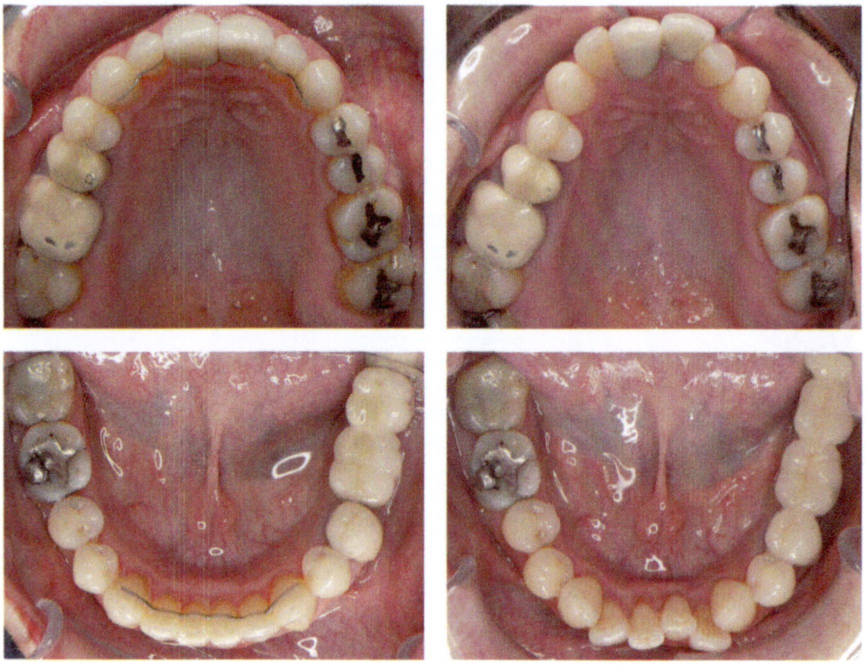

Fig. 21.43 Initial (left) and final occlusal (right).

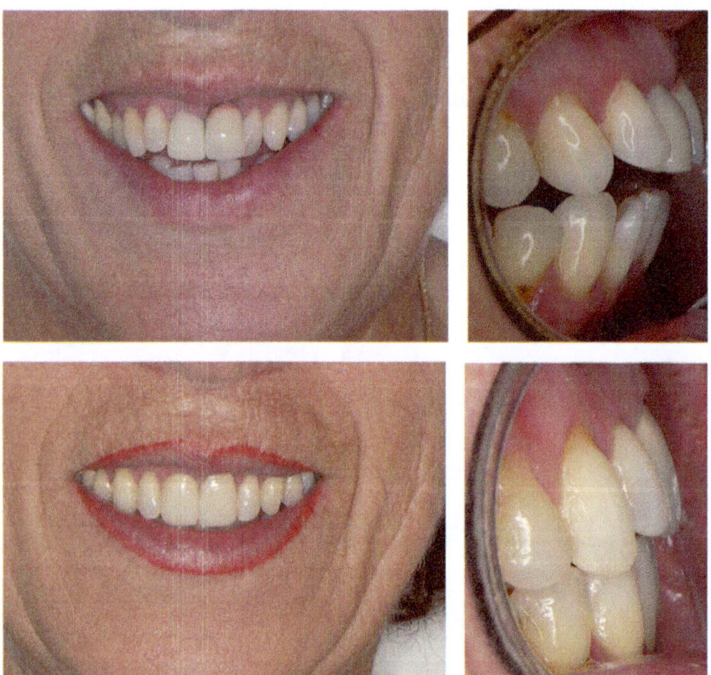

Fig. 21.44 Initial and final smiles and overjet.

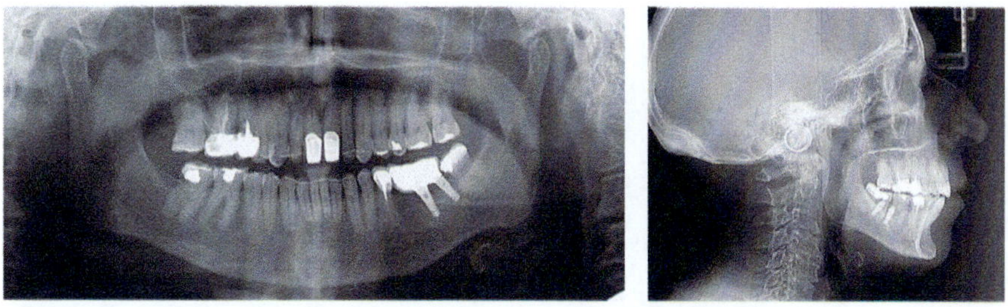

Fig. 21.45 Final panoramic and lateral X-rays.

21.1.3 Open Bite: Vertical Cause Treated with TADs

Diagnosis

A 60-year-old diabetic patient presented with an open bite with sagittal and vertical problem. They had hyperdivergent skeletal class III pattern with maxillo-mandibular protrusion, labial incompetence, right-side deviation of upper midline and missing 13 and 36.

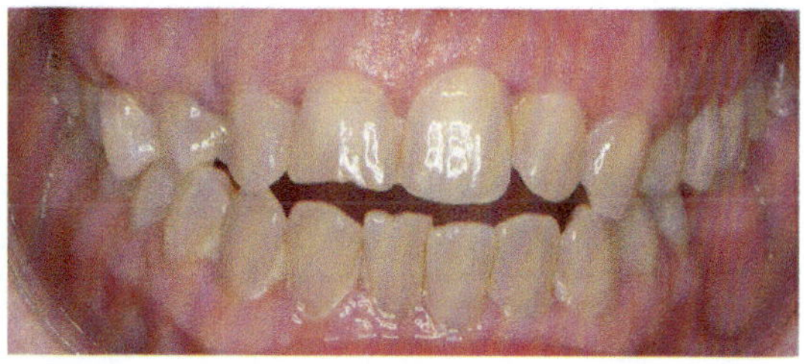

Fig. 21.46 Initial intraoral view.

Treatment Plan

- Close the open bite by expansion and simultaneous distalization and intrusion of molars in order not to create a gummy anterior smile
- Open a space for the missing 13
- Centre both midlines
  - sagittal: correct open bite and open space for missing 13 by simultaneous distalization using TADs in the tuberosity and simultaneous distalization in retromolar zone
  - vertical: close open bite by relative incisor extrusion and by intrusion of upper and lower molars using TADs

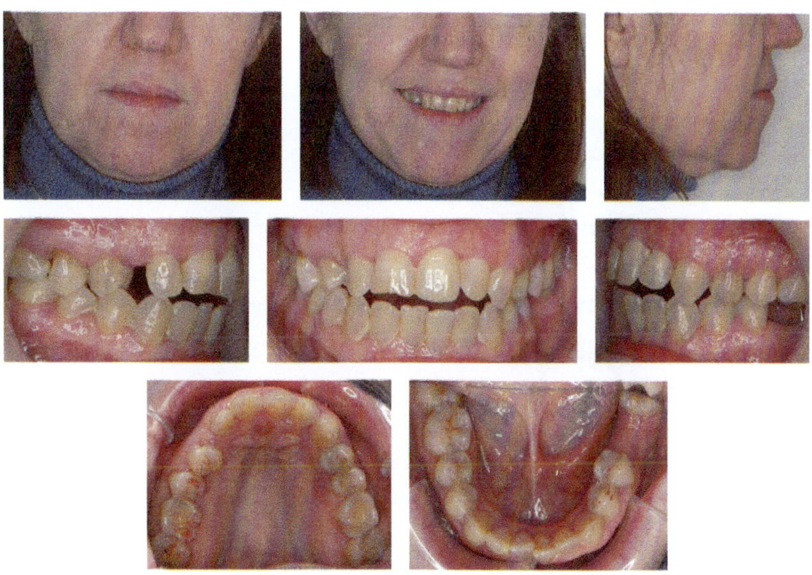

Fig. 21.47 Initial extraoral and intraoral views.

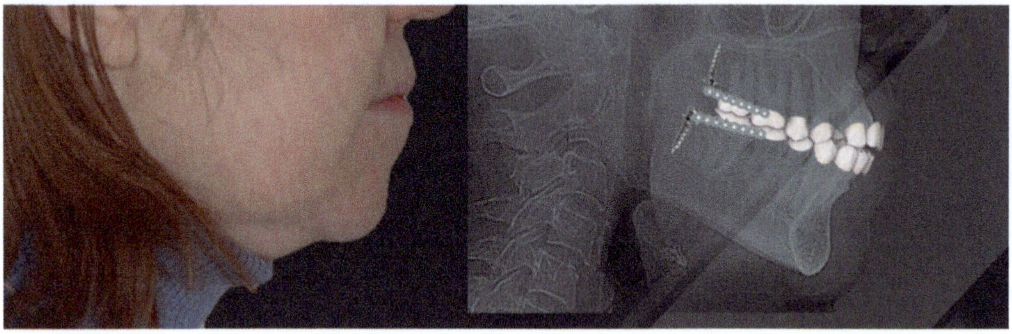

Fig. 21.48 Goal of treatment: close open bite by upper and lower distalization and relative extrusion of upper incisors.

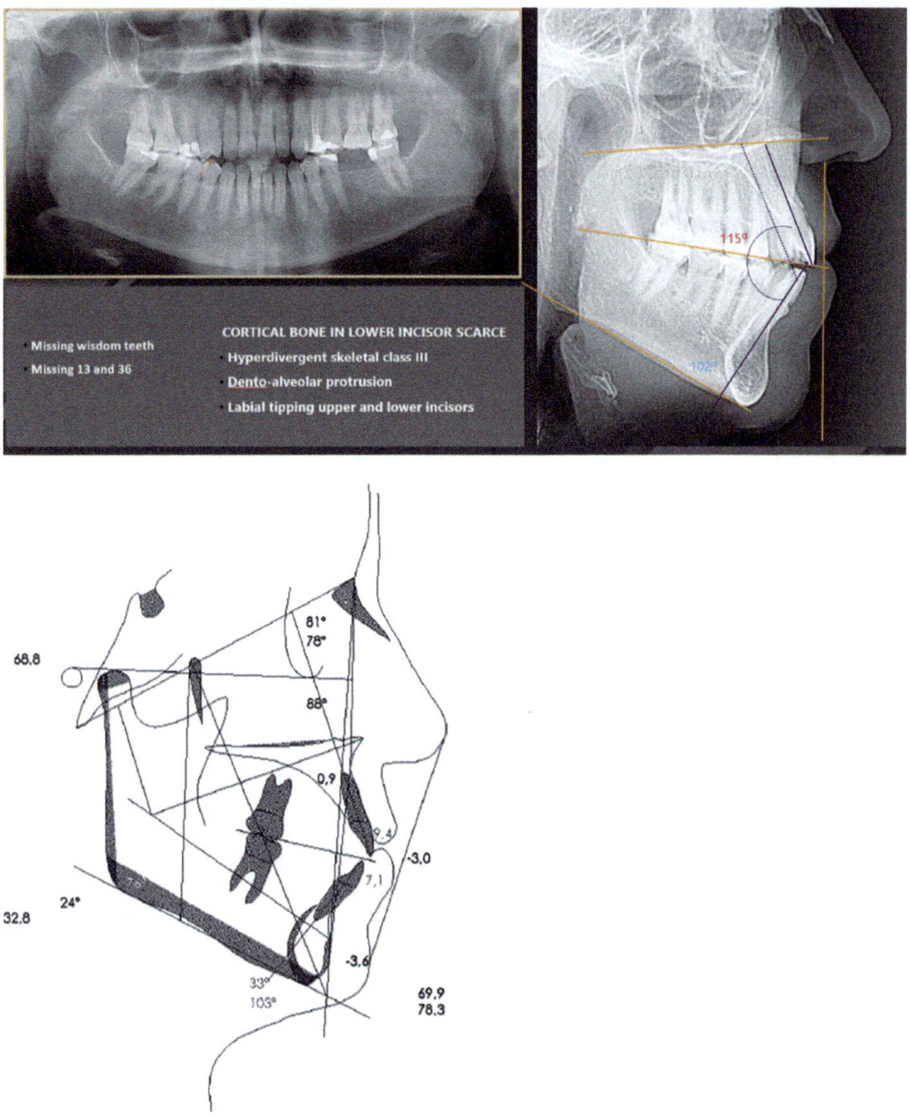

Fig. 21.49 Initial panoramic X-ray, teleradiograph and cephalometry.

Requirements for the Technician

- Provide expansion to the arches by changing torque, applying labial crown torque to premolars and molars of the upper and lower arches during simultaneous distalization
- Simultaneous distalization of molars, and when the molars achieve their final position distalize 5 to 5 in a row

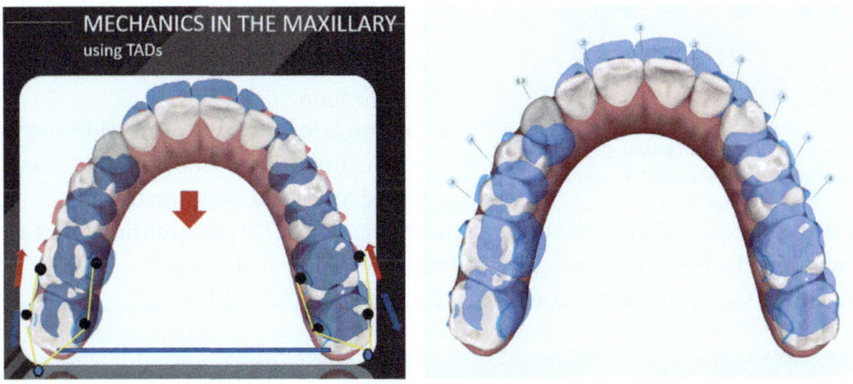

Fig. 21.50 Mechanics of simultaneous distalization from temporary anchorage devices in the tuberosity.

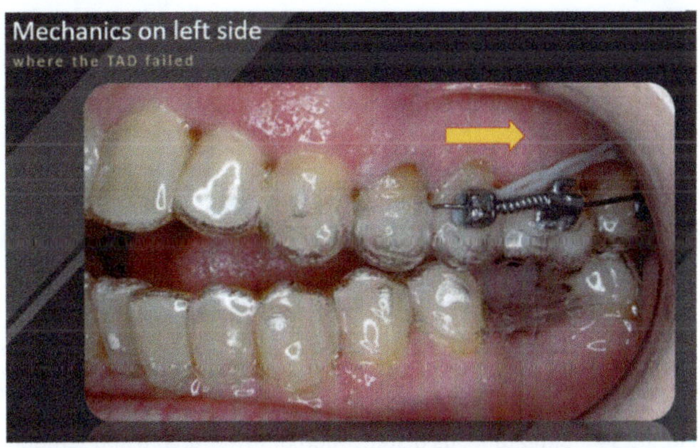

Fig. 21.51 Temporary anchorage devices in left tuberosity failed. It was changed between 26 and 27 to finish the upper left distalization with a sectional wire.

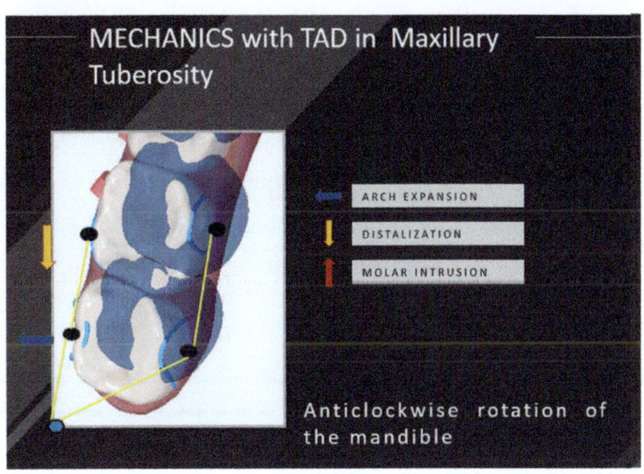

Fig. 21.52 Mechanics with temporary anchorage device in the tuberosity.

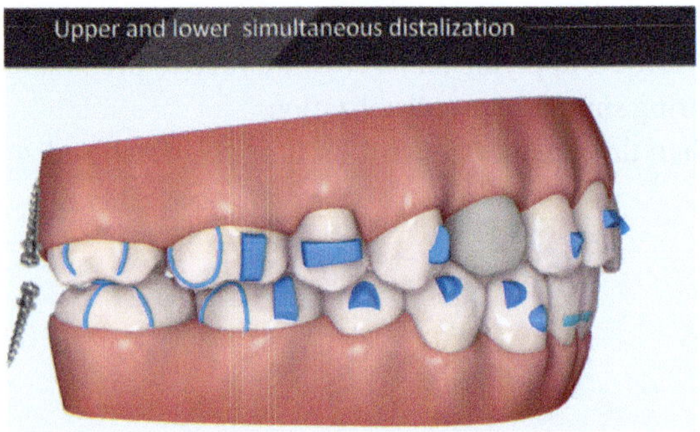

Fig. 21.53 Mechanics for upper and lower simultaneous distalization. Opening space for missing 13.

Treatment Summary

- The treatment was completed in 25 months
- Initially, the patient had 45 aligners which were changed on a 10-day protocol, and a set of additional aligners to settle the final occlusion
- The patient used triangular elastics for night use during the treatment to maintain a class I relationship during the distalization
- The implant for 36 was placed during the treatment and the implant for 13 was placed at the end of the treatment
- A Powerarm was needed to upright the root of upper first right premolar to place the implant of 13
- The open bite was closed without increasing the gummy smile of the patient
- During osteointegration of the implant a composite veneer was placed in 13

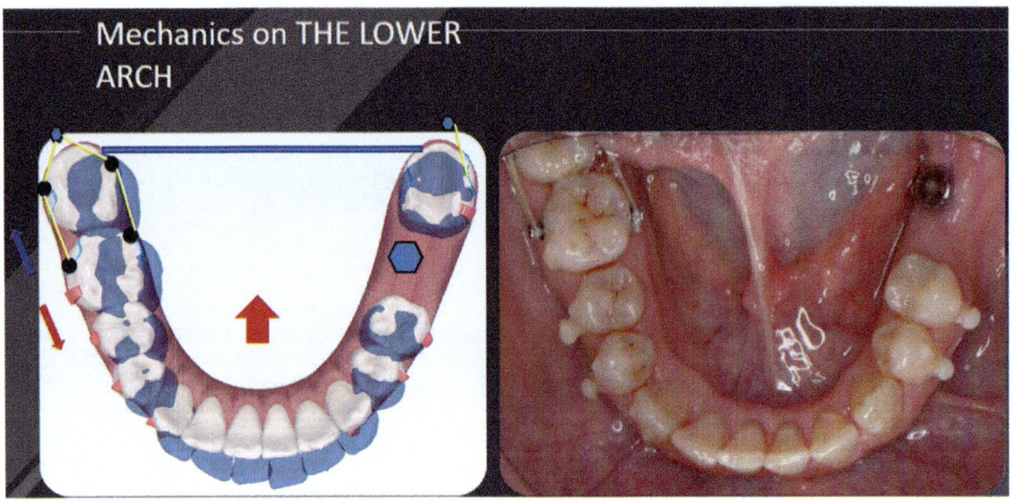

Fig. 21.54 Simultaneous distalization of lower arch using temporary anchorage devices in retromolar zone.

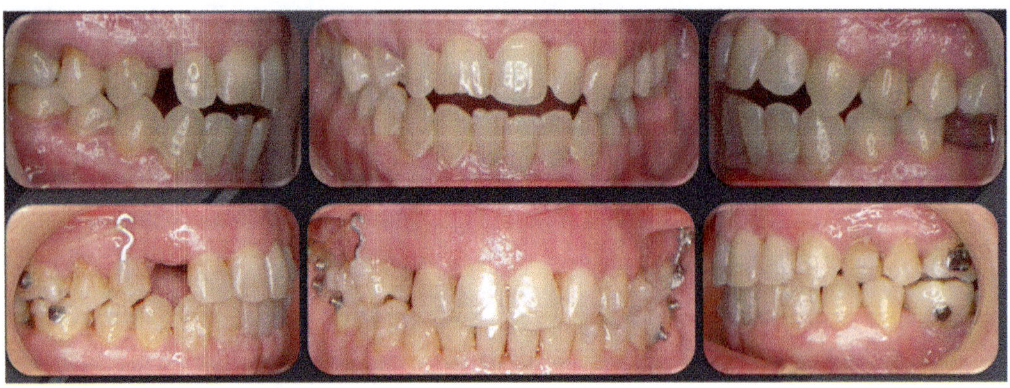

Fig. 21.55 Initial views before refinement. Opening space for missing 13, uprighting 14 to place implant and implanting of 36 and provisional crown.

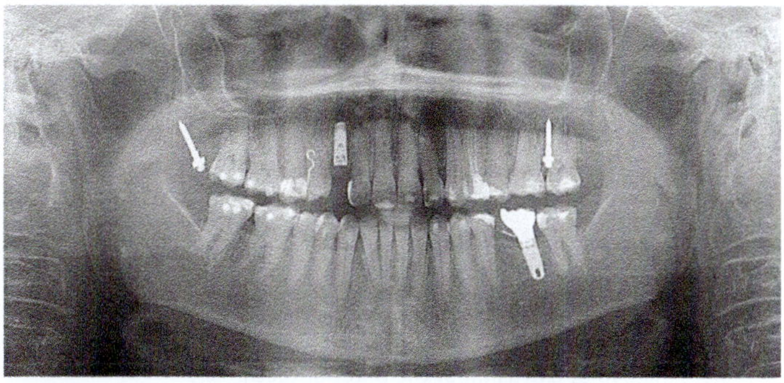

Fig. 21.56 Final panoramic X-ray, after placing the implant for 13 and removing temporary attachment devices.

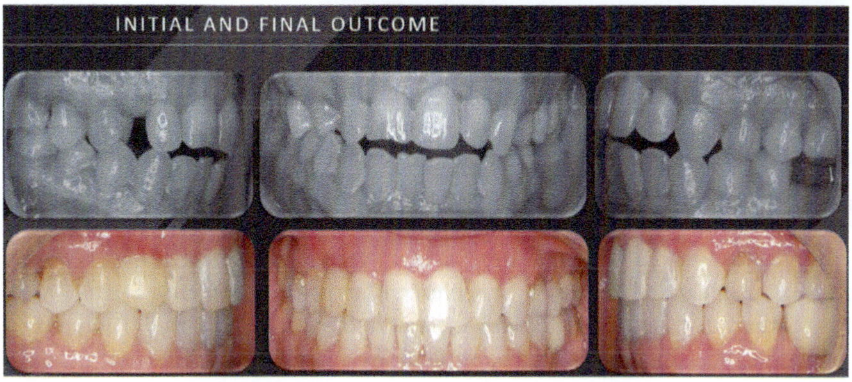

Fig. 21.57 Initial and final intraoral images with composite veneer for 13 inserted while the patient waits for the osteointegration of the implant.

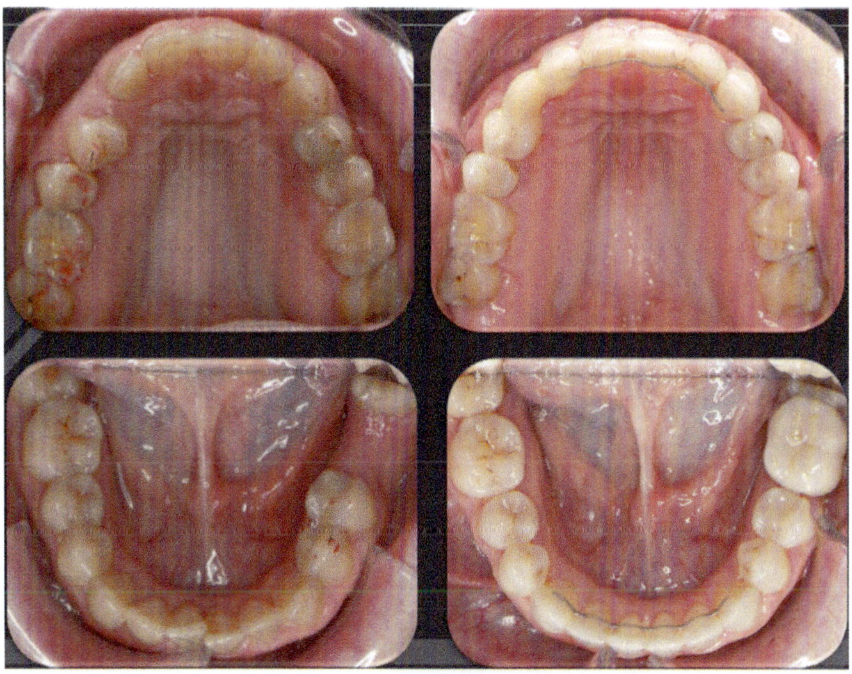

Fig. 21.58 Initial (left) and final (right) occlusal (composite veneer in 13).

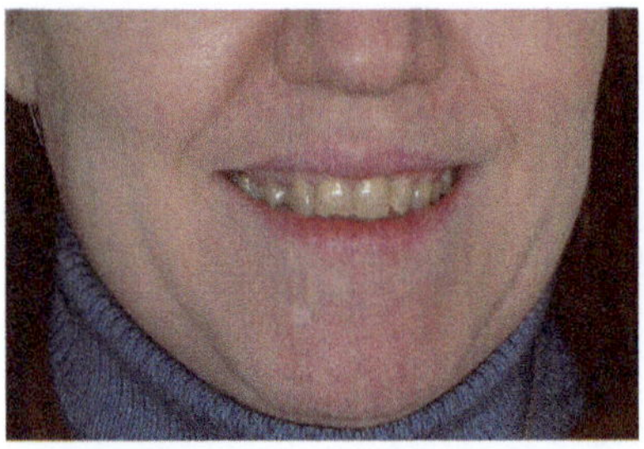

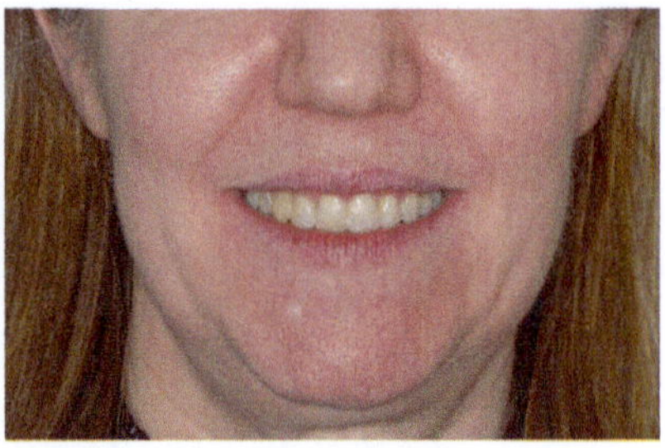

Fig. 21.59 Initial and final smile. Correction of the open bite without creating gummy smile by intrusion of molars instead of extrusion of the anterior teeth.

Tips for Open Bites

- Correct the open bite in all three planes of space (transversal, sagittal and vertical).
- The skeletal and dental diagnosis is extremely important for determining which treatment mechanics should be used to correct the anterior open bite.
- In vertical skeletal patterns, it is desirable to have posterior intrusion as well as anterior extrusion to close the open bite.
- Check for molar fulcrum before sending the case.
- Provide enough posterior anchorage during extrusion of the incisors, do not move molars during absolute anterior extrusion and use anchorage attachments in the posterior zone.
- Pretreatment maxillary and mandibular incisors inclination should be corrected before extrusion, and incisors should be aligned and not in a vertical position before being extruded.
- Evaluate the smile of the patient, as a gummy smile should not be treated by extrusion of upper incisors to close the open bite.
- A posterior gap of 0.5 mm in the molars could help to prevent a possible relapse of the anterior open bite after the treatment.

Communication with the Technician

Maxilla:

- Expansion and simultaneous retraction of upper incisors (relative extrusion)
- At the end of the treatment, absolute extrusion reciprocal to molar intrusion of no more than 0.5 mm

Mandible:

- Expansion + IPR + relative extrusion (upright lower incisor –1 degree)

21.1.4 Open Bite with Tongue-thrusting Habit

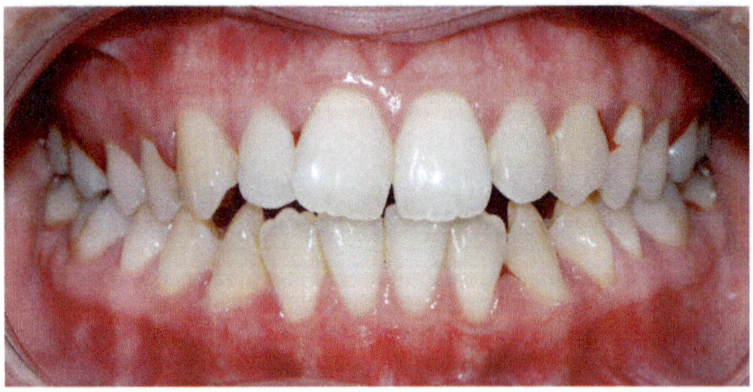

Fig. 21.60 Initial intraoral view.

Diagnosis

- A 26-year-old patient presented with an open bite with sagittal and vertical problems, a tongue thrusting habit, posterior compression and gummy smile. They had a mild right side class II, upper central incisors had a short display and left-side deviation of upper midline

Treatment Plan

- Close the open bite by expansion and arch depth loss causing an anterior relative extrusion
- Distalization combined with posterior intrusion to reduce posterior gummy smile and close the bite by mandibular anterior rotation
- Asymmetric expansion to improve posterior torques
- Anterior extrusion to improve central incisor display
- Manual lingual precision cuts on 11–21 to allow tongue tamers to be placed, preventing the tongue thrusting habit

ClinCheck 1: Requirements for the Technician

- Expand right side, using left side as anchorage
- Sequential distalization on right side
    - at same time as expanding
    - at same time as anterior torque correction to create a counterforce movement
- Class II elastics placed on manual precision cuts
- Lower IPR to
    - allow retrusion (anterior extrusion) while levelling the Spee curve (by intrusion)
    - facilitate anterior alignment
- Although IPR is usually set at initial stages to avoid round-tripping of lower incisors, in this case it was delayed because there were no proper contact points between them, as would have been achieved in the past with brackets and wires: start with a round NiTi archwire, align and then perform the IPR, closing the spaces with a Powerchain

Treatment Summary

- The treatment was completed in 22 months.
- Initially, the patient had 43 aligners changed on a 7-day protocol, a set of 40 additional aligners, and a final 12 refinement aligners for settlement.
- The patient used right class II elastics during the distalization.
- End of the treatment revealed a gum recession on 43 resulting from a final root position that was not carefully planned; patient therefore sent for a soft tissue graft.

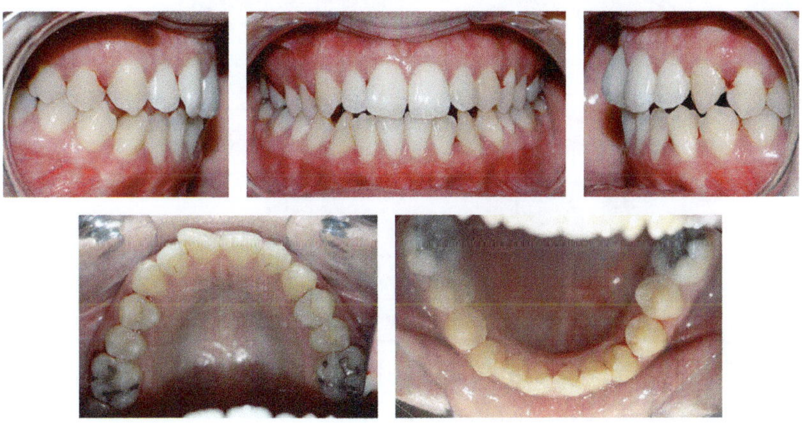

Fig. 21.61 Initial intraoral views: right, front, left, upper, lower.

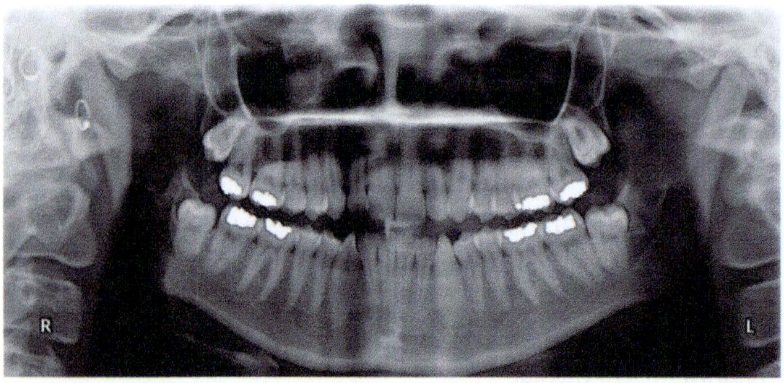

Fig. 21.62 Initial panoramic X-ray.

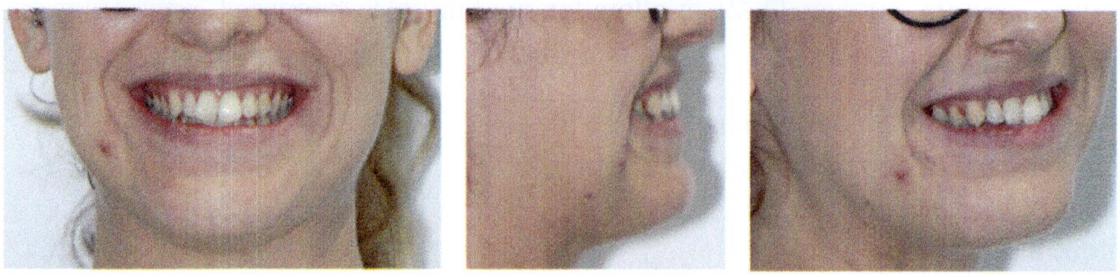

Fig. 21.63 Initial extraoral views.

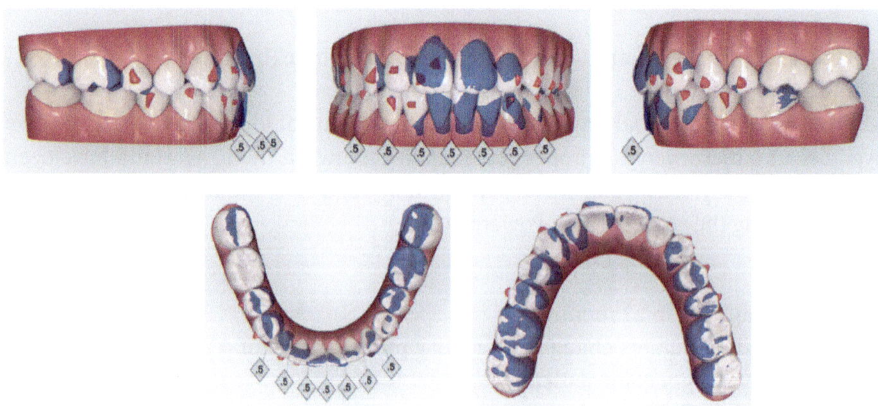

Fig. 21.64 Initial ClinChecks (right, front, left, upper, lower).

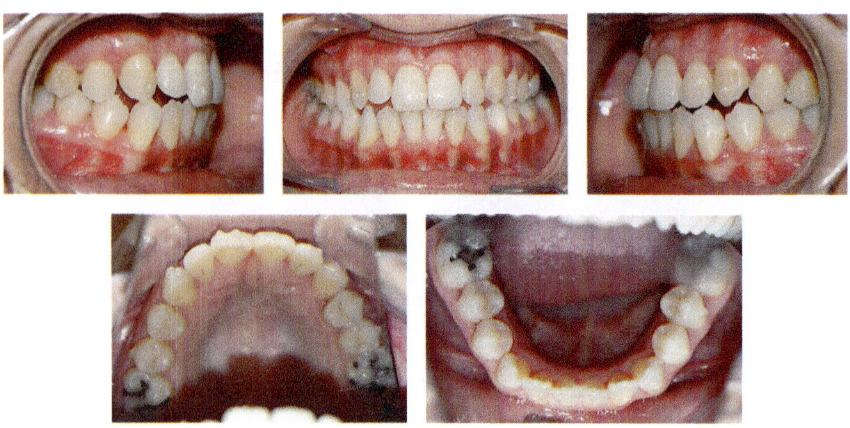

Fig. 21.65 Refinement intraoral views (right, front, left, upper, lower).

ClinCheck 2: Requirements for the Technician

Before the end of first set of aligners, clinical examination showed anterior interferences and lack of overjet associated with arch depth loss and right distalization, which made us re-scan the patient and order additional aligners with additional IPR in lower arch to create overjet and keep the initial mechanics.

- Perform IPR in lower arch
- Add extra LRT to 33–43 to create an 'en masse' movement and avoid recessions
- Add precision cuts on right side for class II elastics mechanics
- Centre the midline simultaneously with expansion and arch shaping

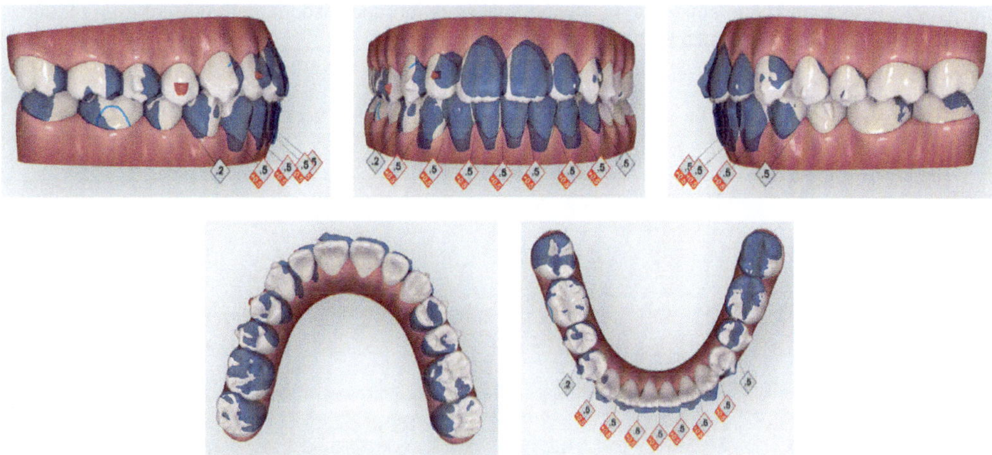

Fig. 21.66 Refinement ClinChecks: right, front, left, upper, lower.

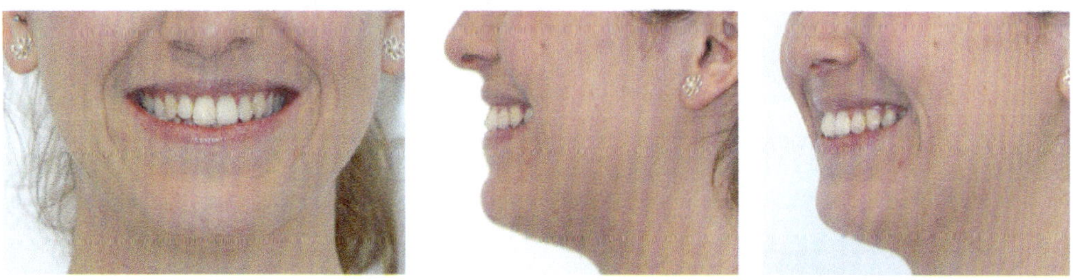

Fig. 21.67 Refinement: extraoral views.

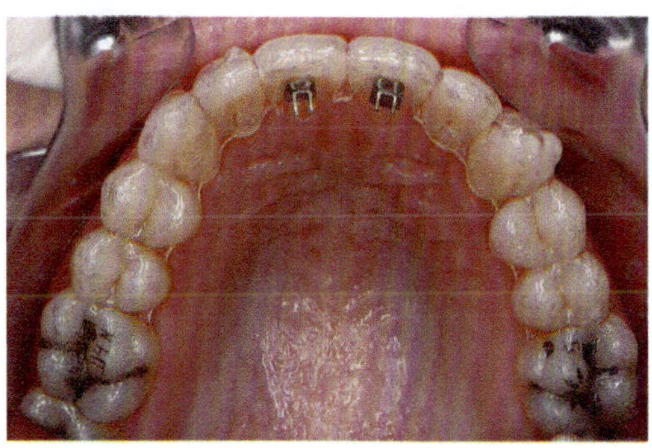

Fig. 21.68 Refinement: a third set of aligners was ordered for final settlement and aesthetic, in which the patient kept wearing tongue tamers to prevent relapse from tongue thrusting habit.

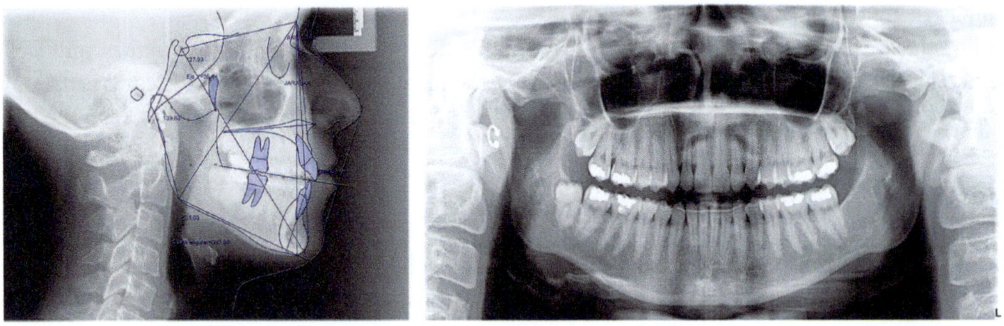

Fig. 21.69 Lateral and panoramic X-rays showing final situation, and wisdom teeth present even though saggital correction was performed with upper distalization.

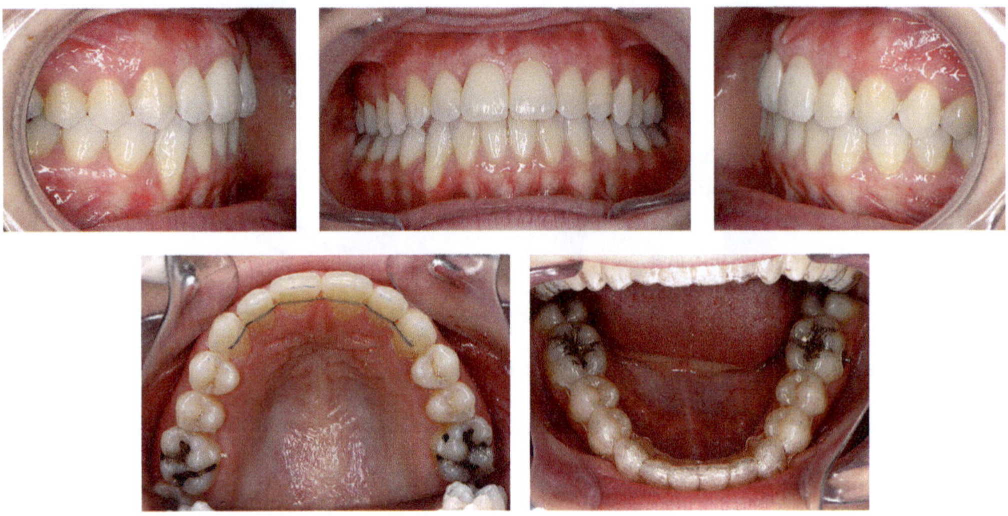

Fig. 21.70 Final intraoral views (right, front, left, upper, lower).

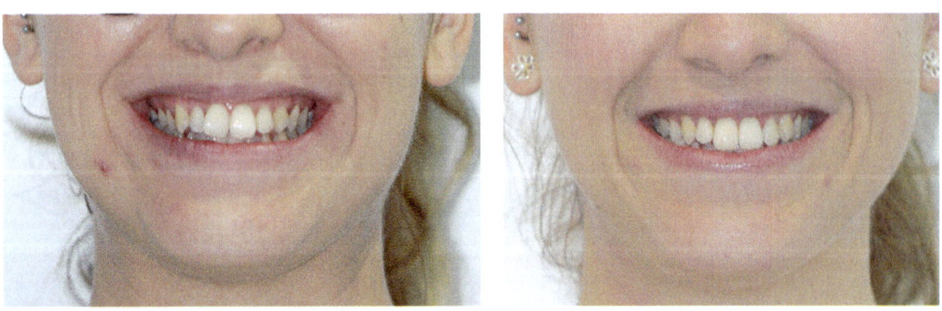

Fig. 21.71 Before and after smiles.

21.1.5 Open Bite with Insufficient Incisor Display

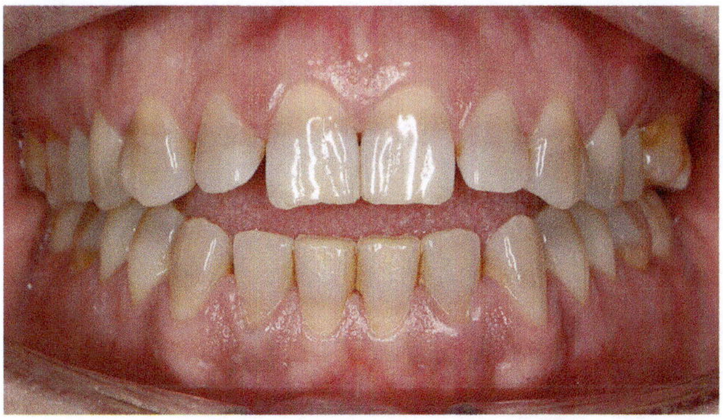

Fig. 21.72 Initial intraoral view.

Diagnosis

A 44-year-old patient presented with an open bite with sagittal and vertical problems. They had mild left side class II, a tongue-thrusting habit, and a posterior compression and short upper display.

Treatment Plan

- Close the open bite by arch depth loss causing an anterior relative extrusion as a result of:
  - Expansion
  - Anterior space closure and retrusion
- Improve 27 position, help create space for an implant on 26
- Intrude posterior sectors to rotate the mandible and solve open bite
- Anterior extrusion to improve central incisors display
- Manual lingual precision cuts on 11–21 to allow tongue tamers to be placed, preventing tongue-thrusting habit

ClinCheck 1: Requirements for the Technician

- Occlusal attachments to increase posterior bite forces and intrusion
- Sequential distalization on left side
- Class II elastics were placed on manual precision cuts
- Lower IPR to:
  - allow retrusion (anterior relative extrusion)
  - improve size relationship owing to Bolton discrepancy

Treatment Summary

- The treatment was completed in 12 months.
- For a first set of aligners the patient initially had 31 aligners which were changed on a 7-day protocol, followed by a set of 14 additional aligners.
- The patient used right class II elastics.
- The patient wore tongue tamers to help solve the tongue-thrusting habit, preventing future relapse.

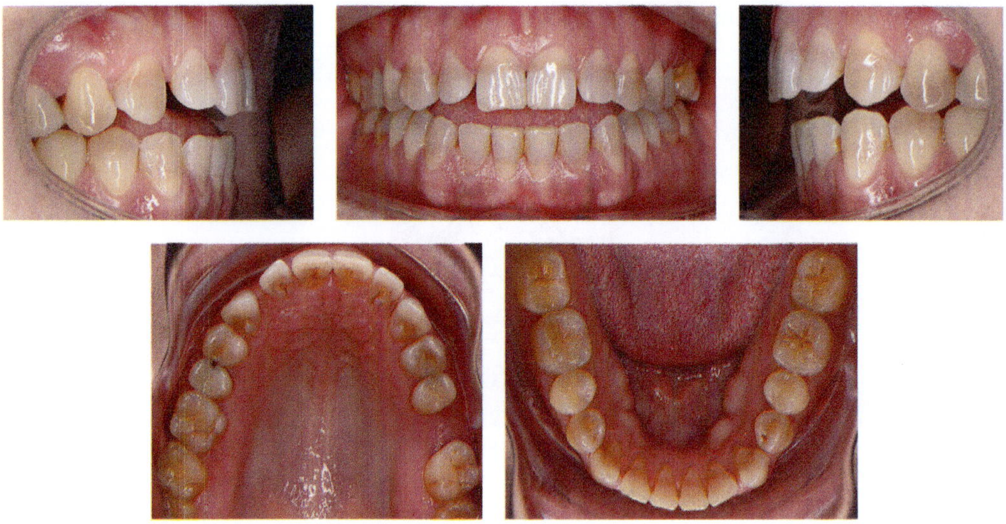

Fig. 21.73 Initial intraoral views (right, front, left, upper, lower).

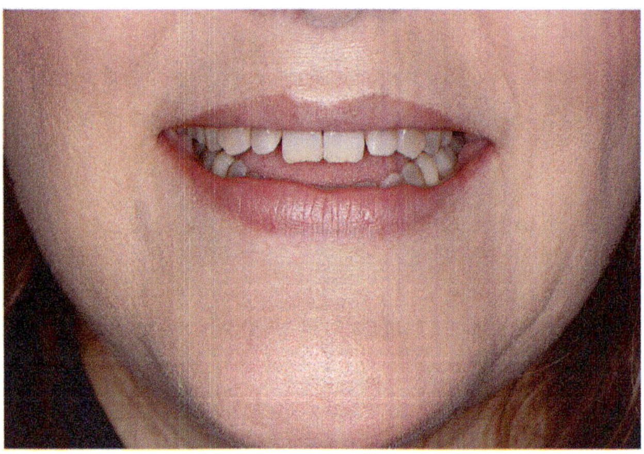

Fig. 21.74 Initial smile: short incisor display required aesthetic improvement together with anterior bite closure.

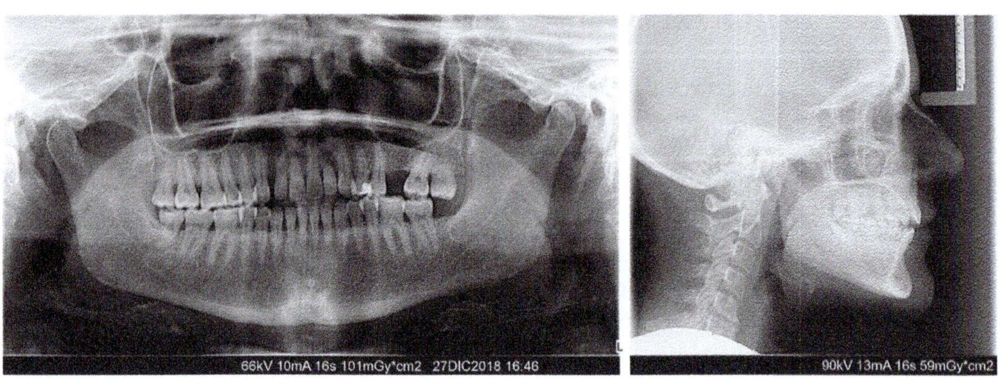

Fig. 21.75 Initial panoramic and lateral X-rays.

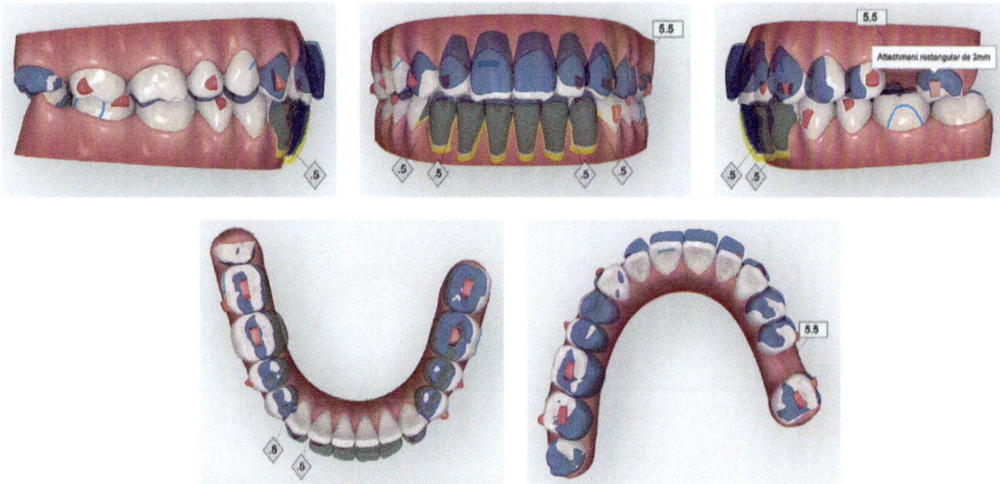

Fig. 21.76 Initial ClinChecks (right, front, left, upper and lower).

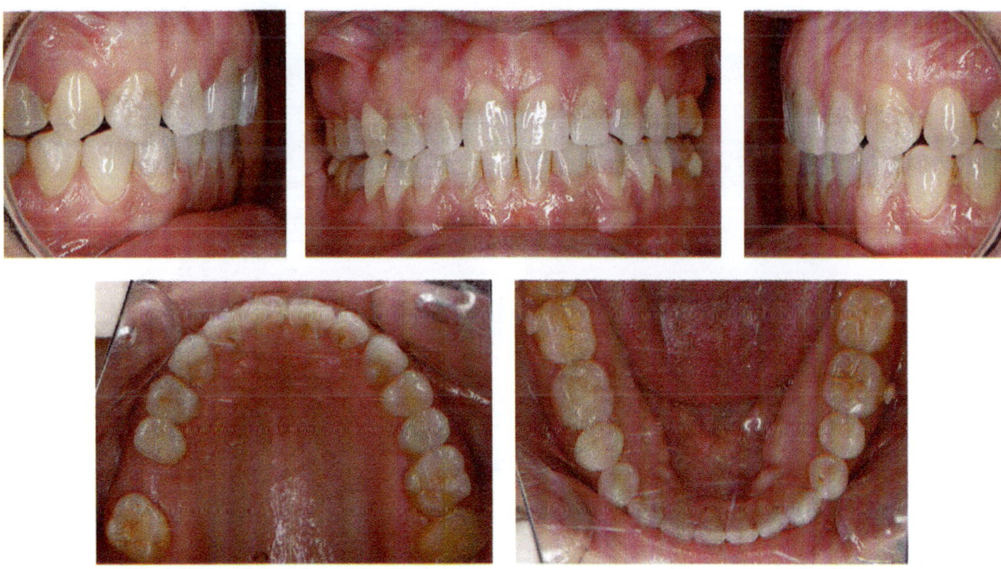

Fig. 21.77 Refinement: intraoral views (right, front, left, upper and lower).

ClinCheck 2: Requirements for the Technician

- Right posterior button cutouts for V-shaped elastics to extrude premolars
- Class II elastics, left side, with button cutout on canine for less interference on anterior torque
- Anterior torque improvement by extra palatal root torque on 12–22 with power ridges on 11-22
- Extra LRT to lower incisors, together with IPR to retrude them, improving overbite and creating an 'en masse' movement

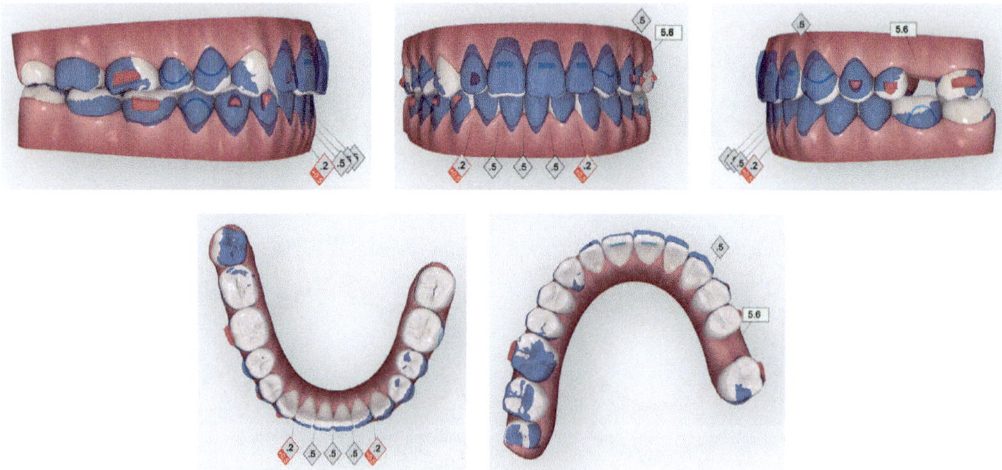

Fig. 21.78 Refinement ClinChecks (right, front, left, upper and lower).

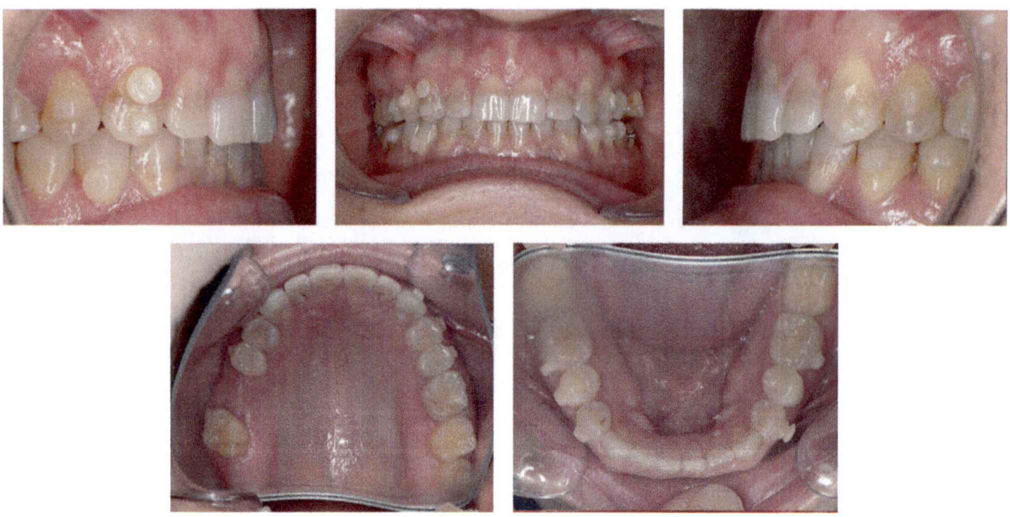

Fig. 21.79 Final intraoral views (right, front, left, upper with tongue tamer and lower).

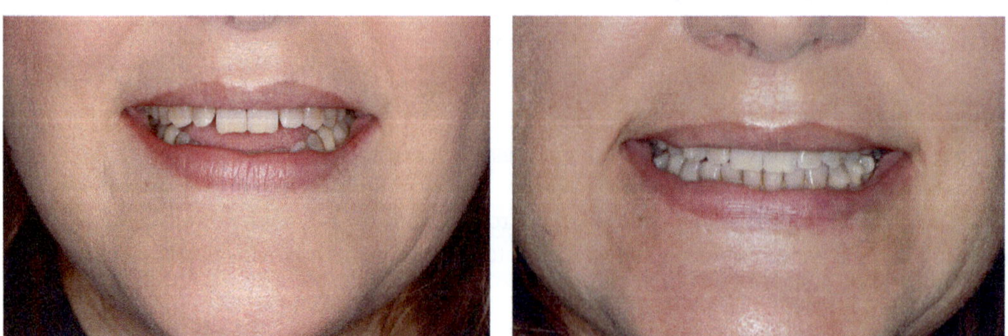

Fig. 21.80 Smile before and after treatment.

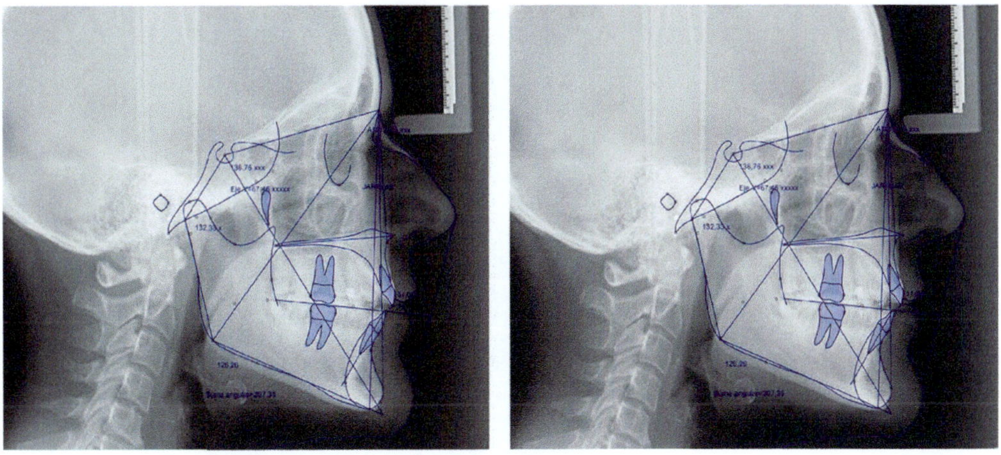

Fig. 21.81 Final lateral X-rays.

21.1.6 Open Bite with 4 Day Aligner Change

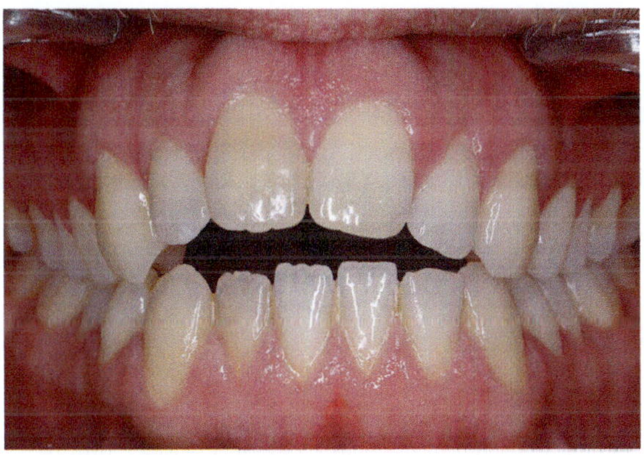

Fig. 21.82 Initial intraoral view.

Diagnosis

A 29-year-old patient presented with an open bite with sagittal and transverse problems. They had a tongue-thrusting habit, bilateral mild class II, posterior compression and short upper display.

Treatment Plan

- Close the open bite by arch depth loss causing an anterior relative extrusion as a result of:
  - expansion
  - anterior space closure and retrusion
- Virtual jump as a result of posterior intrusion

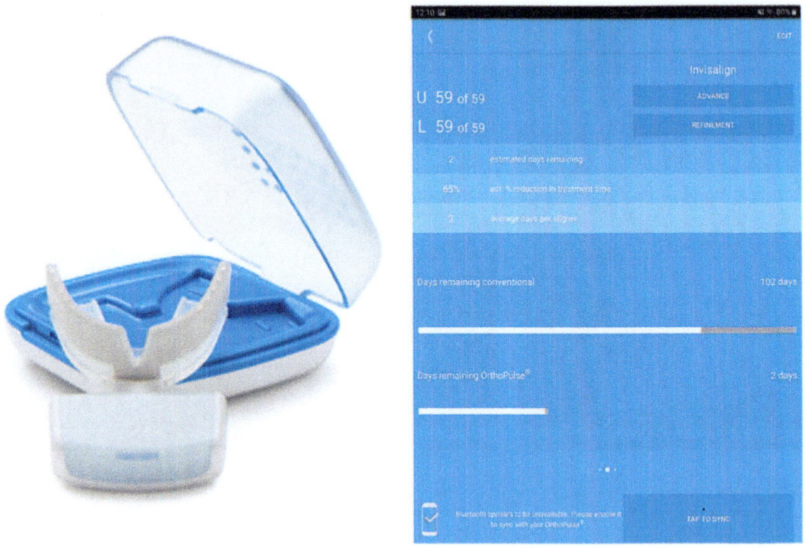

Fig. 21.83 The Orthopulse device was used by the patient to accelerate treatment and improve results. The device (top) is linked to a SmartPhone App that controls patient daily compliance and offers the doctor really valuable information.

- Anterior extrusion to improve central incisors display
- Manual lingual precision cuts on 11–21 to allow tongue tamers to be placed, preventing the tongue-thrusting habit
- Use Orthopulse according to the manufacturer's instructions

ClinCheck 1: Requirements for the Technician

- Bilateral half sequential distalization with class II mechanics
- When retruding 12–22 apply extra LRT to avoid torque loss
- Class II elastics to be placed on precision cuts
- Lower incisors extrusion combined with posterior intrusion to create a posterior open bite

Treatment Summary

- The treatment is expected to finish in 15 months
- The patient initially had 59 aligners which were changed on a 4-day protocol, followed by a set of 49 additional aligners, with a 2-day change interval protocol
- The patient used class II elastics on the right side

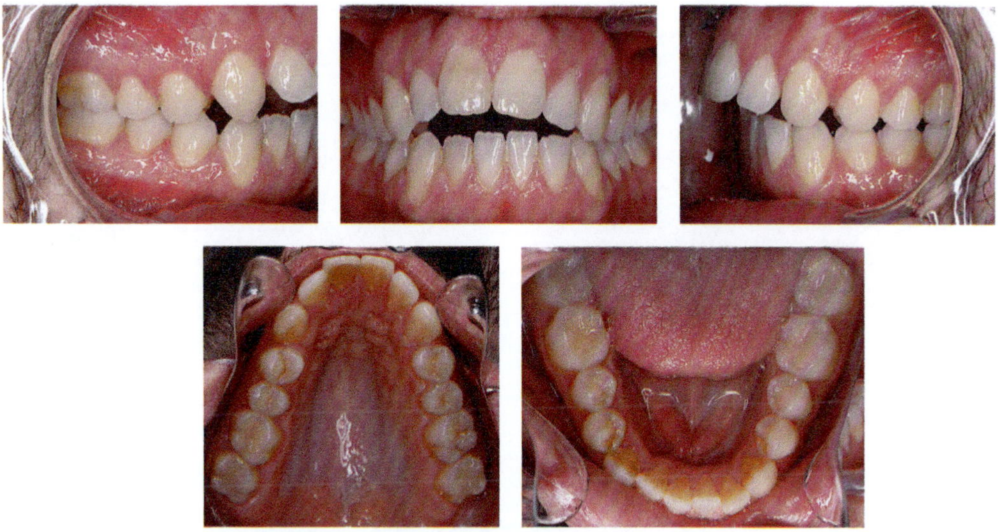

Fig. 21.84 Initial set of intraoral views (right, front, left, upper and lower).

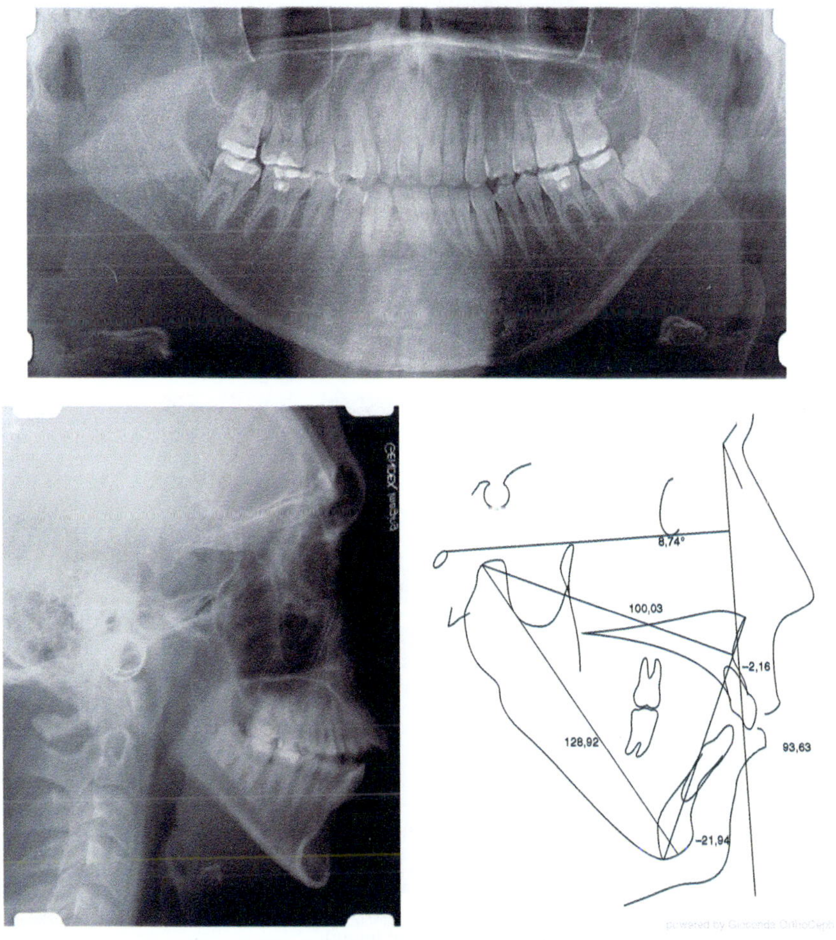

Fig. 21.85 Initial panoramic and lateral X-rays and cephalometric measurements.

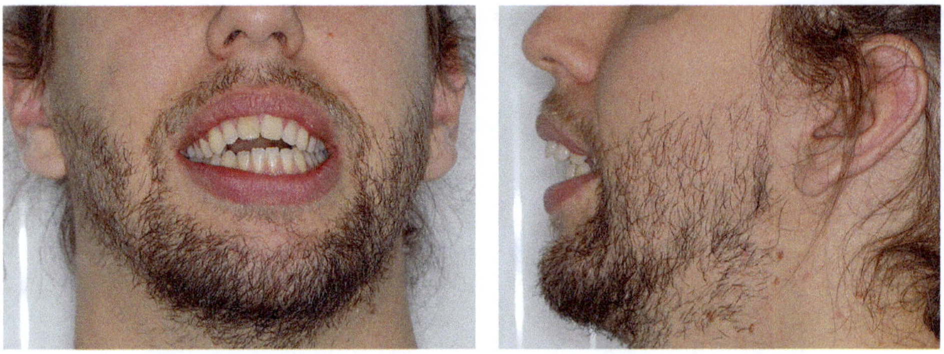

Fig. 21.86 Initial extraoral views.

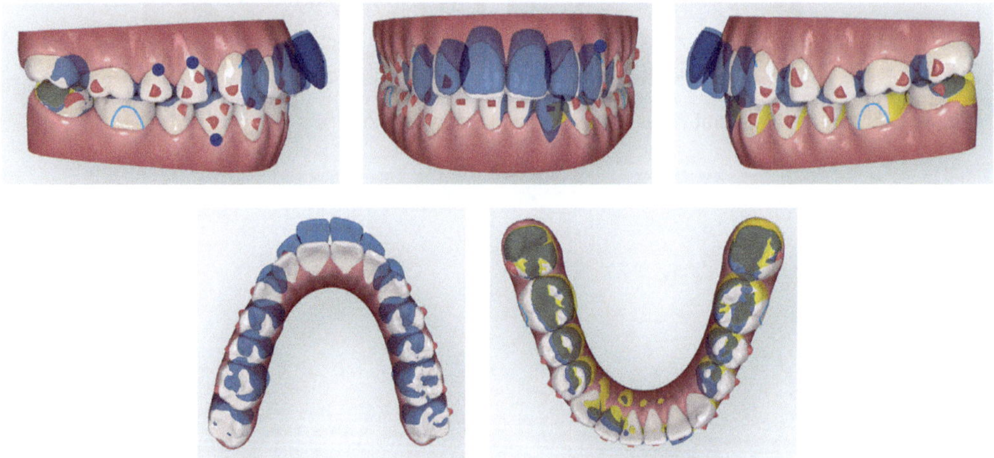

Fig. 21.87 Initial ClinChecks (right, front, left, upper and lower) with virtual jump in yellow.

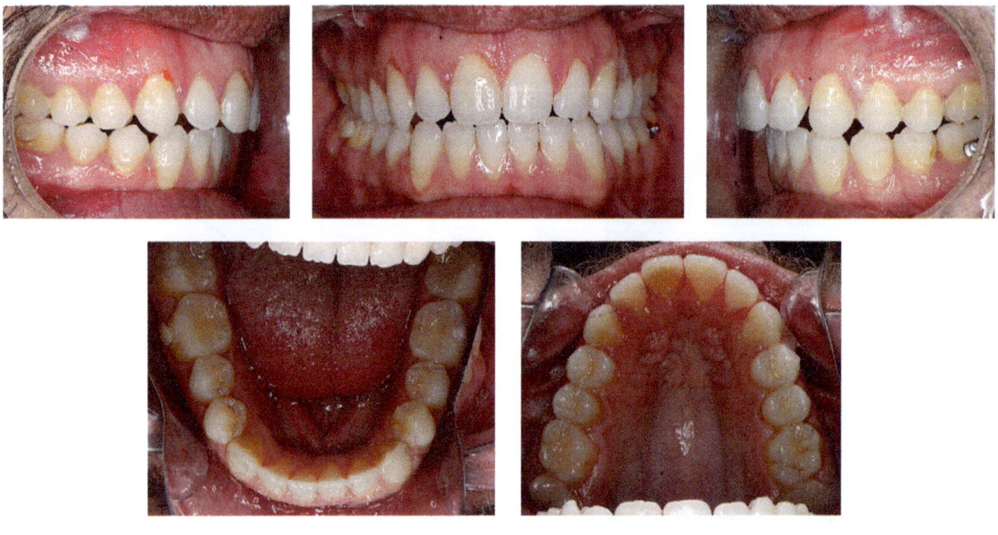

Fig. 21.88 Refinement: intraoral views (right, front, left, upper and lower).

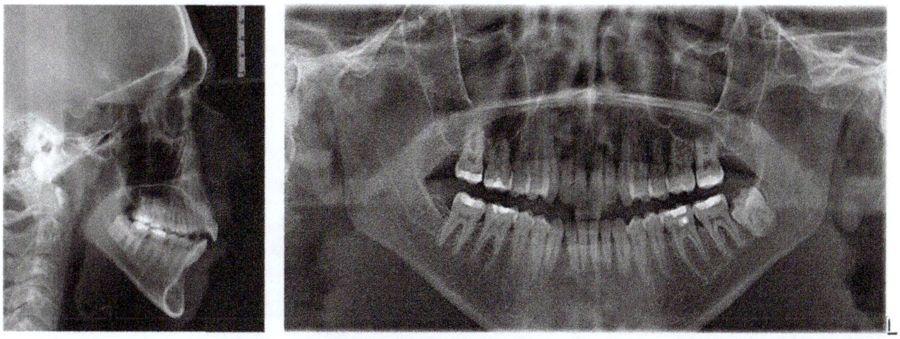

Fig. 21.89 Refinement: lateral and panoramic X-rays.

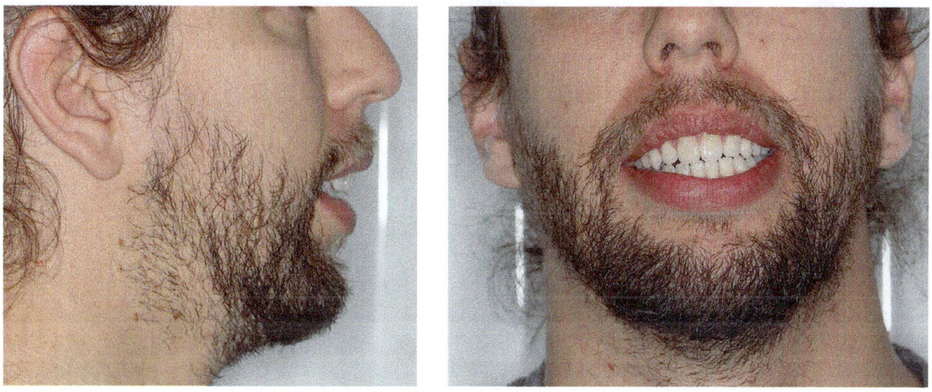

Fig. 21.90 Refinement: profile and smile.

ClinCheck 2: Requirements for the Technician

- Use remaining anterior space for distalization before starting on posterior
- When retruding 12–22 apply extra LRT to avoid torque loss
- Class II elastics placed on precision cuts

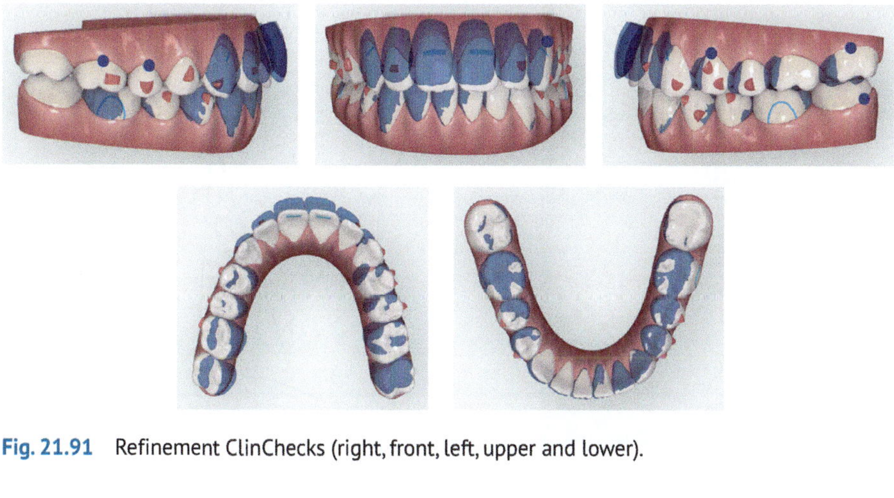

Fig. 21.91 Refinement ClinChecks (right, front, left, upper and lower).

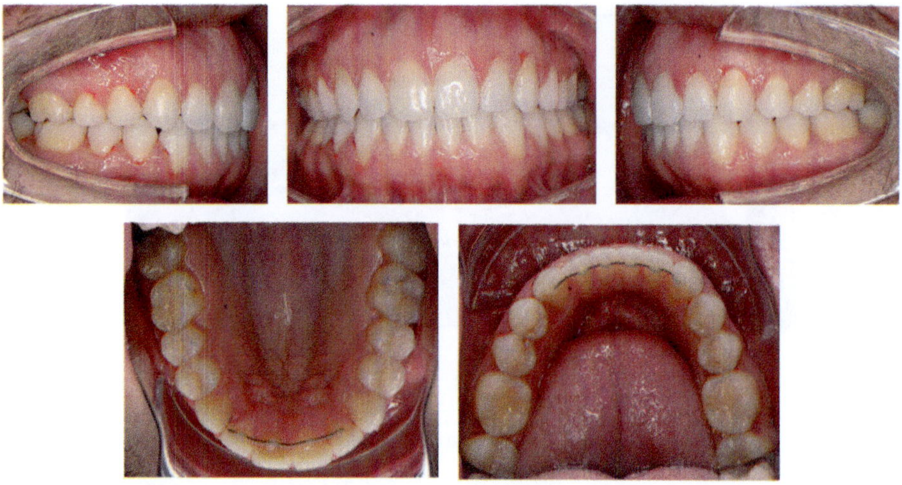

Fig. 21.92 Current intraoral views (right, front, left, upper and lower).

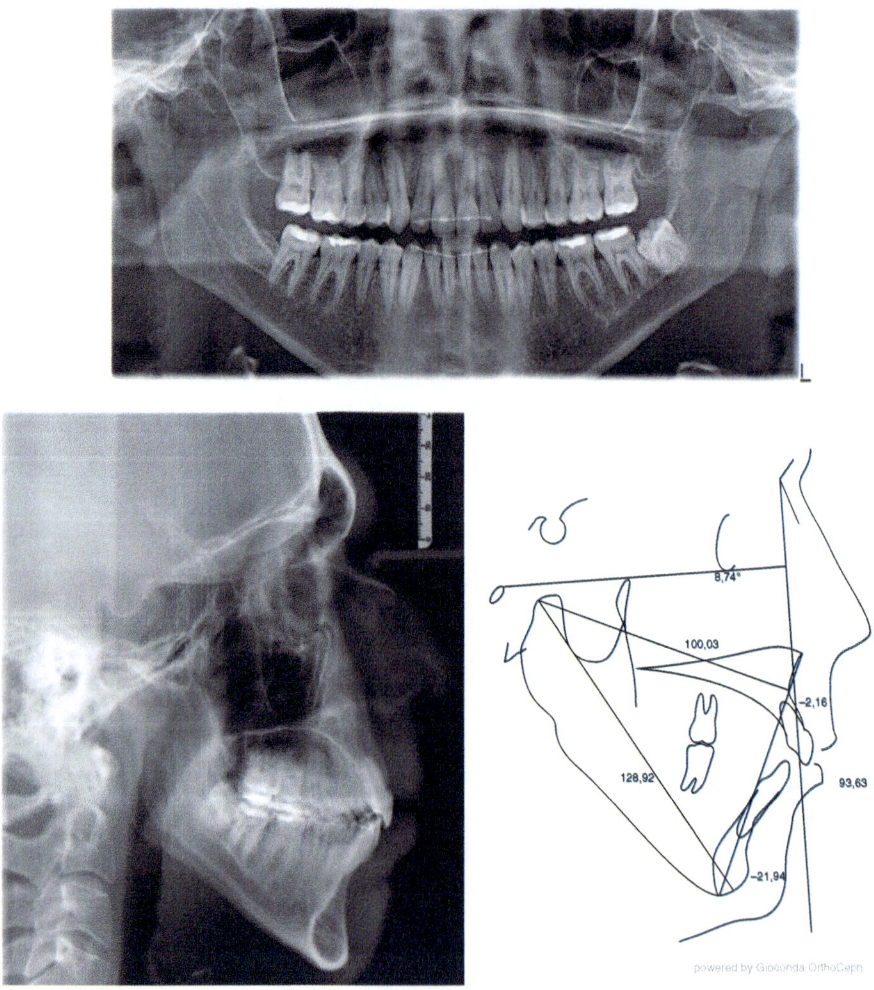

Fig. 21.93 Current lateral and panoramic X-rays and cephalometry.

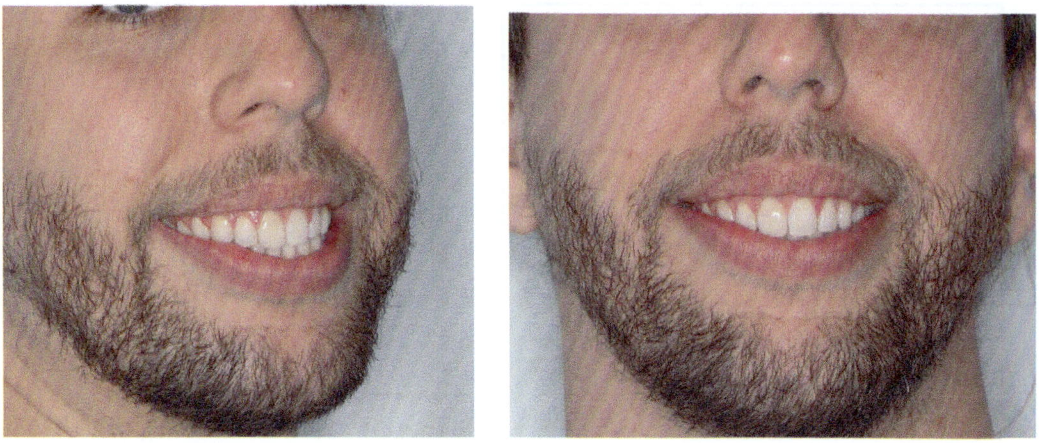

Fig. 21.94 Final smile.

21.2 Deep Bite: Classification According to Complexity

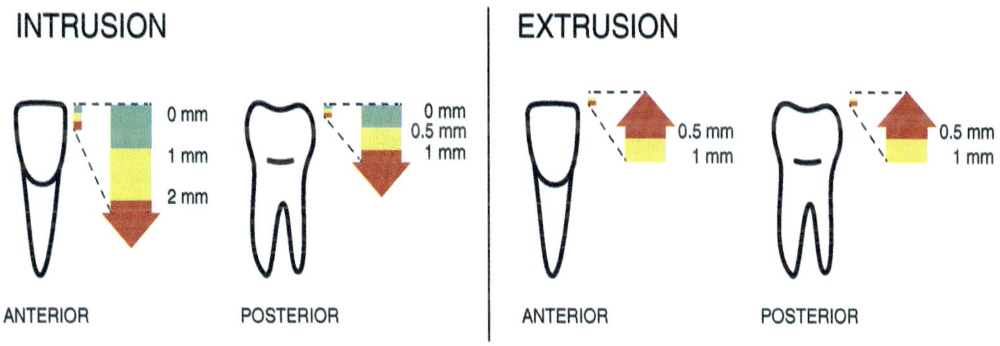

Fig. 21.95 Predictability of vertical movements is important in order to plan auxiliary techniques or in deciding not to use them.

Deep Bite Prescription Form

Question 6, correct deep bite:

- Only by anterior intrusion
- By anterior intrusion and posterior extrusion
- Others (surgical, special instructions)

Question 7: bite ramps (incisors optimized/ canines not optimized).

Specific Features for Deep Bite

Pressure Areas

- Designed to level the curve of Spee by improving control of anterior intrusion and premolar extrusion for more predictable deep bite treatments

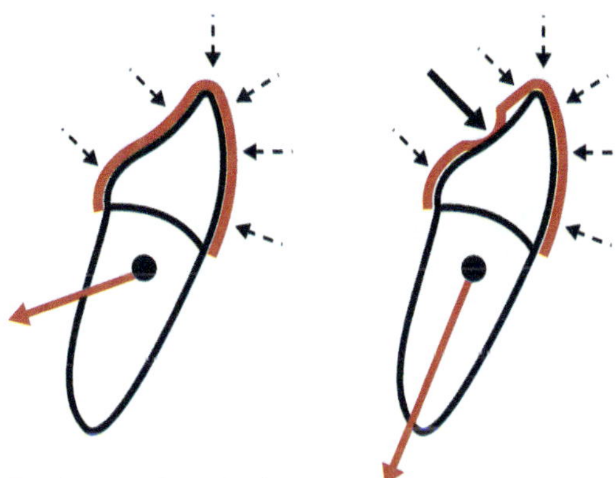

Fig. 21.96 Optimized pressure areas help intruding anterior teeth by combining their forces with those related to optimized attachments.

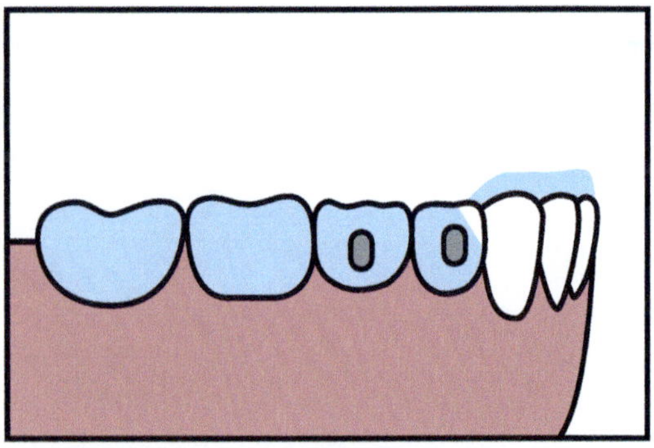

Fig. 21.97 Optimized extrusion attachments on premolars create a counterforce when aligner is exerting an intrusion force on anterior.

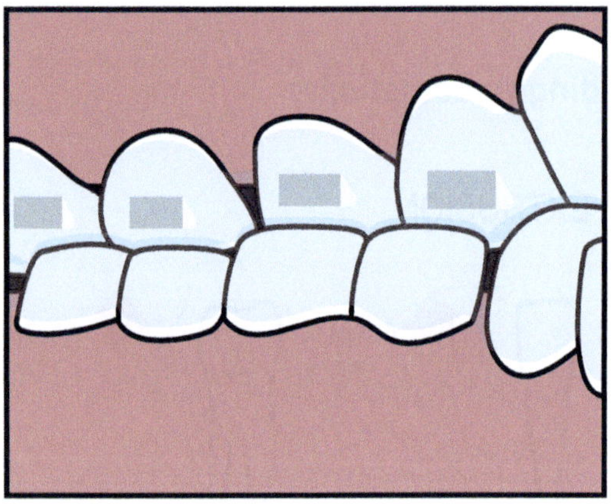

Fig. 21.98 Precision bite ramps are designed to dissoclude posterior sectors and exert an intrusive force on anterior incisors.

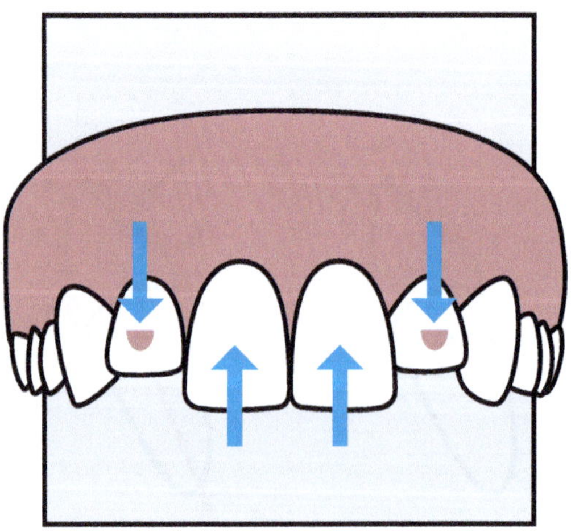

Fig. 21.99 Optimized support attachments are designed to help intruding upper central incisors.

Optimized Deep Bite Attachments

- Designed to support incisors or canines intrusion through a counterforce exerted on premolars.
- HBO attachments are bevelled to occlusal if the software does not place optimized deep bite attachments in first and second premolars.

Precision Bite Ramps

- Designed to disocclude the posterior teeth for improved efficiency in deep bite treatments with Invisalign
- They can be placed on the lingual surface of the upper incisors to maintain anterior occlusal contact, in a way that they help in exerting an intrusive force on upper and lower incisors
- They also disocclude the posterior zone allowing the extrusive forces on premolars to act easier
- When there is an increased overjet, bite ramps should be placed on the canines instead

Optimized Support Attachments

- Placed on lateral incisors when 1 mm or more intrusion is planned on adjacent canine or central incisor

Deep Bite Diagnosis

The main causes of deep bite are:

- Upright or retroclined incisors (in these cases the deep bite will have a better prognosisc as it will be possible to ask for relative intrusion)
- Hypererupted maxillary incisors (absolute intrusion will be needed)
- Steep curve of Spee in the lower arch
- Short face syndrome or hypodivergent skeletal pattern

That said, diagnosis should be based on.

- Smile analysis:
  - Low smile: do not intrude upper incisors, correct by intrusion of lower incisors.
  - Gummy smile: correct by intrusion of upper incisors.

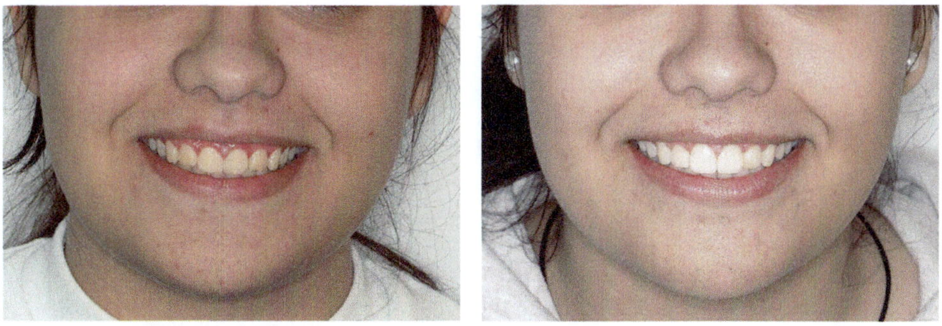

Fig. 21.100 Patient with a gummy smile and deep bite. Expand + procline incisors + upper incisors intrusion.

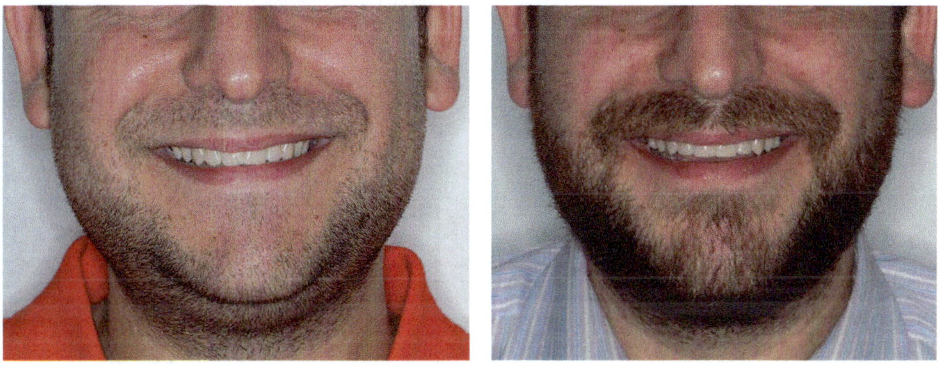

Fig. 21.101 This patient (before and after views) presented low smile with deep bite. Expand + procline incisors + lower incisors intrusion (in growing patients: simultaneous movement of anterior intrusion of lower incisors and posterior extrusion of premolars).

- Facial skeletal pattern:
  - hyperdivergent: incisors intrusion
  - hypodivergent: bite ramps, combination of anterior intrusion and posterior extrusion
- Severity of the deep bite:
  - 100%: sagittal priority: start proclining upper incisors without expansion
  - mild: start the treatment with lateral positive torque, then go for anterior proclination
- Possibility of transversal arch development:
  - the more dentoalveolar compression (negative posterior torque), the better to correct deep bite
- Incisor torque:
  - relative intrusion: is the intrusion obtained when retroclining incisors. In these cases, the deep bite is caused by lingual tipping of incisors

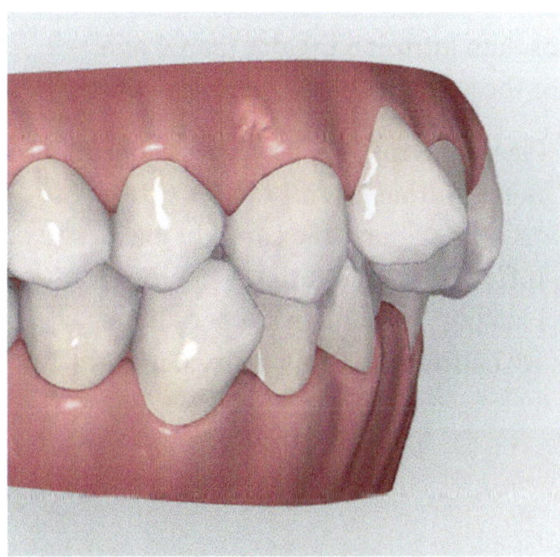

Fig. 21.102 When anterior torque is negative, relative intrusion might be easily performed.

- Absolute intrusion: the incisor intrusion when the intrusive force is directed along the long tooth axis. Incisors have a normal or a labial torque. Intrusion, lingual root torque and retrusion need to be applied. The contact points (IPR strips) need to be softened during the intrusion and the intrusion overtreated.

Incisor Retraction Protocol

Incisors, in order to be intruded, cannot be retroclined, so it is necessary to remove the root from the cortical bone before starting the intrusion:

- Procline
- Intrude
- Retrude applying lingual root torque simultaneously

This is also applicable on lower arch as, in many occasions, the ClinCheck starts the correction of the curve of Spee in the lower arch by intruding lower incisor without removing first the root from the cortical bone.

The staging of movement to correct effectively the curve of Spee should be:

- Procline lower incisors until the labial surface is perpendicular to the bone
- Once the root has been removed from the cortical bone, make an IPR to soften the contact points
- Apply absolute anterior intrusion
- Overtreat the anterior intrusion until edge to edge occlusion is achieved
- Finish the occlusion with a heavy posterior occlusal contact in posterior zone (red occlusal point)

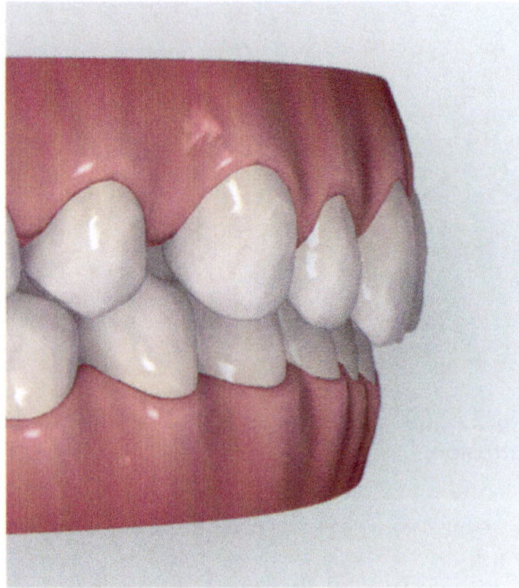

Fig. 21.103 When pure intrusion is needed, interproximal reduction will help in softening contact points.

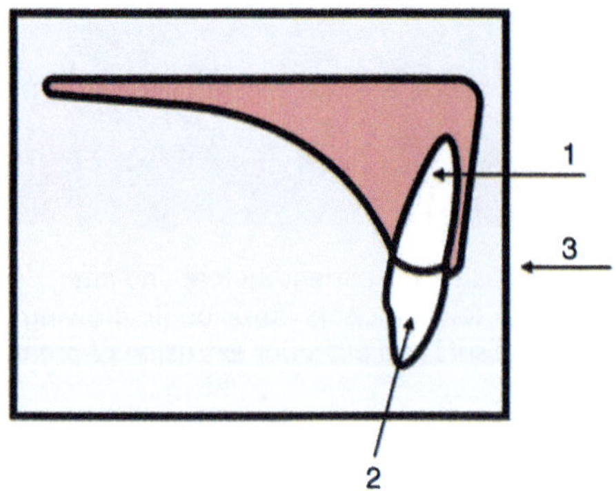

Fig. 21.104 Incisors protocol in deep bite is: procline crown, intrude, then retrude applying LRT simultaneously.

Absolute Intrusion Greater than 4 mm

For these cases:

- Place an 8 mm TAD between laterals and canines
- Bond buttons from 12 to 22
- Ask the patient to wear light elastics (2 oz)
- Inform the patient that a gingivectomy might be required during treatment
- Plan 0.25 mm intrusion per aligner
- Take intraoral X-rays every 6 months to check root status

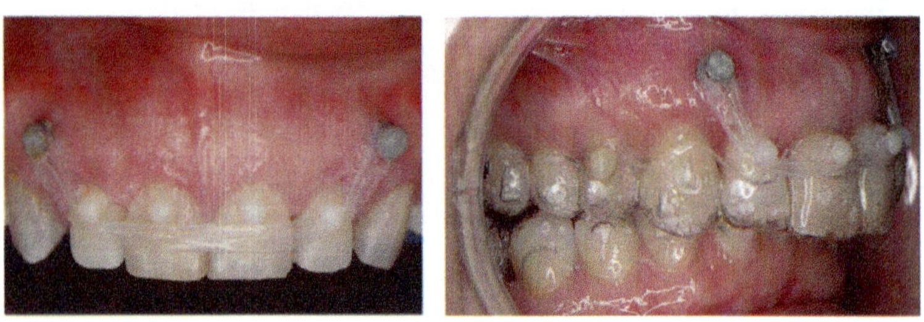

Fig. 21.105 Anterior temporary anchorage devices will help with this case.

Final Suggested Incisor Torque

To overcorrect deep bite, procline upper and lower incisors (relative intrusion).

Biomechanics for Deep Bite Correction

- Procline retroclined maxillary and mandibular incisors
- Overtreat the levelling of the curve of Spee
- Selective extrusion of premolars (in growing patients with hypodivergent skeletal pattern)

Deep bite must be treated in three planes:

- Transversal: expansion until the tooth axis becomes perpendicular to the bone.
  - Leave posterior teeth upright with its bone
  - Final torque 0 degrees
- Sagittal: proclination
  - We must avoid root contact with the cortical bone before intruding
  - Ask for labial crown torque and lingual root torque
  - Ask for reciprocal compression of second molars during incisors proclination

For this, Power ridges are mandatory, as correcting anterior torque is a movement that needs two forces to be fully developed.[1] In cases where there is only one Power ridge on buccal side of the aligner, risk of aligner misfitting is higher than with both buccal and palatal power ridges.

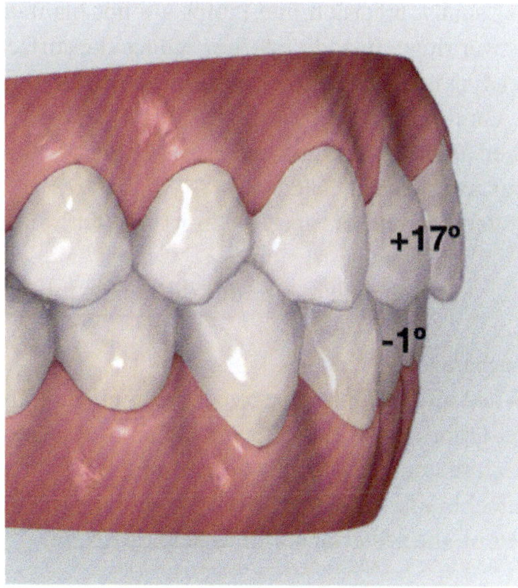

Fig. 21.106 Suggested torque for upper (+17 degrees) and lower incisor (−1 degree) to avoid anterior interference.

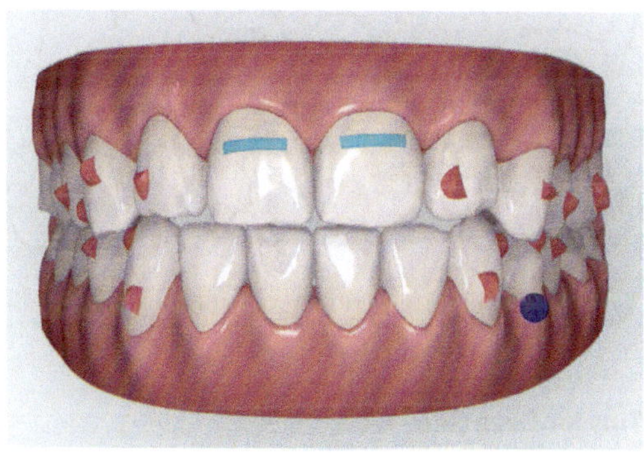

Fig. 21.107 Hypercorrection of the curve of Spee usually creates an open bite tendency.

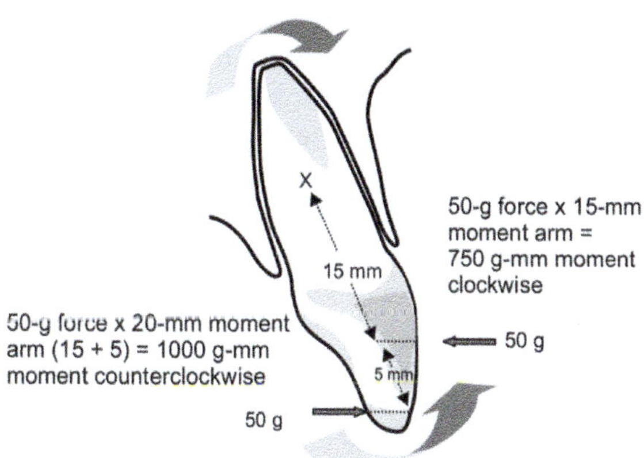

Fig. 21.108 A single buccal or palatal power ridge (left and middle) creates disinsertion of the aligner from the tooth, while double Power ridges (right) create torque properly.

1 Hahn *et al.* Torquing an upper central incisor with aligners—acting forces and biomechanical principles. *Eur J Orthod* 2010: **32;** 607–613.

Usually, precision bite ramps are not planned because they are incompatible with the palatal power ridge. In addition, they reduce the surface of contact on palatal side of anterior teeth, thus leading to a lack of anterior torque correction.

For this reason, Power ridges are preferable to ensure torque correction is properly achieved, and then anterior intrusion and retrusion are performed: this creates a correct deep bite solution, without any bite ramp needed.

- Vertical: incisors absolute intrusion (with simultaneous posterior extrusion)
  - IPR during intrusion
  - Apply lingual root torque during the intrusion and reciprocal posterior extrusion

Anchorage

When anterior intrusive forces are applied on the anterior zone, a reciprocal force tends to lift the posterior part of the aligner away from the teeth. This is why support/extrusion attachments are required on the first and second premolars to prevent the aligner from lifting up. Without these attachments the intrusive force would not be effective. However, we can also use buttons and elastics on the posterior sector to help extrusion.

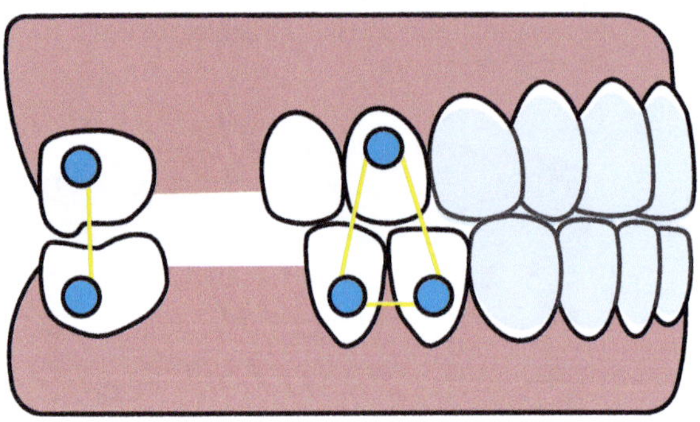

Fig. 21.109 Posterior extrusion might be achieved with optimized extrusion attachments or button cutouts and intermaxillary elastics (1/8, 6.5oz).

Tips for Deep Bite

- Correction of a deep bite with Invisalign is done through transversal and sagittal arch development, expansion and proclination of incisors with a strong posterior anchorage and with an adequate staging of movement of the incisors
- First the roots are removed from the cortical bone and then movement of intrusion, retrusion and simultaneous lingual root torque is applied
- Diagnosis determines the treatment mechanics to solve the deep bite. If there is a gummy smile the upper incisors will be intruded, whereas if there is a low smile in a brachyfacial patient it will be corrected by lower intrusion and premolar extrusion
- It is essential to provide anchorage to intrude the incisors. If the technician does not place an optimized attachment, use a horizontal attachment on the distal teeth (premolars) to assist the anterior intrusion
- Ensure the incisor's root is outside of the cortical bone before starting the intrusion movement. Bite ramps can be used during proclination but eliminate them before intrusion so that pressure areas may be placed for intrusion along the long axis of the tooth
- Vivera retainers will be very efficient retention devices because they prevent eruption of previously intruded teeth. Nevertheless, in bruxism a bruxism splint is the best option
- Ask for reciprocal compression of second molars to assist the effectivenes of incisors proclination

21.2.1 Deep Bite and Bruxism: Skeletal Class I with Crowding

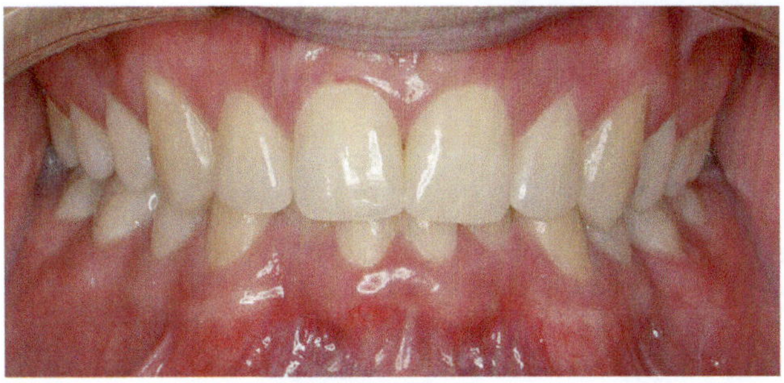

Fig. 21.110 Initial intraoral view.

Diagnosis

A 32-year-old man with symmetric hypodivergent skeletal class I presented with a low smile, centred upper midline and an 80% deep bite. He had been treated with brackets and four premolar extractions when he was a child, and had bruxism and lower crowding with a steep curve of Spee and lingual tipping of upper and lower incisors.

Treatment Plan

The deep bite would be addressed in the three planes:

- Transversal: expansion from first molar to first molar (using second and third molars as anchorage)
- Sagittal: proclination and lingual root torque to remove the root from the cortical bone and for relative intrusion
- Vertical correction: by anterior intrusion and posterior extrusion (using intermaxillary vertical elastics)

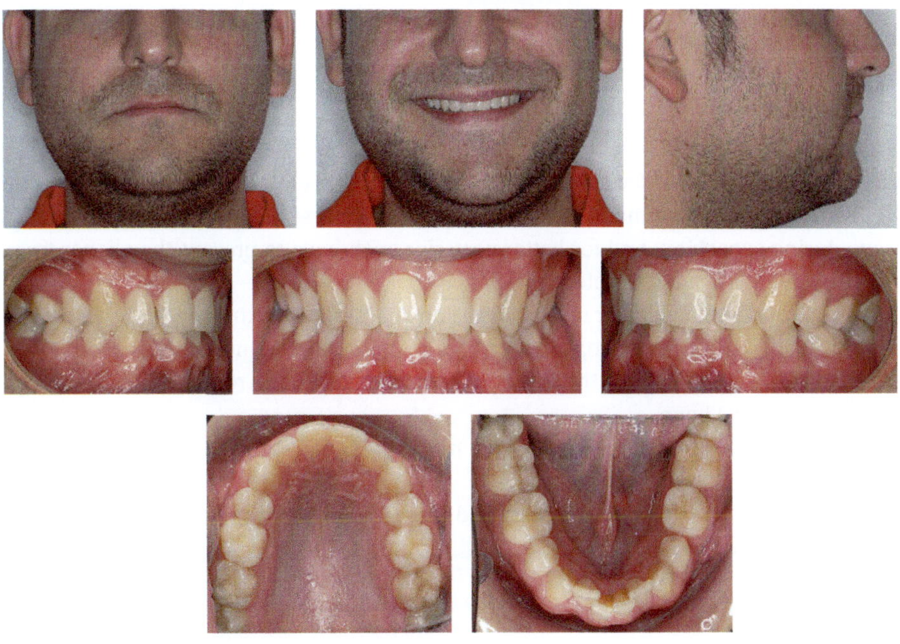

Fig. 21.111 Initial extraoral and intraoral views.

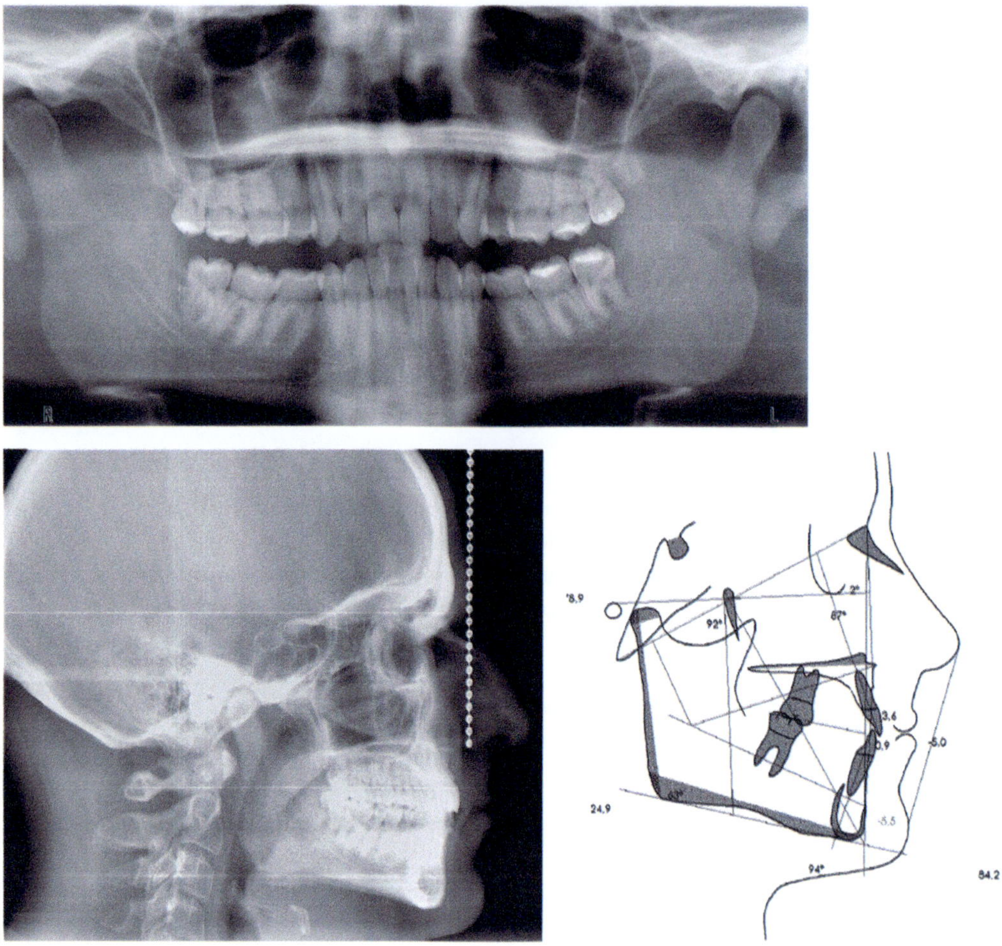

Fig. 21.112 Initial panoramic and lateral X-rays and cephalometry.

Requirements for the Technician

- AT anchorage attachments bevelled to occlusal in first premolars (second premolars were missing) and HBG horizontal attachments bevelled to gingival in first molars to control posterior molar torque during expansion, and for better posterior anchorage to prevent the aligner from lifting up when the intrusive forces acted on the incisors.
- Apply: expansion, proclination, lower incisor intrusion and posterior extrusion.
- Make as little IPR as possible to develop the arches more transversally and sagitally.
- Staging on incisors: do not start with the intrusion movement until the roots of the incisors are removed from the cortical bone.
- Make the posterior extrusion of premolars and molars reciprocal to the anterior intrusion movement.
- Overtreat incisors intrusion (0 mm overbite) and overtreat posterior extrusion (red contact points on the posterior teeth).

- Transversal arch development: Expansion (changing torque of lateral teeth)
- Sagittal development: Proclination (relative intrusion)

- Vertical correction: anterior intrusion + simultaneous posterior extrusion (using posterior elastics)
- AT HBO U4/ L4 and AT HBG U6/L6

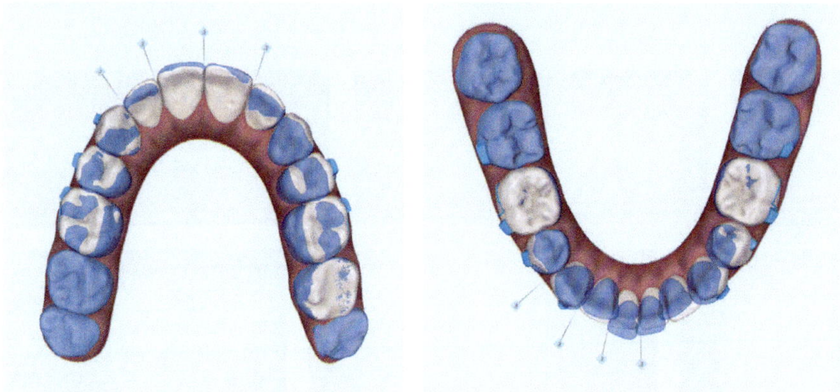

Fig. 21.113 Initial occlusal upper and lower superimposition ClinCheck views.

- Expansion + proclination + lower intrusion and posterior extrusion
- Try to do as little IPR as possible to increase transversal and sagittal arch development

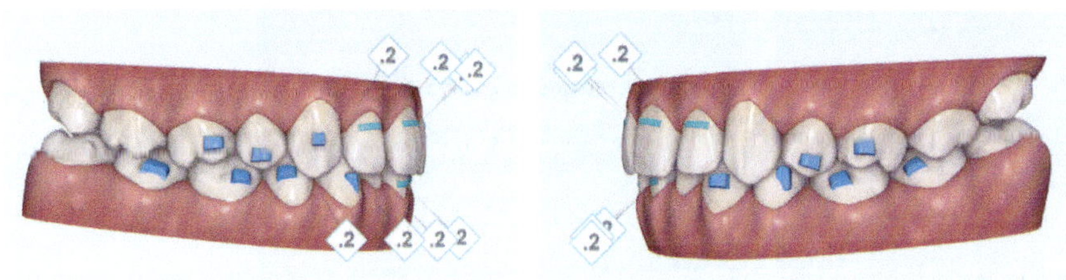

Fig. 21.114 Initial right and left ClinCheck views.

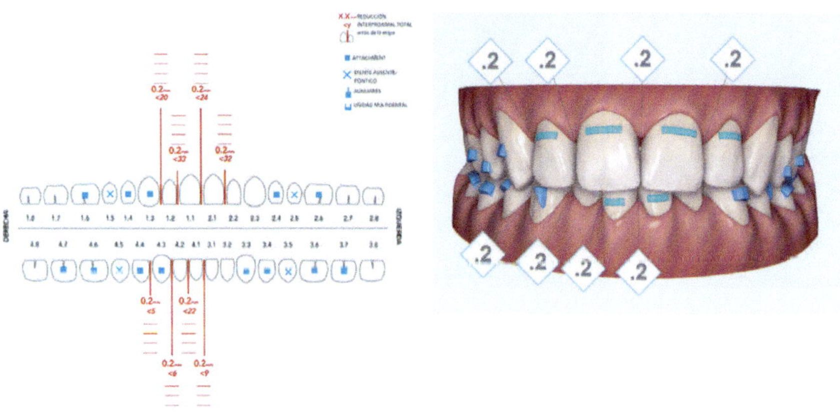

Fig. 21.115 Interproximal reduction.

Treatment Summary

- The case was treated with 43 aligners changed on a 2-week intervals
- A new set of additional aligners was needed to overtreat the deep bite
- Total treatment time was 25 months
- For retention, a bruxism splint was applied for night use

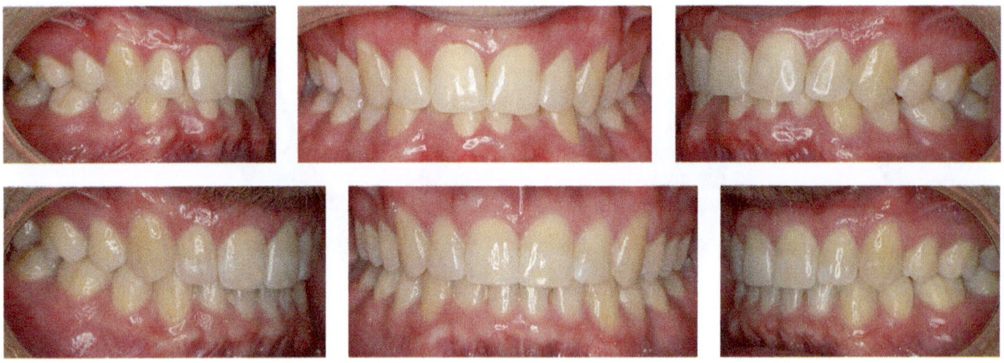

Fig. 21.116 Initial (upper) and final intraoral views (lower).

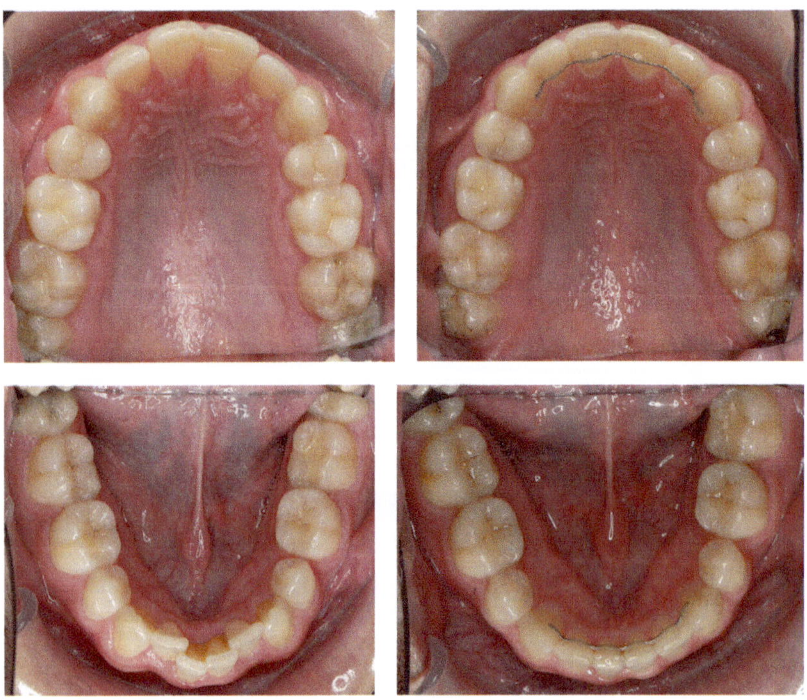

Fig. 21.117 Initial (left) and final occlusal (right).

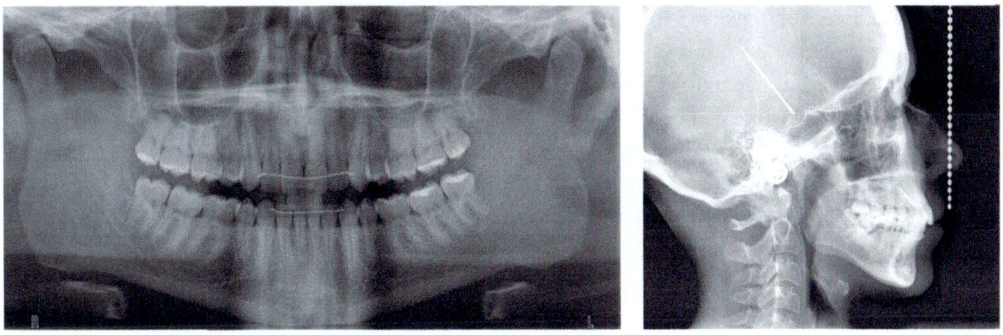

Fig. 21.118 Final panoramic and lateral X-rays.

21.2.2 Deep Bite, Class II: Skeletal Class II with Deep Bite and Lower Severe Crowding

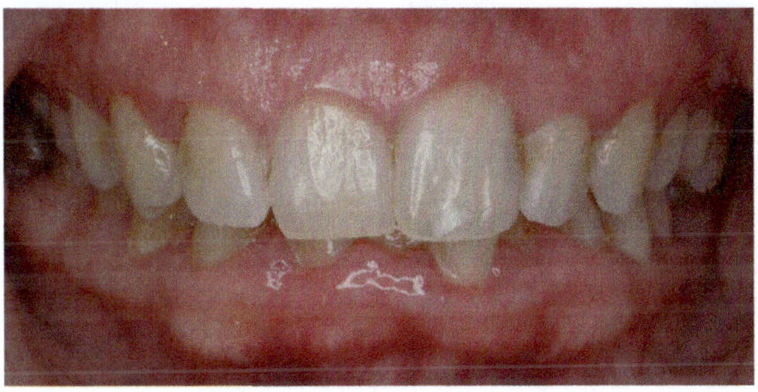

Fig. 21.119 Initial intraoral view.

Diagnosis

A 42-year-old woman with normodivergent skeletal class II presented with a 90% deep bite, class II division 2 and an extruded 26. She had a class II profile, symmetric with labial competence, lower midline deviated to the left. There was negative torque on the lateral segment, severe crowding and mesial tipping of 37 with impacted 47 and 48.

Treatment Plan

The original treatment plan included placing and implanting of 36 with a provisional crown to assist the intrusion of 26 or two TADs and the extraction of 48 to upright 47. Patient refused the treatment plan as she only wanted to wear aligners and elastics and did not want to receive any surgical treatment. An alternative plan, which consisted of two phases of treatment was accepted by the patient.

- First phase: make expansion 5 to 5 and procline the upper incisors. No movement on the molars would be performed, in order to have enough posterior anchorage for the upper torque correction. In the lower arch, expansion 5 to 5 and IPR would be performed to solve the crowding and centre the lower midline
- Second phase (additional aligners): intrusion of 26 would be addressed, using the contact point between 27 with 37 and horizontal attachments on the adjacent teeth as anchorage for the intrusion. The uprighting of 47 was not a goal of this treatment as the patient did not want 48 extracted

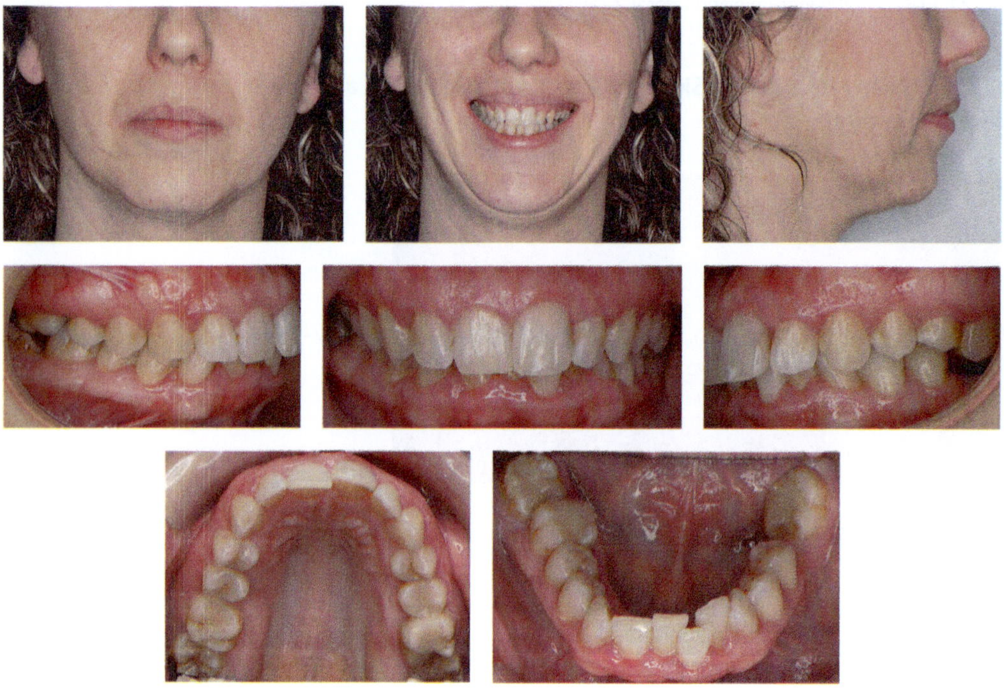

Fig. 21.120 Initial extraoral and intraoral views.

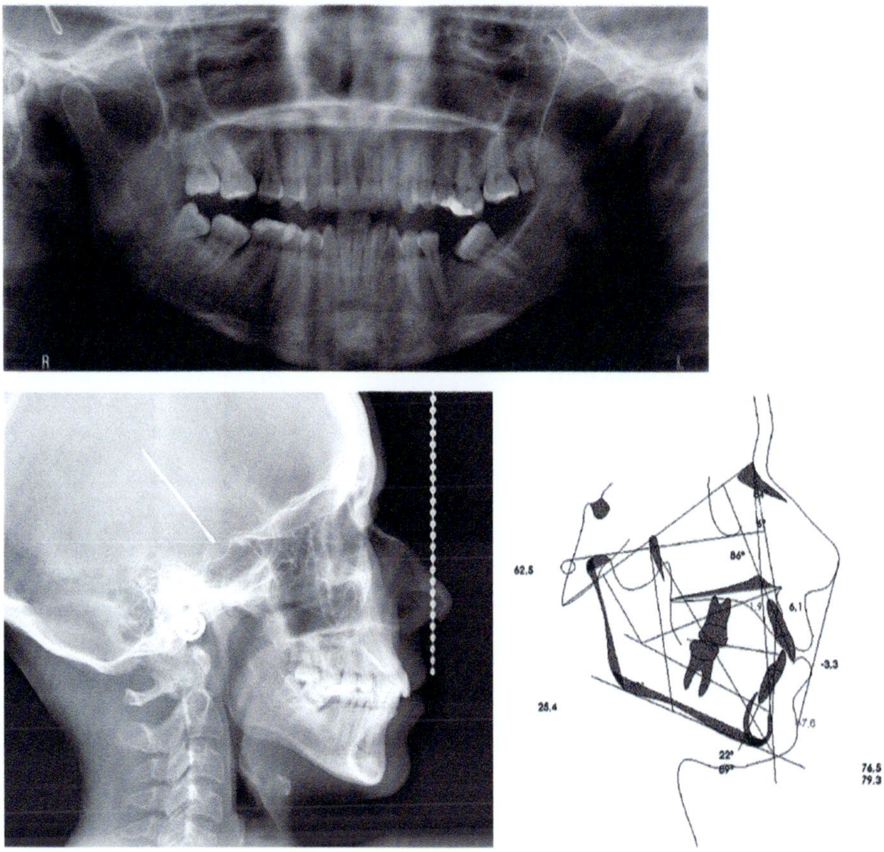

Fig. 21.121 Initial panoramic X-ray, teleradiograph and cephalometry.

Requirements for the Technician

- Do not move upper molars during upper incisors expansion and proclination.
- In the lower arch, centre the lower midline at the same time as the proclination of the lower incisors.
- The deep bite solved by upper and lower proclination of incisors and intrusion of the lower incisors.
- Precision cut in upper canines and button cutouts in lower molars is required for additional anchorage to correct the class II dental relationship.

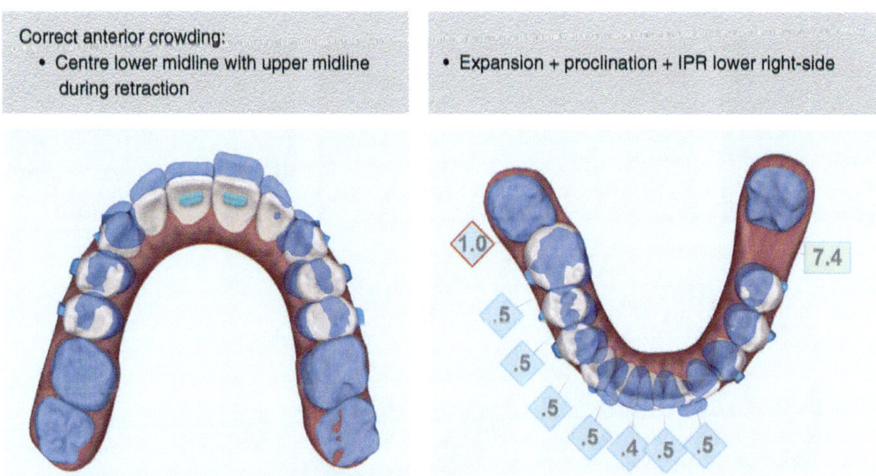

Fig. 21.122 Initial upper and lower ClinCheck views.

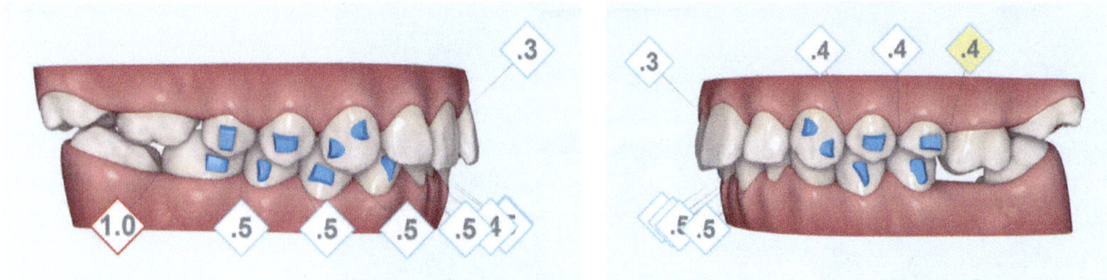

Fig. 21.123 Initial right and left ClinCheck views.

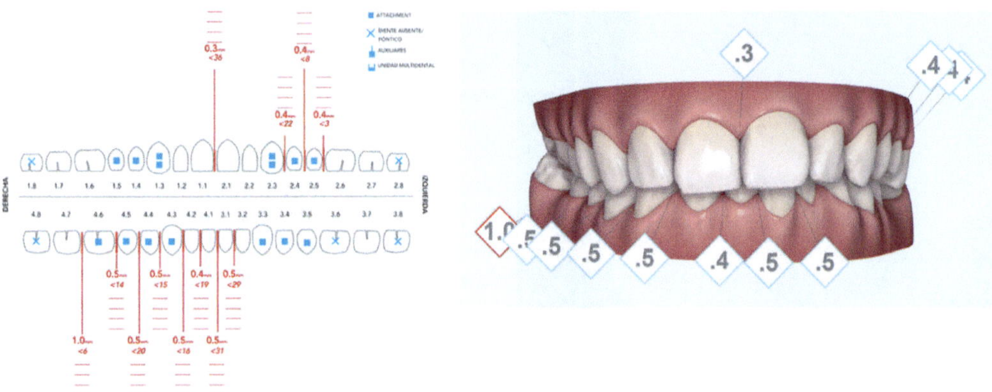

Fig. 21.124 On the additional aligners set, distal tipping of the crown in 37 was planned to achieve occlusion with 27 and to intrude 26. Uprighting 47 was not an option as patient refused extraction of 48.

Treatment Summary

- Total treatment time was 30 months.
- The first phase of aligners was 49 aligners with 2-week change intervals. Additional aligners were requested for further correction of the deep bite and to intrude 26.
- Sequencing the movement into two treatment phases was crucial for efficient correction of the deep bite.
- Crowding was resolved by expansion and IPR.

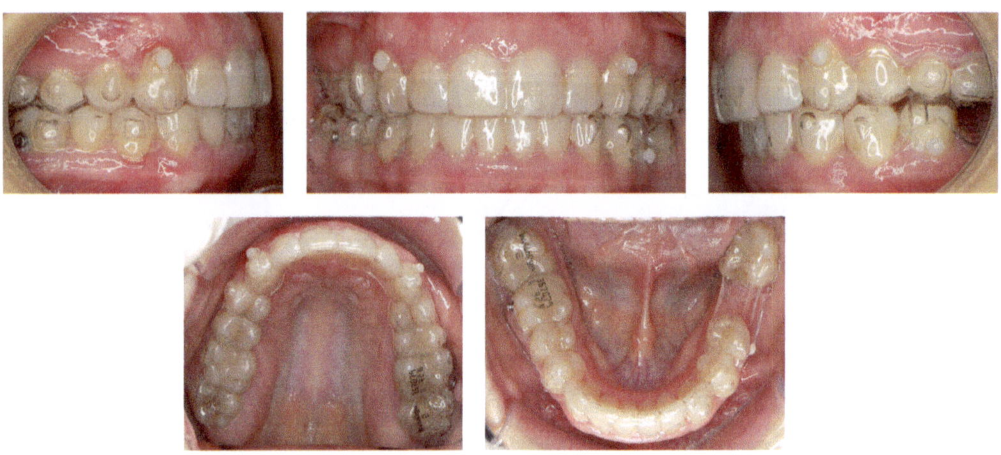

Fig. 21.125 Evolution in last aligner before refinement.

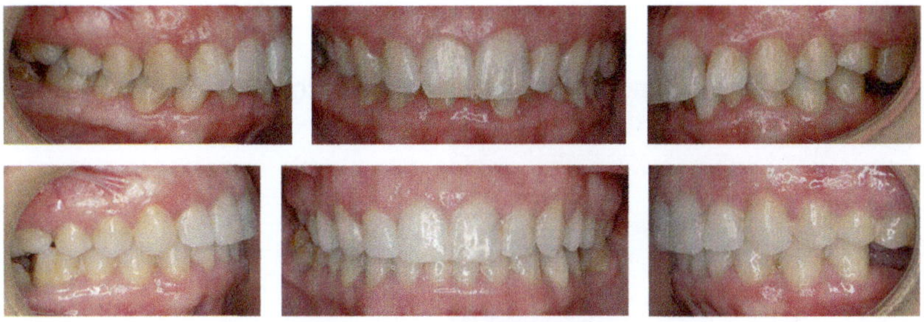

Fig. 21.126 Initial (upper) and final (lower) intraoral views.

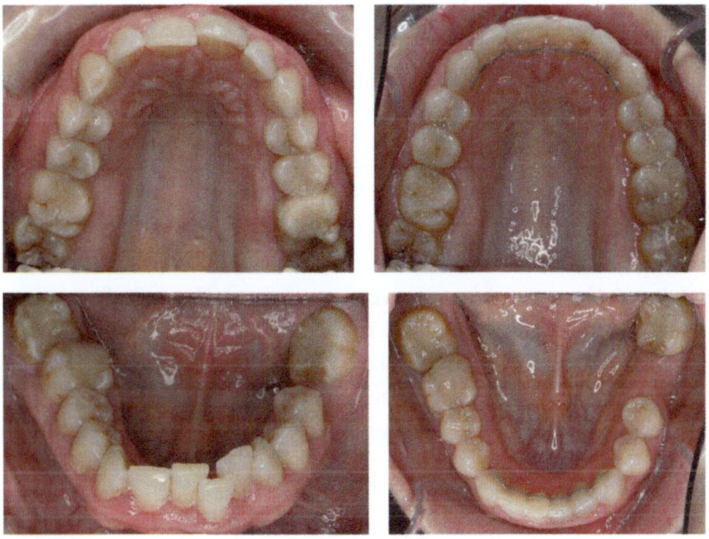

Fig. 21.127 Initial (left) and final (right) occlusals.

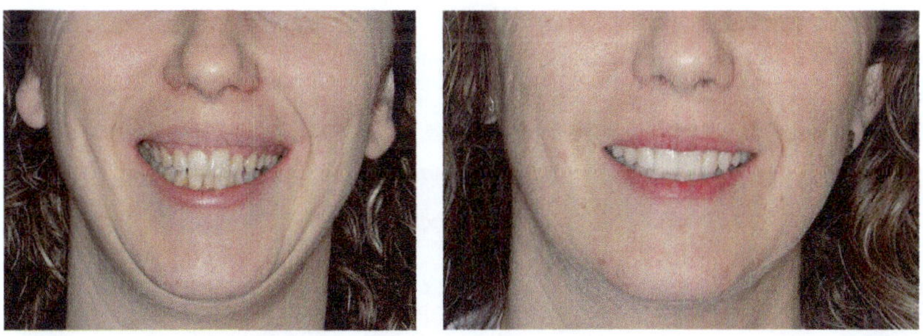

Fig. 21.128 Before and after smile.

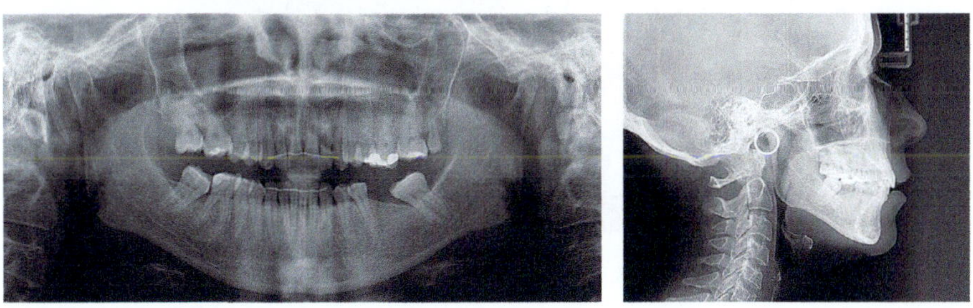

Fig. 21.129 Final panoramic and lateral X-rays.

21.2.3 Deep Bite: Skeletal Class I

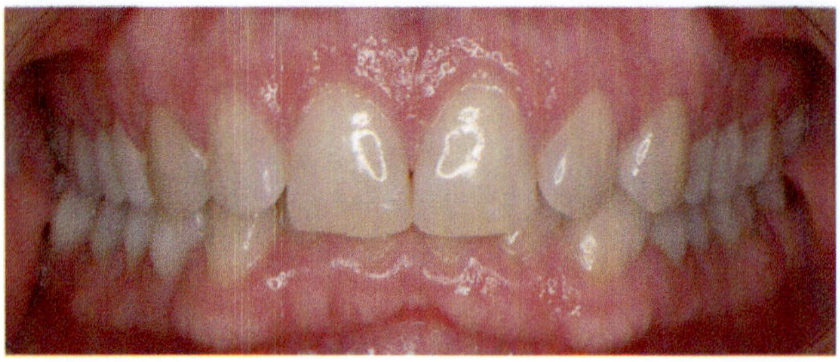

Fig. 21.130 Initial intraoral view.

Diagnosis

A 43-year-old woman presented with a 90% deep bite, low smile, lower moderate crowding and lingual tipping on upper and lower incisors.

Treatment Plan

The deep bite would be treated in the three planes:

- Transversal: expansion from first molar to first molar
- Sagittal: proclination and TRL lingual root torque to remove the root from the cortical bone and for relative intrusion. Also, for correction it was planned to move distally the teeth on the upper left quadrant during the expansion assisted by class II elastic to get a buccal class I on the left side. To visualize the elastics effect a virtual jump was requested at the end of the treatment
- Vertical correction: by anterior intrusion to level gingival margins and posterior premolar extrusion

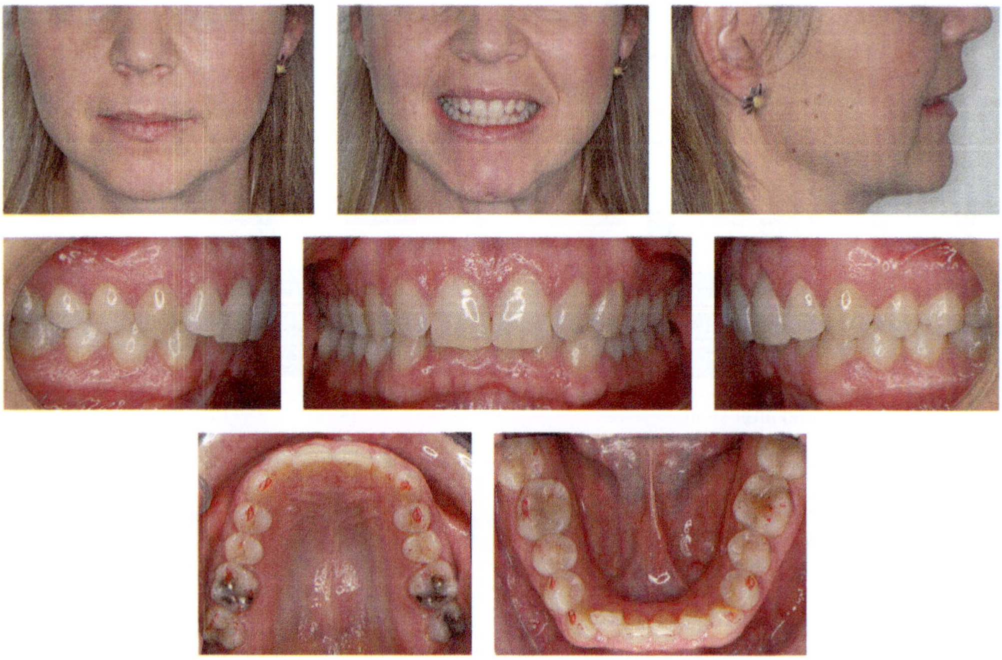

Fig. 21.131 Initial extraoral and intraoral views.

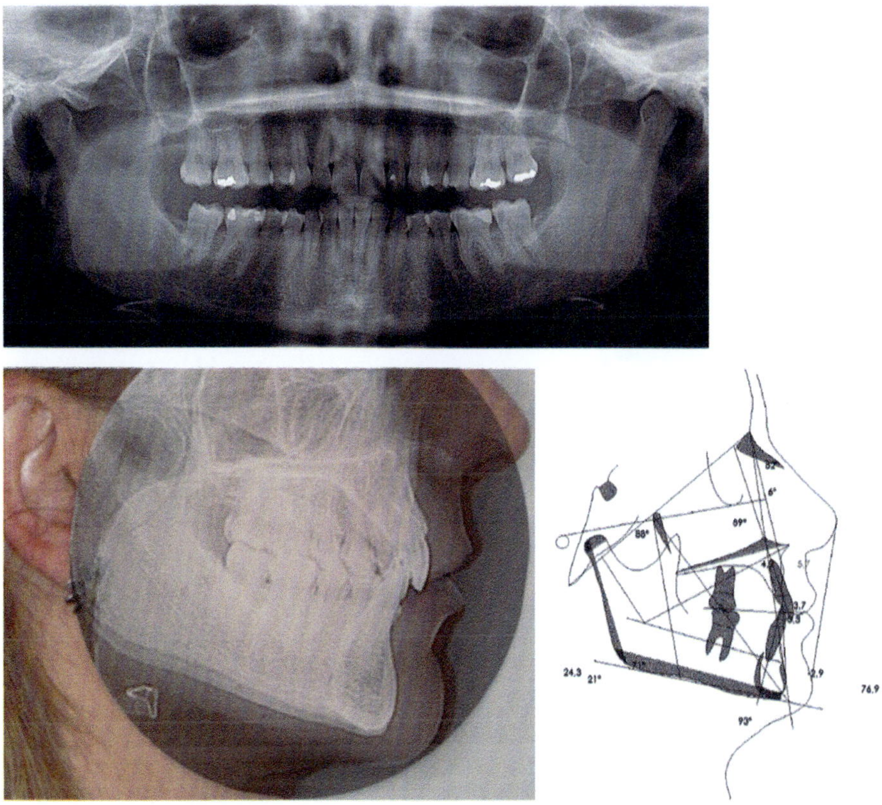

Fig. 21.132 Initial panoramic X-ray, teleradiograph and cephalometry.

Requirements for the Technician

- Make the expansion and the proclination in a simultaneous way, as the expansion is going to be made by changing the torque, providing labial crown torque to premolars and molars (if the expansion had been a body expansion, the proclination would have been postponed after the expansion)
- Use the space gained by the expansion to move the upper right teeth into a distal position to achieve a class I relationship

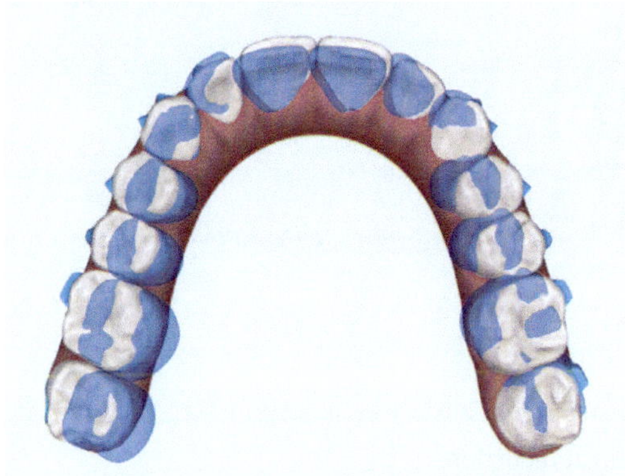

Staging maxillary:

- Expansion and upper proclination (relative intrusion)

Fig. 21.133 Initial upper occlusal superimposition ClinCheck view.

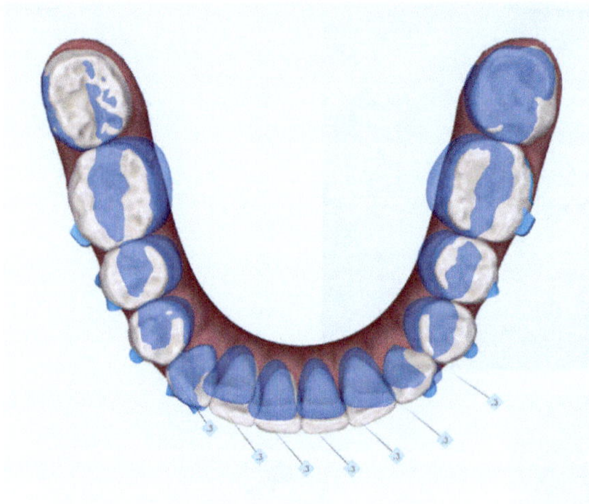

Staging mandible:

- Expansion + proclination + IPR

Fig. 21.134 Initial lower occlusal superimposition ClinCheck view.

- Upper and lower proclination (relative intrusion)
- Lower absolute intrusion

Virtual jump to simulate class II elastic effect on left side

→

- Overtreat anterior intrusion, edge to edge anterior occlusion
- Overtreat posterior intrusion (red-contact posterior ponit at the end of the treatment)

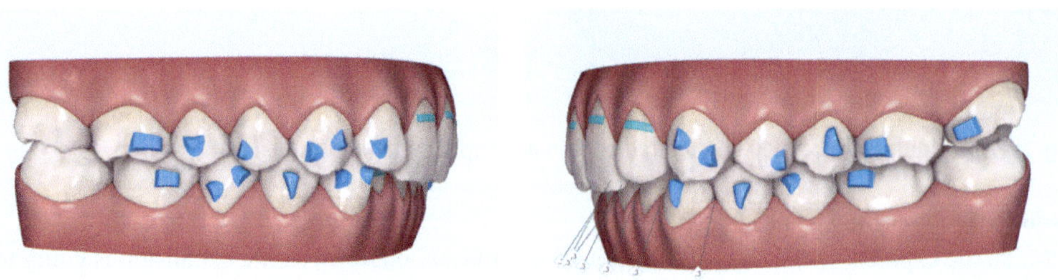

Fig. 21.135 Initial right and left ClinCheck view.

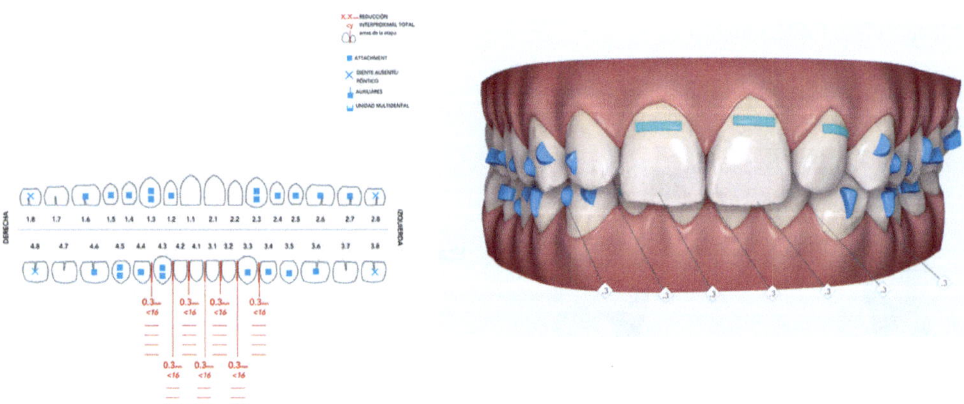

Fig. 21.136 Initial front ClinCheck view with interproximal reduction.

Treatment Summary

- Total treatment time was 15 months.
- The case was treated with 26 aligners replaced on a 10-day interval.
- The gingival margins were levelled in this first set of aligners.
- A new set of additional aligners were needed to overtreat the deep bite.
- The deep bite has been totally corrected without reducing the exposure of the upper incisors at rest.
- For retention, fixed retainers were bonded and Vivera retainers made for night use.

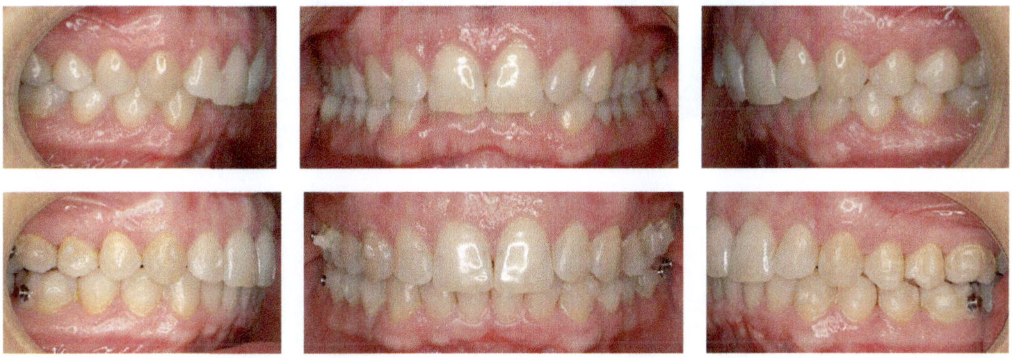

Fig. 21.137 Initial views (upper) and evolution after 12 months (lower).

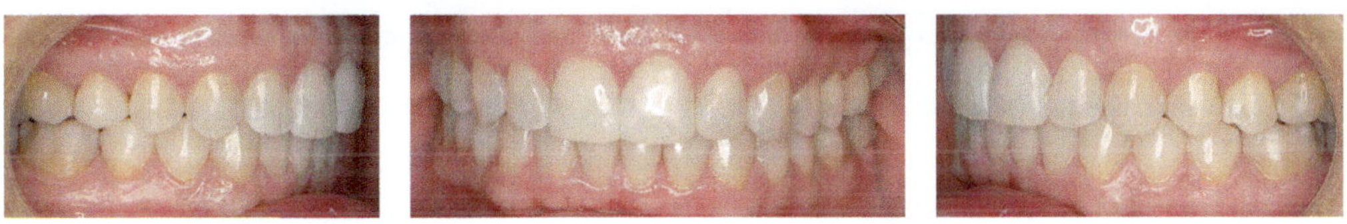

Fig. 21.138 Final intraoral views.

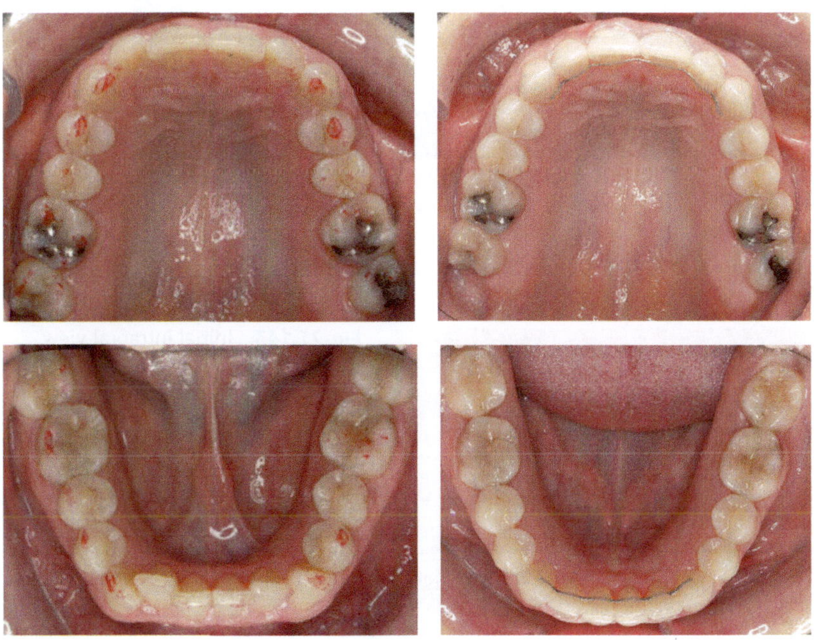

Fig. 21.139 Initial (left) and final occlusal (right).

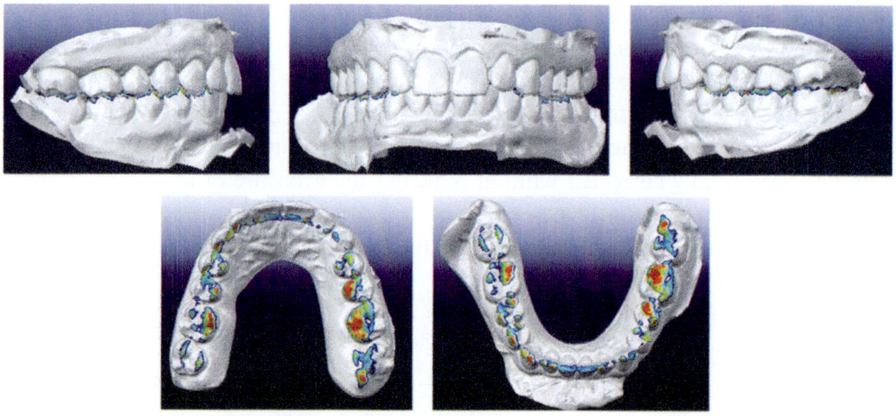

Fig. 21.140 Occlusal contact point at the end of the treatment.

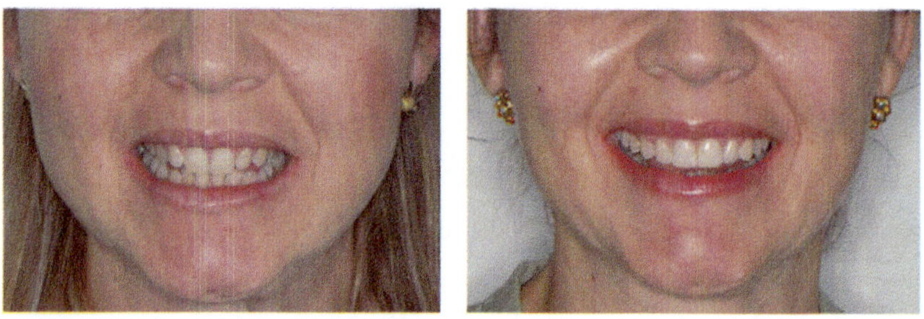

Fig. 21.141 Initial and final smile.

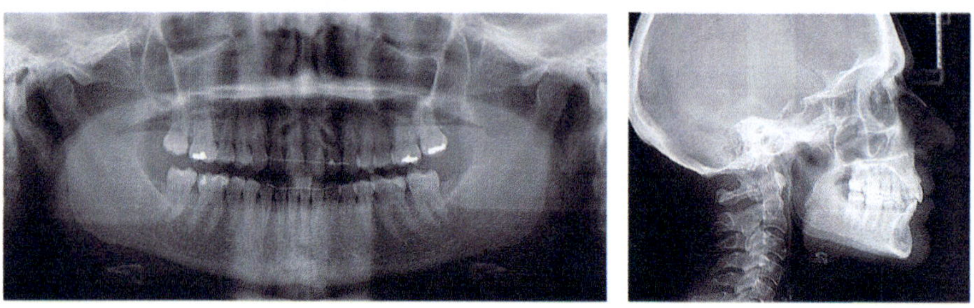

Fig. 21.142 Final panoramic and lateral X-rays.

21.2.4 Deep Bite: Skeletal Class II with TADs

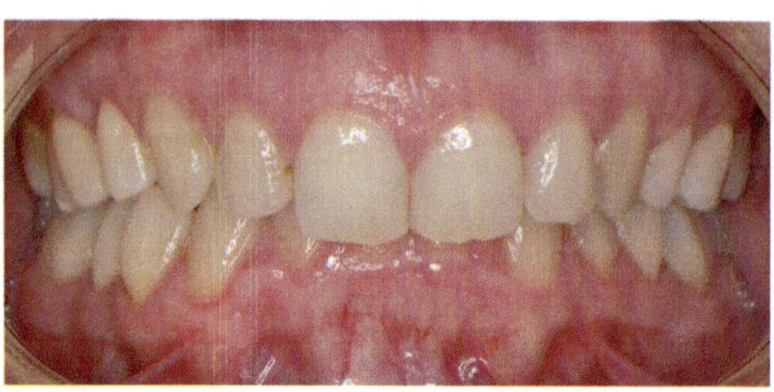

Fig. 21.143 Initial intraoral view.

Diagnosis

A 41-year-old woman with symmetric hypodivergent skeletal class I presented with centred upper midline and a 90% deep bite. As a child the patient had been treated with brackets and two upper premolar and a lower incisor extraction had been done in the previous treatment. On arrival, she had lower crowding with a steep curve of Spee and lingual tipping of upper and lower incisors with a relapse in the overbite.

Treatment Plan

The deep bite would be treated in three planes:

- Transversal: expansion from first molar to first molar.
- Sagittal: proclination and TRL lingual root torque to remove the root from the cortical bone and for relative intrusion.
- Insert TADs between upper first and second molar and indirect anchorage to first molar to provide enough posterior anchorage to create an effective intrusive force in the anterior zone.
- Vertical correction: by anterior intrusion and posterior extrusion (using intermaxillary vertical elastics).

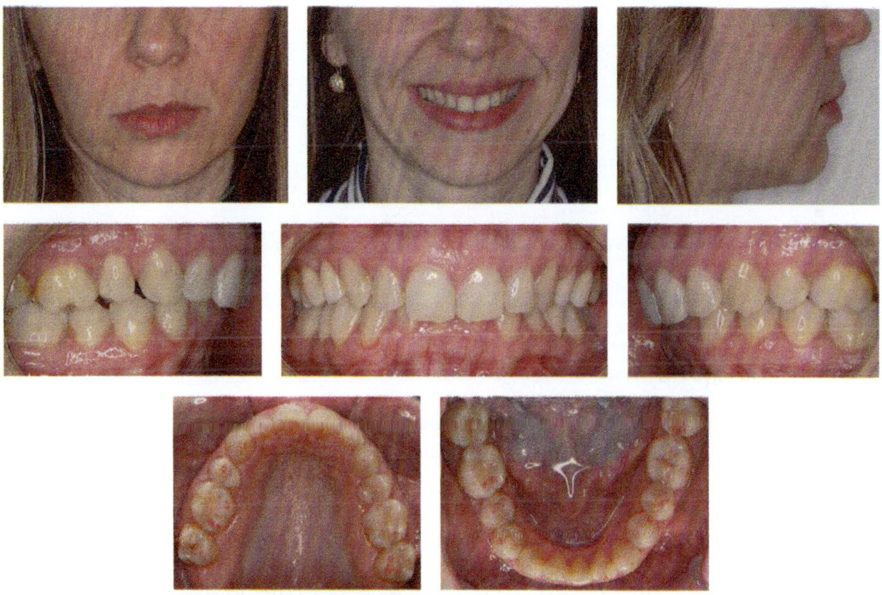

Fig. 21.144 Initial extraoral and intraoral views.

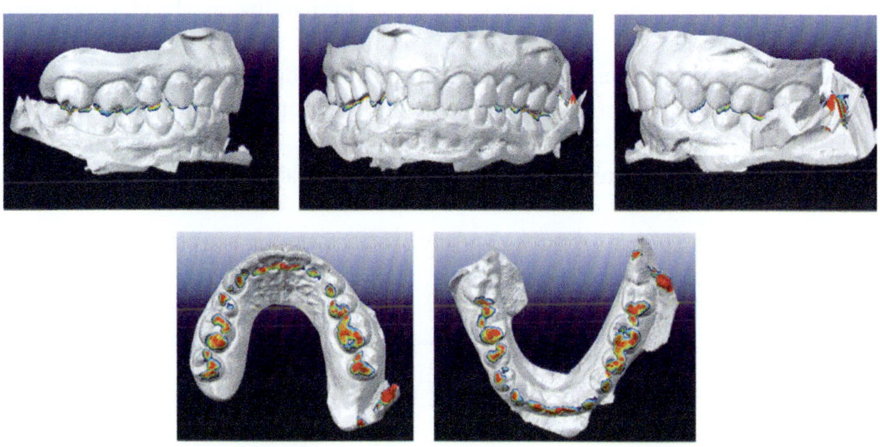

Fig. 21.145 Initial occlusal contact.

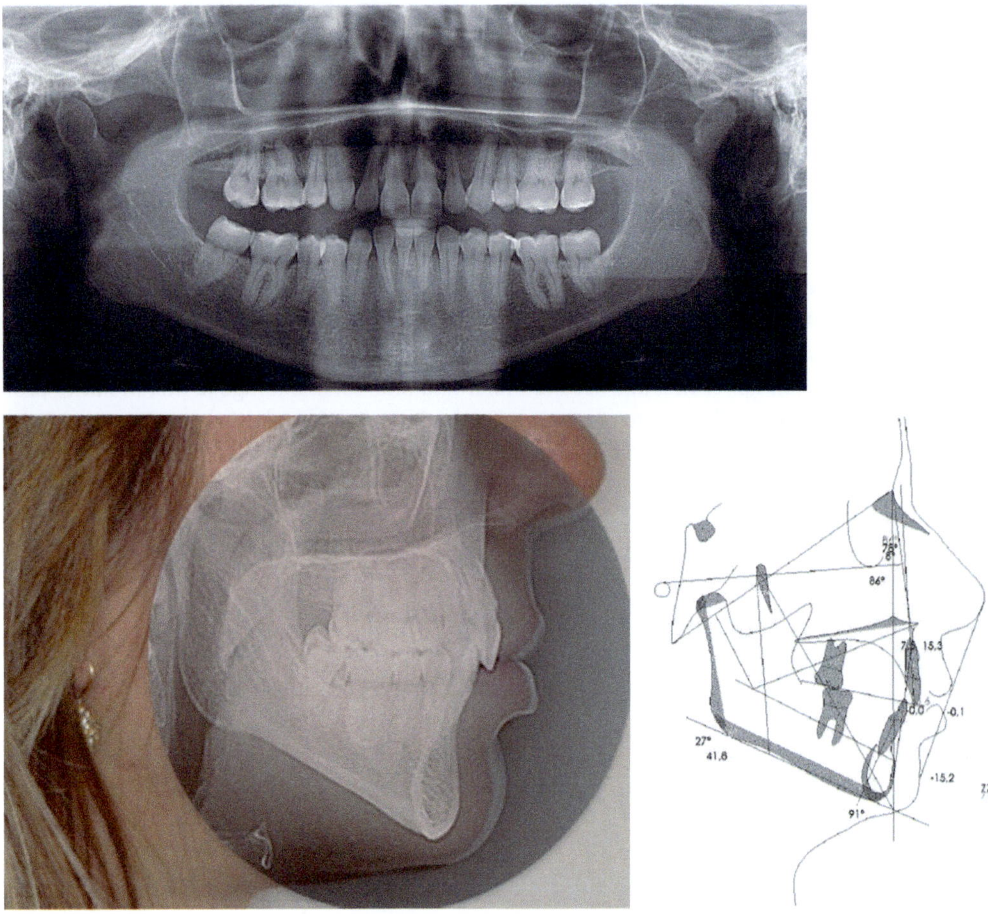

Fig. 21.146 Initial panoramic X-ray, teleradiograph and cephalometry.

Requirements for the Technician

- AT anchorage attachments bevelled to occlusal in premolars and HBG horizontal attachments bevelled to gingival in first molars in order to control posterior molar torque during expansion, and provide better posterior anchorage to prevent the aligner from lifting up when the intrusion forces acted on the incisors
- Apply: expansion, proclination, lower incisor intrusion and posterior extrusion
- Staging on incisors: do not start the intrusion movement until the root of the incisors are removed from the cortical bone
- Make the posterior extrusion of premolars and molars reciprocal to the anterior intrusion movement
- Overtreat incisors intrusion (0 mm overbite) and overtreat posterior extrusion (red contact points on the posterior teeth)

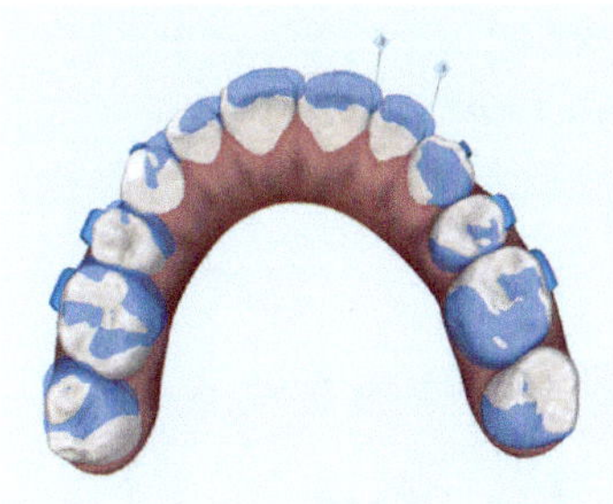

Staging maxillary:

- Expansion + mesial-out rotation of 1.6 and 2.6
- Lingual root torque of upper incisors + labial crown torque of upper incisors

Fig. 21.147 Initial upper occlusal superimposition ClinCheck view.

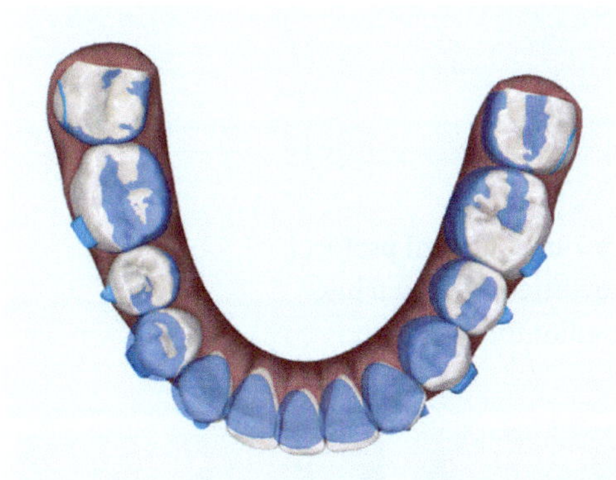

Staging mandible:

Expansion

Relative intrusion through proclination

Lower incisors intrusion

Fig. 21.148 Initial lower occlusal superimposition ClinCheck view.

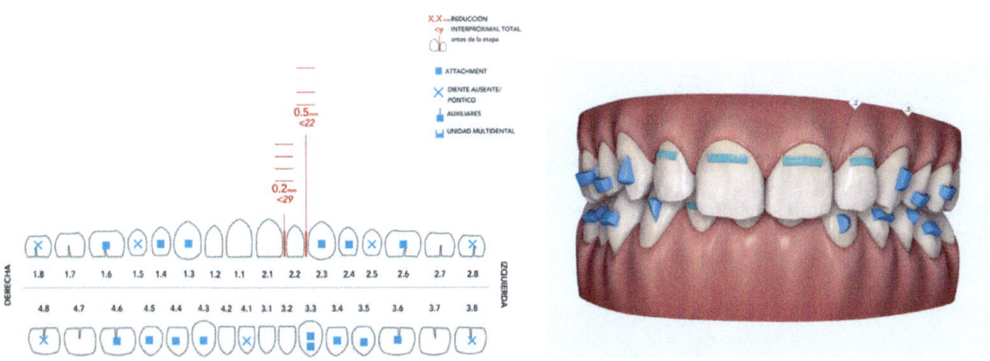

Fig. 21.149 Interproximal reduction is only needed mesial and distal to 22 to make the shape equal to that of 12.

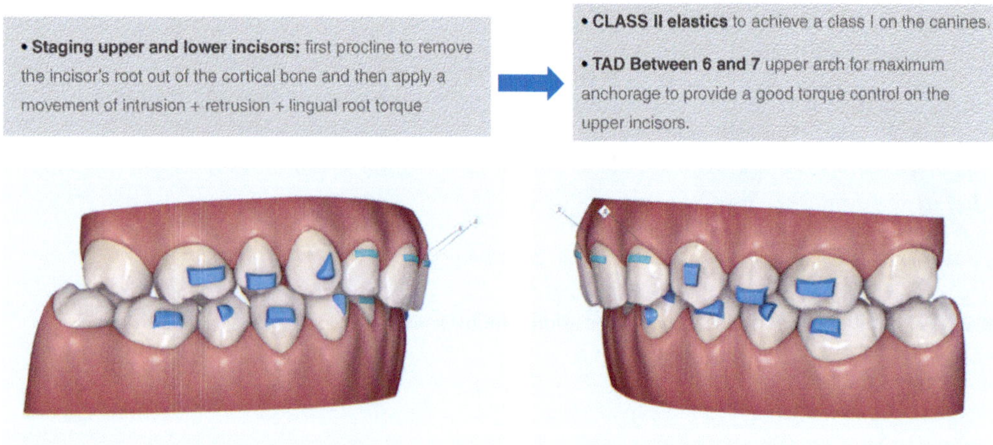

Fig. 21.150 Initial right and left ClinCheck view.

Treatment Summary

- Total treatment time was 18 months
- The case was treated with 50 aligners changed on a 7-day interval protocol
- A new set of 21 additional aligners was needed to overtreat the deep bite
- For retention, it used fix retainers and an occlusal splint for night use

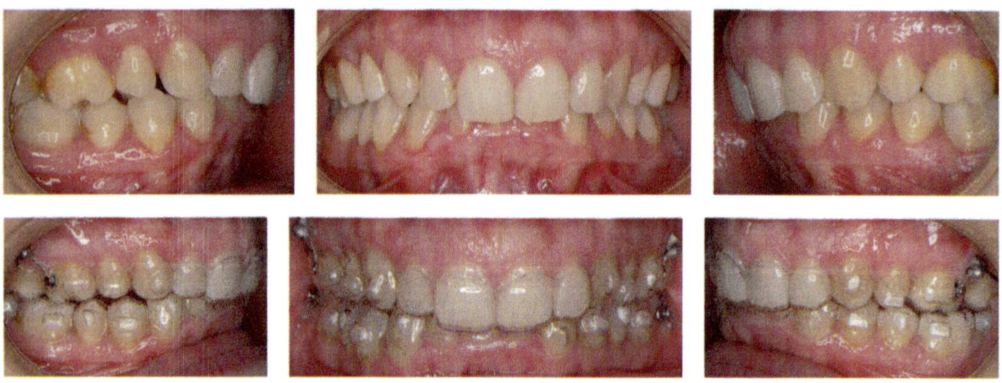

Fig. 21.151 Temporary anchorage devices to provide enough posterior anchorage in order to create an effective anterior intrusive force.

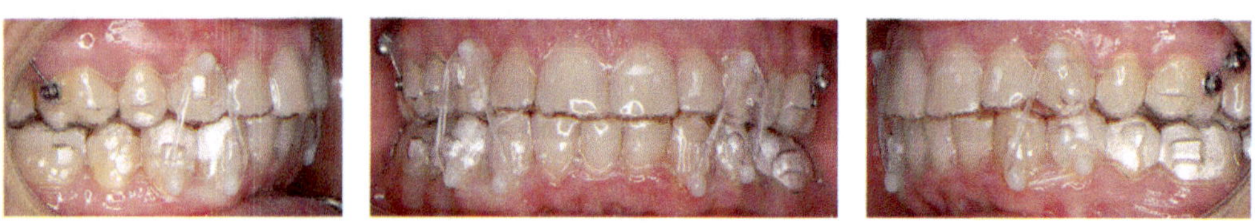

Fig. 21.152 Evolution at the end of additional aligners. Intermaxillary elastic was used to settle the occlusion.

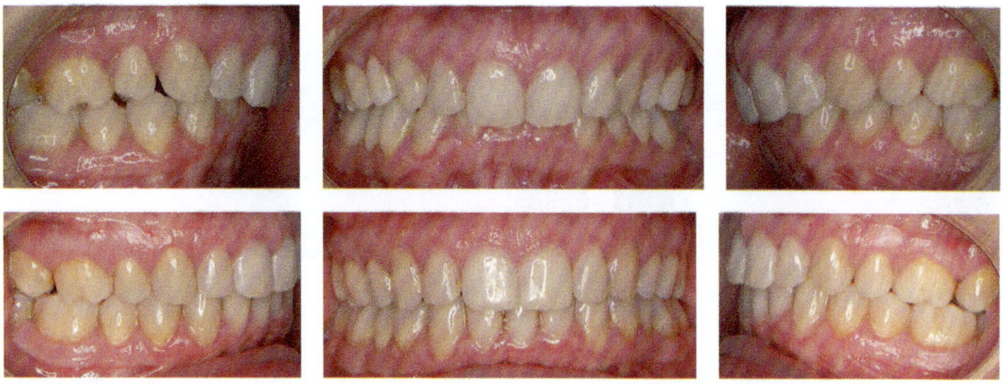

Fig. 21.153 Initial (upper) and final (lower) intraoral views.

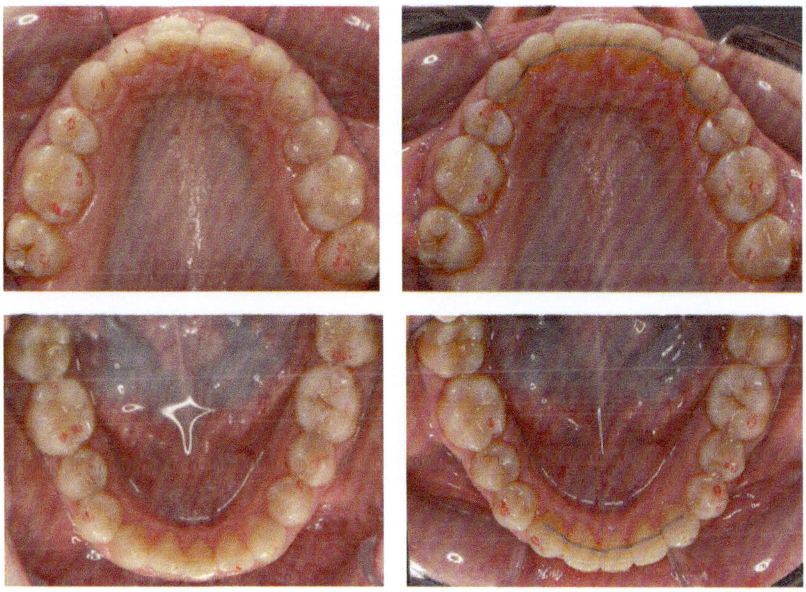

Fig. 21.154 Initial left) and final (right) occlusal.

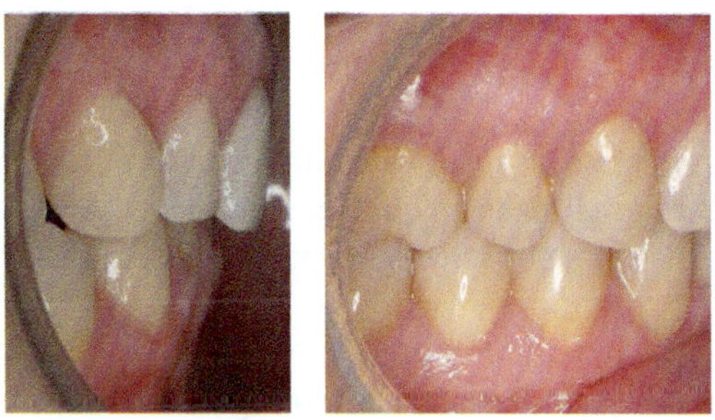

50 Aligners (+ 21 of refinement) were changed every 7 days
(18 months of treatment)

Fig. 21.155 Initial and final overjet and final correction of the deep bite.

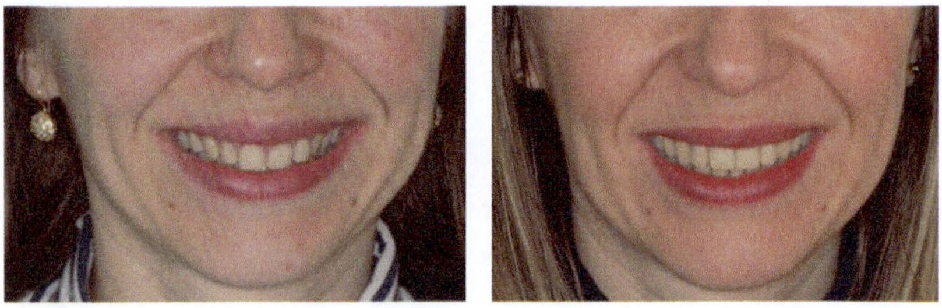

Fig. 21.156 Initial and final smile.

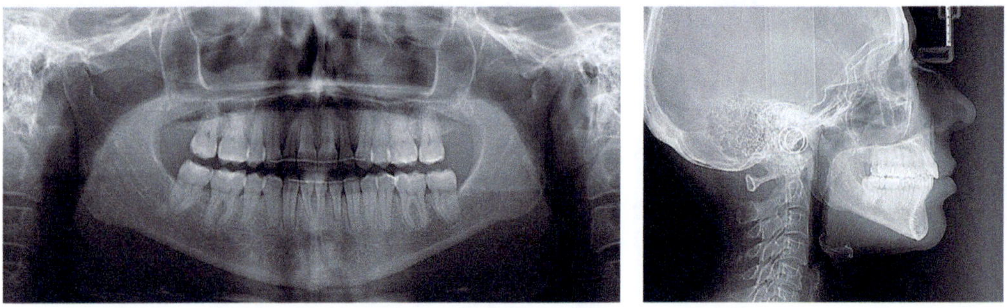

Fig. 21.157 Final panoramic and lateral X-rays with an appropriate inclination of lower incisor.

21.2.5 Deep Bite with Lite Treatment

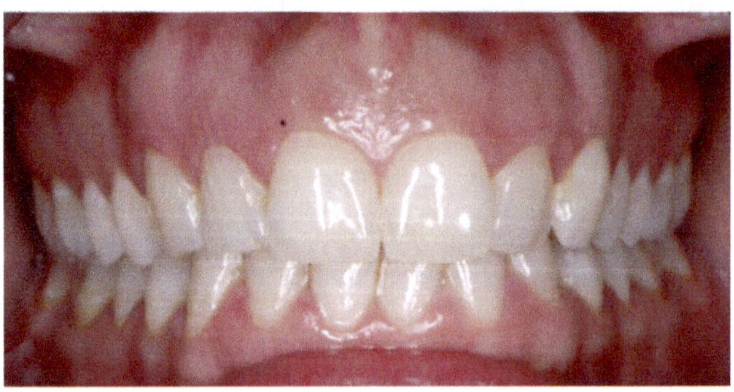

Fig. 21.158 Initial intraoral view.

Diagnosis

A 31-year-old woman presented with a relapse from previous treatment with mild crowding. She had a symmetric hypodivergent skeletal class I, centred upper midline, a 50% deep bite and a gummy smile caused by increased lip mobility (which was not a treatment goal).

Treatment Plan

- The deep bite would be corrected with a Lite treatment, knowing that in 14 aligners the anterior intrusion sequence is not predictable
- For this reason three ClinChecks with an anterior open bite were planned, hypercorrecting occlusion from a vertical perspective, so as to achieve the maximum vertical result without upgrading the treatment option

Requirements for the Technician

- Extrusion attachments on the posterior sector to prevent the aligner from lifting up when the intrusion forces act on the incisors
- Apply expansion, proclination, lower incisor intrusion and posterior extrusion simultaneously
- Hypercorrect incisor intrusion (as maximum as possible intrusion in 14 aligners)
- Set posterior sectors as unmovable

Treatment Summary

- The case was treated with 14 + 14 + 14 aligners changed on a 7-day interval protocol
- Total treatment time was 14 months
- Vivera was used for retention, with increased posterior thickness

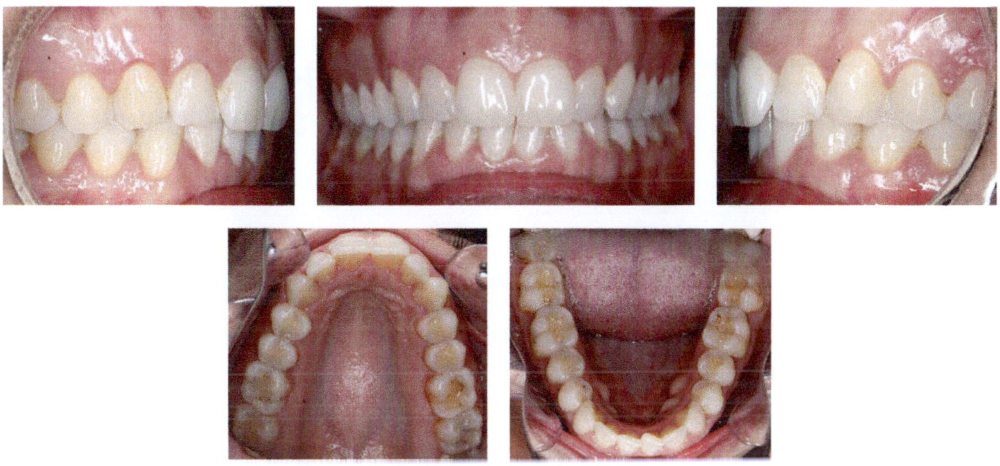

Fig. 21.159 Initial intraoral pictures (right, front, left, upper and lower).

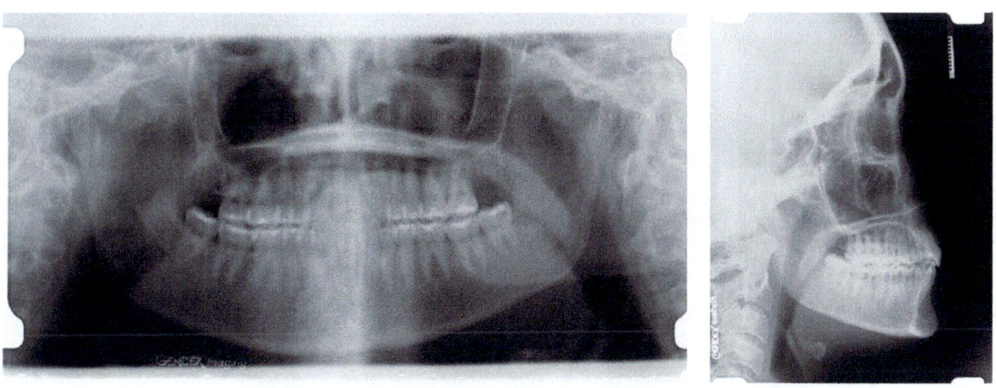

Fig. 21.160 Initial panoramic and lateral X-rays.

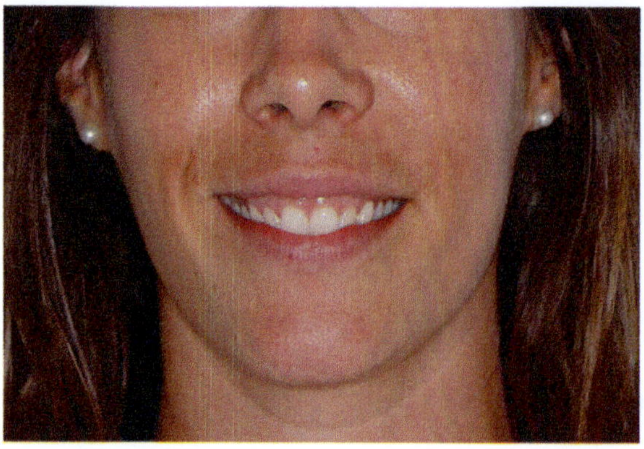

Fig. 21.161 Initial smile.

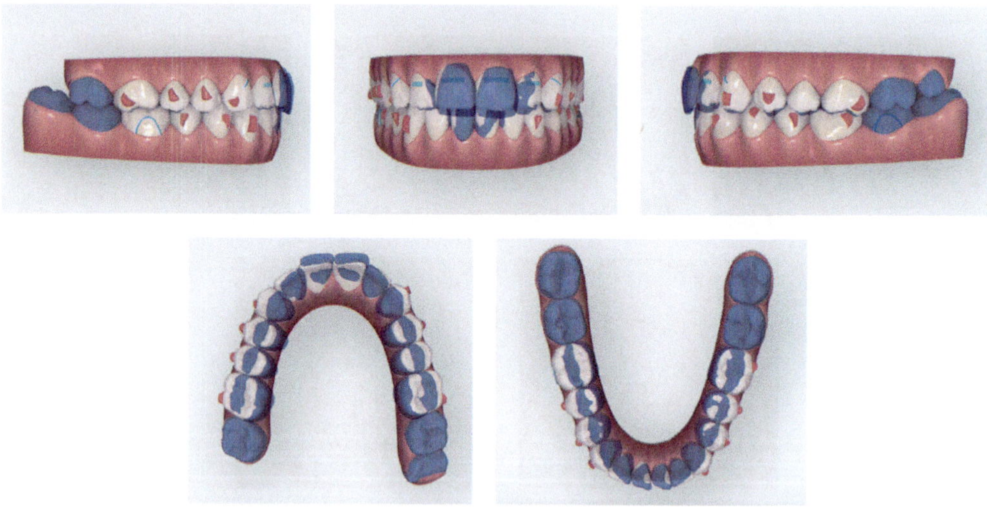

Fig. 21.162 Initial ClinChecks (right, front, left, upper and lower).

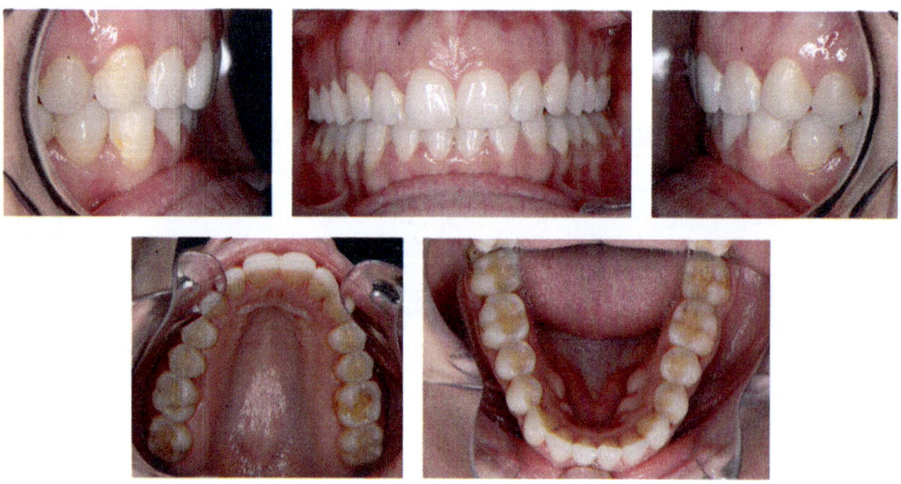

Fig. 21.163 Refinement 1: intraoral views (right, front, left, upper and lower). Alignment has improved but the deep bite stays almost the same owing to simultaneous anterior movement, which makes it less predictable.

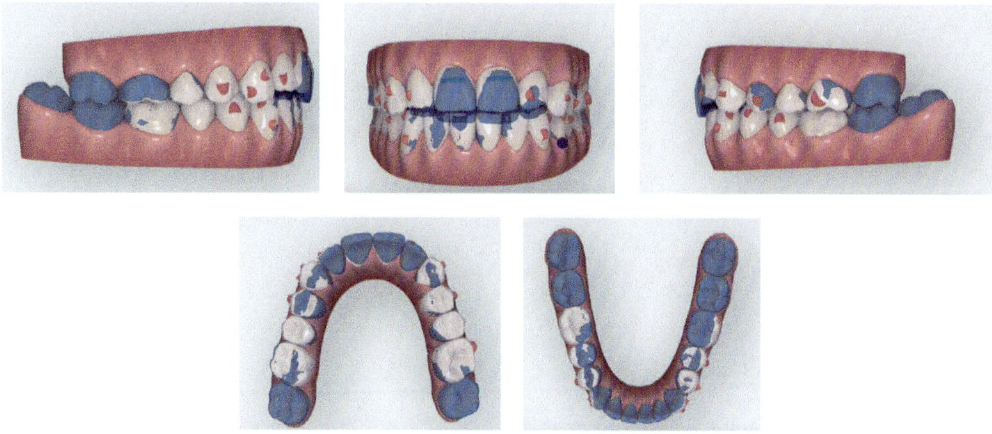

Fig. 21.164 Refinement 1 ClinChecks (right, front, left, upper and lower). Anterior open bite is requested once again from the technician, knowing that 14 aligners will be enough for a proper anterior deep bite correction.

Fig. 21.165 Refinement 2 (aligner): at the end of first refinement, the aligner fits perfectly, even though intrusion does not happen because of simultaneous anterior movements.

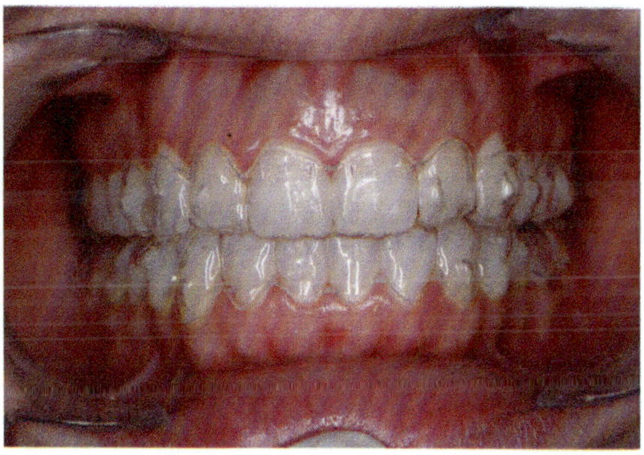

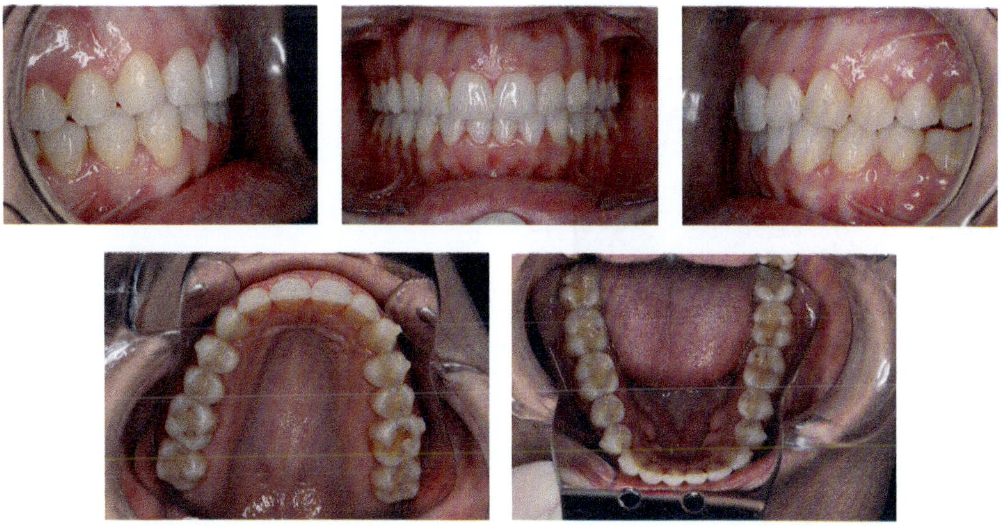

Fig. 21.166 Refinement 2 (aligner: right, front, left, upper and lower). Alignment has improved but the deep bite stays almost the same because of simultaneous anterior movement, which makes it less predictable.

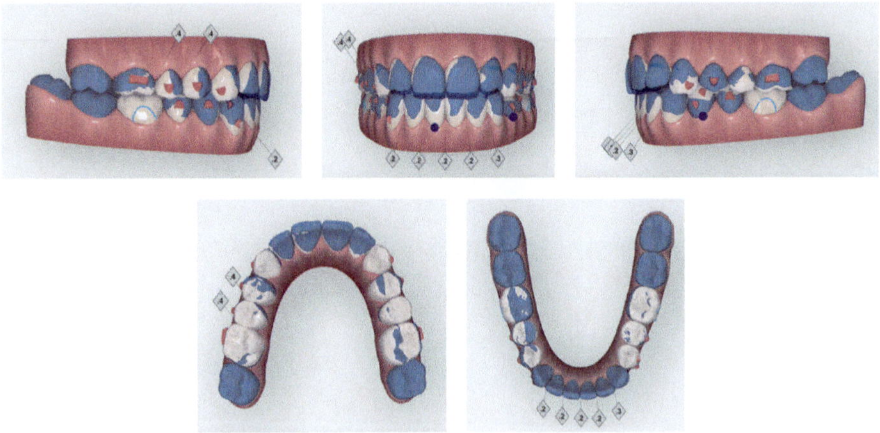

Fig. 21.167 Refinement 2 ClinChecks (right, front, left, upper and lower). Anterior open bite is requested once again from the technician, knowing that 14 aligners will not be enough for a proper anterior deep bite correction.

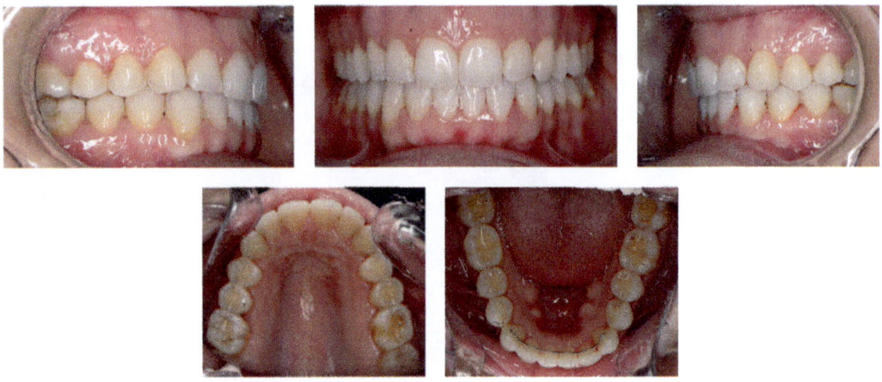

Fig. 21.168 Final intraoral pictures: right, front, left, upper and lower. Deep bite has improved with Lite treatment thanks to hypercorrection.

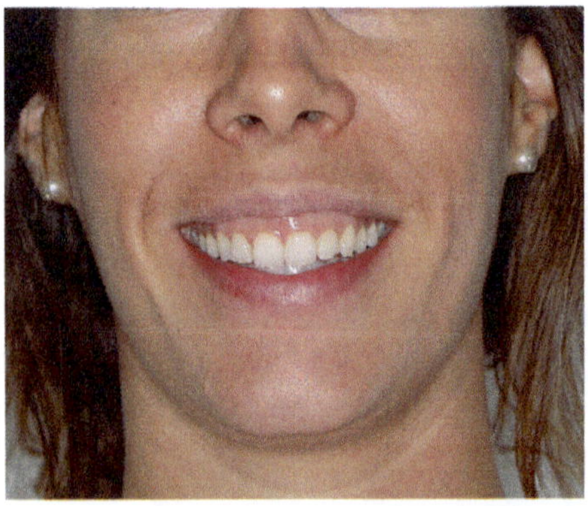

Fig. 21.169 The smile has widened but still gummy, as initially predicted.

22

Asymmetries

After its introduction in 1997, the Invisalign system has been continually developed and improved thanks to considerable investment in research and development, including new attachment designs – SmartTrack material – designed to enable additional treatment biomechanics such as those seen in this book.

Invisalign aligners can perform major tooth movements, such as derotation up to 50 degrees and intrusions, but despite the efficiency of the treatment, its clinical development remains controversial among professionals, some arguing that there are significant limitations, especially in the treatment of complex malocclusions.

For this reason, complex cases are covered at the end of this book in order to show how any patient might benefit from this technique, the advantages of which have already been described.

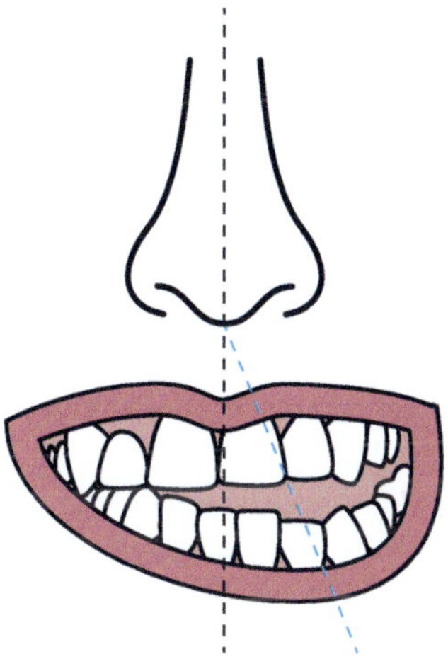

Fig. 22.1 Asymmetries can be managed with specific aligner biomechanics.

22.1 Growing Patients with Asymmetry

22.1.1 Skeletal Class II with Asymmetry

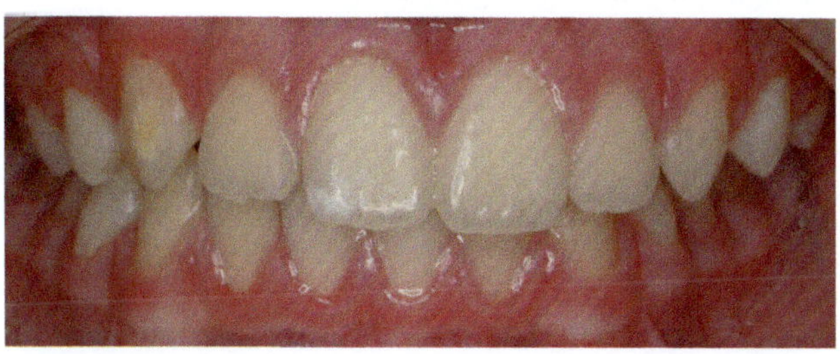

Fig. 22.2 Initial view.

Aligner Techniques in Orthodontics, First Edition. Susana Palma Moya and Javier Lozano Zafra.

Companion website: www.wiley.com/go/lozano-zafra/aligner-techniques

Diagnosis

A 14-year-old boy with hyperdivergent skeletal Class II presented with a dental Class II right subdivision, midfacial asymmetry with slight canted occlusal planes, canted maxillary occlusal plane, left-side deviation of the upper midline (the deviation of both midlines was equal to the width of one lower incisor) and a unilateral scissor bite on left side that led to a facial asymmetry. The patient had unilateral right side mastication.

Treatment Plan

Maxilla:

- Compress left premolars to coordinate both arches
- This movement of compression allows increasing arch length simultaneously, so for that reason it was planned to make the compression and the right sequential distalization simultaneously

Mandible:

- Uprighting of lower incisors to create positive overjet to correct the Class II
- Mesialize the fourth quadrant in order to reduce the amount of upper right distalization needed

Functional treatment:

- The patient was asked to use the left side for mastication during all the treatment.

Requirements for the Technician

Maxilla:

- Compress the upper left quadrant simultaneously to the upper right sequential distalization

Mandible:

- Reciprocal movement of lower incisors retraction and 4s-7s mesialization to correct the Class II on the right side
- Centre the lower midline at the same time as the retraction of the lower incisors to make it more predictable

Treatment Summary

- Total treatment time was 18 months.
- Patient wore two series of aligners replaced at 10-day intervals.
- Patient used Class II 24-hour elastic on right side and only night use on the left.
- Buccal occlusion was corrected into a Class I relationship.
- Careful management of the reciprocal staging of movements were critical for a successful treatment outcome.

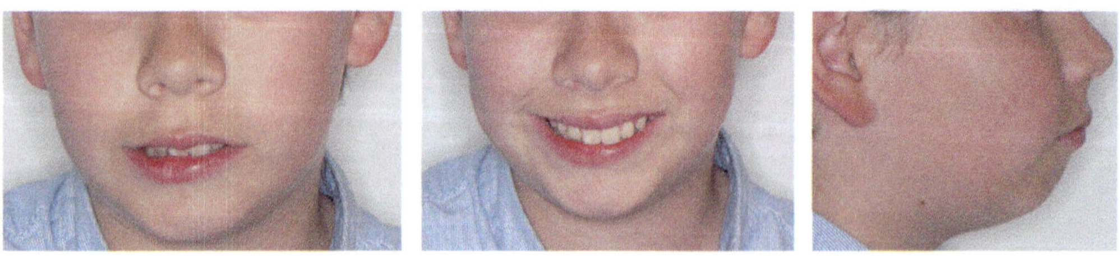

Fig. 22.3 Class II subdivision on right side, deviation of both midlines equal to the width of one incisor. There is a unilateral scissor bite on left side that leads to facial asymmetry.

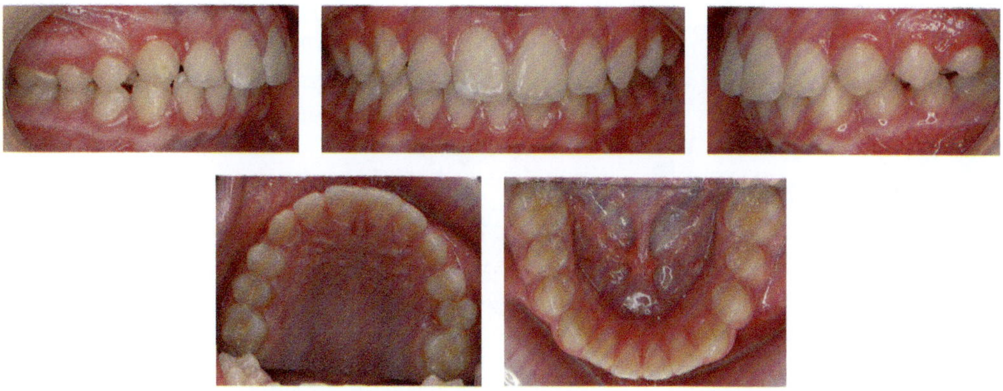

Fig. 22.4 Pretreatment intraoral views.

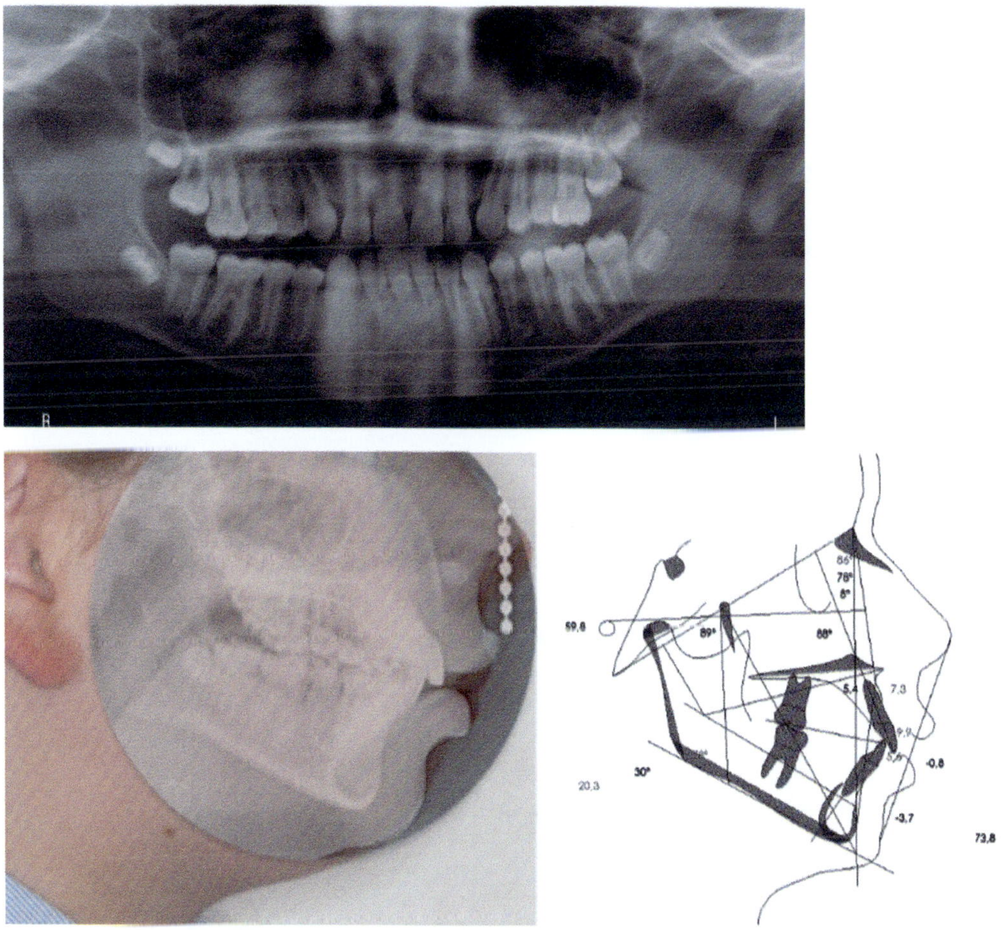

Fig. 22.5 Initial panoramic X-ray, teleradiograph and cephalometry.

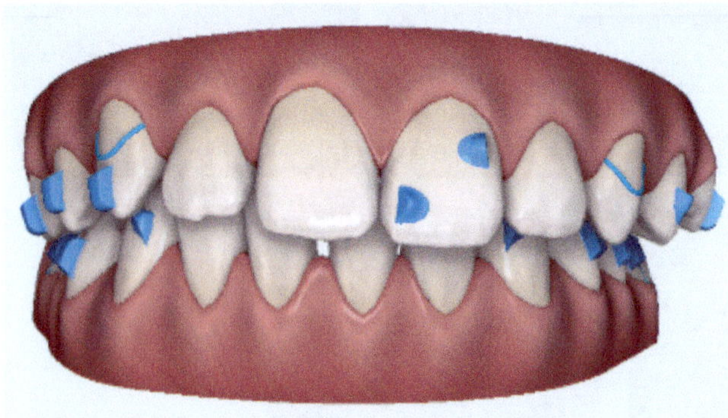

Fig. 22.6 Initial frontal ClinCheck view.

Maxillar:

- Left premolars compression favourable to right distalization (do both movements simultaneously)

Mandible:

- Reciprocal movement: lower incisors retrusion + lower premolar and canine mesialization (all movements are done simultaneously)

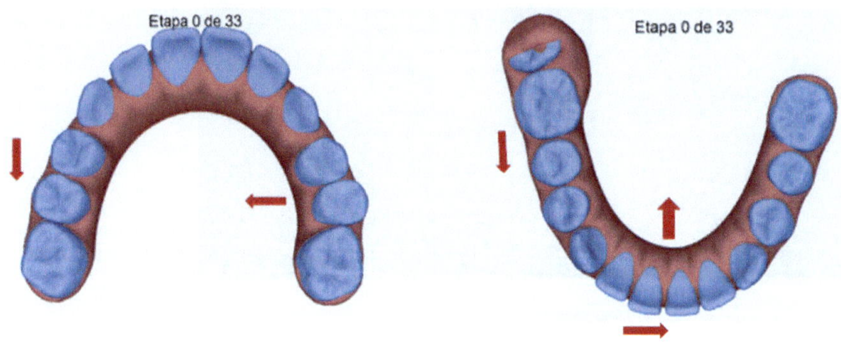

Fig. 22.7 Upper and lower ClinCheck archshape changes and instructions to CAD designer.

- Place vertical attachments in lower premolars and molars to avoid tipping during mesialization
- Class II elastic (right side 24 hours and left side night use)
- Maintain upper incisors torque during retraction

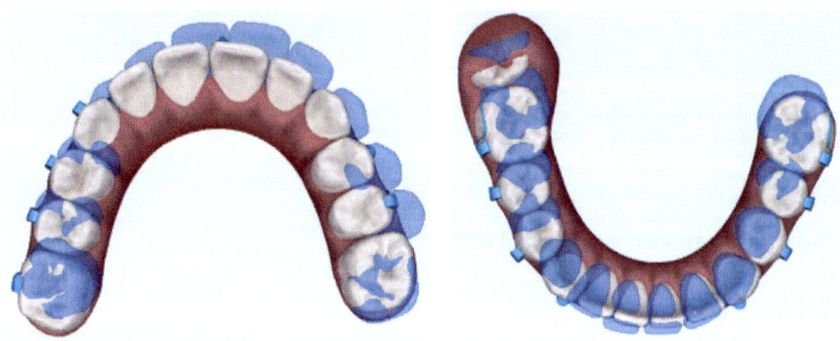

Fig. 22.8 Upper and lower CC superimposition and instructions to CAD designer.

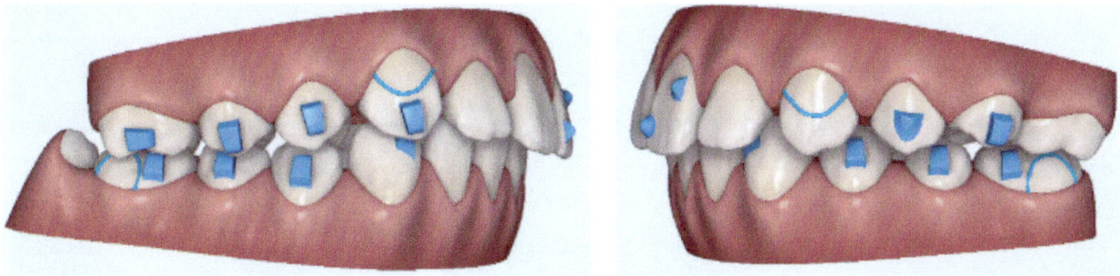

Fig. 22.9 Lateral ClinCheck views.

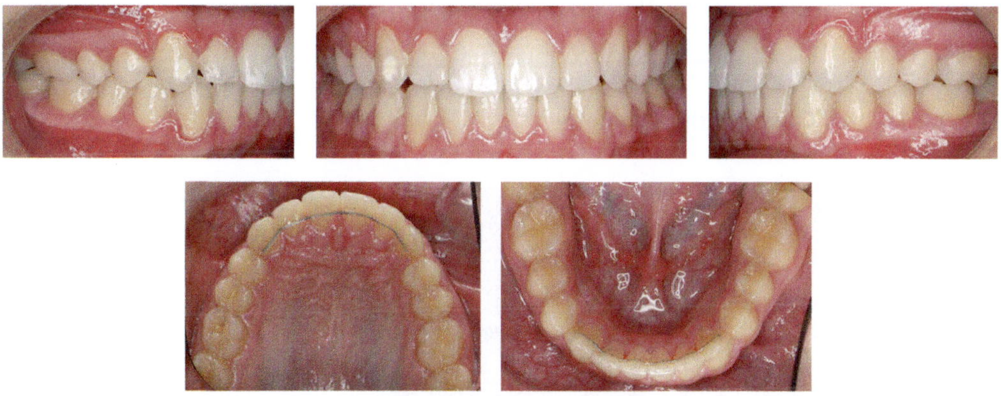

Fig. 22.10 Final intraoral views.

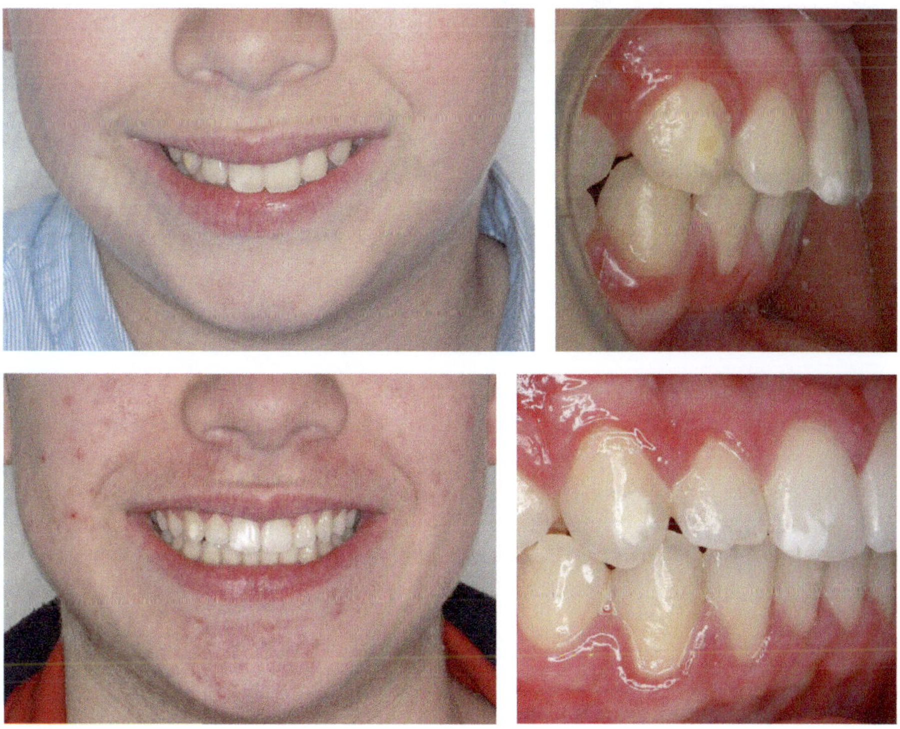

Fig. 22.11 Initial and final smile and overjet.

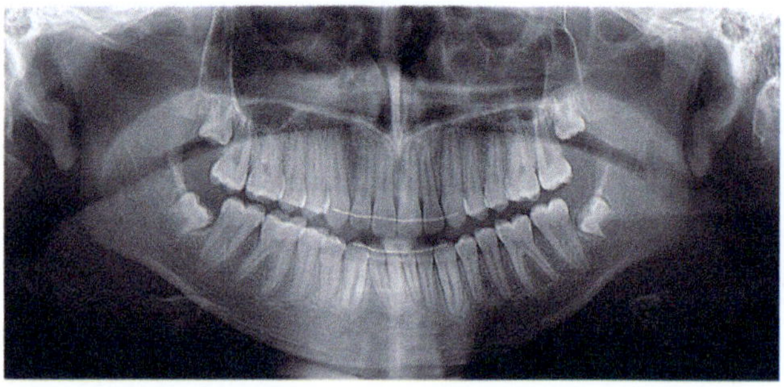

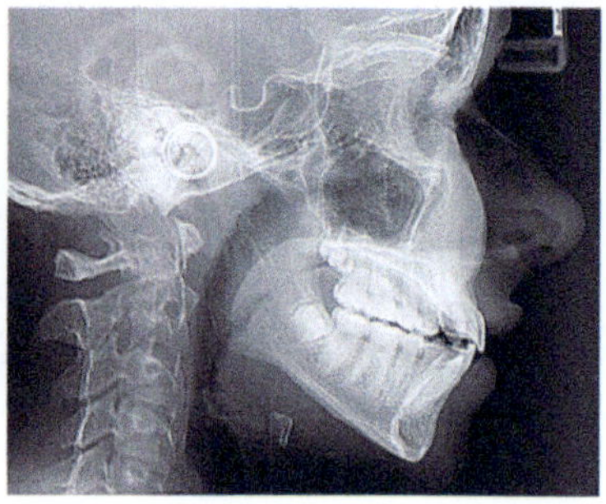

Fig. 22.12 Final panoramic and lateral X-rays.

22.1.2 Skeletal Class II with Asymmetry

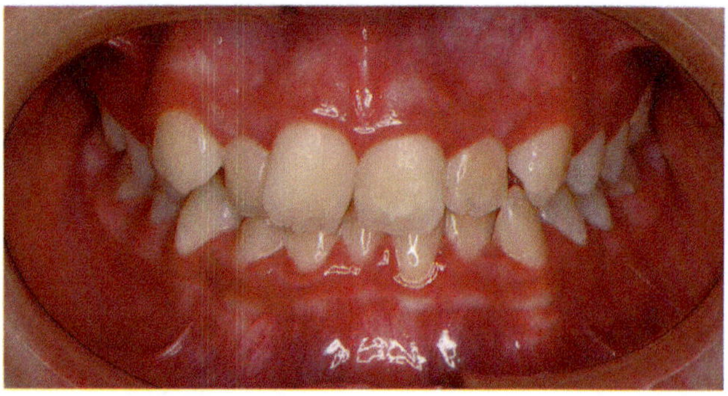

Fig. 22.13 Initial intraoral view.

Diagnosis

A 13-year-old girl with a hypodivergent skeletal Class III pattern presented with mandibular asymmetry, left-side deviation of the lower jaw, dental unilateral class III on right side and a class I on left side. The upper midline was centred with facial midline and she had a deep bite with mild upper and lower crowding

Treatment Plan

Maxilla:

- Symmetrical expansion and proclination of upper incisors
- Tipping and rotation of 11 to be corrected during the anteroposterior movement of the incisor

Mandible:

- Expand and use the retraction movement of the incisors to move lower midline to the right
- Virtual jump (elastic simulation) to centre both midlines, simulating the asymmetric elastics to be used (Class III on right side and Class II on left side)

Requirements for the Technician

Correct the rotation and tipping of 11 in two steps:

- First, procline and rotate mesial-out
- Second, make IPR between 11 and 12 to make room for the intrusion, rotation distal-in and mesial crown tipping of 11

A vertical attachment was placed in the labial surface of 11 to increase predictability (double attachment was not placed by the software as it was a crown tipping, not a root one).

Treatment Summary

- Total treatment time was 26 months.
- Patient used 35 aligners replaced at 2-week intervals.
- After the first set of aligners the patient had a relapse in the asymmetry because of interruption in the use of the elastics and asymmetric growth. At that time a series of additional aligners replaced at 10-day intervals was requested.
- Patient used Class II elastic on left side and Class III elastics on right side (both full-time wear) until 6 weeks before the end of the treatment.
- Buccal occlusion was corrected into a class I.
- Careful management of the sequential movement of 11 made the correction of the incisor's rotation and tipping possible.
- Mandible was centred, as retainer patient is using a Damon splint that maintains the lower midline centred with the upper midline.

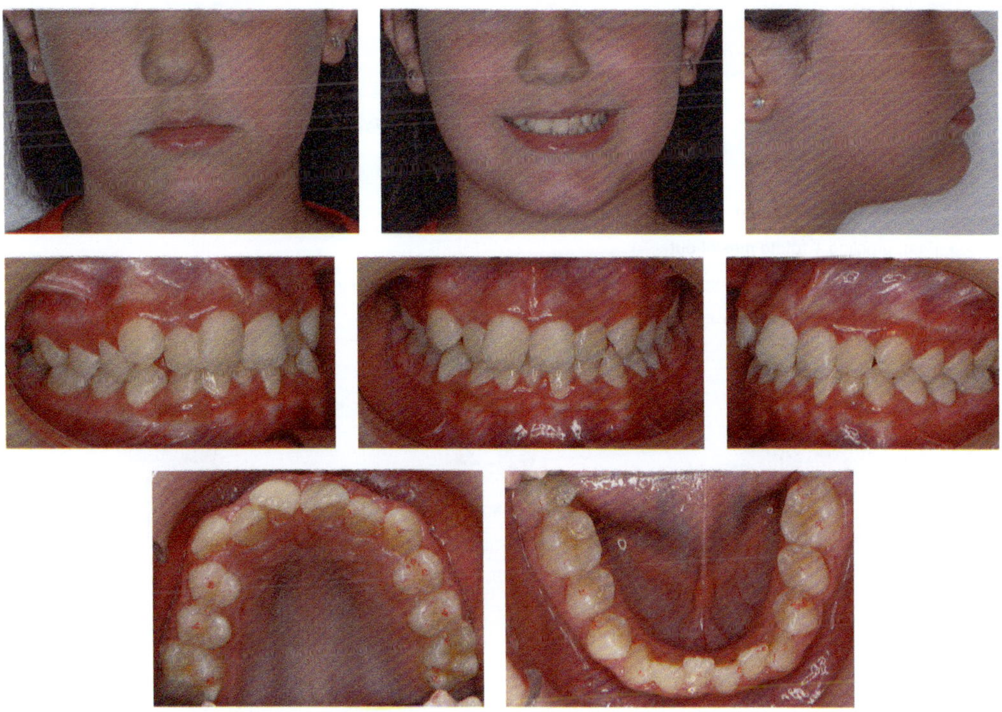

Fig. 22.14 Pretreatment extraoral and intraoral views.

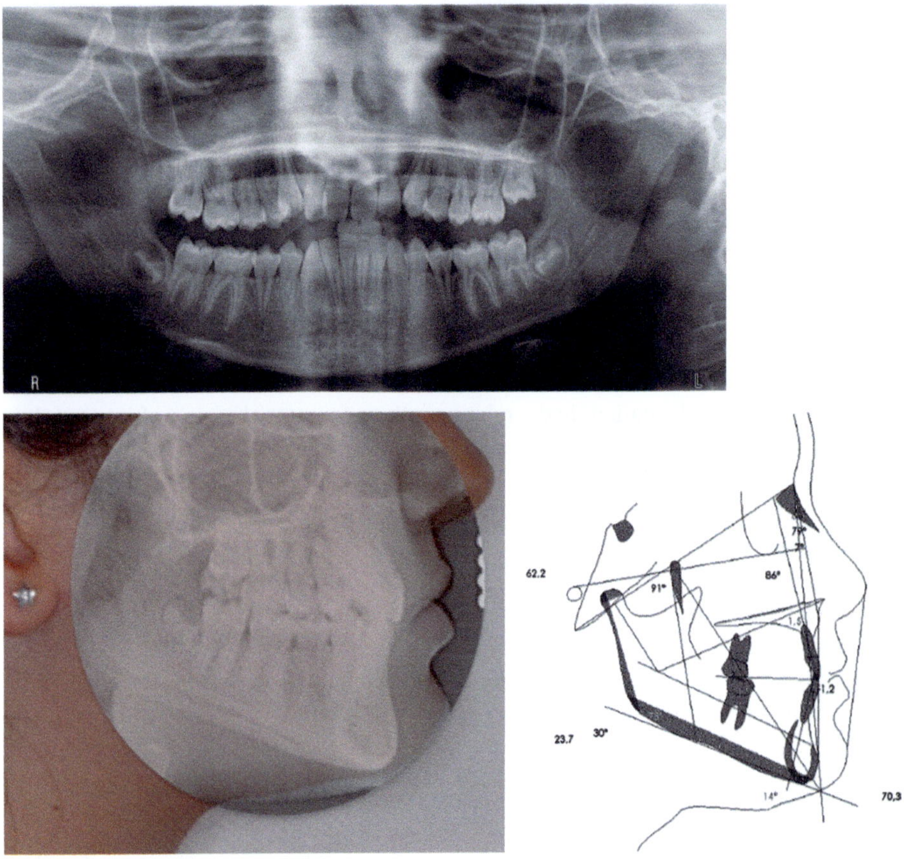

Fig. 22.15 Initial panoramic X-ray, teleradiograph and cephalometry.

Tipping 11 (movements staging):

- First: procline + rotate mesial-out
- Second: 10 degree mesial tipping of the crown + intrusion + rotate distal-in
- Whenever there is rotation + tip, do not start correcting tipping

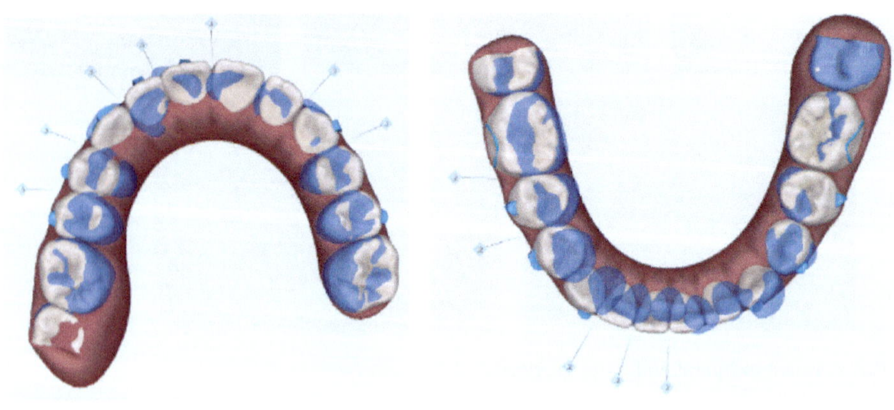

Fig. 22.16 Upper and lower CC superimposition and instructions to CAD designer.

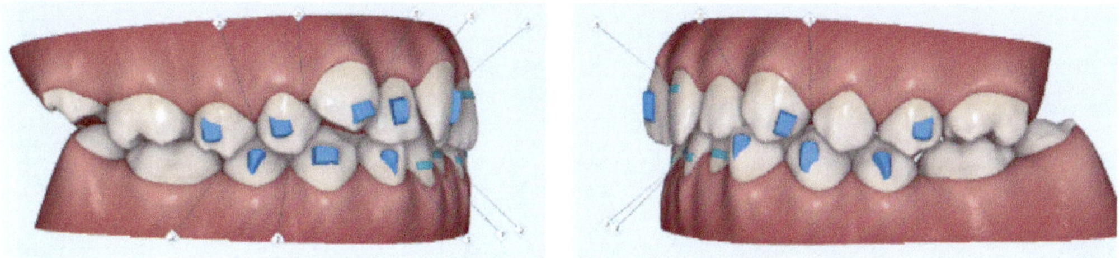

Fig. 22.17 Lateral ClinCheck views.

Fig. 22.18 Initial frontal ClinCheck view.

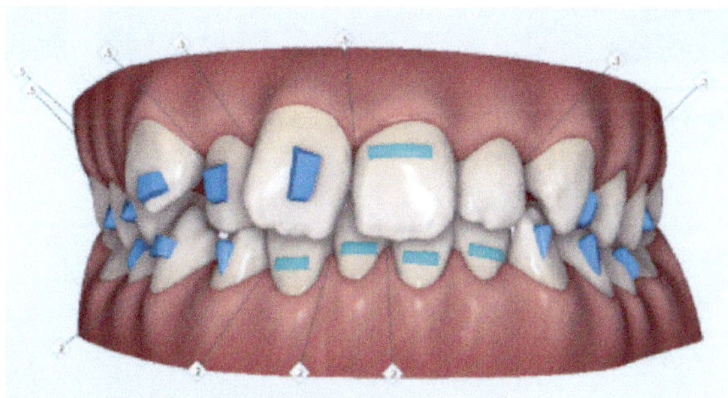

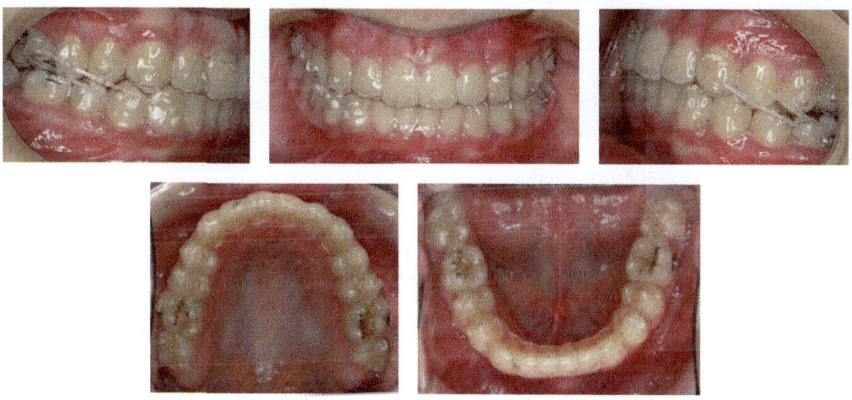

Fig. 22.19 Intermaxillary elastics to correct asymmetric mandibular growth. Use of asymmetric elastics: Class III on the right and Class II on the left.

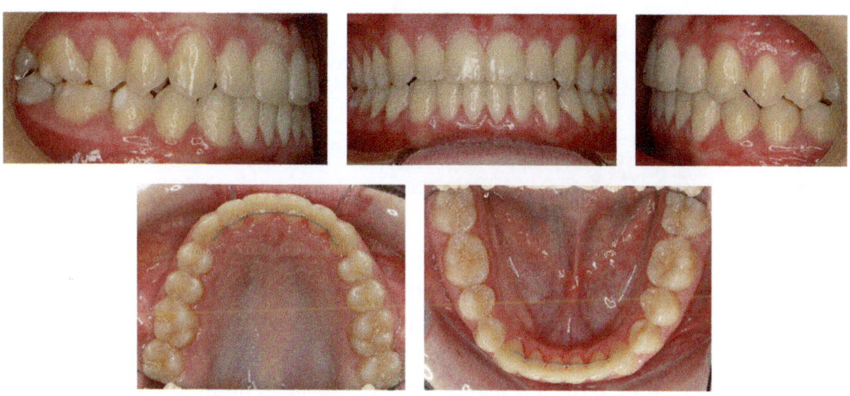

Fig. 22.20 Final occlusion.

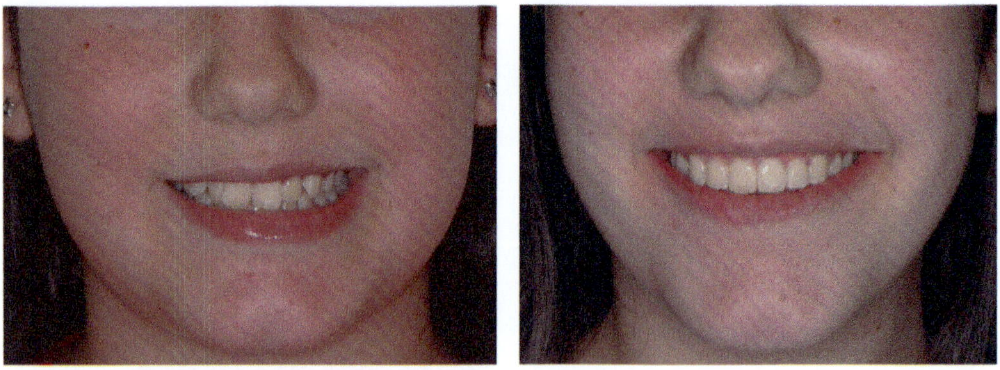

Fig. 22.21 Initial and final smile.

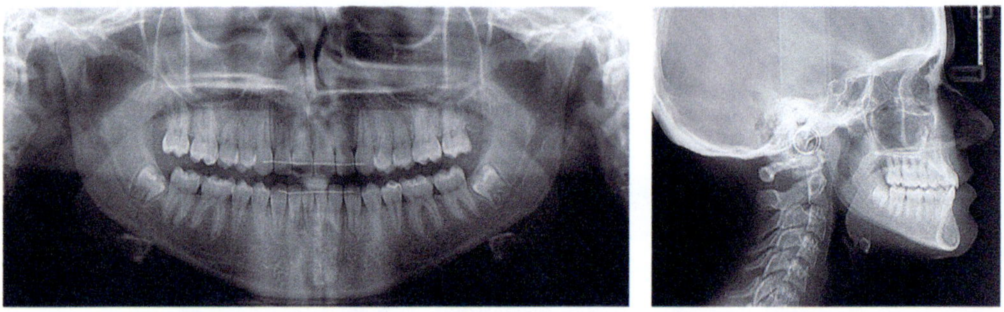

Fig. 22.22 Final panoramic and lateral X-ray.

22.2 Non-growing Patients with Asymmetry

22.2.1 Skeletal Class III with Maxillomandibular Asymmetry

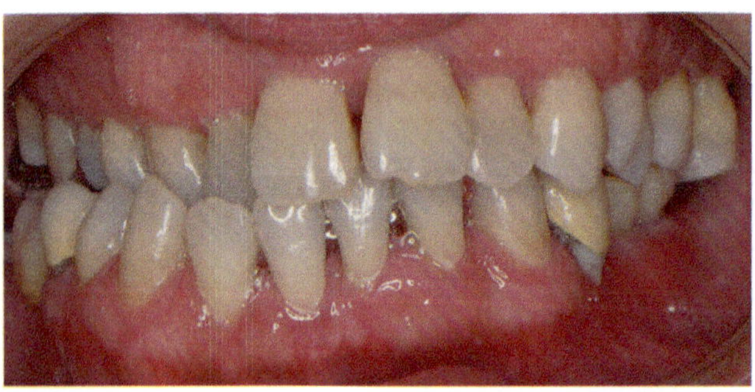

Fig. 22.23 Patient with maxillomandibular asymmetry.

Diagnosis

A 45-year-old woman with normodivergent skeletal Class III presented with mandibular asymmetry, unilateral crossbite on right side, an anterior crossbite of 12 and periodontal disease. Buccal occlusion was Class III on right side and a Class II on the left. There was molar extrusion in 27 and the upper midline was deviated 2 mm to the left with respect to the facial midline.

In the TMJ examination there was a Centric Occlusion (CO)-Centric Relationship (CR) shift, in CR occlusion there was an open bite and premature posterior contacts. Deviation of both midlines was maintained in CR. In the X-ray examination the dentoalveolar protrusion of the incisors could be seen. A dental bridge in the lower right between 45 and 47 was removed before treatment.

Treatment Plan

- Maxilla: remove the dental bridge on the lower right side to expand the upper arch and make a simultaneous upper right distalization to centre upper midline with facial midline using a TAD in upper right tuberosity
- Mandible: asymmetric compression to help correct the posterior crossbite. During the treatment an implant for 37 was planned with a provisional crown to assist the intrusion of 27

Requirements for the Technician

Maxillary:

- Asymmetric expansion and distalization
- Expansion on the upper right side and simultaneous distalization on the right

Mandible:

- Compression of the lower right arch and virtual jump to close the open bite

Biomechanics of the Case

- Maxillary: simultaneous distalization was assisted by a TAD on the right tuberosity and a 'rein horse power chain' to assist the movement of all the teeth of the upper arch simultaneously. To close the open bite, relative extrusion of the upper incisors and a virtual jump to coordinate both arches would be needed
- Mandible: compression of the lower right arch tent performed to create a mesial movement of the lower left side compensated by implants on 37 and 36. A TAD mesial to 47 is placed to upright the root of 47 and to hold the molar as anchorage for the criss-cross elastics

Treatment Summary

- Initially, the patient had used 38 aligners replaced at 10-day intervals
- After the first set of aligners the posterior crossbite had been corrected and the upper midline was centred with the facial midline, so a series of additional aligners replaced at 7-day intervals was requested
- The patient had used Class II elastic full-time worn on right side and triangle elastics on right side. Criss-cross elastics were used on the right side for night use. The buccal occlusion has been corrected into a class I
- Careful management of the anchorage with the microscrews and the implants has been critical to the successful correction of the malocclusion
- It is very important in asymmetric patients to explore the CR position, if the CO is not the same as CR we must scan all patient's photograph records in CR and check with the technician that the initial position of the ClinCheck corresponds with the position in CR of the patient
- A bilateral Class I was achieved with normal overjet and overbite and with the full correction of the posterior crossbite

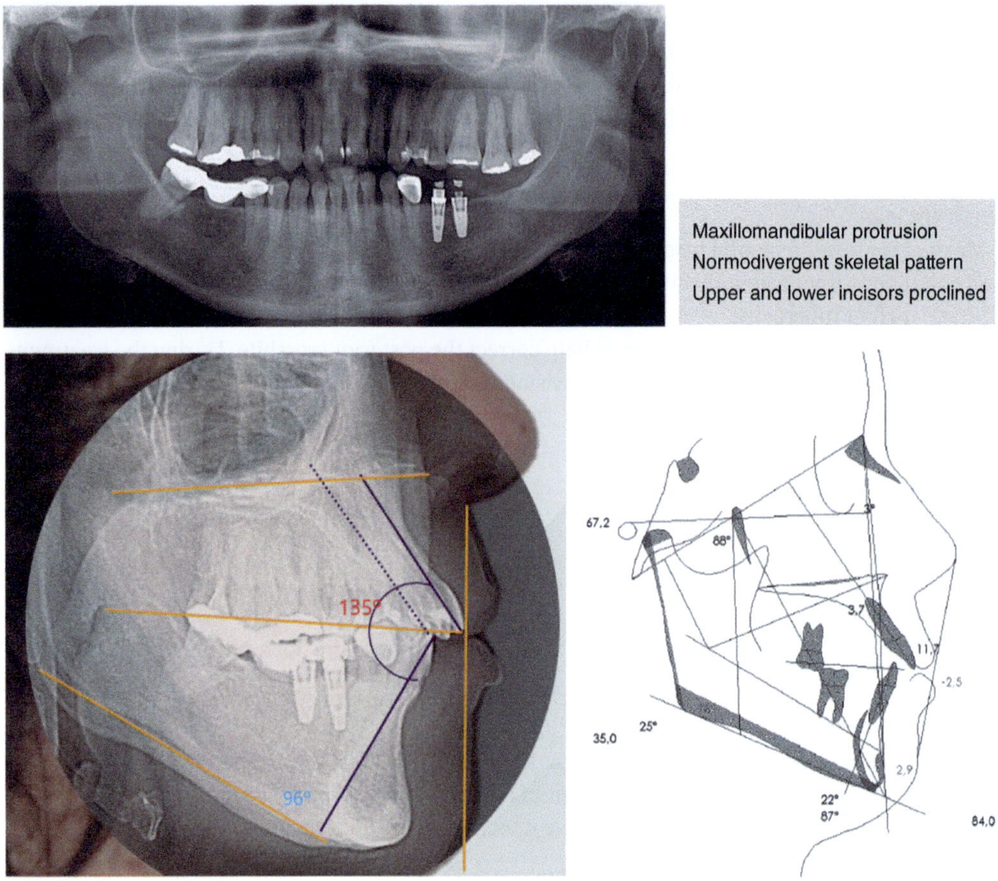

Fig. 22.24 Initial panoramic X-ray, teleradiograph and cephalometry.

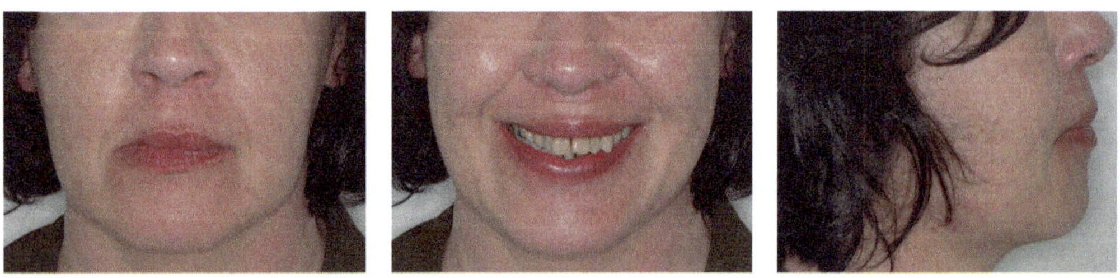

Fig. 22.25 Pretreatment extraoral views.

Intraoral Analysis

- Unilateral Class III
- Unilateral posterior crossbite on the right side
- Right-side mandibular deviation
- Extrusion of 27
- Symmetric maxillary compression

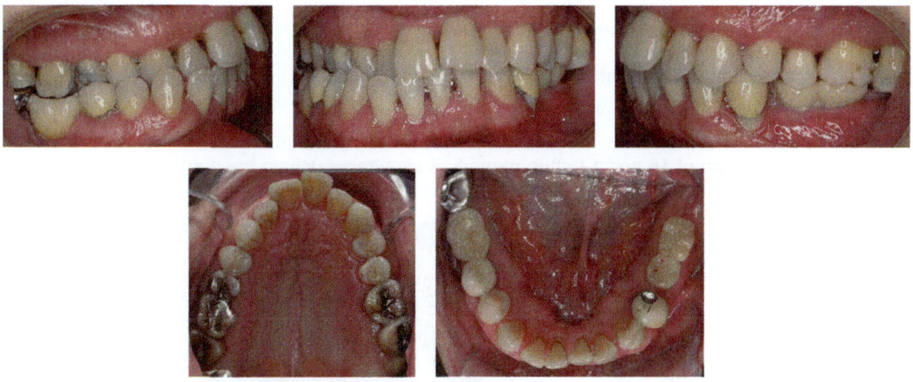

Fig. 22.26 Occlusion in centric occlusion (CO).

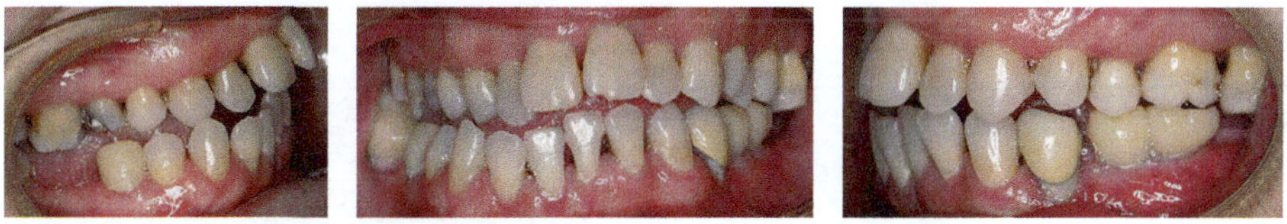

Fig. 22.27 Occlusion in centric relation (CR). In this situation, photographing and scanning must be done.

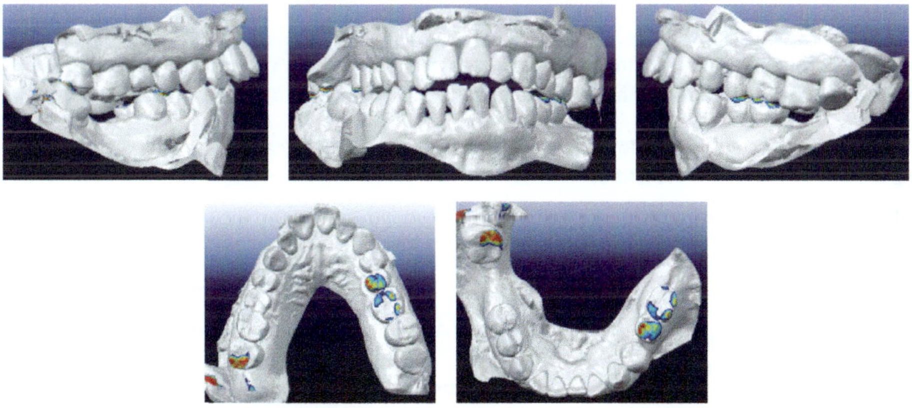

Fig. 22.28 iTero occlusion analysis.

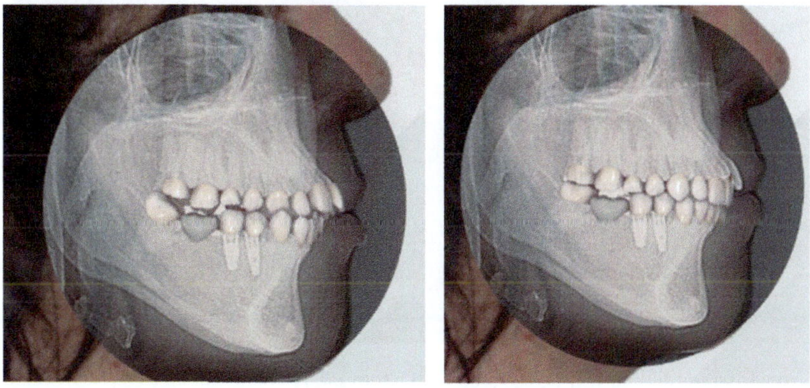

Fig. 22.29 The treatment goal is asymmetric expansion of the maxilla to correct a unilateral posterior crossbite.

- Asymmetric maxillary expansion: use left side as anchorage
- Centre both midlines: upper right distalization
- TAD 10 mm in maxillary tuberosity
- Simultaneous distalization of 16 and 17, then move 5–5 simultaneously to the right

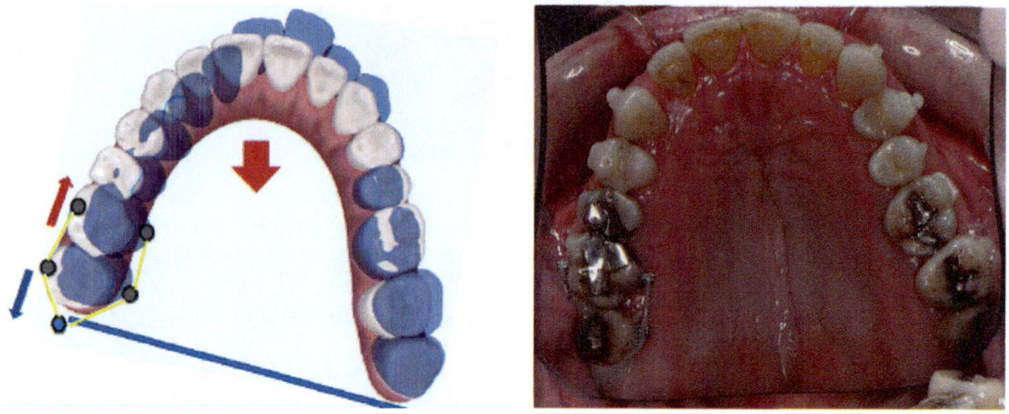

Fig. 22.30 A temporary anchorage device on the tuberosity will assist the movement.

- **Coordinate arches though a virtual jump**: to correct a full class II in a non-growing patient aligners must be accompanied by additional anchorage as TADs.
- **Unilateral crossbite on right side:** it will create a left-side force of mesialization which will be compensated by implants in 36 and 37
- **Vertical attachment in molars**

- **Unilateral crossbite on right side** – it will create a left-side force of mesialization which will be compensated by implants in 36 and 37

→

- **Vertical AT in molars**
- **TAD in mesial of 47,** to apply mesial root tipping and to use 47 as anchorage to use criss-cross elastics on right side

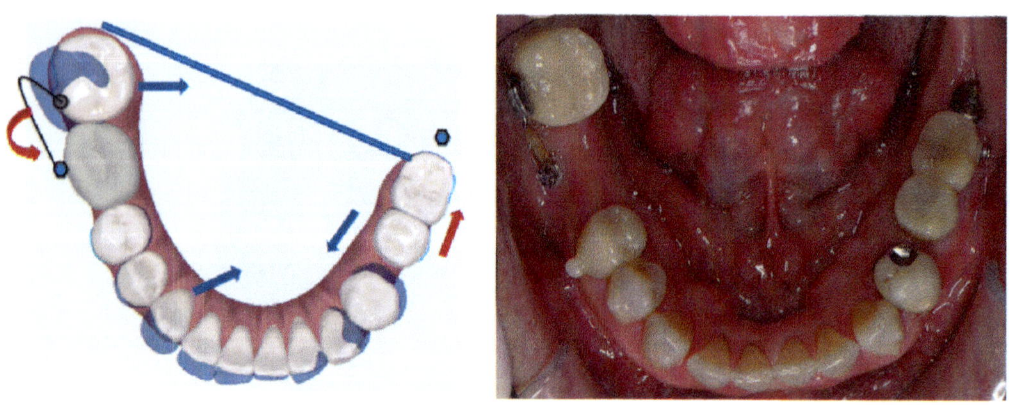

Fig. 22.31 Lower arch molar straightening will be assisted with a temporary anchorage device (TAD) and a sectional wire.

- **Maxilla:** expansion of right side, using teeth on the left side as anchorage. (sequence movements on upper arch)
- Palatal attachments AT HBG 3 mm in four upper incisors (anterior anchorage during expansion)

- Unilateral expansion of right side
- Cutting lower right dental bridge
- Lower right compression to correct crossbite (using implants as anchorage on left side)
- AT must not be very retentive (periodontal disease)

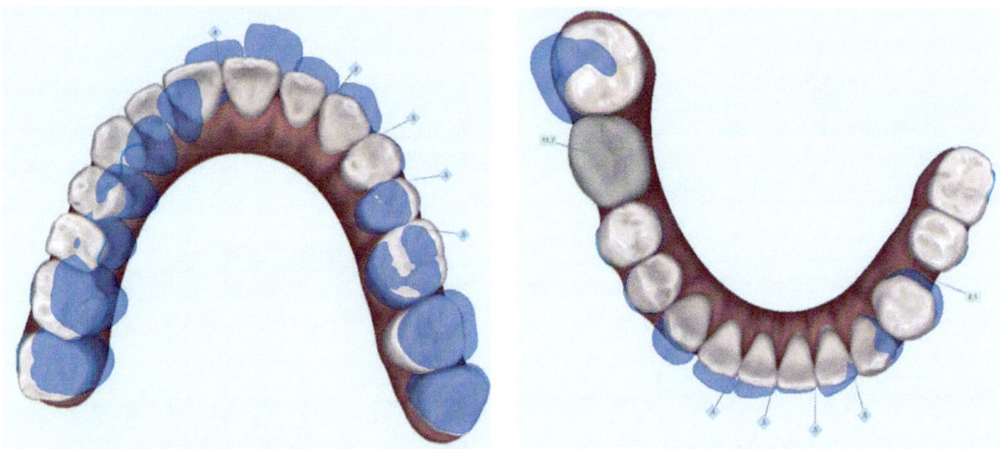

Fig. 22.32 Occlusal ClinCheck views.

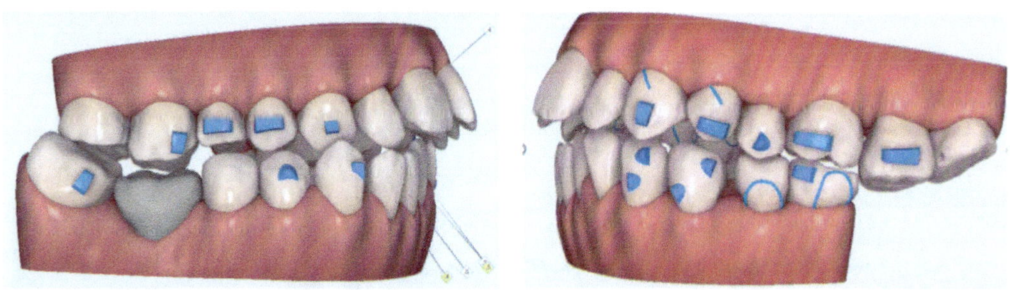

Fig. 22.33 Lateral ClinCheck views.

Fig. 22.34 Frontal ClinCheck view.

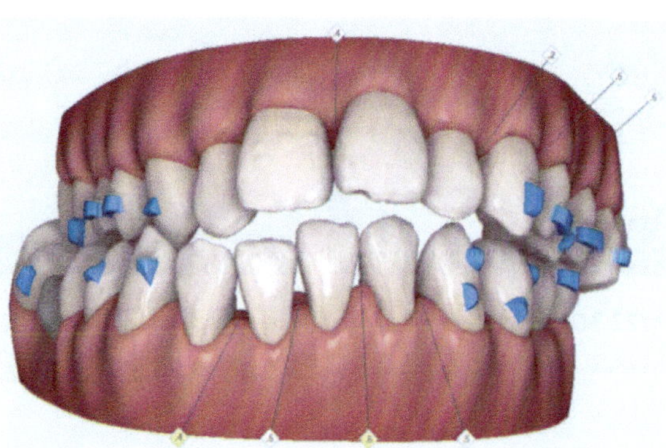

Biomechanics

- Correct unilateral posterior crossbite
- Centre both midlines
- Mesialize 3.4 and 3.3 to Class I (lower left implants as anchorage)
- Asymmetric expansion on upper right side
- IPR + lower right compression, applying lingual root torque (criss-cross elastic during the night)
- Make all incisors, torque equal, followed by retrusion and relative extrusion of upper incisors + virtual jump

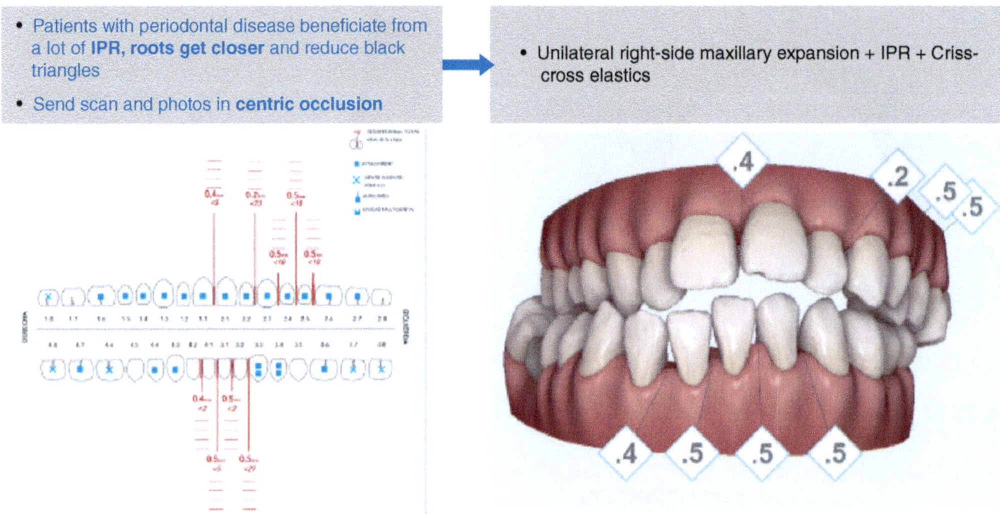

Fig. 22.35 Interproximal reduction.

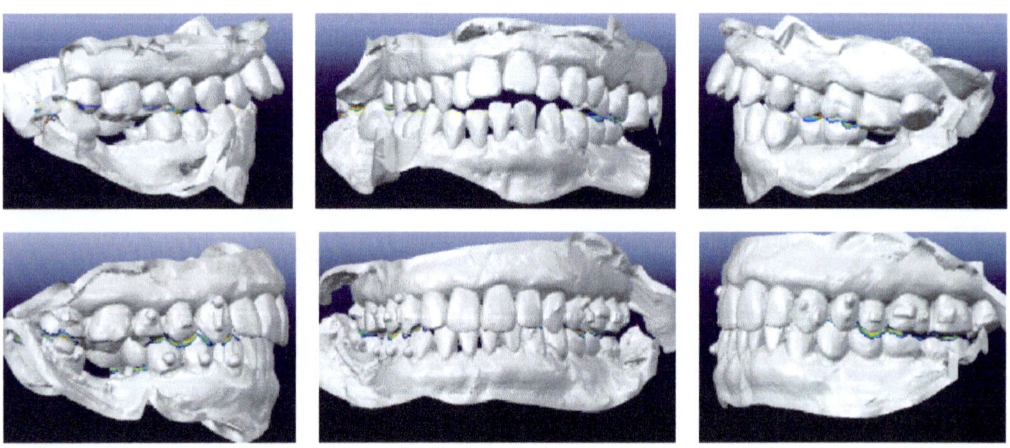

Fig. 22.36 Evolution in the occlusal contact.

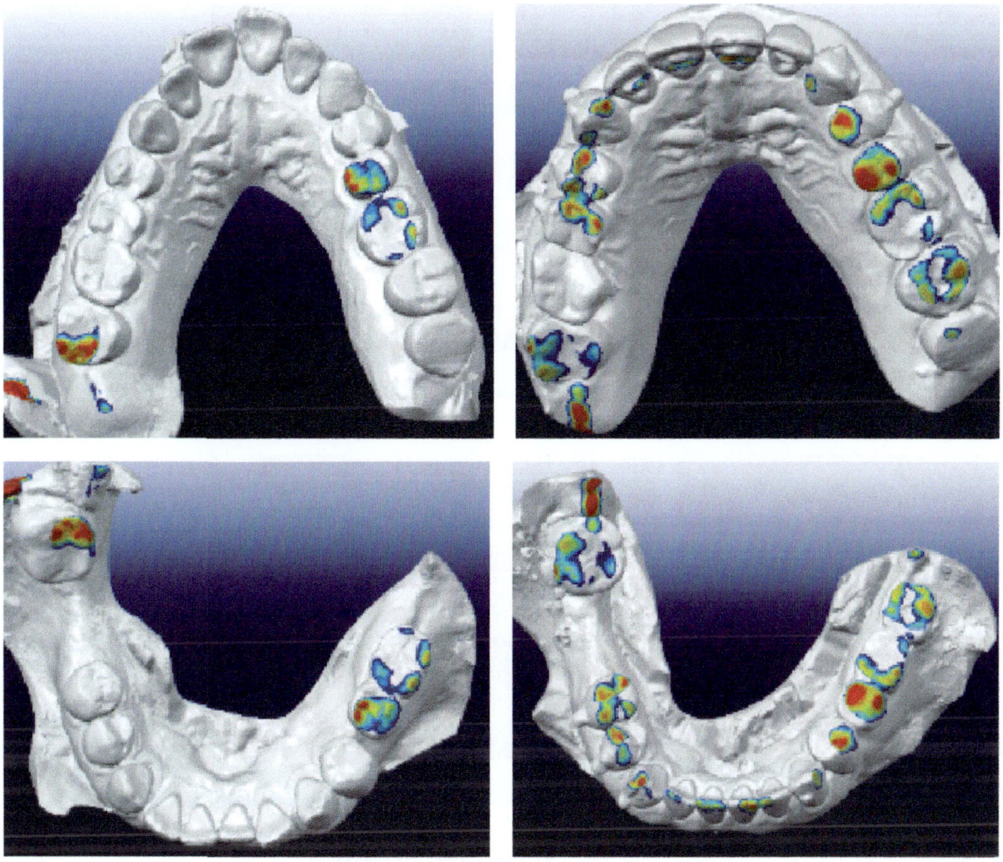

Fig. 22.37 Arch development.

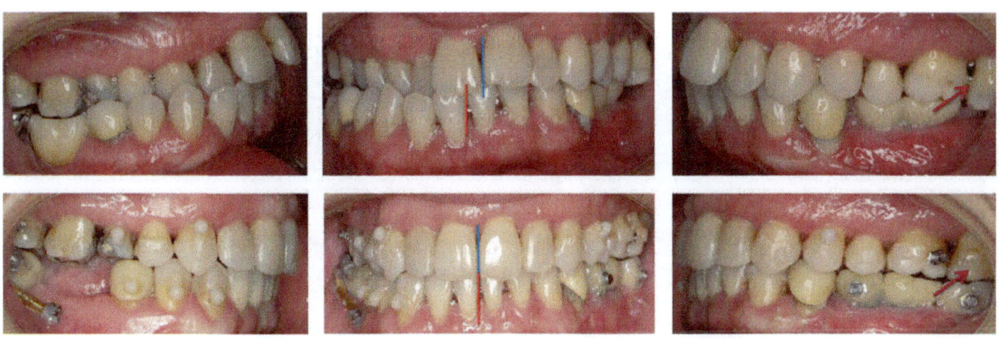

Fig. 22.38 Initial (upper) views and evolution at month 18 of treatment (lower).

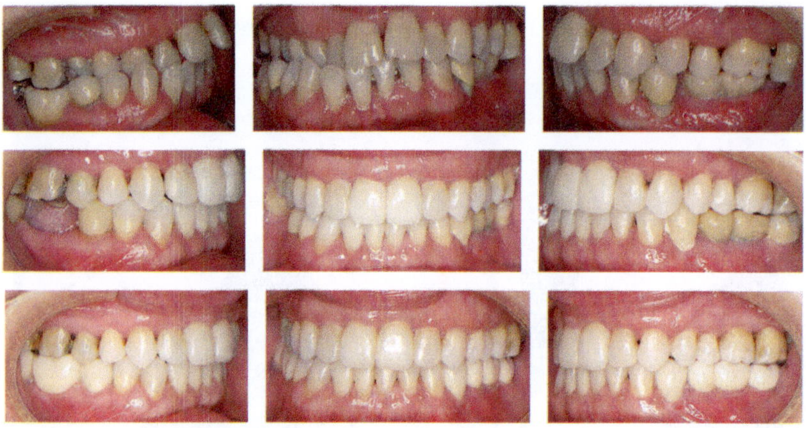

Fig. 22.39 Initial (upper), after Invisalign and before prosthesis (middle) and final views (lower).

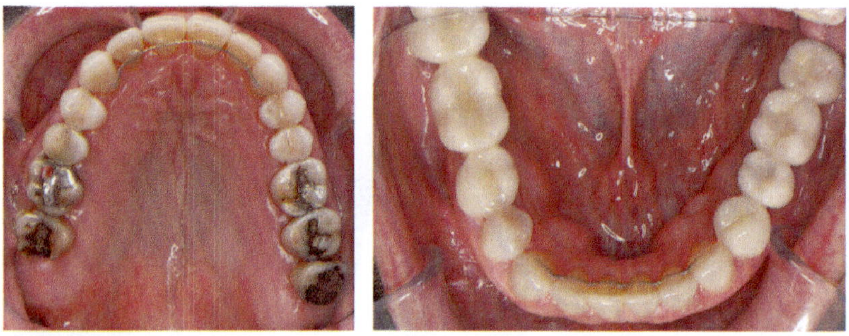

Fig. 22.40 Final occlusal.

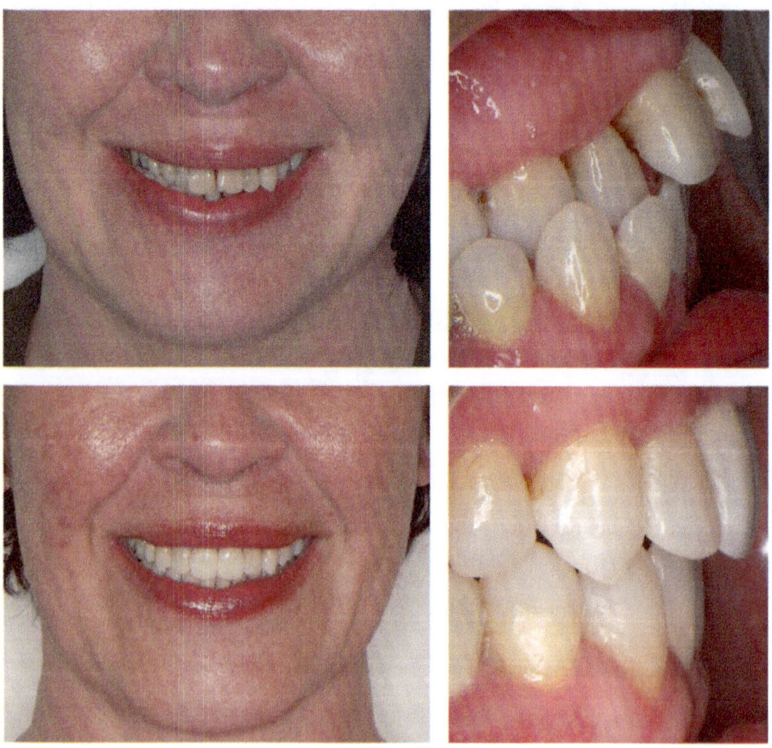

Fig. 22.41 Comparison of initial and final smile and overjet.

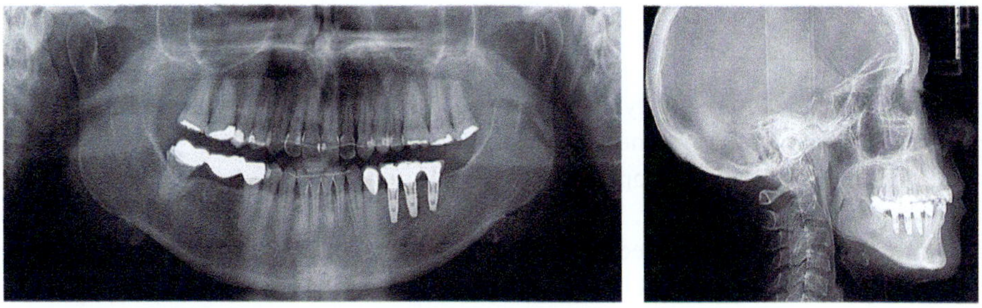

Fig. 22.42 Final panoramic and lateral X-rays.

22.2.2 Skeletal Class III with Mandibular Asymmetry

Fig. 22.43 Initial intraoral view.

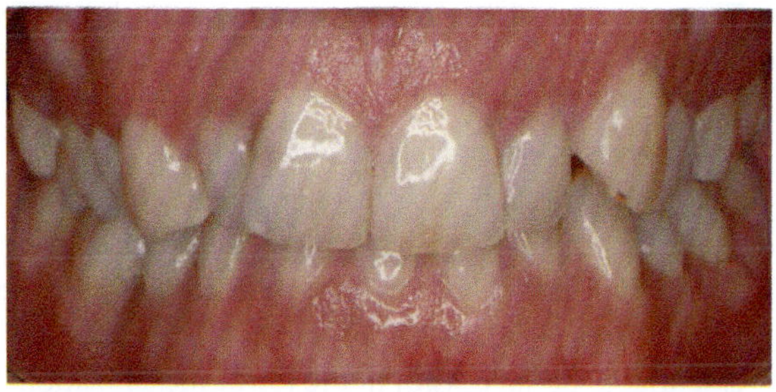

Diagnosis

A 40-year-old patient with hyperdivergent skeletal Class II presented with Class II left subdivision, missing 14/35 and 45 from a previous orthodontic treatment. There was a vertical asymmetry with canted occlusal plane and left-side deviation of the mandible and the upper midline is centred with facial midline. They had a 90% deep bite, over extruded upper incisors and lingual tipping of upper and lower incisors.

Treatment Plan

- Asymmetric expansion of the upper arch to coordinate the upper and lower arches and provide upper incisors with labial torque
- In the lower arch, level the curve of Spee through lower incisor proclination and intrusion and correct the unilateral Class II on the left side (for this a lower left mesialization was planned as the upper midline was centred with the facial midline)

Requirements for the Technician

Maxillary:

- Make upper arch symmetric in size, form and shape, (asymmetric expansion) labial torque to upper incisors
- Level right and left side vertically to correct canting

Mandible:

- Make a sequential mesialization of the lower arch, first proclining lower incisors until the labial surface becomes perpendicular to the bone
- With the lower incisor's root anchored to the cortical bone, mesialize both premolars 33 and 34 and finally both molars 36 and 37

Biomechanics for Lower Mesialization

Staggered sequential mesialization:

- First, procline lower incisors until they are perpendicular to their bone, using proclination to simultaneously centre the lower midline to the right
- While proclining the lower incisors apply mesial tipping to the roots of the molars, preparing them for the posterior mesialization
- At this stage lower incisors are anchored to the cortical bone; this is when the lower canine and the premolar can start their movement to a mesial position (mesialize 33 and 34)
- Once the premolars are on a mesial position, reposition the microscrew distal of 33 and mesialize both molars simultaneously applying mesial tipping to the root during all the mesialization movement

Treatment Summary

- The treatment was completed in 28 months.
- The patient used 49 aligners replaced at 10-day intervals.
- After the first set of aligners canting on the occlusal plane had already been corrected by intrusion on the upper right premolars and canines, arches were coordinated and the lower left canine and premolar were mesialized into a Class I.
- The patient needed two sets of additional aligners that were replaced at 7-day intervals.
- In the first set a virtual jump was planned to centre both midlines at the end of the treatment. She used Class II elastic with full-time wear on the left and night use on the right.
- Careful management of the anchorage and the staging of movements in the lower arch was essential to be successful in the lower mesialization.
- The microscrews in this case provided the necessary anchorage for the uprighting and mesialization of the lower molars.
- A bilateral class I was achieved with normal overjet and overbite, and symmetric arches in size and torque. The patient smile has improved considerably.

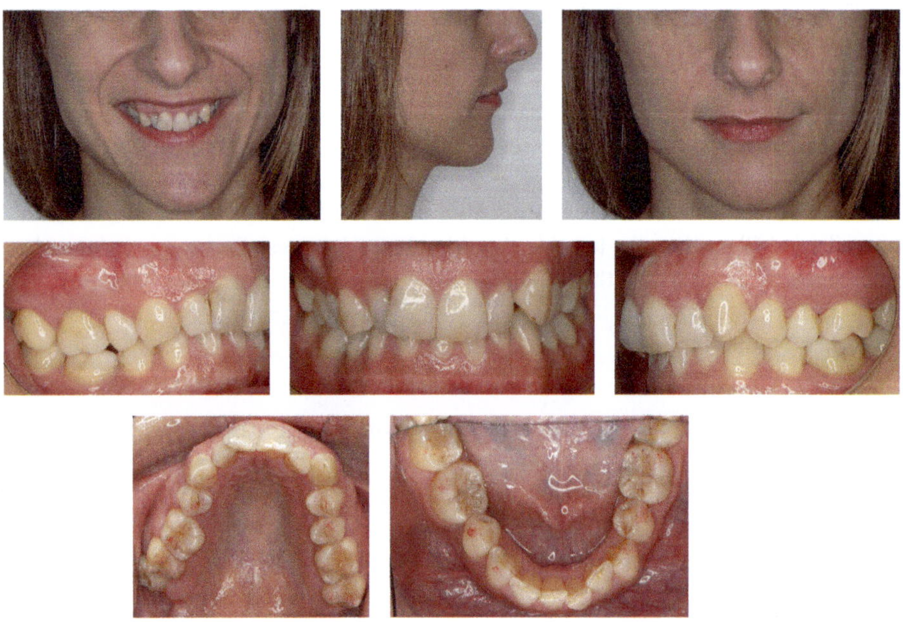

Fig. 22.44 Pretreatment extraoral and intraoral views.

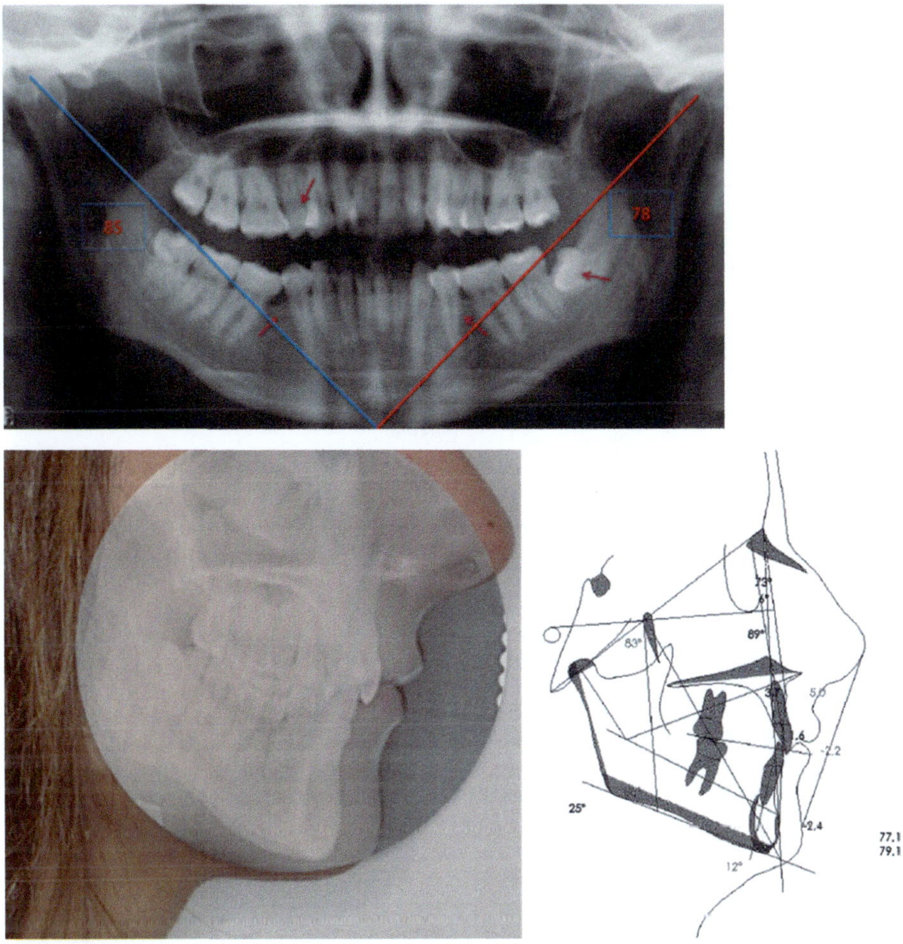

Fig. 22.45 Initial panoramic X-ray, teleradiograph and cephalometry.

- Upright 36 and 46, with mesial tipping to the root
- Planning lower molar distalization with the tooth tied to a TAD will make an 'en masse' mesialization from 5 to 5
- Use the TAD to upright 36 and 46, create anchorage to protrude lower incisors and level the curve of Spee

- Upper proclination
- Anchorage attachment HBO bevelled to occlusal in 4s and 5s, and horizontal attachment in 6s, combined with class II elastics

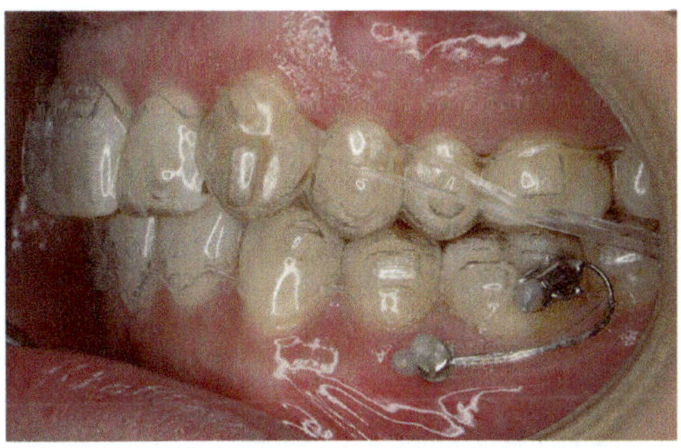

Fig. 22.46 Lateral sectional wire applied based on a temporary achorage device (TAD).

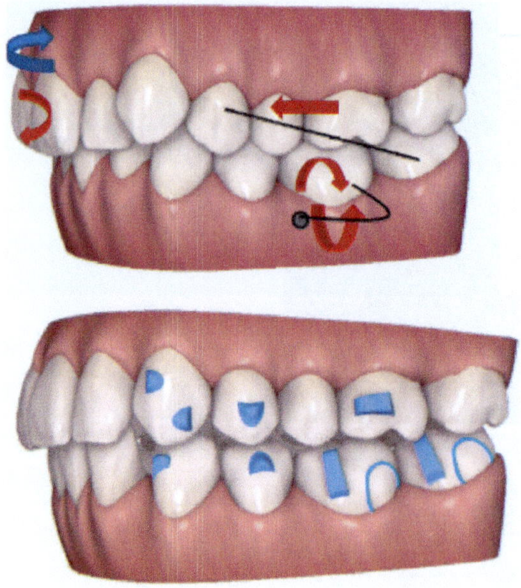

ClinCheck with virtual jump

Maxilla:

- Provide labial torque to upper incisors
- Class II elastics to provide posterior anchorage

Fig. 22.47 Lateral ClinCheck views showing forces applied.

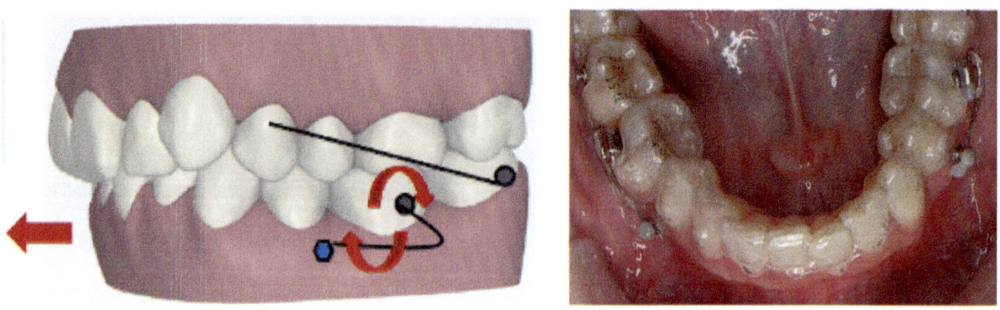

Fig. 22.48 Lateral ClinCheck view showing forces applied with the temporary anchorage device (TAD) and sectional wires, and intraoral view.

Maxilla:

Procline and apply upper lingual root torque **TRL to upper incisors**

- Upper asymmetric expansion
- Correct overjet and overbite
- Final occlusion: bilateral Class I on both canines and Class I molar on the right and Class III on the left

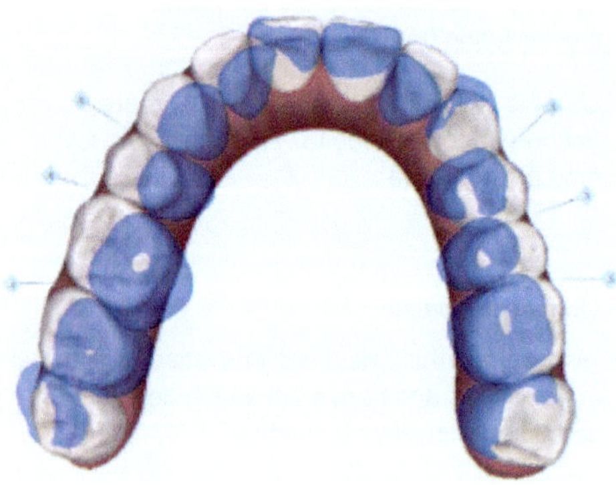

Fig. 22.49 Upper ClinCheck view superimposition.

Mandible:

- Sequential mesialization on lower left side (first, incisors, second L3 and L4 and third L6/L7) using TADs mesial to first molars.
- Centre lower midline with upper midline (at the same time of incisors proclination)
- Lower incisor intrusion during proclination (relative intrusion) to level curve of Spee

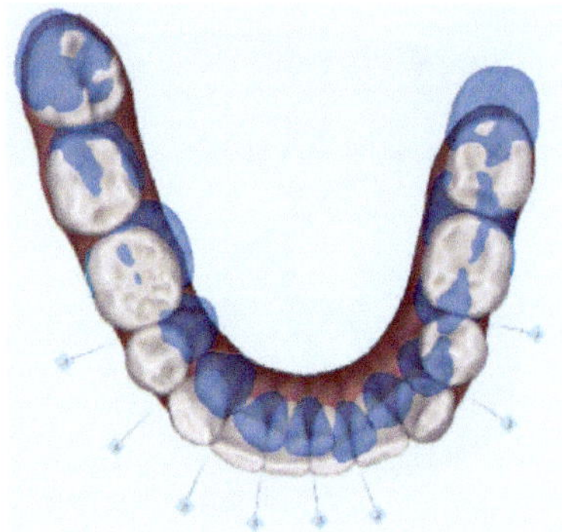

Fig. 22.50 Lower ClinCheck view superimposition.

- Centre lower midline with upper midline
- Level curve of Spee (relative intrusion of lower incisors)

- IPR + proclination + upper and lower intrusion

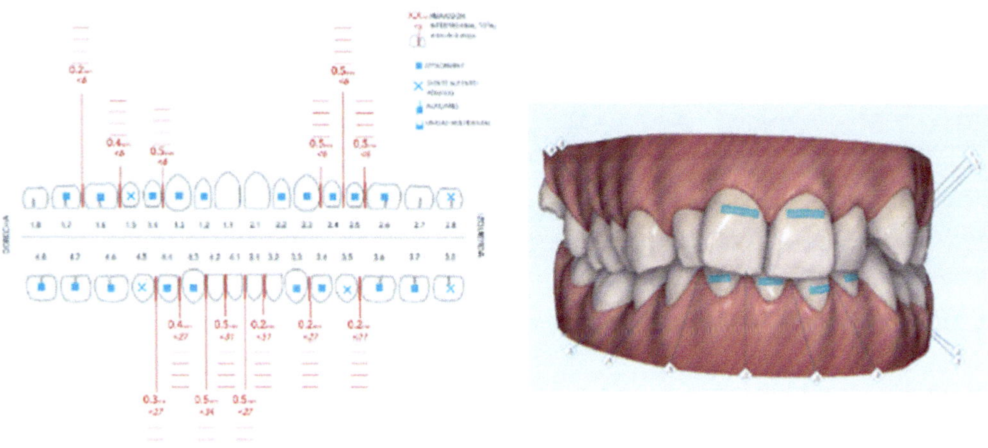

Fig. 22.51 Second set of aligners. Frontal ClinCheck view.

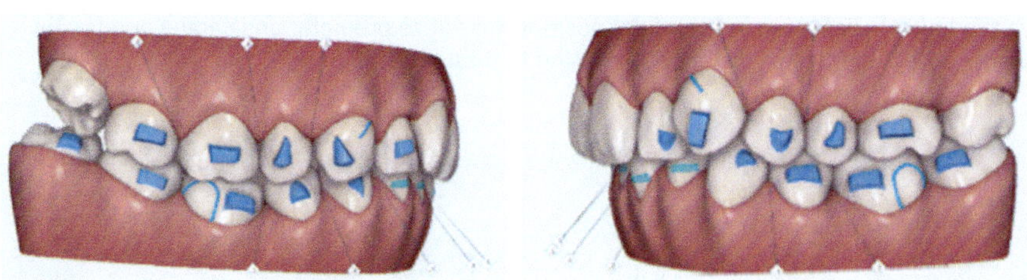

Fig. 22.52 Second set of aligners. Lateral ClinCheck views.

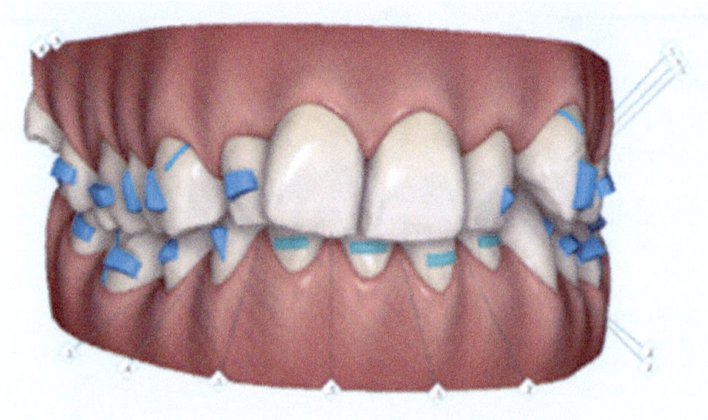

Fig. 22.53 Second set of aligners. Frontal ClinCheck view.

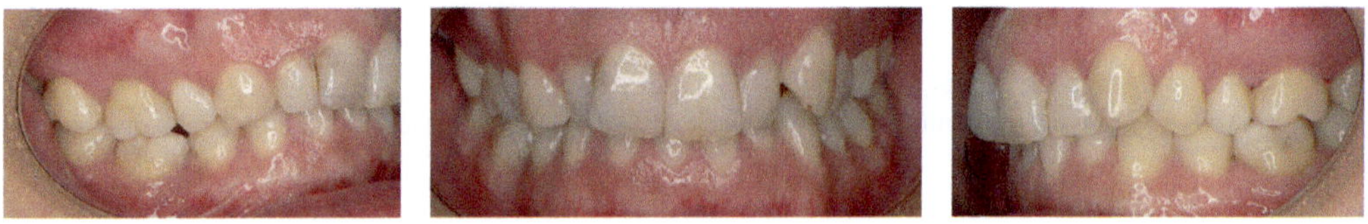

Fig. 22.54 Initial occlusion.

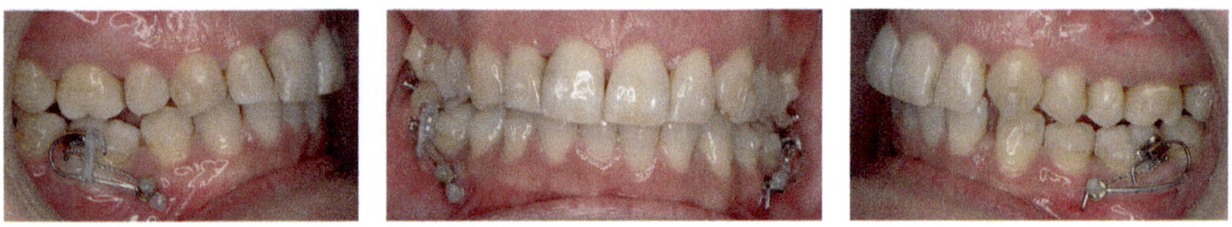

Fig. 22.55 Evolution at 3 months with sectional wire to anchor 36 and 46 to protrude the lower incisors.

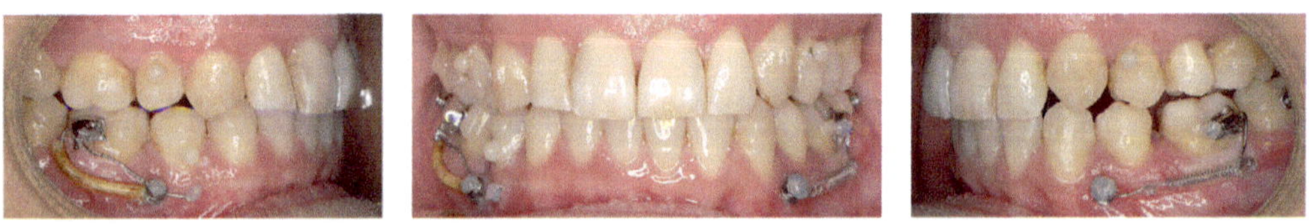

Fig. 22.56 When the lower incisors are in their final position, mesialize premolar and canine and finally change the temporary anchorage device distal to the canine to mesialize the molars.

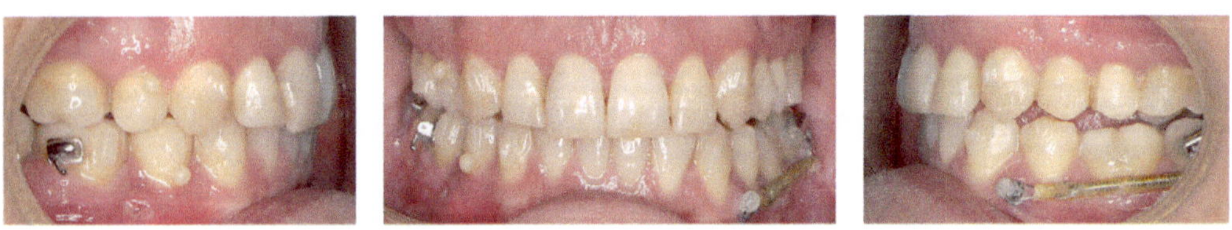

Fig. 22.57 Completing mesialization of second lower molar.

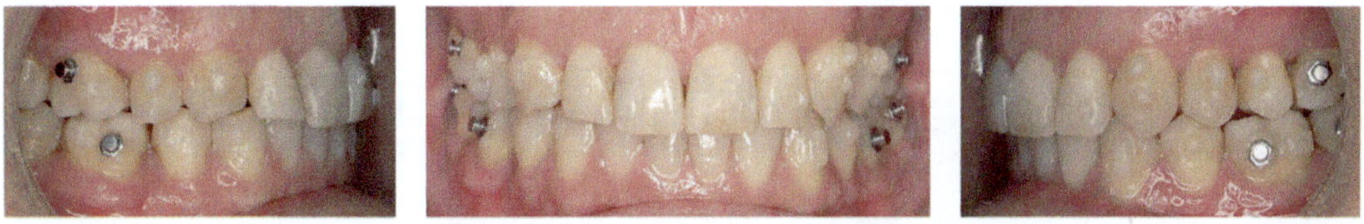

Fig. 22.58 Settle the occlusion with elastics.

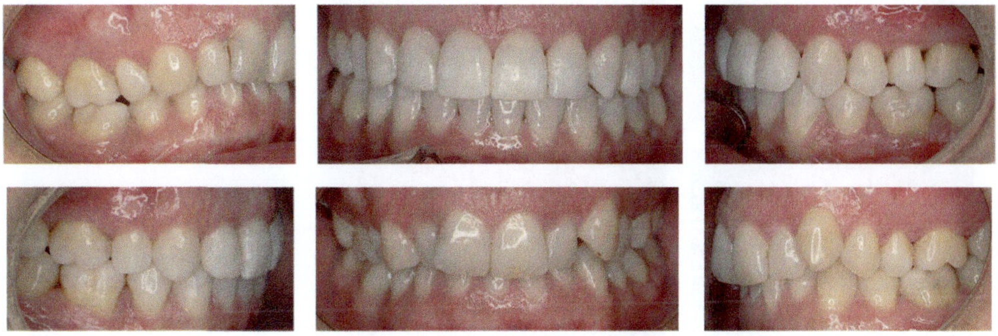

Fig. 22.59 Initial (upper) and final occlusion (lower) views. The full class II on left side is totally corrected and both midlines are centred by mesialization of third quadrant.

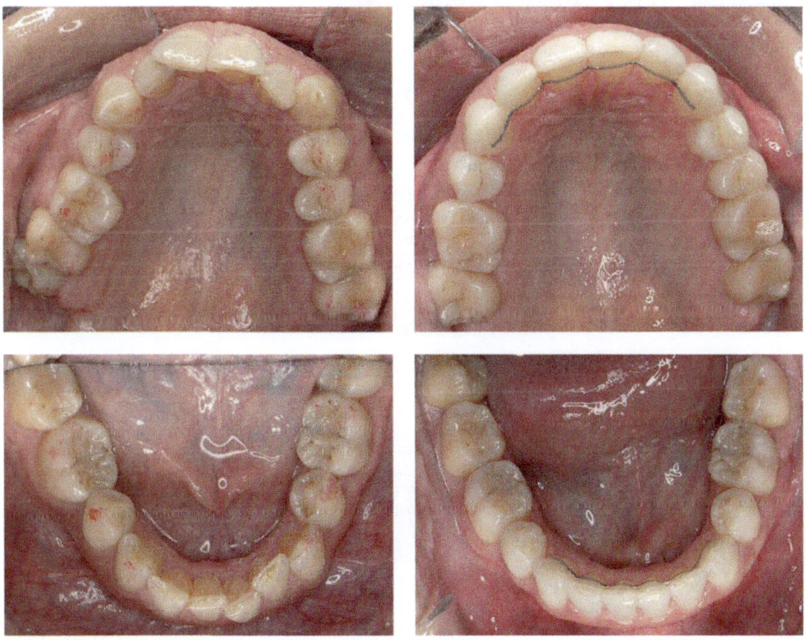

Fig. 22.60 Initial (left) and final (right) occlusal.

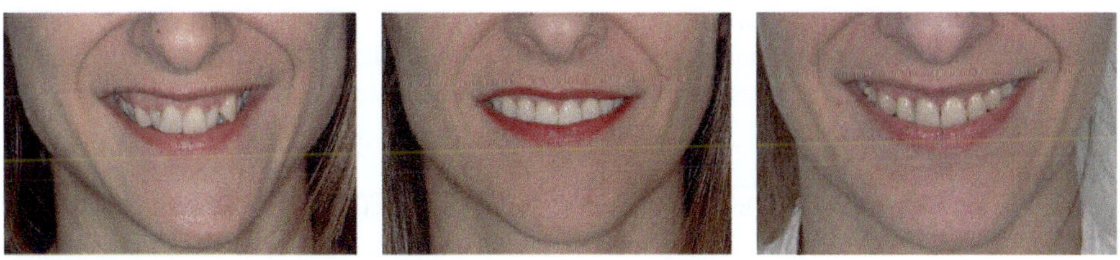

Fig. 22.61 Initial, smile in 22 months and final smile.

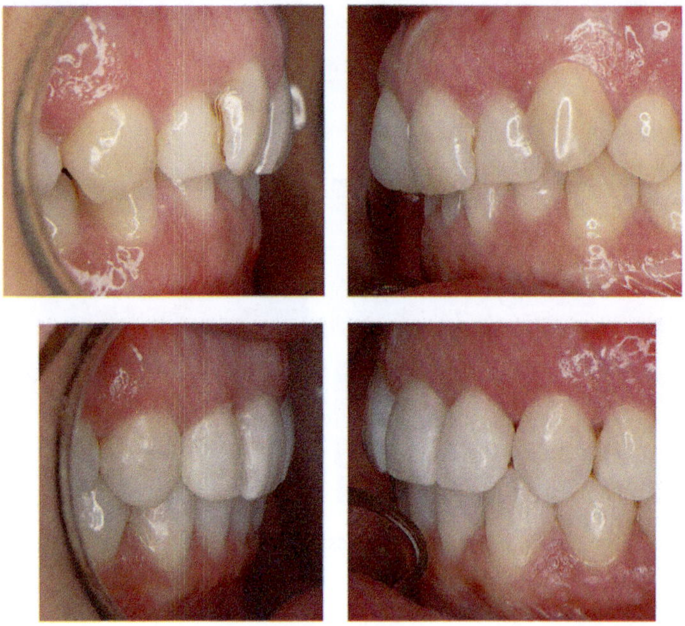

Fig. 22.62 Initial and final overjet (right and left side).

22.2.3 Midline Shift with Anterior Open Bite Tendency, Posterior Crossbite, Left Class II, Right Class III

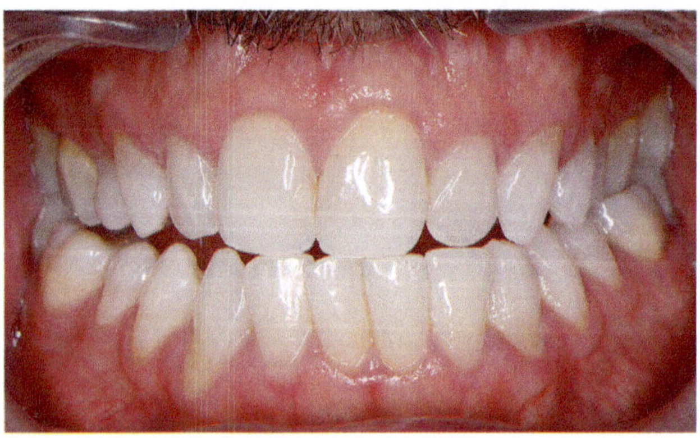

Fig. 22.63 Initial intraoral view.

Diagnosis

A 40-year-old man with hyperdivergent skeletal Class II pattern presented with constricted dental arches, a narrow smile with posterior gummy smile a result of negative lateral torque and upper dental midline deviated to the right.

The intraoral view was one of half cusp Class II division on the left side, half cusp Class III division on the left side, posterior crossbite on the left side and an anterior open bite tendency.

Treatment Plan

- Mandible: anterior IPR to enable compression of archwidth together with criss-cross elastics on third quadrant

- Maxilla: Class II correction on the left side, having the right side as anchorage, centring the midline simultaneously to the expansion. After this, start with Class III right side correction

ClinCheck 1: Requirements for the Technician

Maxilla:

- Start movement on second quadrant using first as anchorage, distalizing and expanding upper arch with 24 hours elastics, simultaneous to anterior extrusion thanks to the vertical component of elastics
- When Class II is resolved use left quadrant as anchorage to solve right Class III

Mandible:

- Anterior IPR to be able to compress archwidth together with criss-cross elastics on third quadrant

Treatment Summary

- Total treatment is estimated at 24 months
- The patient wore two sets of aligners with full-time wear Class II elastic on the left side and full-time wear Class III elastic on the right side, regardless of whether distalization was happening in the ClinCheck or not, as some 'virtual jump' was expected
- First set of aligners had a lack of coincidence between ClinCheck and the anatomical relationship problem after 40 aligners (Class II was meant to be already solved on the left side, but was not)
- Rescan was done for a new series of additional aligners after around 10 months of treatment (same mechanics were applied)

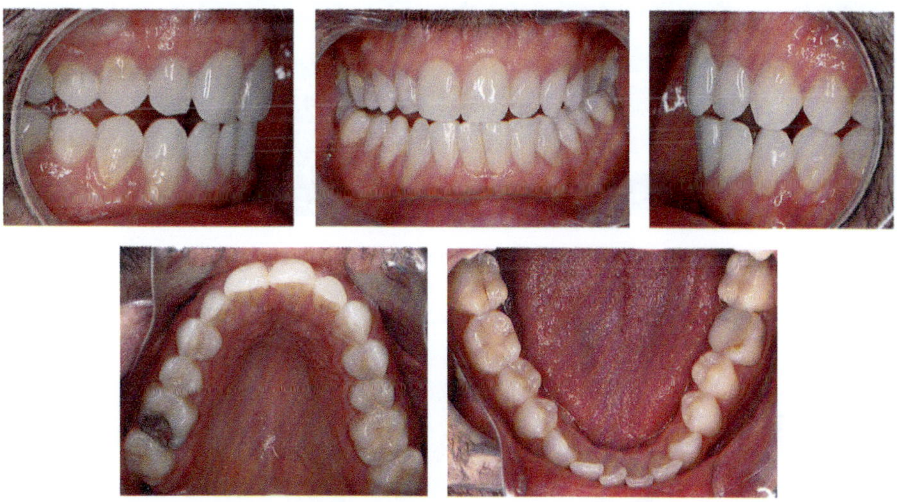

Fig. 22.64 Initial intraoral views.

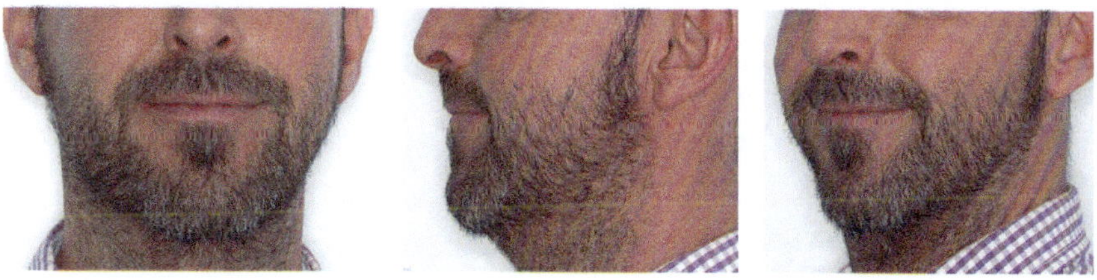

Fig. 22.65 Initial extraoral views.

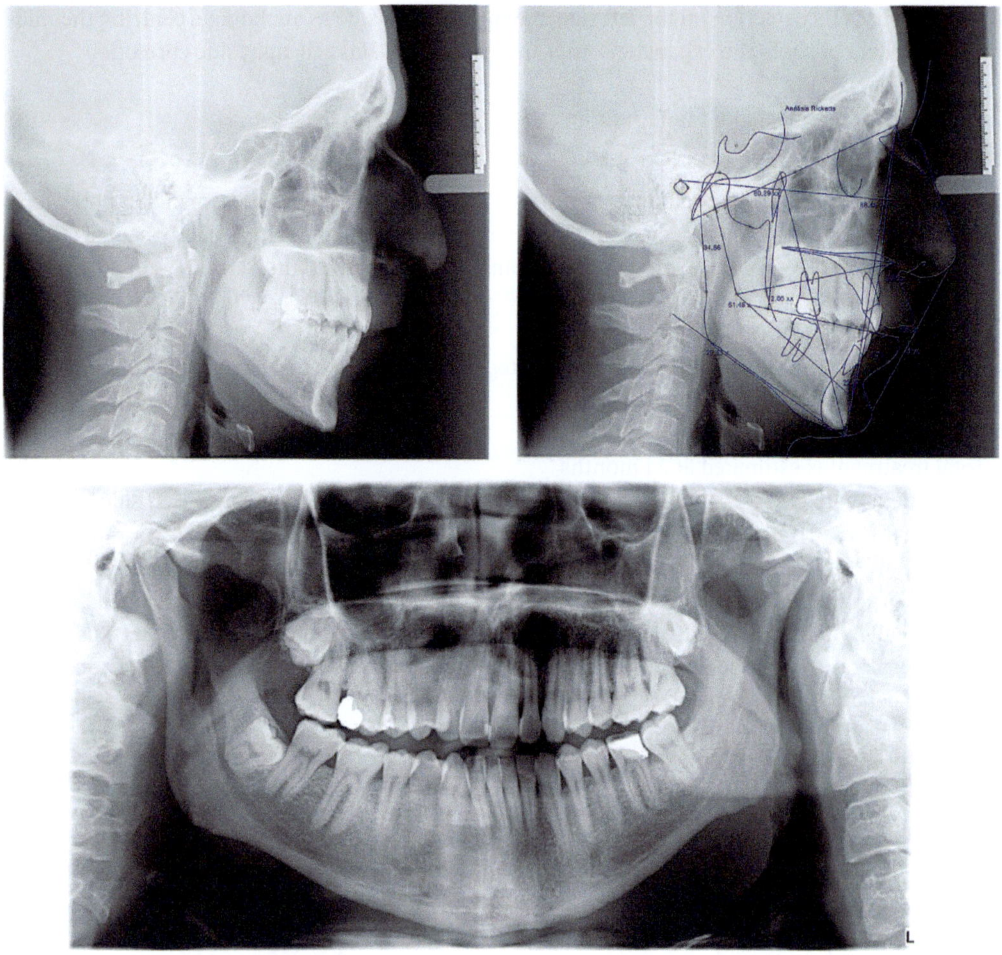

Fig. 22.66 Initial lateral and panoramic X-ray and cephalometric analysis.

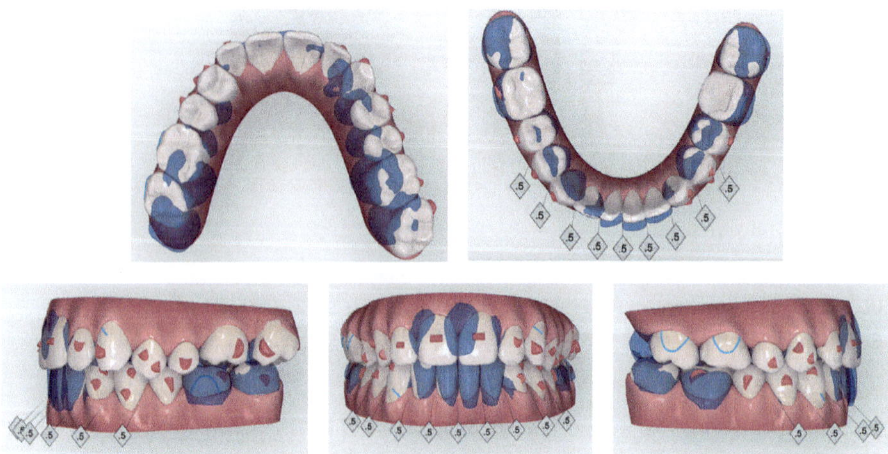

Fig. 22.67 Initial Clinchecks: the left side should be in a Class II relationship on aligner 40, but was found not to be, so an additional set of aligners was added.

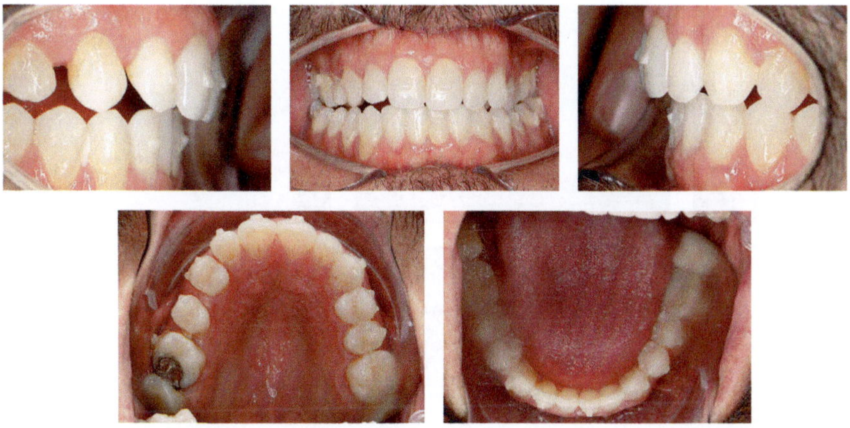

Fig. 22.68 After 10 months of treatment, the intraoral situation was good, but not as predicted on ClinCheck, which necessitated a rescan of the patient and requesting additional aligners.

Fig. 22.69 Extraoral view after 10 months.

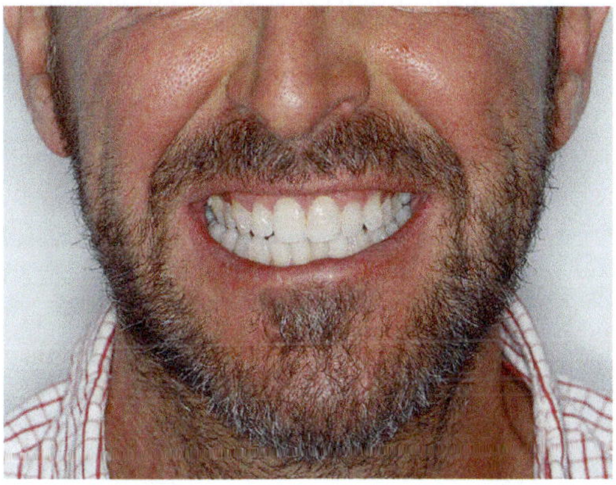

ClinCheck 2: Requirements for the Technician

Same mechanics are used as in ClinCheck 1, adding:

- Additional distalization on second quadrant
- Additional compression on third quadrant
- Overcorrection of upper molar intrusion, in order to ensure anterior bite closure by posterior fulcrum reduction
- Virtual jump to simulate full-time wearing of Class II/III elastics

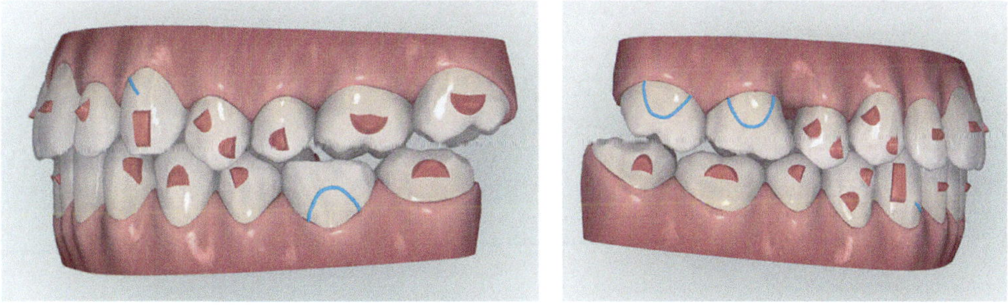

Fig. 22.70 After 10 months, the ClinCheck had vertical overcorrection and virtual jump.

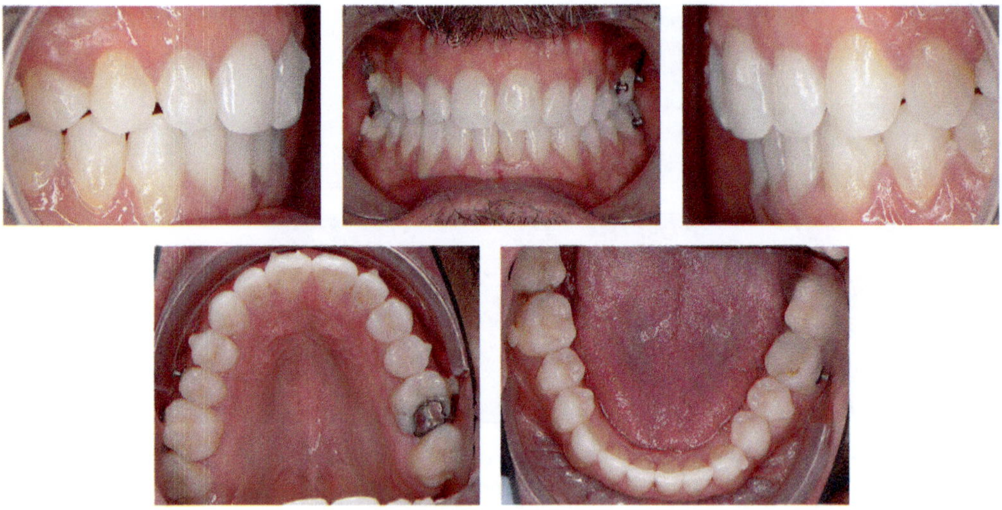

Fig. 22.71 Current views after 20 months of treatment, but expected at 24 months.

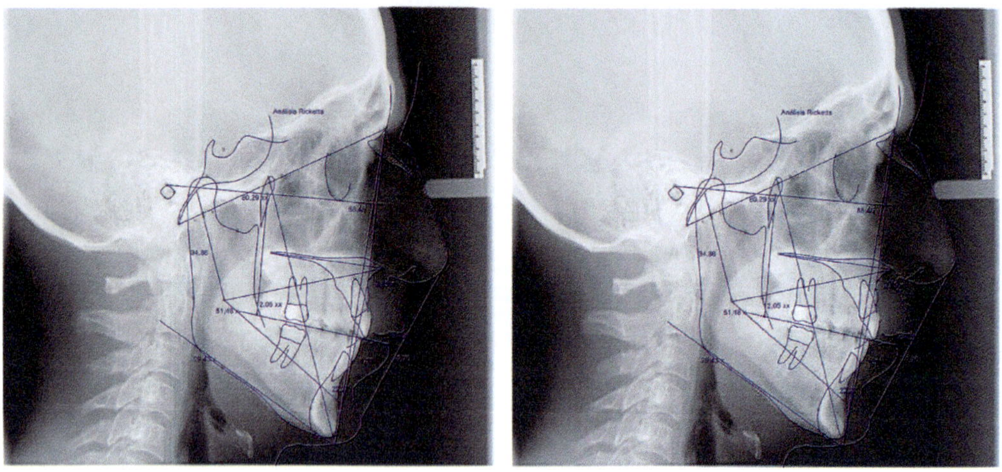

Fig. 22.72 Pretreatment and current X-rays.

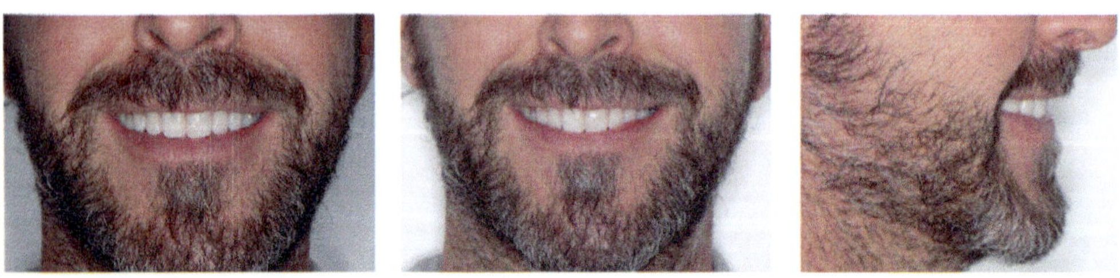

Fig. 22.73 Extraoral pictures after treatment.

23

Extraction Cases

23.1 Incisor Extraction

Extraction of incisors is indicated in:

- Dental Class III with lower crowding and microdontia of upper lateral incisors
- Dental Class I with significant mandibular incisors crowding
- Acceptable soft tissue profile
- Minimal growth potential
- Minimal to moderate overjet and overbite

Prescription for Extraction Cases

Question 10: Select the teeth you are going to extract, among these three options:

- First: extraction of a lower incisor
- Second: extraction of 4s with maximum anchorage (up to 2 mm posterior mesialization)
- Third: extraction of 4s with minimum anchorage or extraction of 5s (more than 2 mm posterior mesialization)

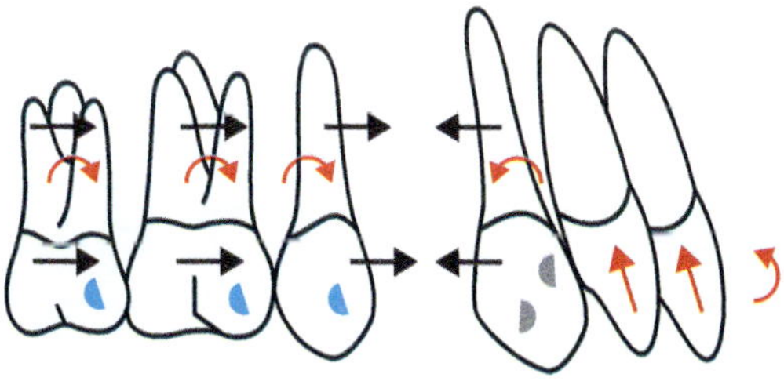

Fig. 23.1 First premolar extraction, G6 protocol.

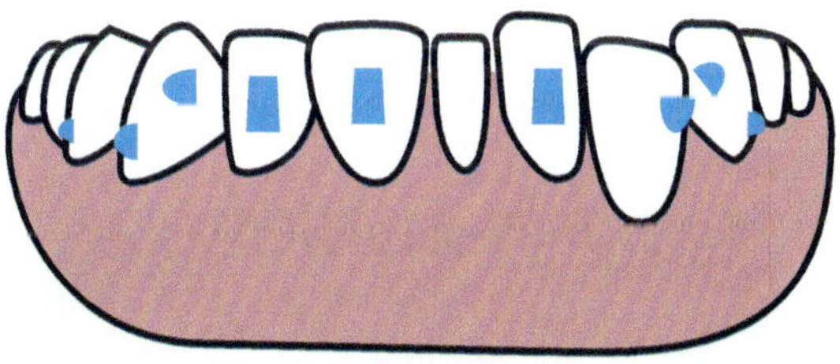

Fig. 23.2 Lower incisor extraction, with vertical attachments on the remaining lower incisors.

Factors to Choose the Incisor to be Extracted[1]

- Periodontically compromised mandibular incisor
- Most severely displaced mandibular incisor
- Mesiodistal width of the incisor

1 Zawawi *et al. Orthodontic Treatment of a Mandibular Incisor Extraction Case with Invisalign*. Case Reports in Dentistry Volume 2014, Article ID 657657, 4pp.

Aligner Techniques in Orthodontics, First Edition. Susana Palma Moya and Javier Lozano Zafra.

Companion website: www.wiley.com/go/lozano-zafra/aligner-techniques

- Adjacent root inclination: adjacent root inclinations that diverge away from the extraction site will make it difficult to achieve adequate root parallelism at the end of the treatment. In contrast, when the roots of the adjacent teeth are convergent to the extraction site, there will be a highly predictable crown movement with a final parallelism between the roots
- Lateral incisors are usually preferred

Software Consideration on Incisor Extraction Cases

- Vertical attachments should be placed on the three remaining incisors to control tipping during the closure of the extraction site. The software normally only places the vertical attachment in the two incisors adjacent to the extraction site, not in all three
- Ask for a virtual gable bend of 10 degrees across the extraction site
- Pontic can be requested for covering the space of the extraction site, a small pontic should be considered to allow the aligner material to fully cover the adjacent teeth to the extraction site for a better control of the movements of those teeth
- If the adjacent teeth to the extraction site are divergent, aesthetic buttons and Powerchain by labial should be used to help the aligner provide lingual tipping to the roots and achieve a final position that has adequate root parallelism

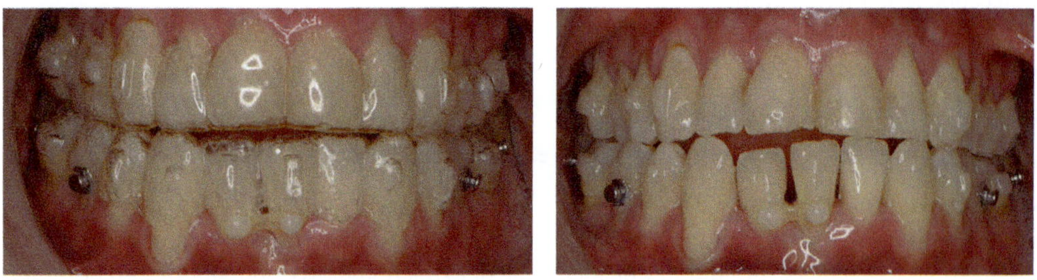

Fig. 23.3 Powerchain helps close final spacing.

- To help achieve perfect root parallelism, Powerarms might be needed in order to get closer to the centre of resistance of the teeth

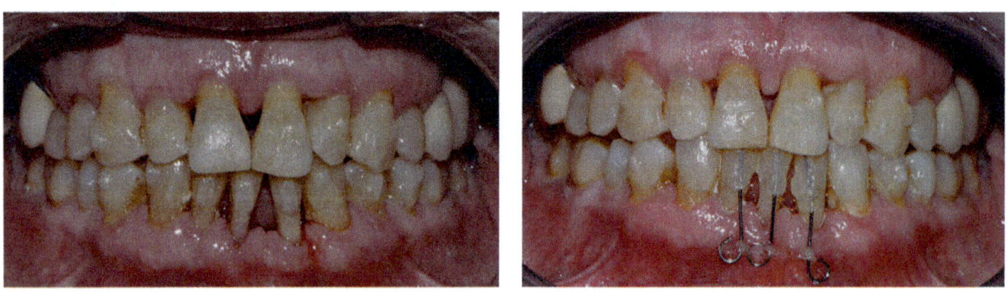

Fig. 23.4 Perfect root parallelism after tooth extraction commonly needs the assistance of Powerarms.

23.1.1 Class III with Lower Incisor Extraction

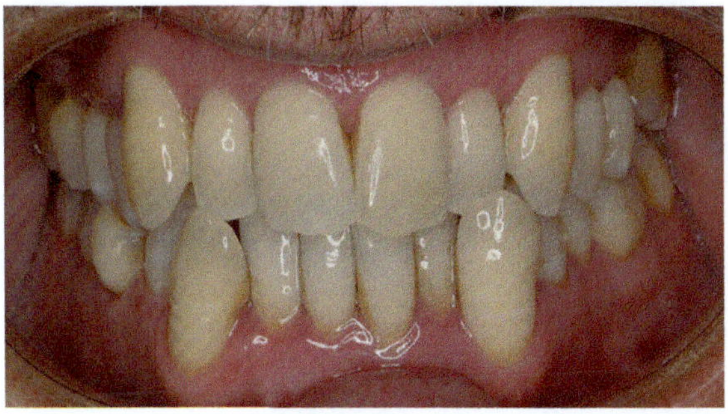

Fig. 23.5 Initial intraoral view.

Diagnosis

A 48-year-old man with a normodivergent skeletal Class III pattern presented with severe lower crowding, centred upper midline, microdontia of 12 and 22, and a missing 26. They had multiple gum recessions but appropriate lip seal posture and exposure of lower incisors when smiling.

Treatment Plan

- Expansion, opening space for missing 26 through sequential distalization of 28 and 27.
- In the mandible, 31 extraction, so final occlusion, in terms of buccal relationship would be similar to the pretreatment condition.
- Microdontia in 12 and 22 prevented much IPR in the upper arch, in order to be able to finish with an appropriate overjet after the lower extraction.

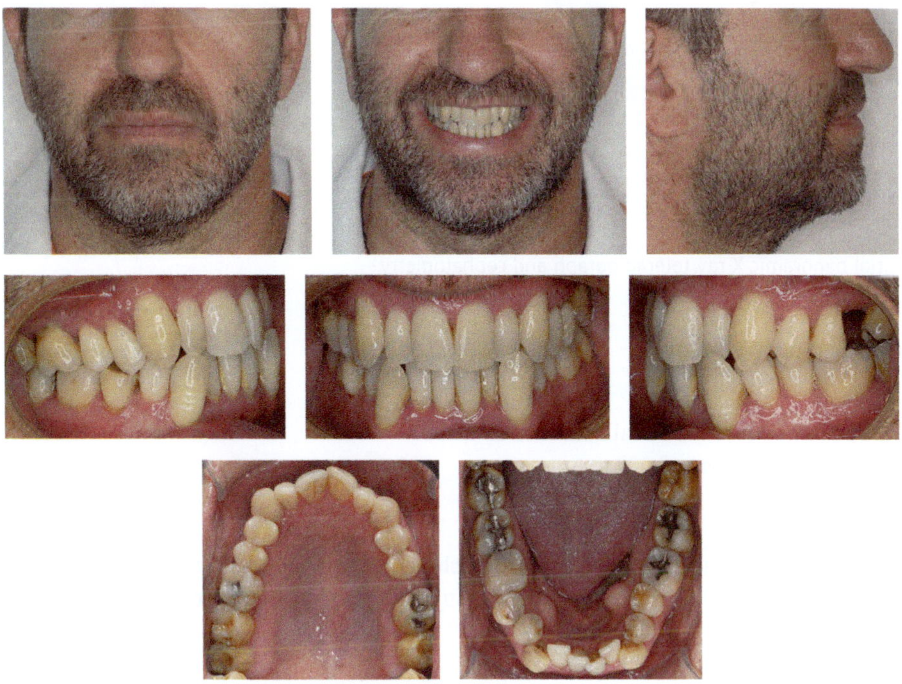

Fig. 23.6 Pretreatment extraoral and intraoral views.

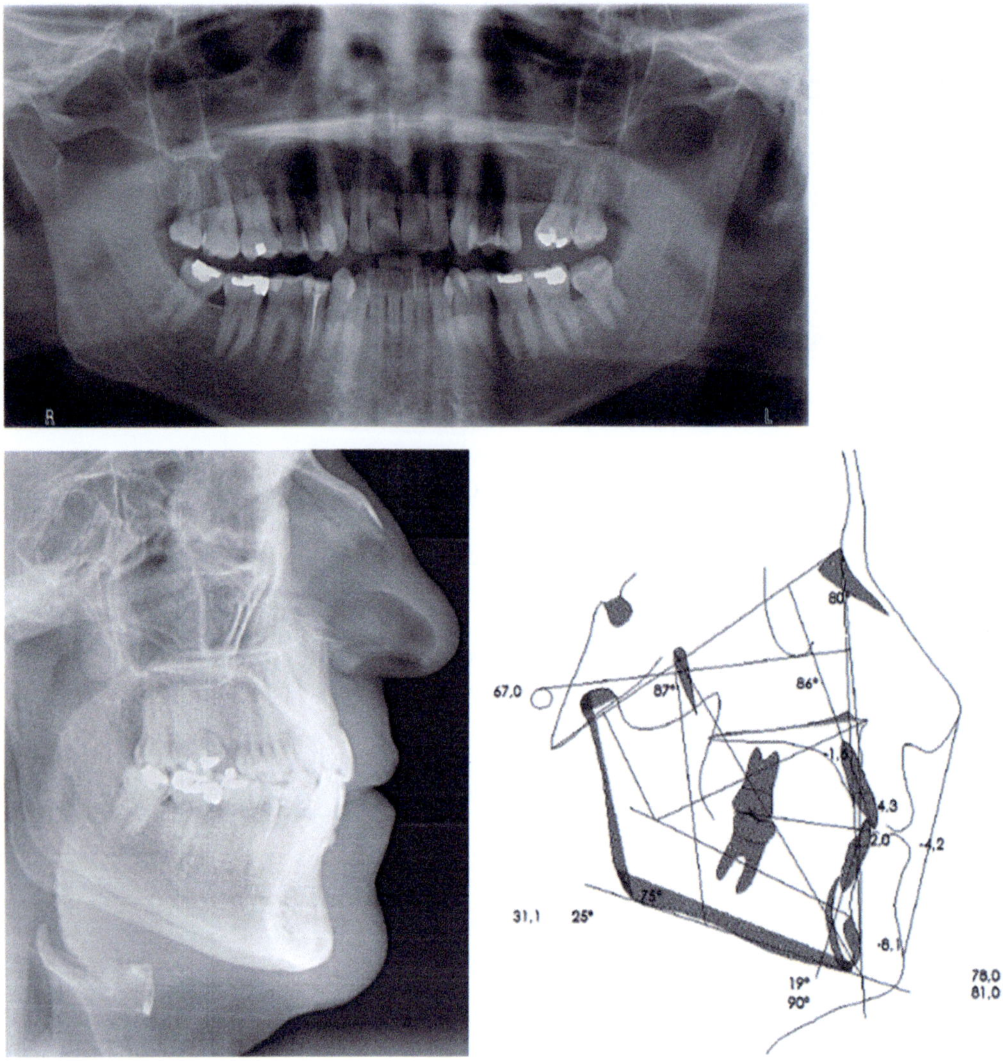

Fig. 23.7 Initial panoramic X-ray, teleradiograph and cephalometry.

Requirement for the Technician

Maxilla:

- Expansion 16 to 25, sequential distalization of 28 and 27
- Proclination of upper incisors

Mandible:

- Expansion of 36 to 46, extraction of 31; vertical attachments in three remaining lower incisors
- Precision cut for class III elastic. Button cutouts in upper 16 and 27 and precision cut in lower 33 and 43
- Apply a gable bend movement of the root of the incisors during the space closure and a small pontic for 31

Symmetric expansion and opening space for missing 26

- Extraction 3.1
- **AT vertical** in remaining lower incisors to prevent tipping

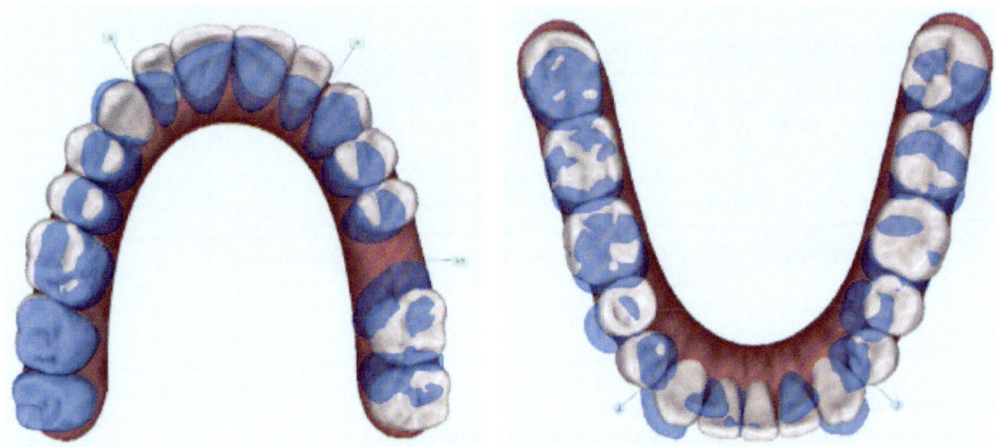

Fig. 23.8 Upper and lower CC superimposition and instructions to CAD designer.

Treatment goals:

- Correct crowding, increase overjet and overbite
- Expansion + 31 extraction + Class III elastics

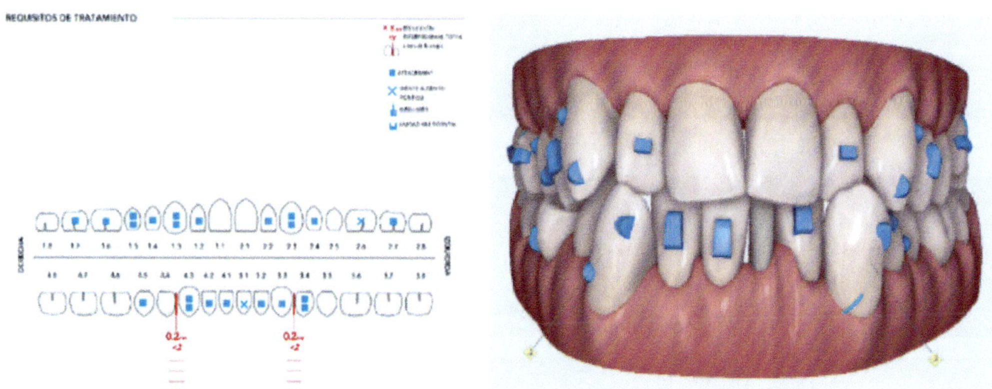

Fig. 23.9 Attachments can be seen in several areas of the ClinCheck software.

- Upper symmetrical expansion: expansion + upper incisors, LRT
- Increase overjet: 31 extraction + Class III elastics
- Correct lower crowding: 27–28 distalization

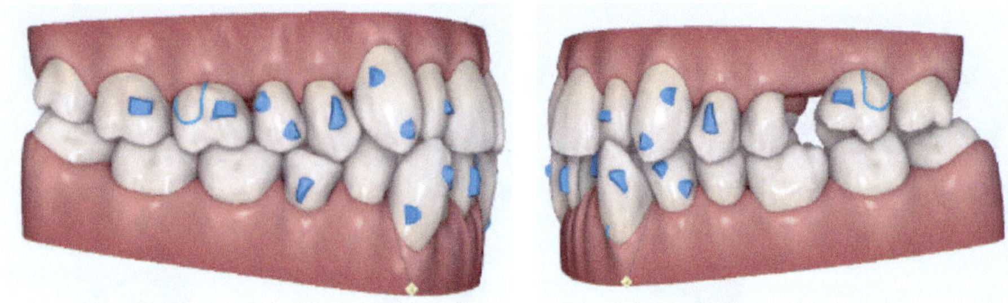

Fig. 23.10 Lateral ClinCheck views.

Treatment Summary

- The patient wore 32 aligners, replaced at 10-day intervals
- First set of aligners closed the space of the 31 completely, but a set of additional aligners was requested to close black triangles and to increase the final overjet
- The whole treatment lasted 18 months and ended with an excellent parallelism between the roots
- An implant was placed for missing 26

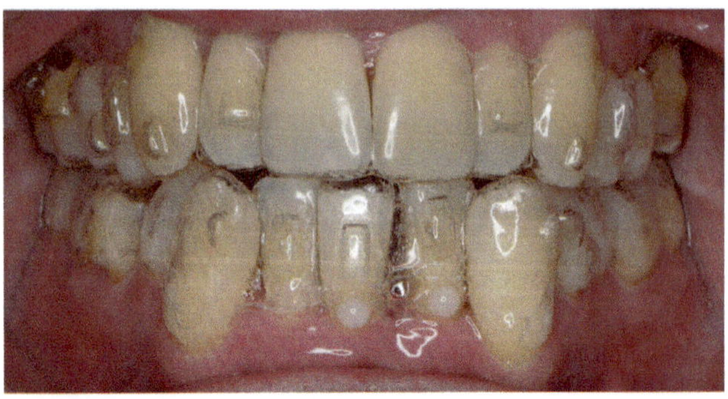

Fig. 23.11 Intraoral view.

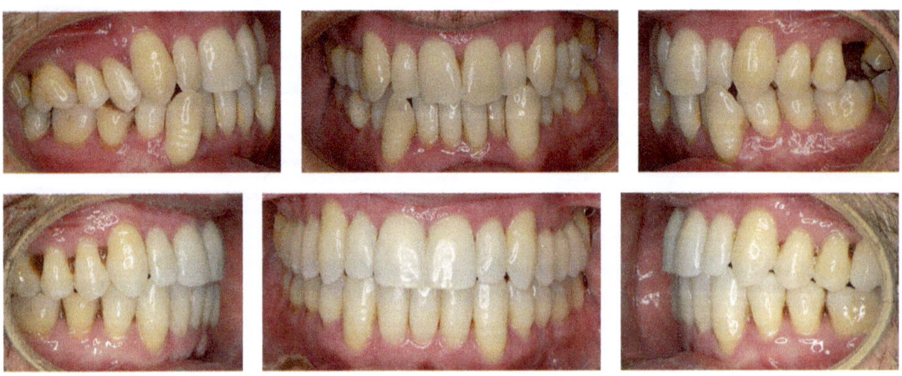

Fig. 23.12 Initial (upper)and final (lower) views.

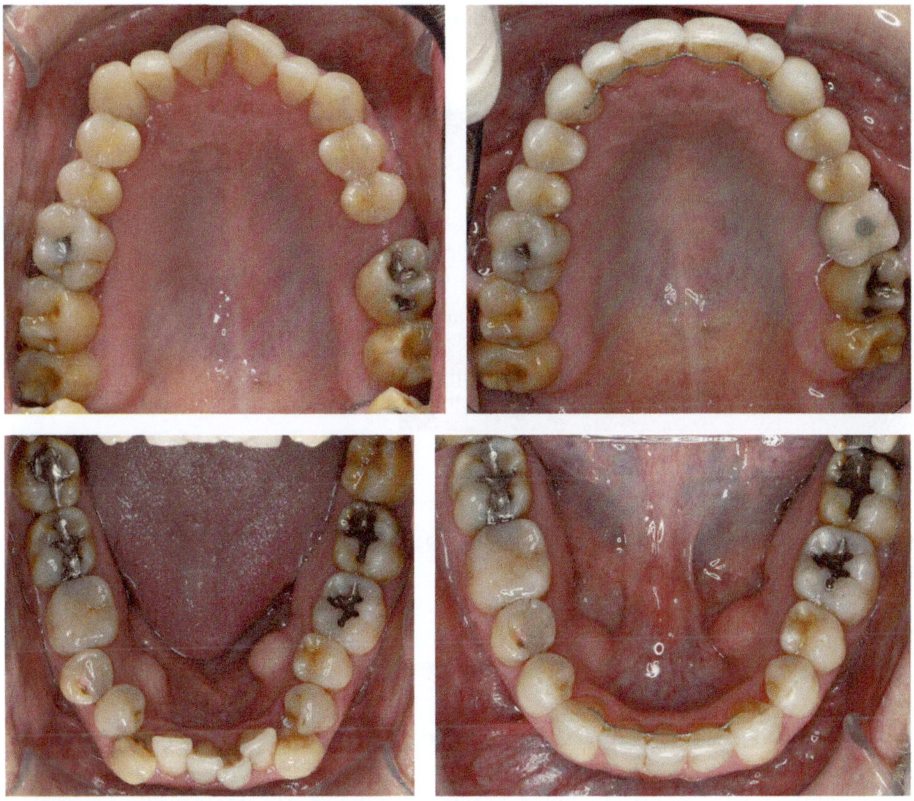

Fig. 23.13 Initial and final occlusal.

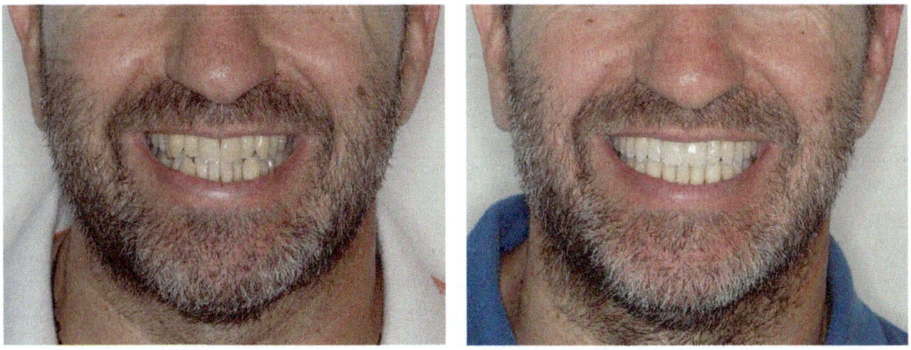

Fig. 23.14 Initial and final smile.

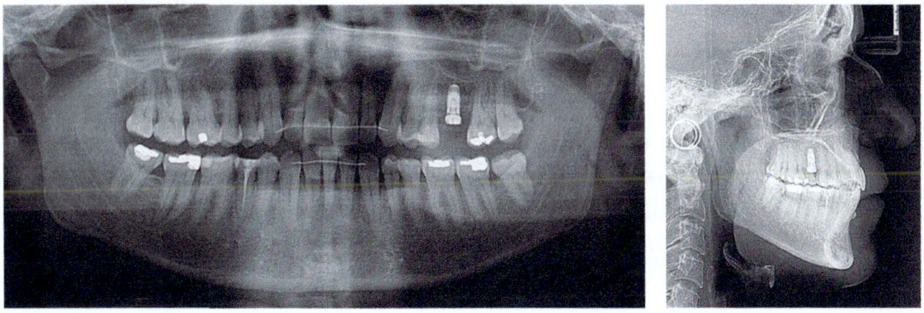

Fig. 23.15 Final panoramic and lateral X-rays: good final parallelism between incisors and adequate interincisal final angle.

23.1.2 Class I with Lower Crowding and Periodontal Problem Lower Incisor Extraction

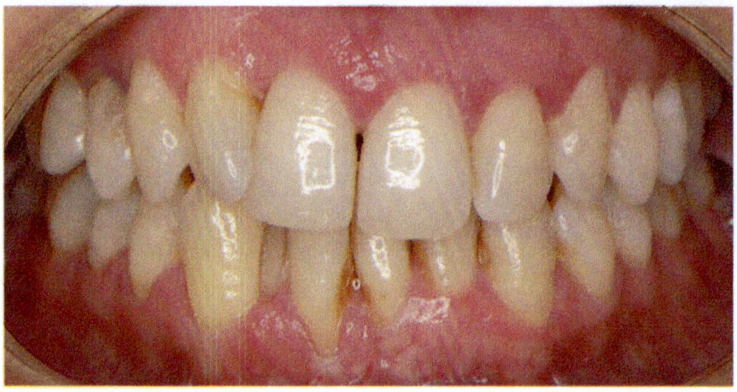

Fig. 23.16 Initial intraoral view.

Diagnosis
A 47-year-old woman with a normodivergent skeletal Class I pattern presented with severe lower crowding and a periodontal problem

Treatment Plan
- Before starting the orthodontic treatment, the patient needed root scaling and planning and periodontal surgery.
- In the maxilla, the periodontal tissue was thin and does not allow much expansion to create space for 12 by proclining and IPR.
- In the lower arch, the treatment plan included 42 extraction in order to create positive overjet.
- Extraction of 42 was chosen because the roots of 43 and 41 were inclined towards the extraction site and only crown tipping would be necessary for closure of the space.

Requirements for the Technician
Maxilla:

- Proclination and IPR to make room for 12.
- Anteroposterior limit for proclination 1 mm.
- IPR in early stages to avoid round tripping of incisors.

Mandible:

- Virtual extraction of 42 in aligner 2 and vertical attachment placed in the adjacent teeth of the extraction site, as well as a pontic for the missing lower incisor.
- A gable bend movement of the root is also required during the closure of the space.
- At the end of the treatment, additional overcorrection of the tipping of the roots in the extraction site.

Treatment Summary
- Patient wore 24 aligners, replaced at 10-day intervals
- The first set of aligners closed completely the space of 42
- A set of additional aligners were requested to close black triangles and to settle the occlusion
- The patient was required to use night wear triangular elastic on the posterior zone
- The whole treatment lasted 17 months and resulted in excellent parallelism between the roots on the extraction site

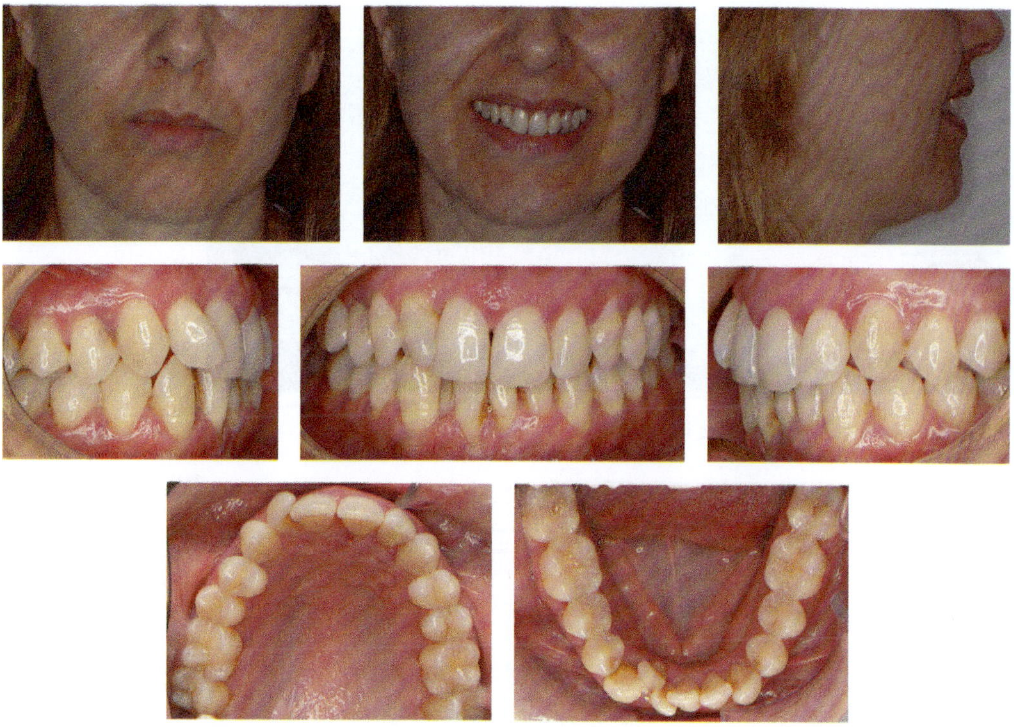

Fig. 23.17 Initial extraoral and intraoral views.

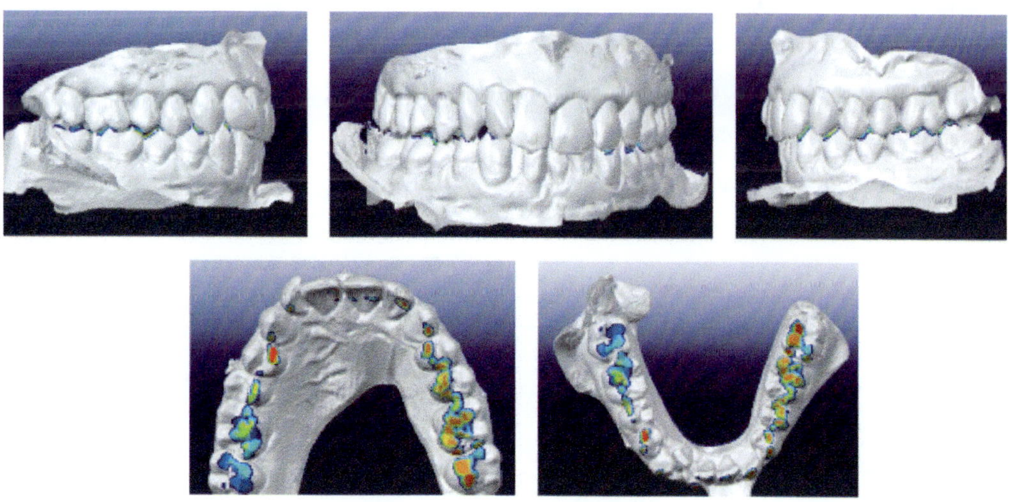

Fig. 23.18 Occlusal contact at the beginning of the treatment.

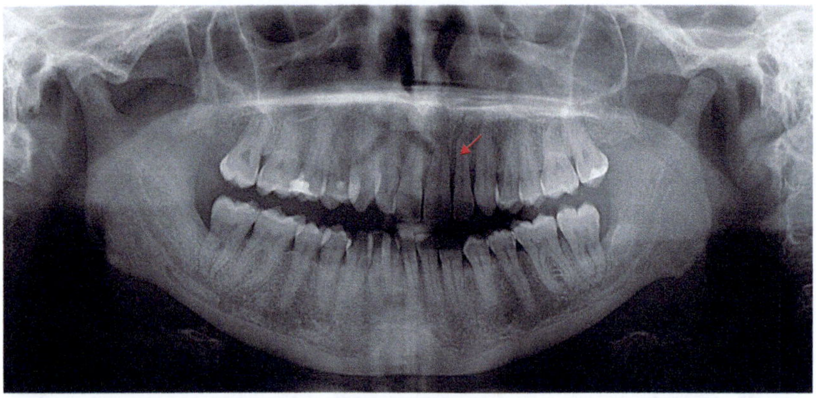

Fig. 23.19 Periodontal bone loss in upper incisors.

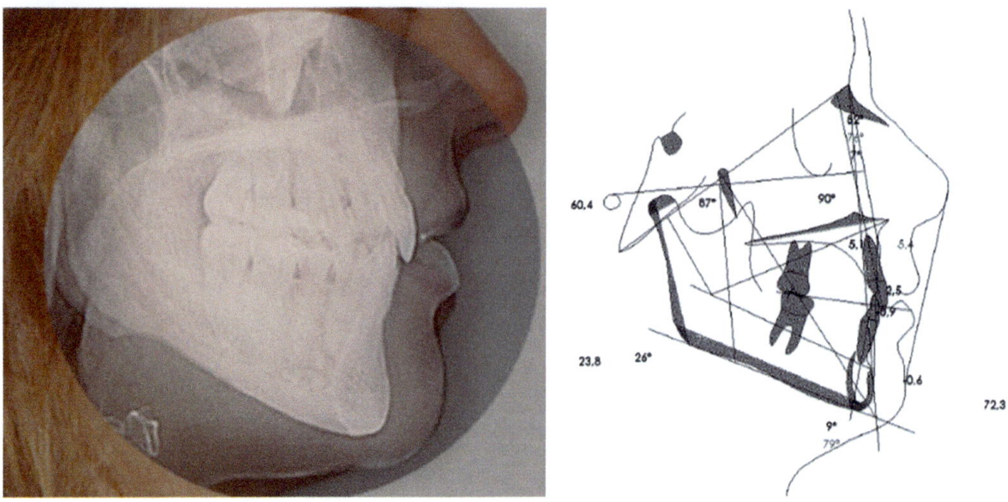

Fig. 23.20 Initial teleradiograph and cephalometry.

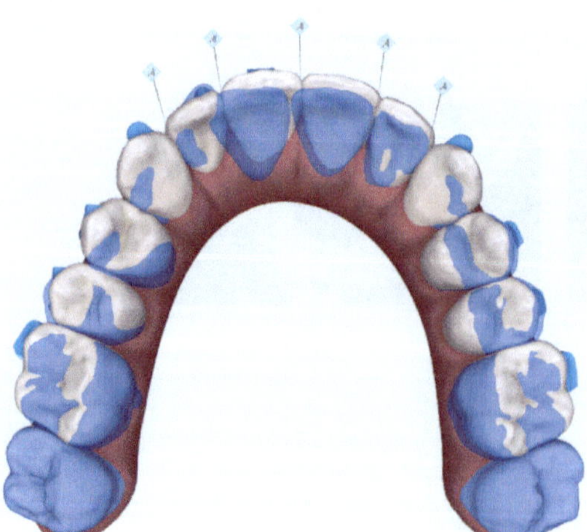

Staging maxillary:

- Expansion 6 to 6
- Do not move second molars to use as anchorage during incisors protrusion

Fig. 23.21 Upper occlusal interproximal reduction to avoid excessive proclination of upper incisors.

Staging mandible:

- Extraction of 42
- Vertical attachment on adjacent lower incisors to control tipping
- Overcorrection at the end of the treatment to have a good parallelism in between the root of lower incisors

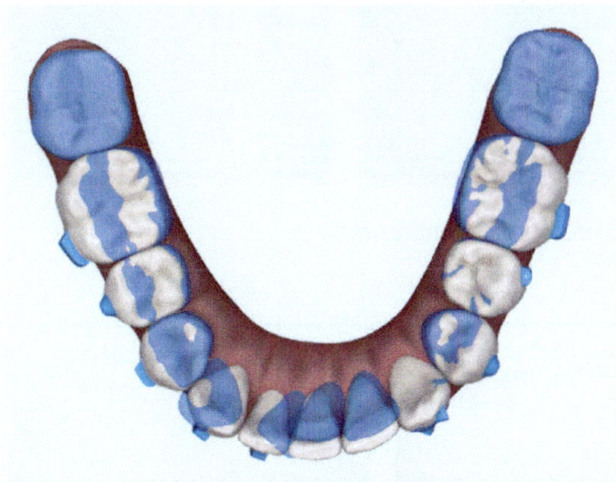

Fig. 23.22 Pontic for extracted 42. Bevelled attachment on lateral incisors to control the lateral torque.

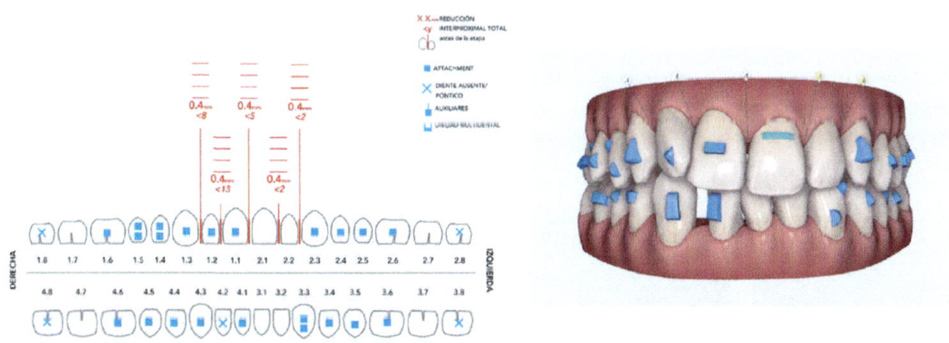

Fig. 23.23 Interproximal reduction of upper arch and lower incisor extraction of 42 in lower arch to solve crowding.

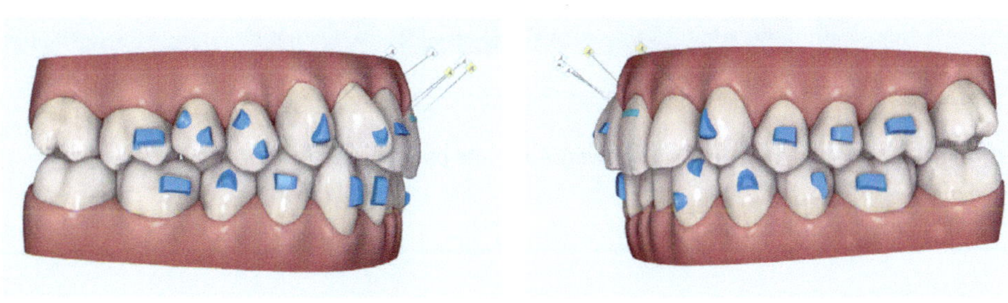

Fig. 23.24 Lateral ClinCheck views.

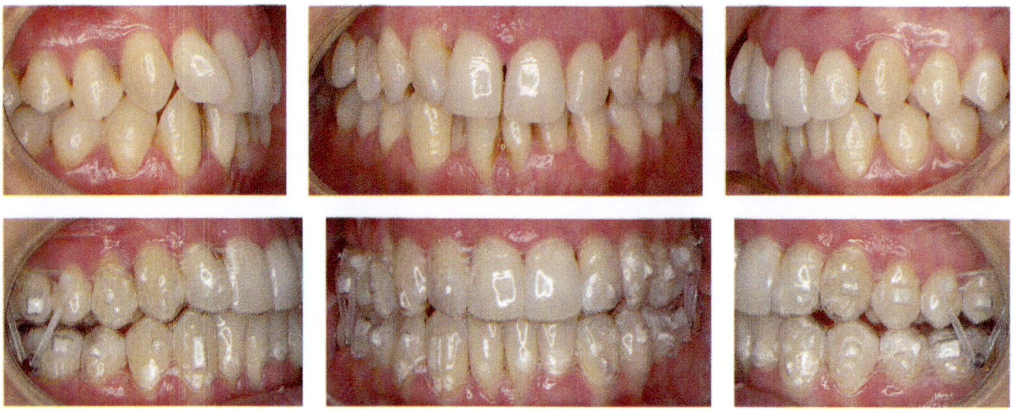

Fig. 23.25 Initial (upper) and evolution after 11 months of treatment (lower).

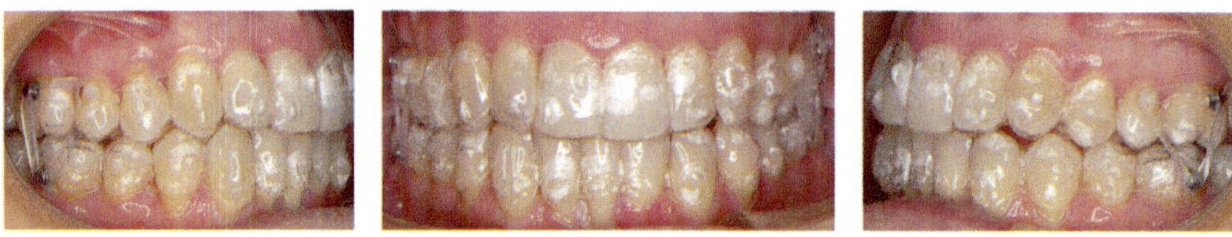

Fig. 23.26 Finishing refinement. Posterior elastic is used to settle the occlusion.

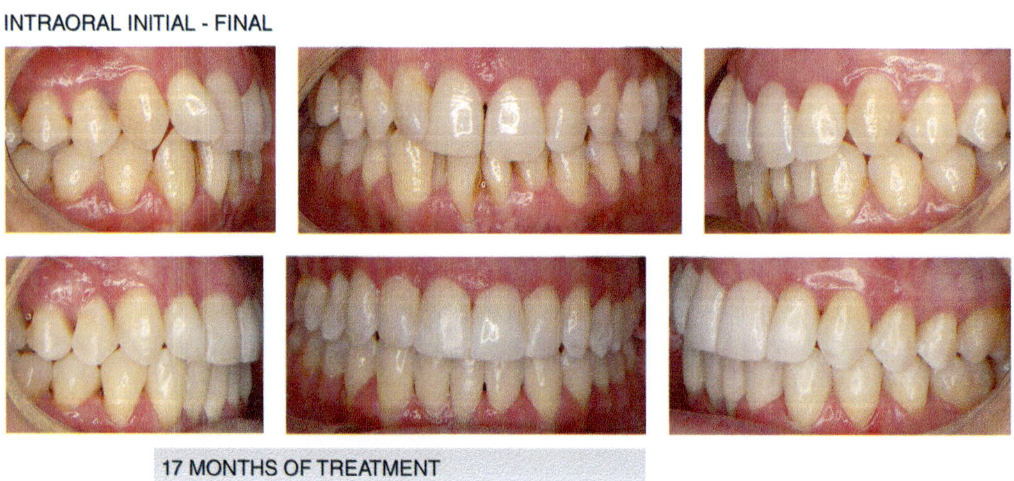

Fig. 23.27 Initial (upper) and final occlusion (lower). Adequate parallelism is achieved between roots of lower incisors.

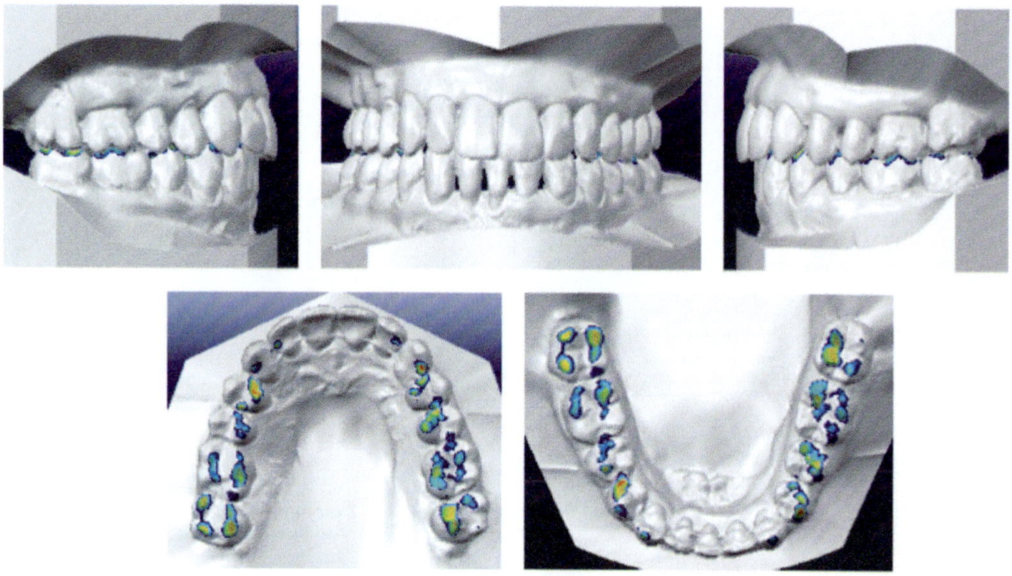

Fig. 23.28 Occlusal contact point at the end of the treatment.

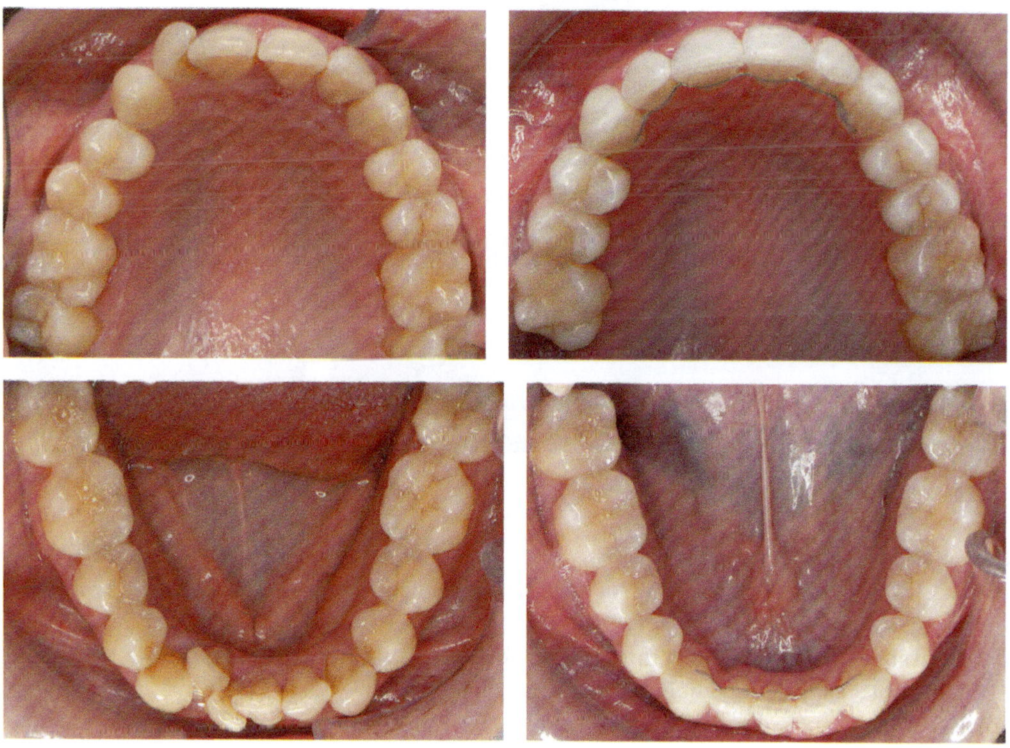

Fig. 23.29 Initial and final occlusal.

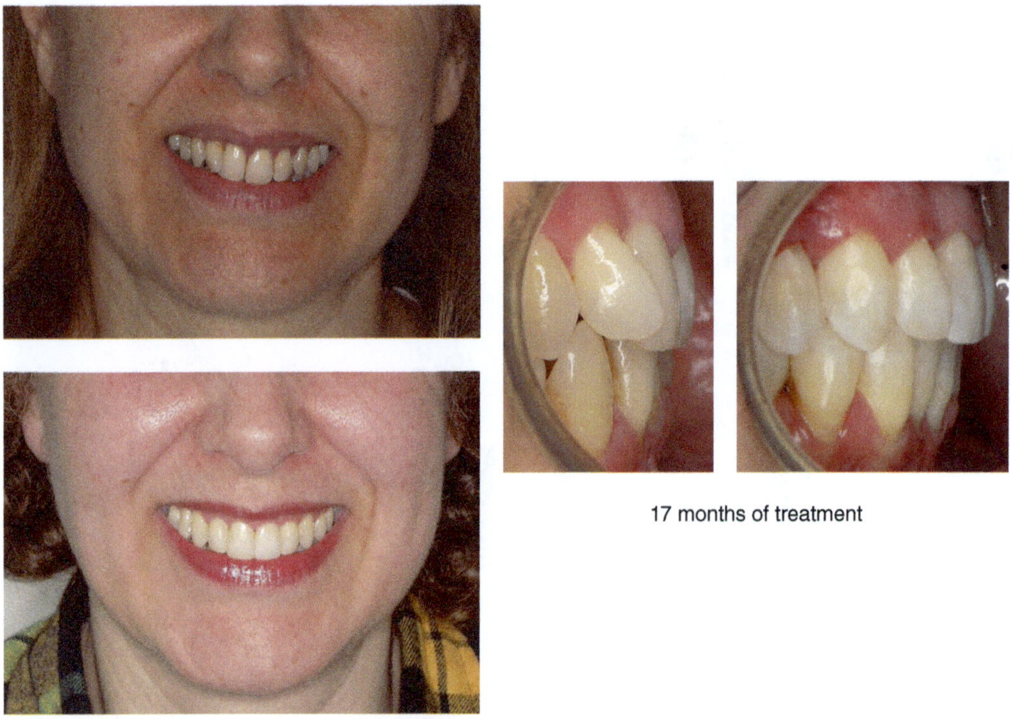

17 months of treatment

Fig. 23.30 Initial and final smile and overjet.

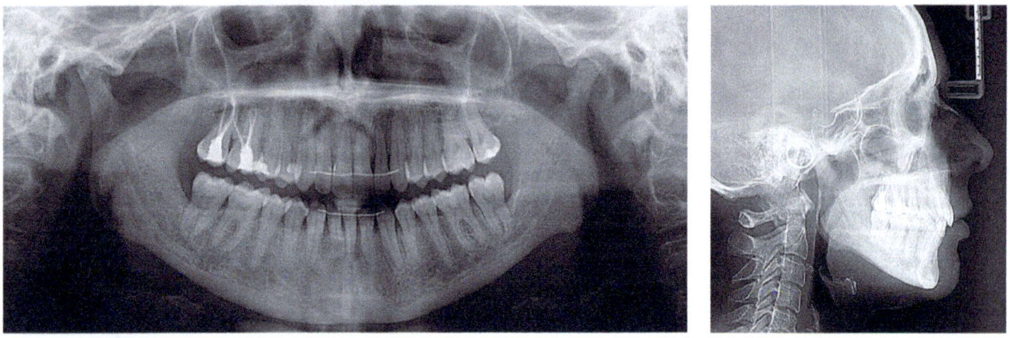

Fig. 23.31 Final panoramic and lateral X-rays.

Tips for Incisor Extraction Treatment

- Check before extracting the incisor, for a favourable root position of adjacent incisors toward the extraction site
- Vertical attachments in the other three incisors for tip control during the space closure. Optimized root control attachment might be used in the canines
- Ask the technician to do a simultaneous intrusion + tipping movement of lower incisors to help parallelism of the roots
- 'Speed of root movement must be half of the maximum permitted' gable bend movement starting by movement of the root. Ask for 10 degrees of virtual gable bends when closing extraction sites

23.2 Extraction of Premolars

Management of the anchorage and understanding of the biomechanics of extraction space closure are of paramount concern in extraction treatments.

Ideal cases for extracting premolars include:

- Dento-alveolar protrusion. Proclined incisors where some loss of torque might be acceptable
- Mesially tipped canines with favourable root inclinations adjacent to the extraction sites
- Severe crowding, where excessive IPR would be necessary to solve alignment of the teeth

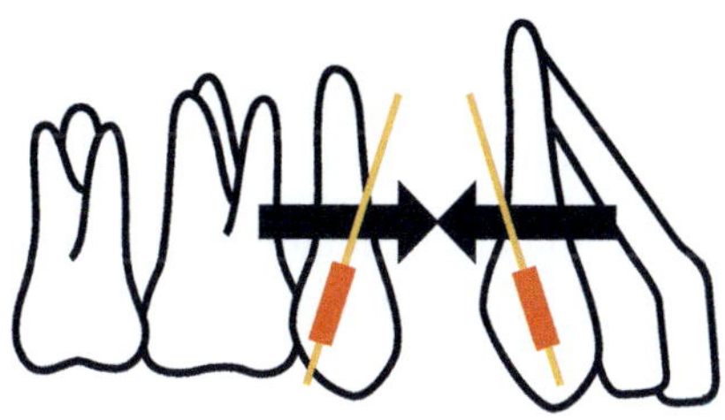

Fig. 23.32 The canine and second premolar in this picture would be ideal for extraction if their axes were parallel to the yellow line, indicating crown movement but with the apex staying in the same position, which makes it a highly predictable movement.

There are four types of anchorage:

- Absolute anchorage
- Maximum anchorage
- Medium or moderate anchorage
- Minimum anchorage: extraction of second premolars (5s)

23.2.1 Absolute Anchorage

This is only achieved when using TADs or implants in the posterior zone. It is possible to create an absolute anchorage situation by ligating the posterior segment to a fixed anchor in basal bone: in this way the posterior segment can be made immovable as an implant, and the entire extraction space can be therefore closed by retraction of the anterior segment.

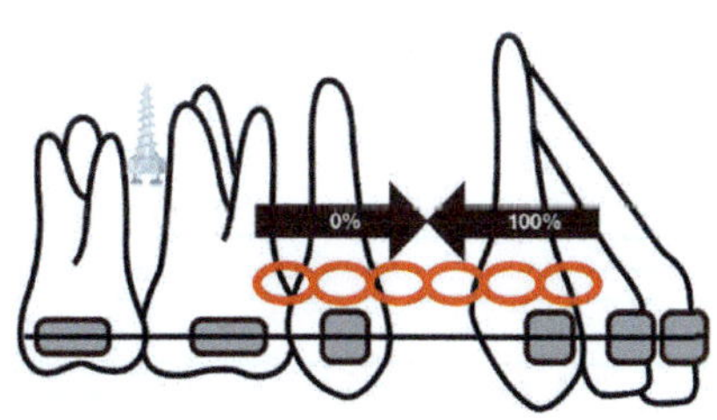

Fig. 23.33 Extraction of first premolars, absolute anchorage: 0 mm posterior mesialization plus all of the space in the extraction site is closed by anterior retraction, which is only possible with posterior TAD anchorage, and exactly the same as with fixed appliances.

23.2.2 Maximum Anchorage

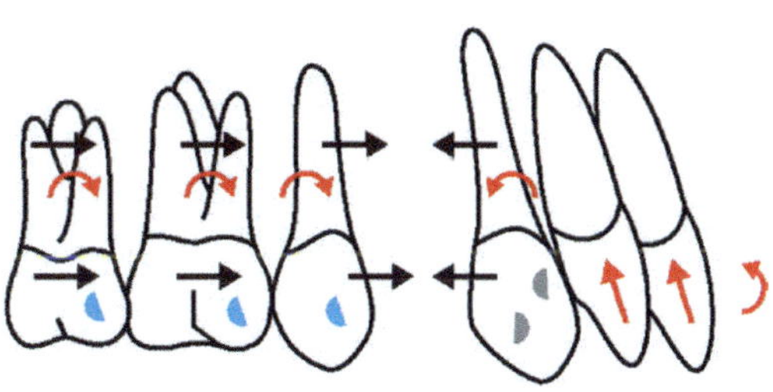

Fig. 23.34 Extraction of first premolars, maximum anchorage: 0–2 mm posterior mesialization and the rest of the space in the extraction site is closed by anterior retraction.

This protocol only applies to first premolar extraction treatments where the posterior loss in anchorage must be 2 mm or less to finish in a cusp-to-fossae relationship. G6 is automatically applied by the software program in quadrants where the criteria for maximum anchorage are met.

Extractions of First Premolars: Maximum Anchorage (Less than 2 mm of Posterior Mesialization)

- SmartForce optimized retraction attachments: in canines for retraction and works at the same time as the activation of Smartstage on the aligner
- SmartForce optimized anchorage attachments: 5s/6s and 7s to increase posterior anchorage and works with the Smartstage activations on the aligners
- Smartstage activations on the upper incisors: to prevent bowing effect (extrusion and lingual tipping of upper incisors during closure of extractions) these are in the aligners and not visible in the ClinCheck

We cannot place or eliminate any of the activations on the tooth or all of the multidental activations will disappear together.

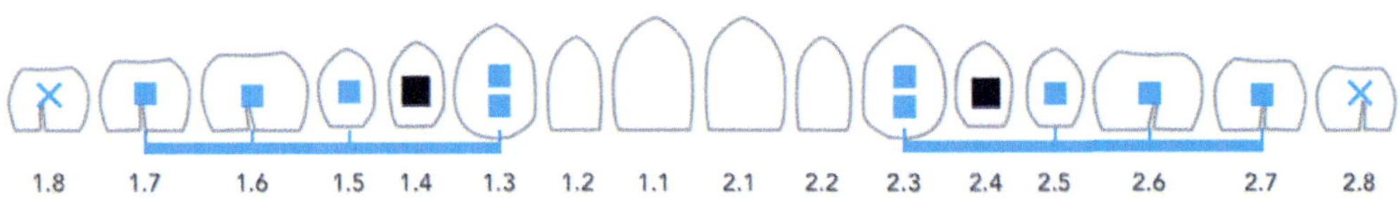

Fig. 23.35 G6 protocol is considered a full system for space closure, therefore does not allow the removal of one attachment without the rest.

G6 Align Protocol

In the G6 protocol, the canine is first retracted one-third of the space into the extraction site, while at the same time the posterior segment is mesialized up to a maximum of 2 mm.

- When the canine has distalized one-third of its total movement, there is a simultaneous retraction of both the canine and the incisors until the extraction site is closed
- The extraction site will not be closed until the end of the treatment
- In order to achieve a maximum anchorage, elastics should be used from the beginning

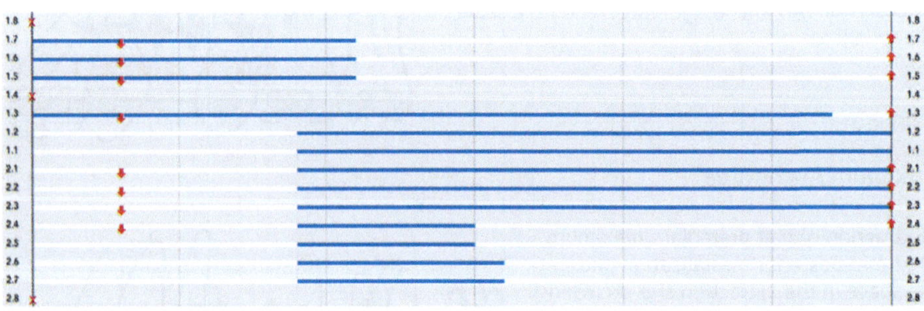

Fig. 23.36 Moderate anchorage protocol will start with canine and posterior segment at the same time, waiting for the canine to move to one-third of its total movement for anterior segment to start moving.

This protocol was designed by Align Technology to maximize posterior anchorage while maintaining root parallelism during retraction and space closure. It also maintains the incisor torque and prevents the overbite from deepening during incisor retraction.

Medium or Moderate Anchorage

- This is also partially solved with G6 protocol, as long as anchorage loss is between 2-5mm
- Mechanics: retraction of anterior teeth and mesialization of posterior teeth to close extraction space
- Staging: reciprocal space closure followed by simultaneous staging
  - Closure of the extraction space begins by moving the canines distally at the same time as the second premolar and first molar moves mesially until one-third of the extraction space is closed
  - The remaining space will be closed simultaneously from both anterior and posterior

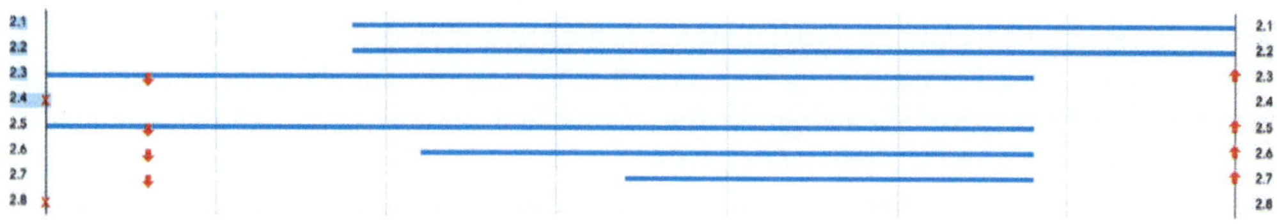

Fig. 23.37 Moderate anchorage protocol will start with canine and second premolar extraction at the same time, waiting for anterior and posterior segment to move until one-third of the space is closed.

How to Prescribe it

- Indicate first premolar extraction on prescription form
- Optional: specify in special instructions preferred solution
- Maximum: 0–2 mm posterior mesial bodily movement
- Moderate: 2–5 mm posterior mesial bodily movement

If no preference or conflicting special instruction is given, Align Technology will set the default to Class I canine occlusion with the appropriate anchorage.

- This reciprocal space closure exists when the posterior teeth act as an anchorage segment for the anterior teeth, and the anterior teeth act as an anchorage segment for the posterior teeth.
- The extraction site will close with the anterior teeth retracting two-thirds into the extraction site and the remaining one-third will be closed by mesialization of the posterior teeth.
- Extractions should be done 7–14 days before insertion of the aligners and space closure of the extraction site should start immediately from the first aligner. Halfway through the treatment the extraction site is closed and the two teeth on the extraction site do not move and thus act as an anchorage segment to retrude the incisors and mesialize the posterior teeth.

Staggered Staging Technique

Another option, very popular in Asia, is the staggered staging technique for extraction of first premolars which consists of:

- First: the canine 3s and the second premolar 5s move first over 8 stages (no movement in molars or incisors)
- Second: the molars 6s mesialize and the incisors retrude another 8 stages (no movement in canines and second premolars)
- Third: the canines 3s and the second premolar 5s move again (no movement in molars or incisors)

This staging pattern continues until all the extraction site is completely closed and the incisors are fully retracted.

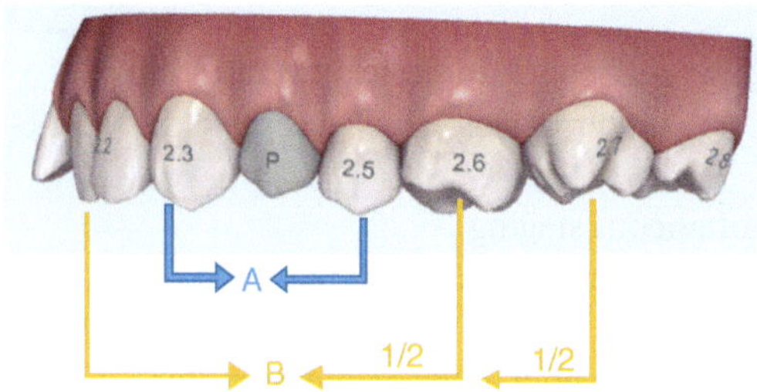

Fig. 23.38 A popular pattern in Asia for extraction space closure.

This technique minimizes tipping of the canines and controls incisor torque. However, a problem with the staggered technique is that it increases the number of aligners.

The attachments used in canines, premolars and molars are rectangular attachments and are placed with 2 mm between the margin of the aligner and the attachment so that the aligner embraces the whole canine and premolars crown.

For a better fitting of the aligner during the space closure, it is important to keep an occlusal contact within the molars 'molar bite control' during the retraction movement. For that purpose, chewies can be used to reinforce the occlusal contacts in the posterior zone during the first stages of treatment. Settling elastics in molars may be used to maintain the posterior occlusal contacts.

For better direction of the elastics during the closure of space instead of button cutouts in the canine, a direct bonding elastic control hook can be used. The bonding hook avoids undesired rotation caused by elastic force.

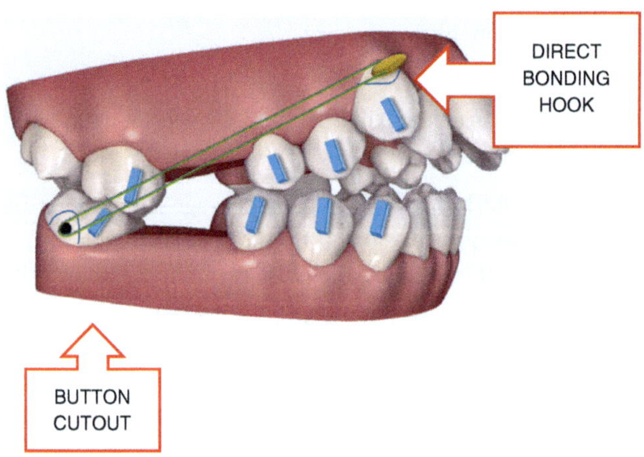

Fig. 23.39 The selection of bonding hooks or buttons has to be carefully planned.

Minimum Anchorage: Extraction of Second Premolars (5s)

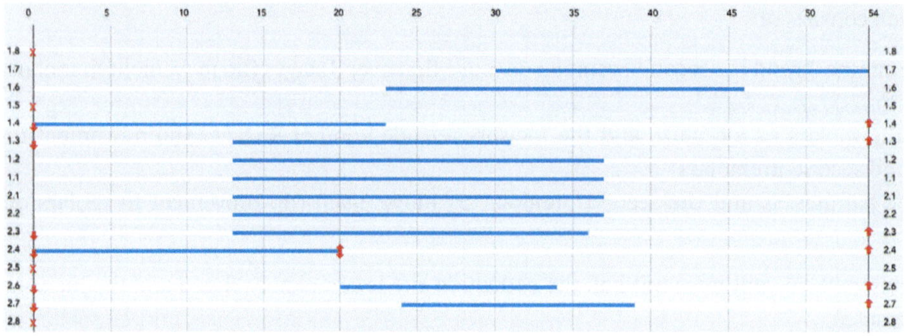

Fig. 23.40 Extraction of 5s with minimum anchorage.

Extraction of 5s, minimum anchorage:

- Place AT in the two mesial teeth (3 and 4) vertical attachments
- Place vertical AT doubled (6 and 7) to prevent tipping of the molars during the mesialization, which is part of the 'bowing effect'

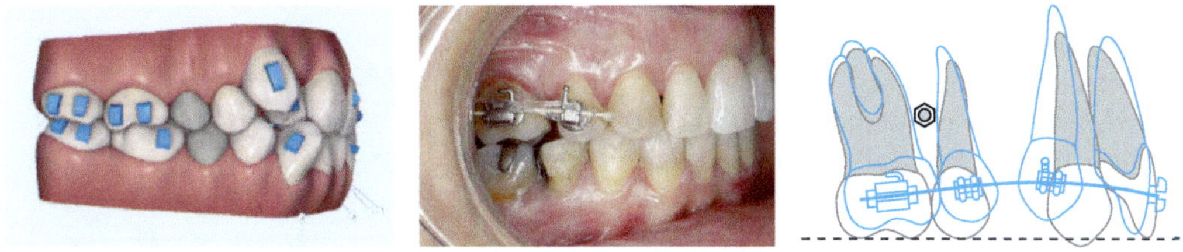

Fig. 23.41 With the double vertical attachment in molars the intrusion of the mesiolabial cuspid of the first molar during the space closure is prevented, and resolved using sectional wires as an auxiliary technique, as seen on the centre and right images.

- In the last three aligners, we can also ask to change the attachments in first premolar and first molar for a Power Arm attachment and ask for overtreatment of the tipping correction of the roots.

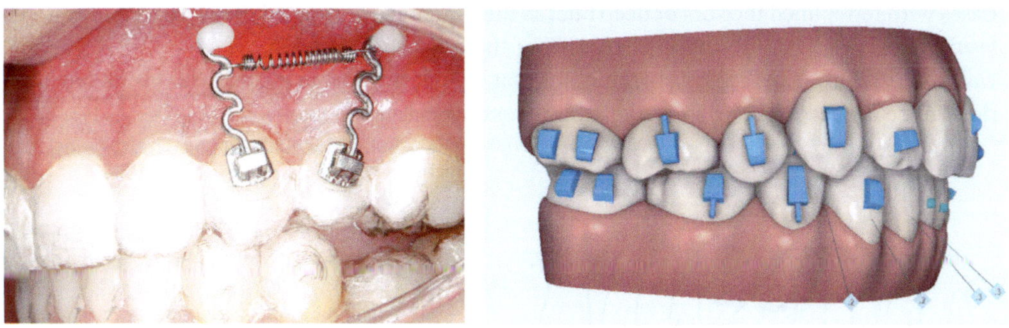

Fig. 23.42 With the Powerarm attachment in molars at the final aligners we can use Powerarms to get closer to the centre of resistance of the teeth adjacent to space closure.

A staggered technique for extraction of second premolars consists of:

- First: the first premolar 4s and the first molar 6s move first for eight stages (no movement in the rest of the teeth)
- Second: the canine 3s and the second molars 7s move another eight stages (no movement in 4s or 6s)
- Third: The first premolar 4s and the first molars 6s move first for eight stages (no movement in the rest of the teeth)

This staging pattern continues until the extraction site is completely closed and the incisors are fully retracted.

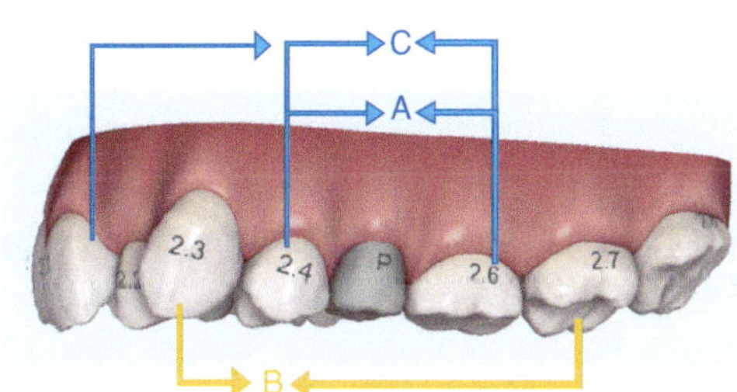

Fig. 23.43 Staggered technique for second premolar extraction.

A Staggered technique for extraction of first molars and mesializing the upper 7s, would consist of:

- The second premolar 5s and the second molars 7s move first for 8 stages (no movement in the rest of the teeth)
- Second: the first premolars 4s and the second molars 7s another 8 stages
- Third: The second premolar 5s and the second molars 7s move first for 8 stages (no movement in the rest of the teeth)
- Fourth: the first premolars 4s and the second molars 7s move another 8 stages

This staging pattern continues until all the extraction site is completely closed and the incisors are fully retracted.

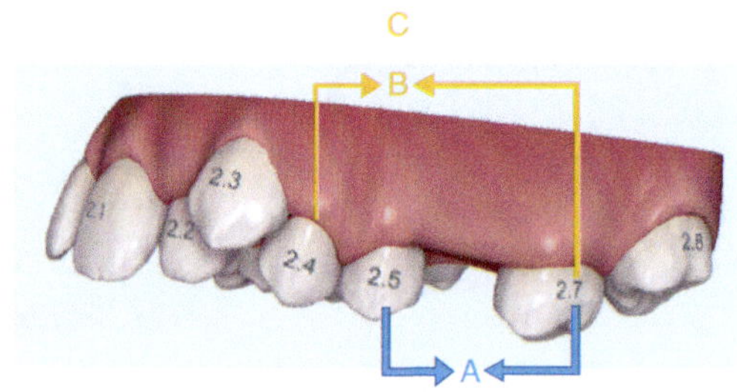

Fig. 23.44 Staggered technique for first molars extraction.

Powerarms Extraction Staging for Space Closure

Powerarms are indicated for some extractions, applying a force in the centre of resistance of teeth, achieving a body movement of the root.

- Cases with retroclined incisors or deep bite: as the incisors are retracted they lose torque and the overbite increases, with resultant deepening of the overbite
- Unfavourable pretreatment root inclinations that diverge away from the extraction sites: auxiliaries will be needed to achieve parallel roots across the extraction site

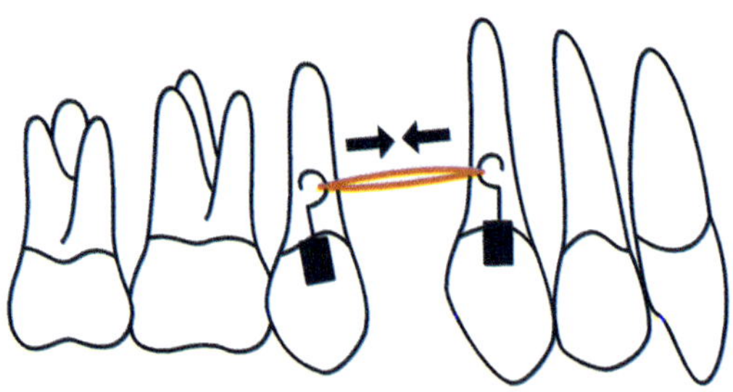

Fig. 23.45 Retroclined incisors might mean increased overbite and need root body movement, which might become more predictable with Powerarms.

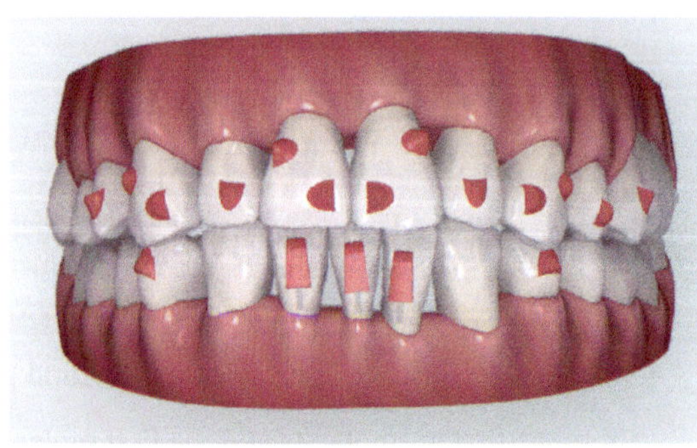

Fig. 23.46 Powerarms are great auxiliaries in achieving root parallelism.

This is an important aspect, as the 'bowing effect' is something that might happen with brackets and wires, and can be managed by getting closer to the centre of resistance of affected tooth:

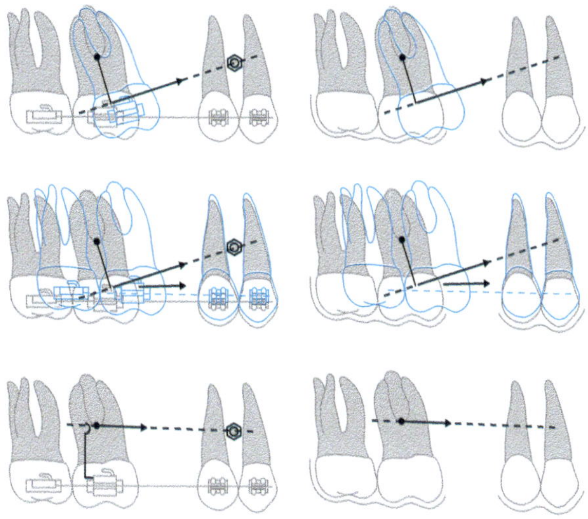

Fig. 23.47 Undesired effects of brackets and wires are quite similar to those found on aligner mechanics, and therefore the solution is also quite similar.

Tips for Extraction Cases with Aligners

- The extraction spaces should be closed with the roots of adjacent teeth converging toward the extraction site rather than away from it.
- The aligner must cover the maximum teeth adjacent to the extraction site; for that purpose use a small pontic or no pontic at all.
- The extractions should be made 7–14 days before the start of treatment and the space should start to close from first aligner.
- In order to maintain incisor torque during retraction and prevent the bowing effect, with the result of deepening the overbite, power ridges should be placed on incisors from the beginning and the clinician should ask the technician to apply intrusion + retrusion + lingual root torque during all the retraction movements.
- Use optimized root control attachment or vertical rectangular attachments on the teeth adjacent to the extraction site to maintain root parallelism. In addition, maintain a virtual gable bend of 10 degrees and ask the technician to close the extraction site with the roots of adjacent teeth converging towards the extraction site.
- To prevent a loss of anchorage, intermaxillary elastic should be used for extra anchorage.
- Overtreat root inclinations on either side of the extraction site and overtreat labial incisors torque.

23.2.3 Class II with 14 and 24 Extraction

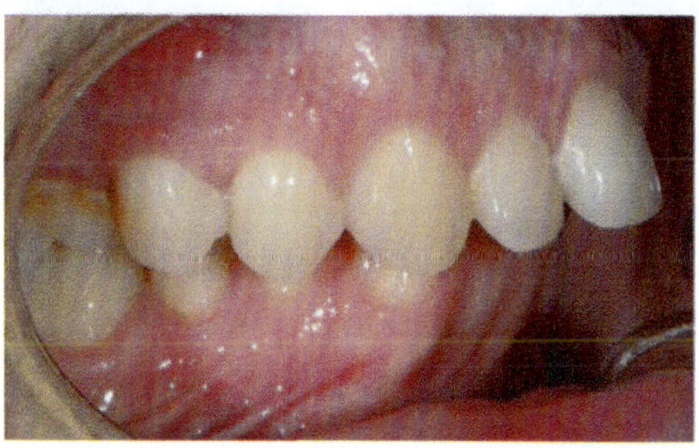

Fig. 23.48 Absolute anchorage with temporary anchorage devices.

Diagnosis

A 39-year-old man with hypodivergent skeletal Class II presented with proclined upper incisors, a 10 mm overjet, a 100% deep bite, scissor bite on right side and a steep lower Spee curve. They had an asymmetric upper arch with a canted occlusal plane and labiomental fold with mentolabial angle closed.

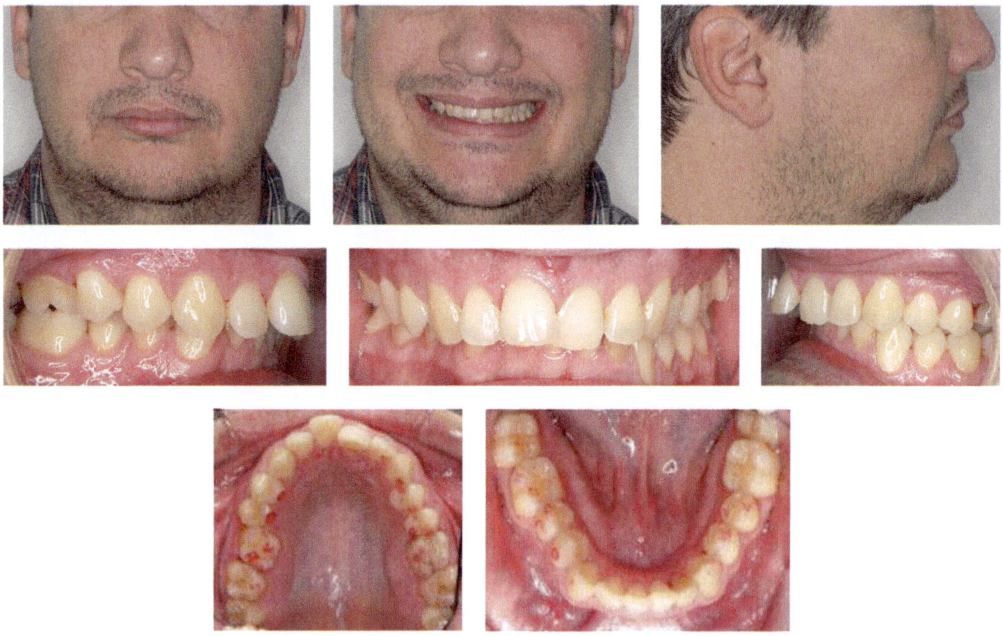

Fig. 23.49 Pretreatment extraoral and intraoral views.

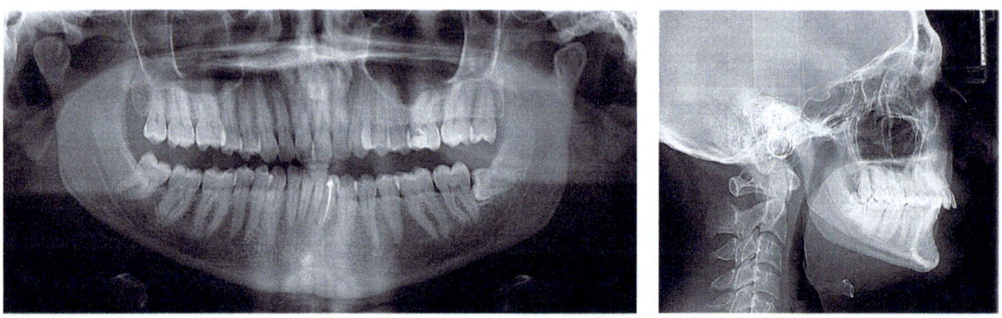

Fig. 23.50 Initial panoramic and lateral X-rays, and cephalometry.

Treatment Plan

Maxilla:

- Do not move third and second molars to use them as anchorage. Extraction of 1.4 and 2.4 to retract upper incisor and correct overjet
- Use TADs between second premolars and first molars to anchor second premolars during the anterior retraction
- Use bite ramps in 13 and 23 to assist the levelling of the curve of Spee

Mandible:

- Use attachments in first and second premolars as anchorage for intrusion of lower incisors. Do not move second or third lower molars, as they will be used as anchorage
- During the intrusion of lower incisors that exceed the predictability limits of alignment, use a lower microscrew between lower lateral incisors and lower canines to assist the intrusion using Powerchain over aesthetic buttons placed on the lower incisors

Requirements for the Technician

- Maximum anchorage G6 protocol on upper right side, on the left side the maximum anchorage protocols requirement was not met, so technician to place vertical attachment on 25 and 26 and double root control attachment on 23
- Button cutouts in 14 and 24 to place buttons from the premolar to the upper microscrews

Maxilla:

- Do not move third and second molar and use them as anchorage
- Extraction of 1.4 and 2.4 to retract upper incisor and correct overjet
- Bite ramps in 13 and 23 to assist the levelling of the curve of Spee with extrusion of premolars

Mandible:

- AT in first and second premolar as anchorage for intrusion of lower incisors. Do not move second or third lower molars as they can be used as anchorage

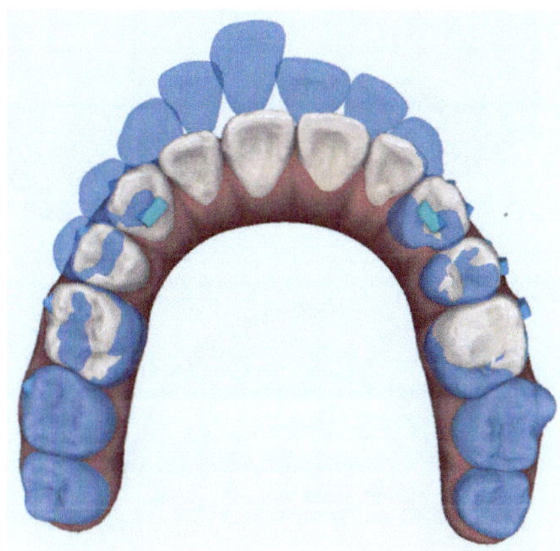

Fig. 23.51 Upper CC superimposition and instructions to CAD designer.

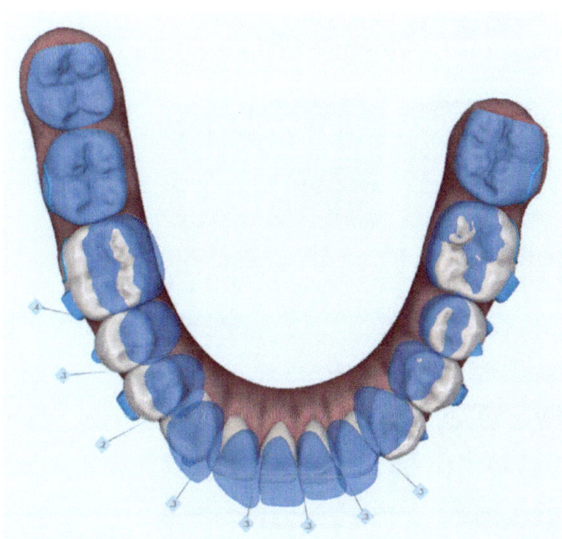

- Maximum anchorage G6 protocol on upper right side
- On the left side vertical attachment on 25 and 26
- Double root attachment on 23
- Class II elastic, full-time wear

Fig. 23.52 Lower CC superimposition and instructions to CAD designer.

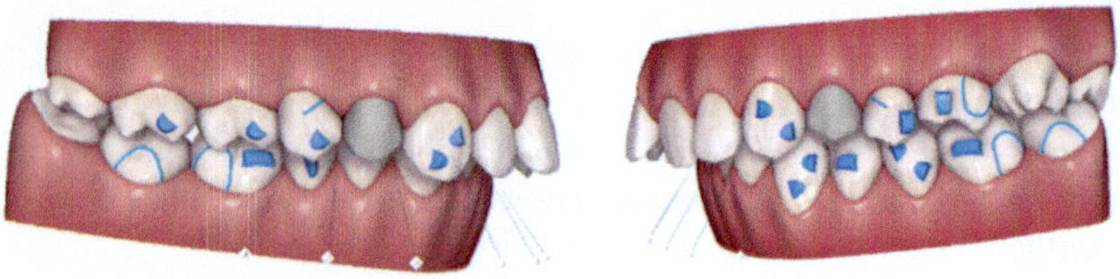

Fig. 23.53 Lateral ClinChecks.

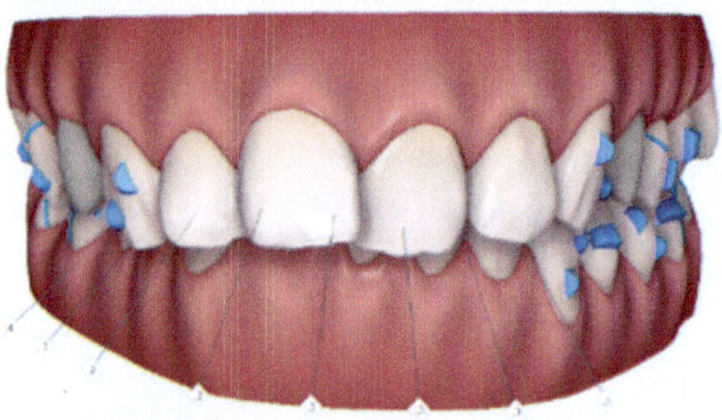

Fig. 23.54 Front ClinCheck view in which we can check deep bite and midline shift.

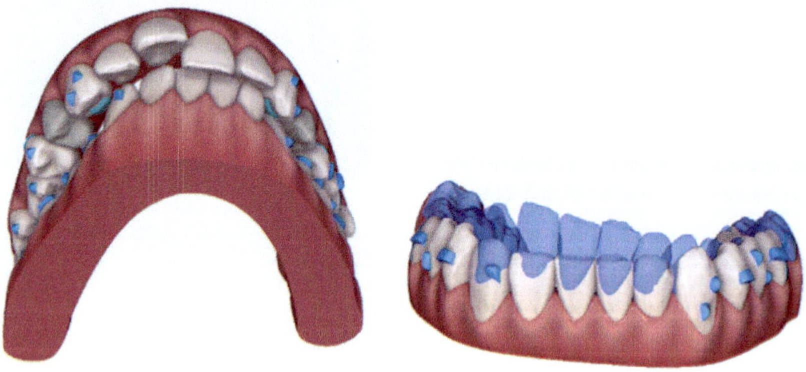

Fig. 23.55 Asymmetry is clear from both a vertical and saggital perspective.

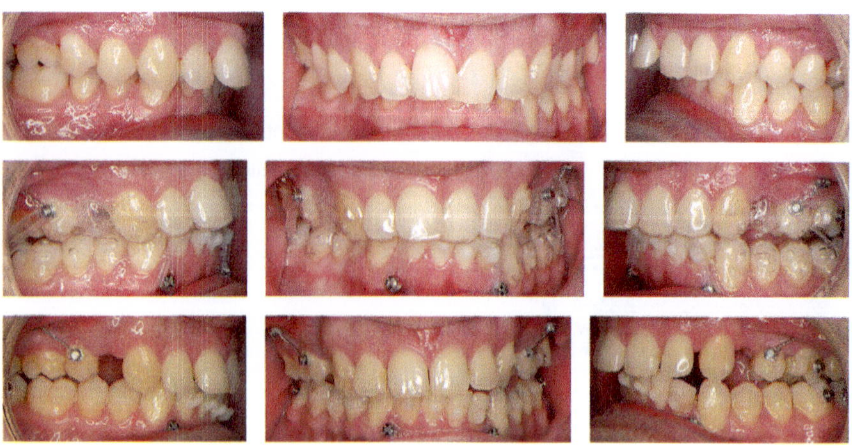

Fig. 23.56 Pure intrusion of lower incisors from TADs (right, front and left). Initial (upper) and evolution at 3 months (middle) and at 6 months (lower).

Treatment Summary

- A total amount of 67 aligners were used, and the patient is currently being treated with a protocol of absolute anchorage on the upper arch assisted with two upper microscrews
- On the lower arch the curve of Spee is being levelled with extrusion of lower premolars and intrusion of lower incisors assisted with lower microscrews between lower lateral incisors and canines
- The patient is using full-time wear class II elastic
- The extractions were realized in aligner two and the patient is using a 10-day interval protocol

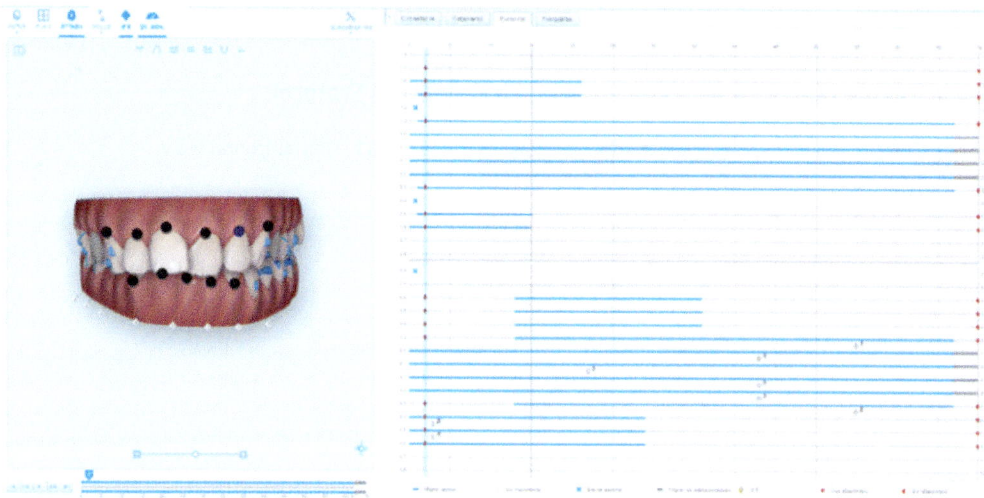

Fig. 23.57 Treatment evolution.

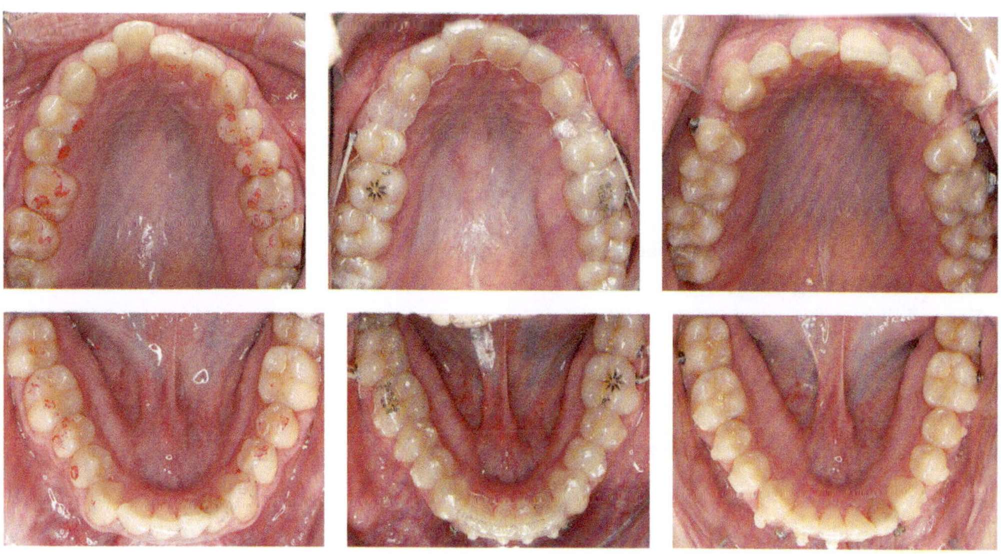

Fig. 23.58 Evolution with aligners. Initial (left) and evolution at 3 months (middles) and at 6 months (right).

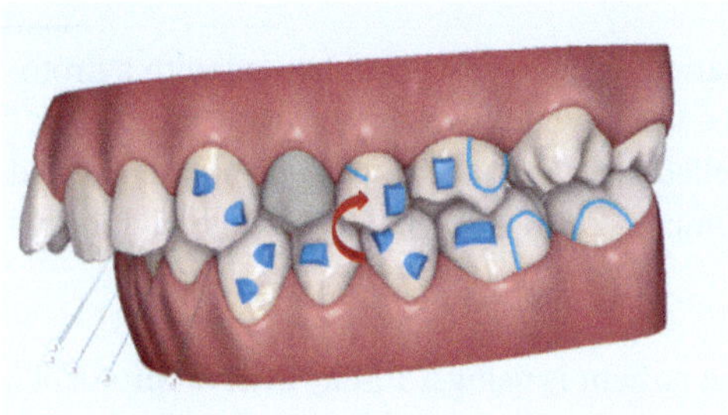

Fig. 23.59 Posterior teeth have distal root tipping movement planned.

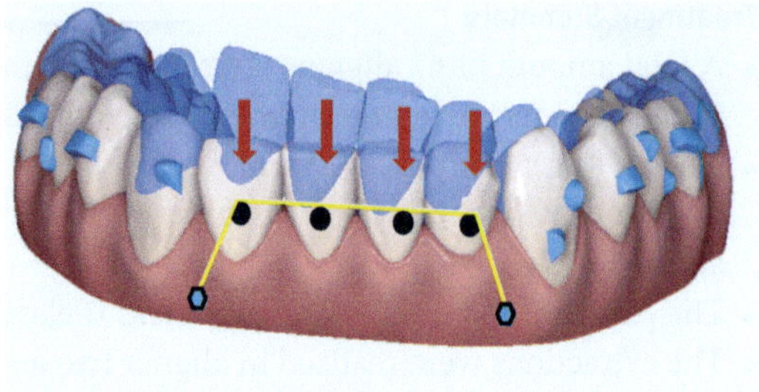

Fig. 23.60 TADs are included in the doctor's treatment plan with these diagram forces.

23.2.4 Extraction of 14 for Right Full Class II Patient, G6 Protocol

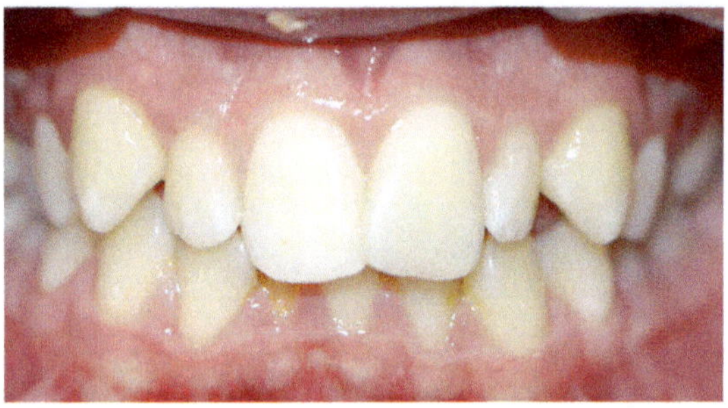

Fig. 23.61 Initial frontal view.

Diagnosis

A 13-year-old boy with no growth potential presented with proclined upper incisors, a 4 mm overjet and midline deviation to the right. He had full Class II right side, Class I left side and short incisor display.

Treatment Plan

Mandibular advancement was rejected because of the patient's skeletal situation and peak growth on CS5.

- Maxilla: reach canine Class I and keep molar full Class II by retruding anterior sector with G6 protocol
- Mandible: lower IPR to maintain overjet caused by upper lateral Bolton discrepancy, as the patient's parent refused veneers

ClinCheck 1: Requirements for the Technician

- Achieve Class I right side
- Expand, improve posterior aesthetics
- G6 protocol, right side
- Expansion on both sides
- Medium anchorage
- Centre midline simultaneously with space closure

Treatment Summary

- A total of 40 aligners used, between first set of 29 aligners and second of set of 11, on a weekly change basis
- On the lower arch the curve of Spee is levelled with extrusion of lower premolars and intrusion of lower incisors
- The extraction was accomplished between aligners two and three
- Incisors display was not improved, as this would require a multidisciplinary surgical approach

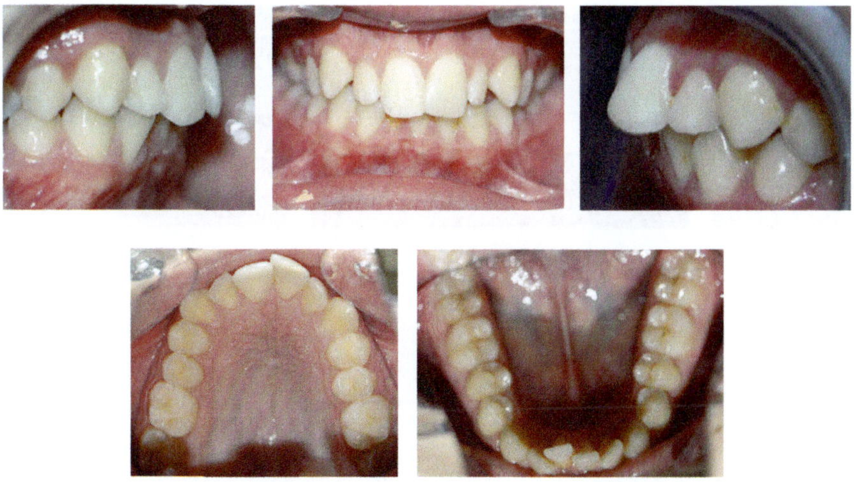

Fig. 23.62 Initial intraoral views.

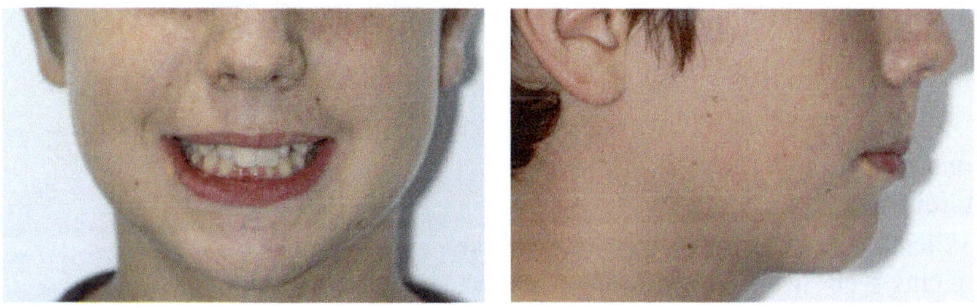

Fig. 23.63 Initial extraoral views.

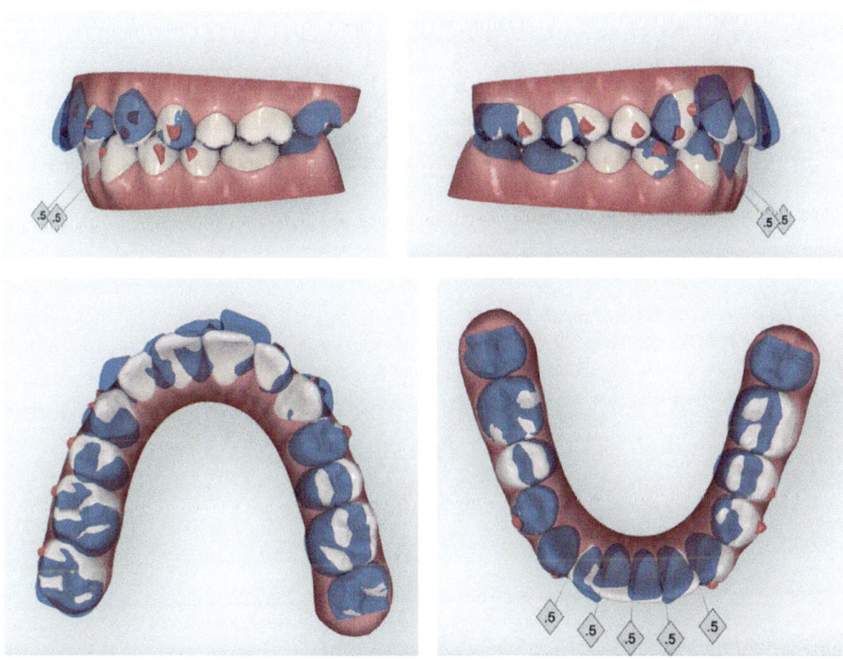

Fig. 23.64 Initial ClinChecks.

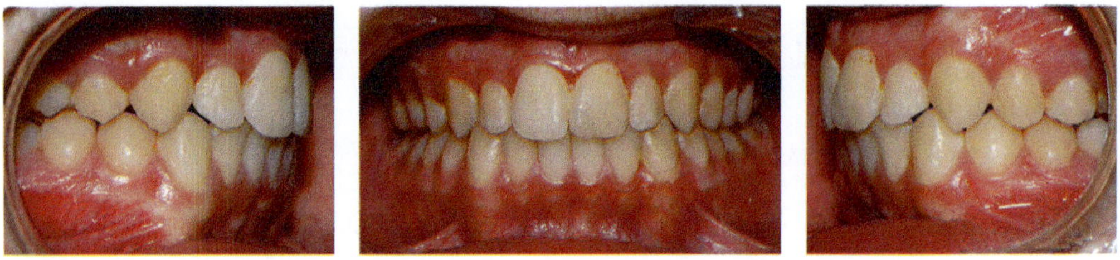

Fig. 23.65 Refinement: intraoral views after first set of aligners.

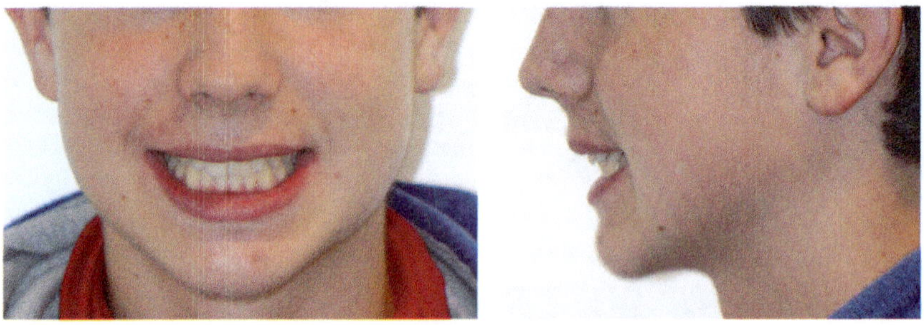

Fig. 23.66 Refinement: extraoral views after first set of aligners.

ClinCheck 2: Requirements for the Technician

- Upper anterior torque improvement
- Attachments bevelled to gingival, that proved to be useless
- Manual precision cuts + elastics for posterior extrusion

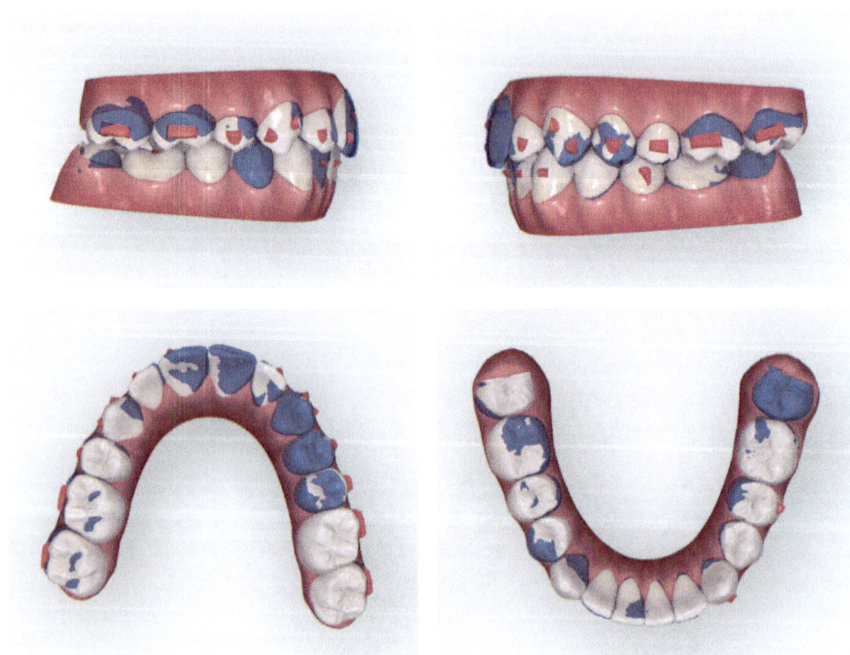

Fig. 23.67 Refinement ClinChecks.

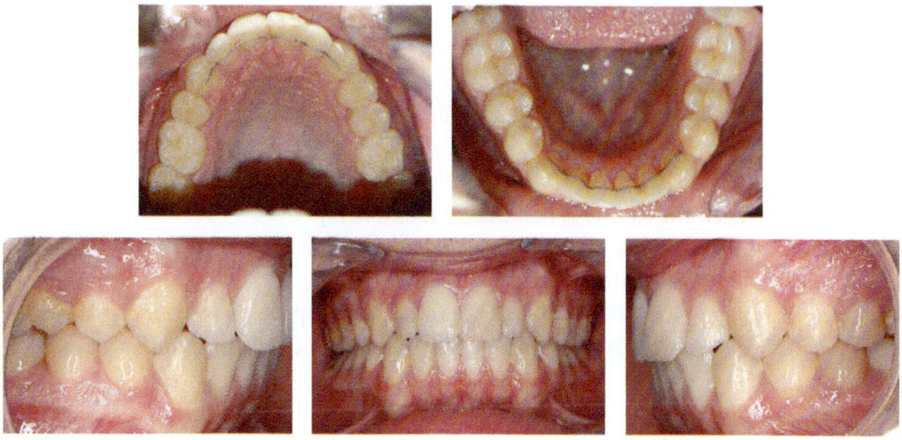

Fig. 23.68 Intraoral views of smile at the end of treatment.

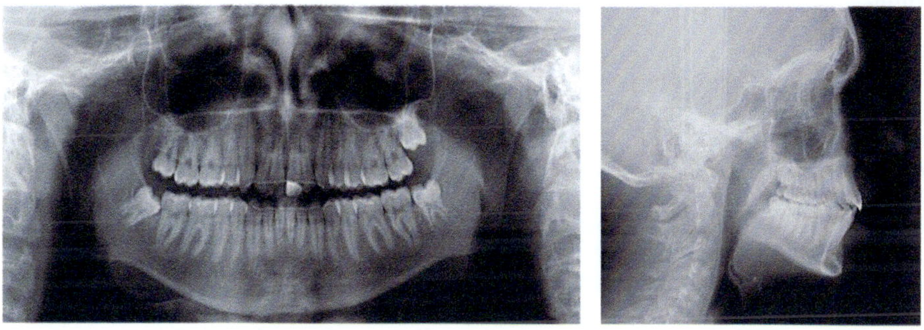

Fig. 23.69 Final panoramic X-ray to check final root paralellism between 13 and 15 after 14 space closure, and lateral X-ray to check final overjet.

23.2.5 Extraction of 14 for Right Full Class II Patient, Modified G6 Protocol

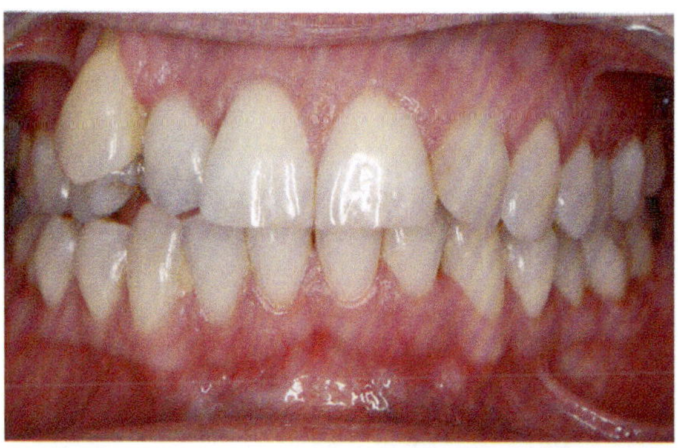

Fig. 23.70 Initial frontal view.

Diagnosis

A 34-year-old female presented with anterior protrusion, short display, a thin gingival biotype and a deep bite. She had full Class II on the right side, crowding, a right crossbite, centred midline and a right premolar crossbite.

Treatment Plan

- Complex extraction cases in which anchorage is moderate might benefit from a two-step space closure approach
- For this, first retrude the anterior sector. As aligner size shrinks on every treatment stage, there is a clear retrusion, but also a mesialization effect on the posterior sector. This last movement might be bigger than expected in the ClinCheck, so it was decided not to plan any mesialization, leaving residual space when the canine is in a Class I relationship
- Scanning or including the wisdom tooth in the PVS impression helps create more posterior anchorage, thereby making the treatment more predictable
- A secondary benefit is that Class III mechanics on a second step helps recover any anterior torque lost in the initial phase, which would not be possible with the simultaneous space closure typical of G6

ClinCheck 1: Requirements for the Technician

- 14 Extraction: G6 protocol
  - 1/3 Canine
  - Anterior
- Keep midline centred
- Expand but do not mesialize 15–17, and leave space between 13 and 15 when 13 is in Class I position
- Use third molars as anchorage, especially for crossbite on the first quadrant
- Class II elastics on right side
- Intrude 33–43 to level curve of Spee

Treatment Summary

- A total of 68 aligners used, distributed in three sets of aligners, changed every 7 days
- On the lower arch the curve of Spee is levelled with extrusion of lower premolars and intrusion of lower incisors
- Patients wore Class II elastics at night to help with anterior distalization
- The extraction was accomplished between aligners two and three

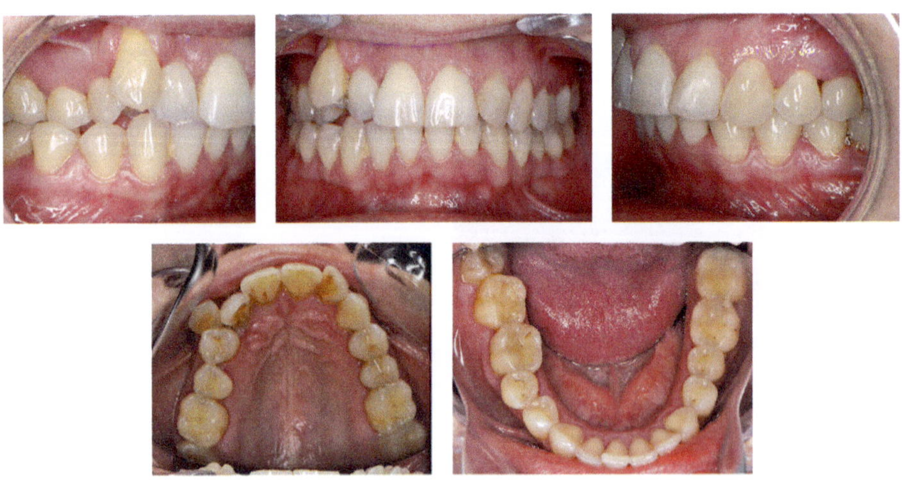

Fig. 23.71 Initial intraoral views.

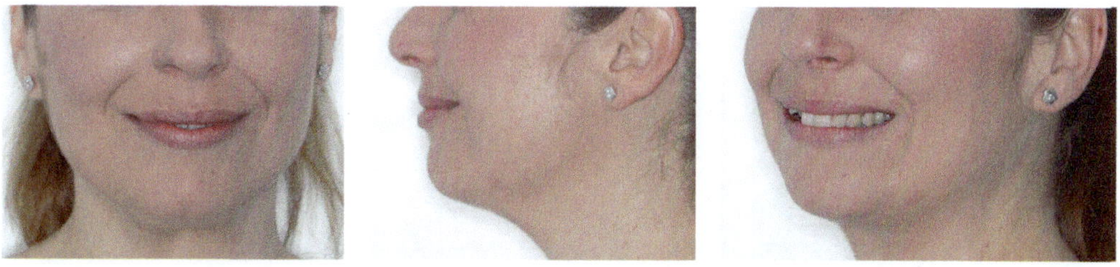

Fig. 23.72 Initial extraoral views.

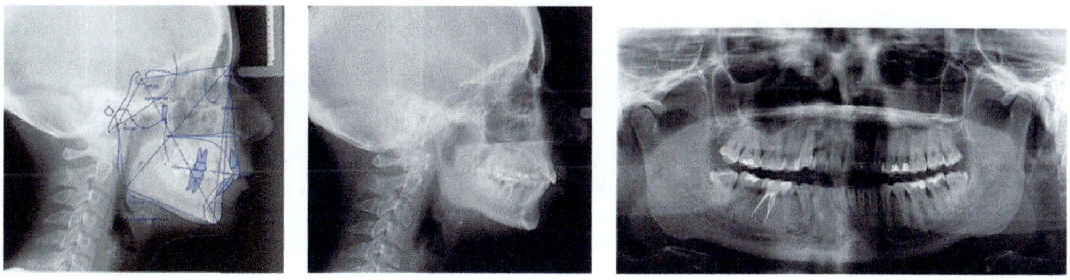

Fig. 23.73 Initial teleradiograph, and lateral and panoramic X-rays.

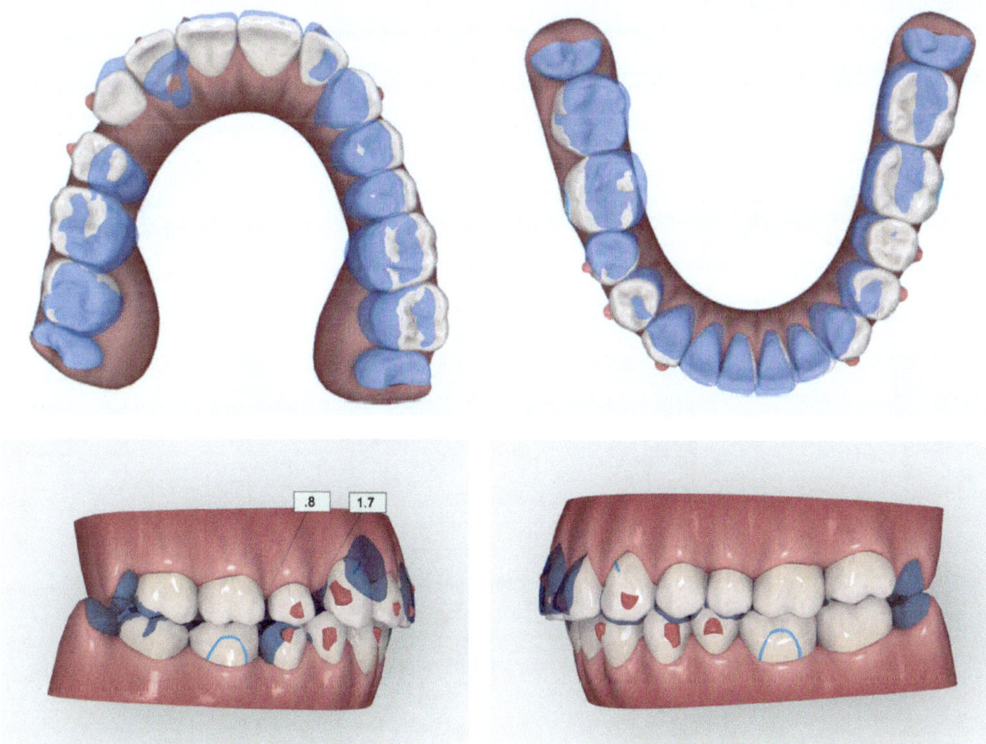

Fig. 23.74 Initial ClinChecks.

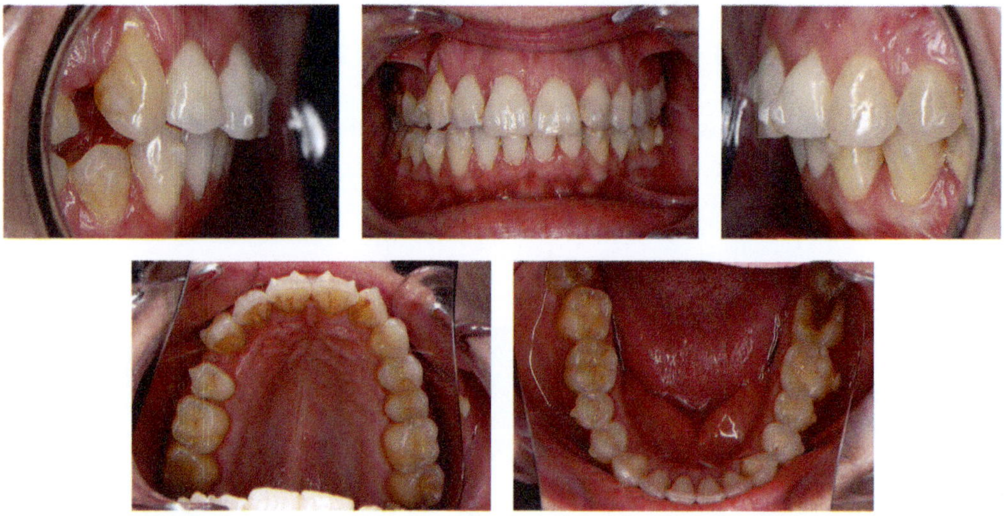

Fig. 23.75 Refinement: intraoral views showing exact position predicted on ClinCheck.

ClinCheck 2: Requirements for the Technician

- Right side
- Class III mechanics
- Anchorage loss first quadrant
- Simultaneous left + right expansion, once right crossbite is solved
- Use 18 as anchorage, opening space distal to it to help mesialize the second quadrant

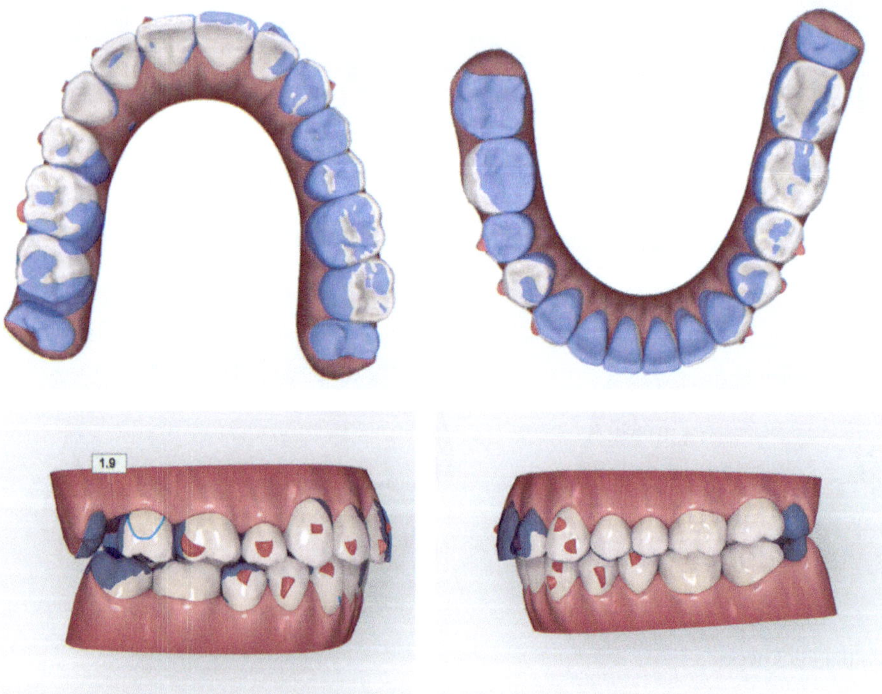

Fig. 23.76 Refinement: ClinChecks showing space mesial to 18.

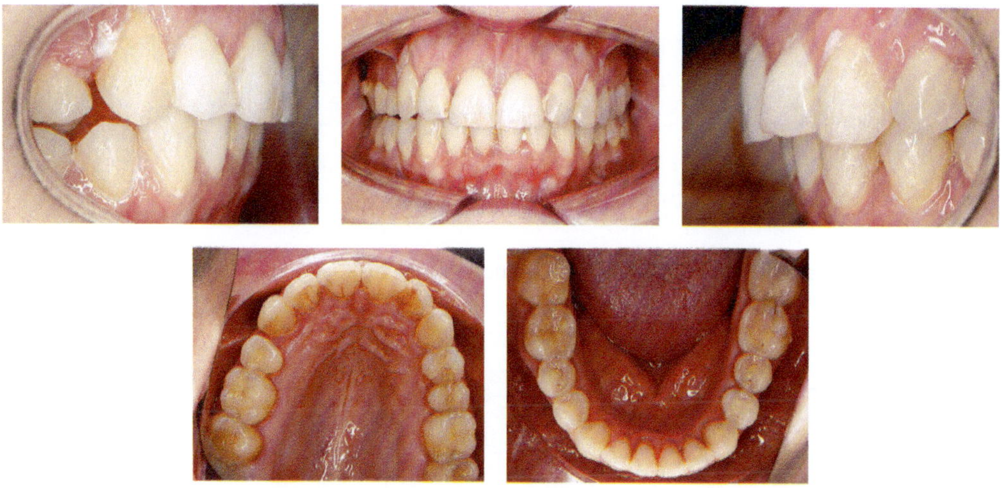

Fig. 23.77 Second refinement: intraoral pictures after two sets of aligners.

Fig. 23.78 Second refinement: smile after two sets of aligners.

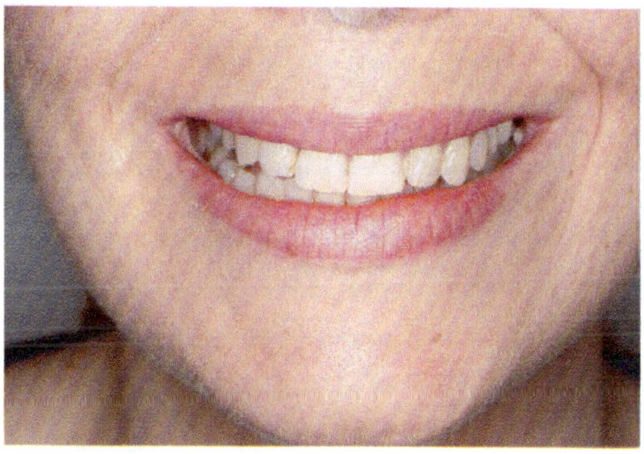

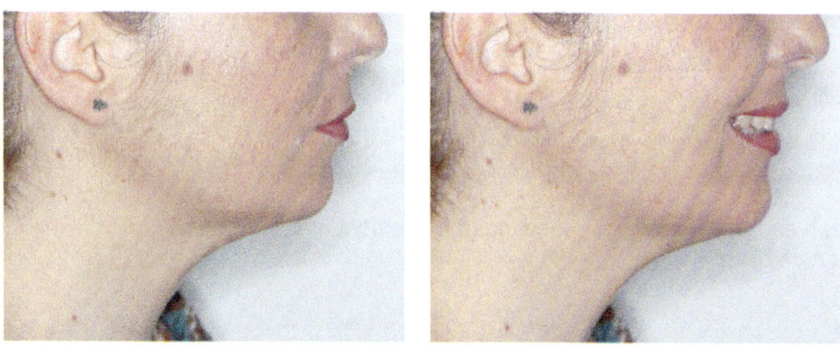

Fig. 23.79 Second refinement: extraoral views after two sets of aligners.

ClinCheck 3: Requirements for the Technician

- B&Es to improve right occlusion
- Expand and mesialize 15–17
- Vertical elastics on right side

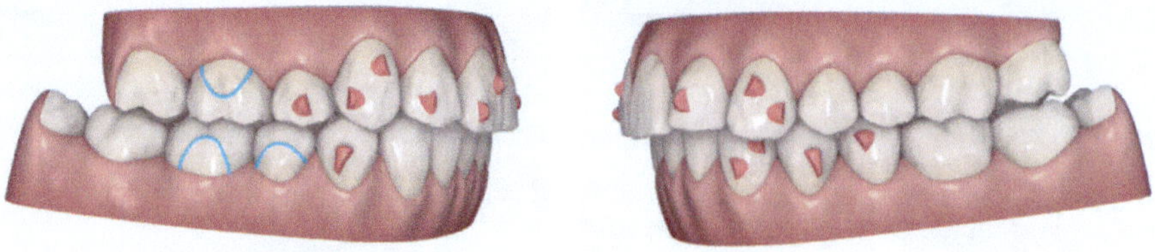

Fig. 23.80 Refinement: ClinChecks showing final vertical engagement.

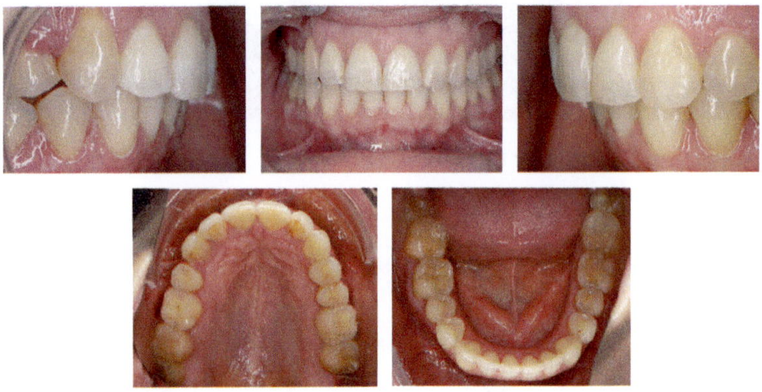

Fig. 23.81 Intraoral views after treatment.

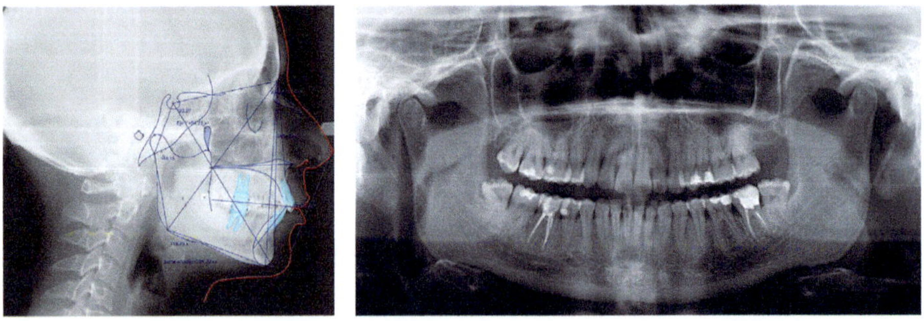

Fig. 23.82 Final teleradiograph and panoramic X-ray showing improvement in profile and root paralellism after extraction of 14.

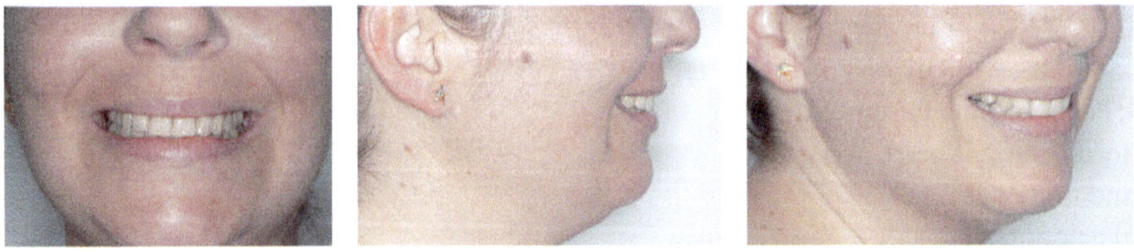

Fig. 23.83 Current extraoral pictures.

23.2.6 Extraction of 14 for Right Full Class II Patient, Modified G6 Protocol and Powerarms for Root Straightening

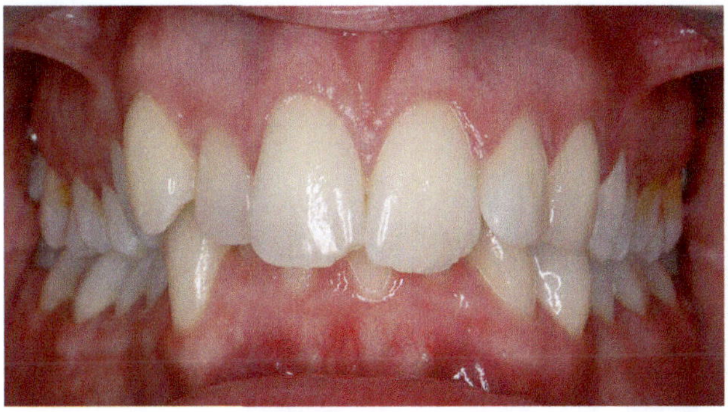

Fig. 23.84 Initial frontal view.

Diagnosis

A 32-year-old female presented with anterior protrusion, proper display, a thin gingival biotype and a deep bite. She had full Class II on the right side, crowding and a midline that deviated to the left.

Treatment Plan

- As this case has an anchorage loss bigger than 2 mm it was decided to go for a two-step space closure approach
- First retrude anterior sector. As aligner size shrinks on every treatment stage, there is a clear retrusion, but also a mesializating effect on posterior. This last movement might be bigger than expected in the ClinCheck, and reason no mesialization was planned, leaving residual space when the canine is in a Class I relationship
- Scanning or including wisdom tooth in the PVS impression helps create more posterior anchorage, therefore making the treatment more predictable by opening space between this and second molar to mesialize quadrant on the second step
- Finally, as space closure is mainly created by crown movements and anchorage loss is large, power arms were planned to straighten roots and achieve proper final root parallelism

ClinCheck 1: Requirements for the Technician

- 14 Extraction: G6 protocol
  - 1/3 Canine
  - Anterior
- Centre midline
- Relative anterior extrusion by retrusion
- Expand but do not mesialize 15–17
- Class II elastics, right side

Treatment Summary

- A total of 85 aligners were used, distributed in three sets of aligners, changed every 7 days
- On the lower arch the curve of Spee is levelled with extrusion of lower premolars and intrusion of lower incisors

- Patient wore Class II elastics at night to help with anterior distalization
- The extraction was accomplished between aligners two and three
- Final precision cuts were made for root straightening with bonded Powerarms

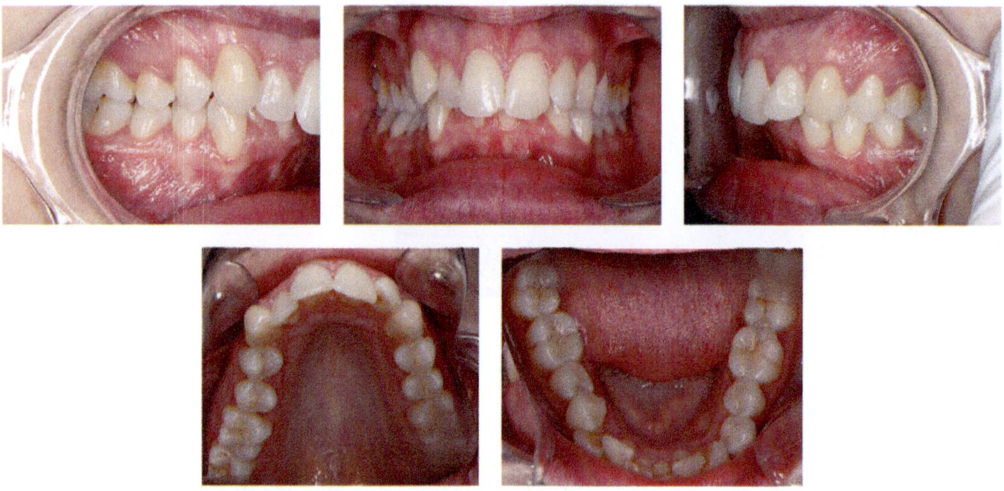

Fig. 23.85 Initial Intraoral views.

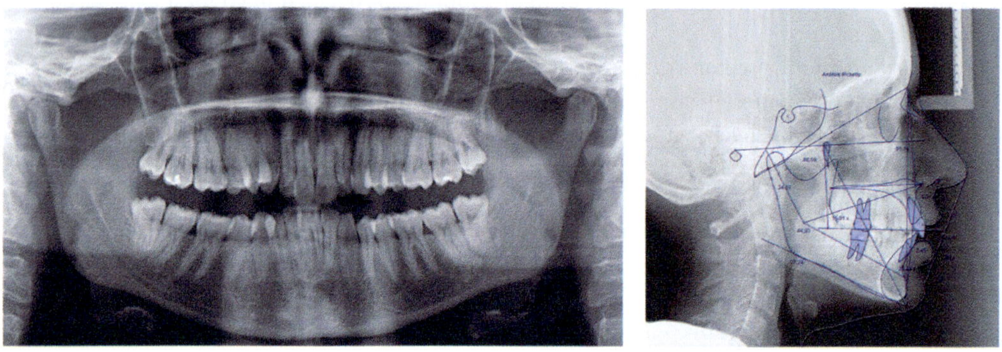

Fig. 23.86 Initial panoramic X-ray and teleradiograph.

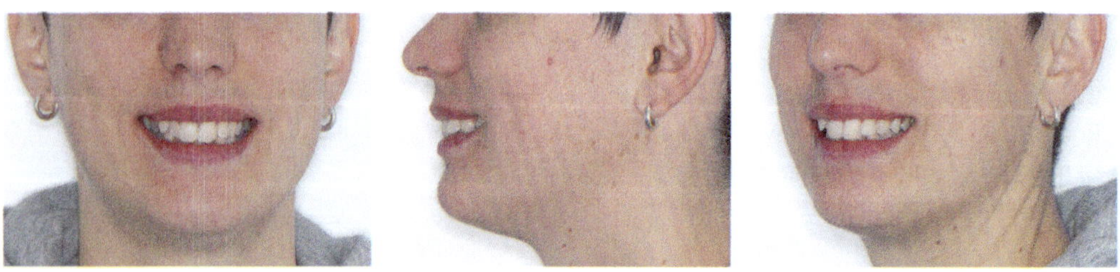

Fig. 23.87 Initial smile.

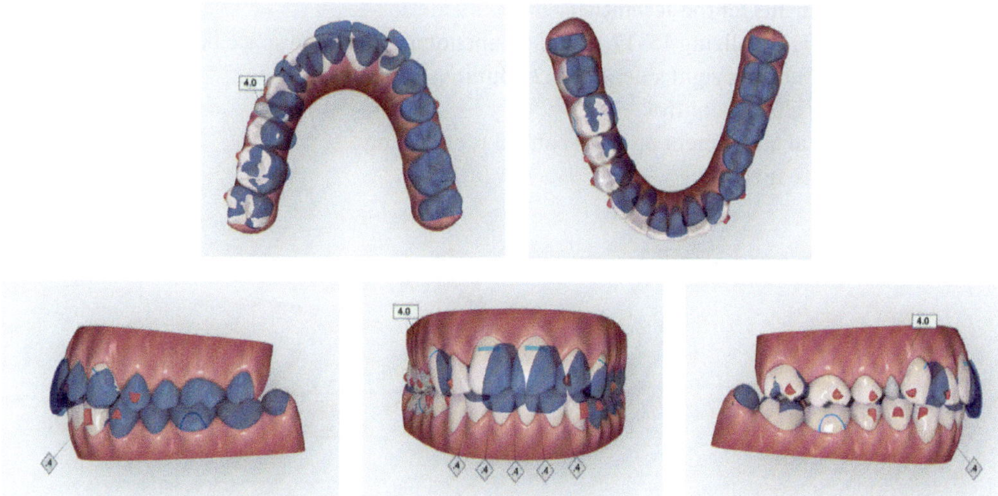

Fig. 23.88 Initial ClinCheck with posterior spacing.

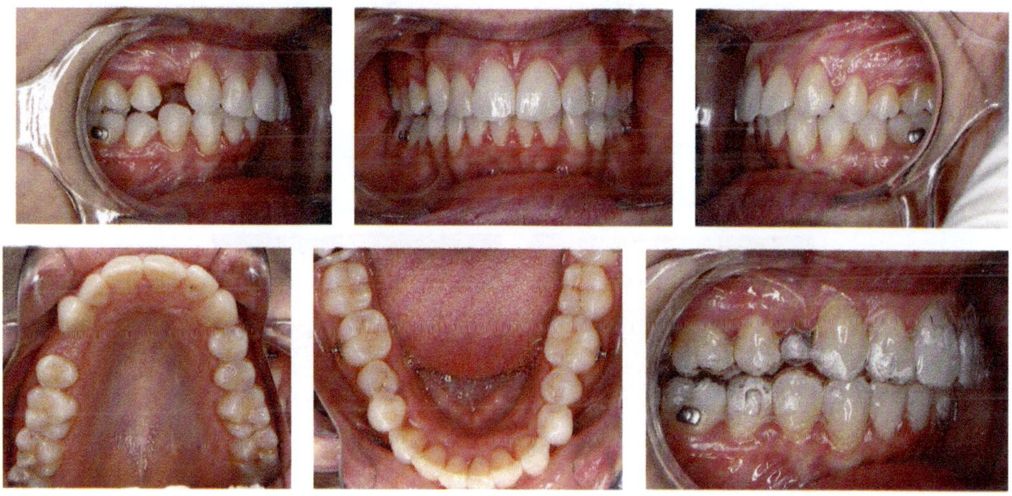

Fig. 23.89 Refinement: ClinCheck with posterior residual spacing, it can be appreciated how the bowing effect occurs even with no posterior mesialization as a result of aligner shrinkage.

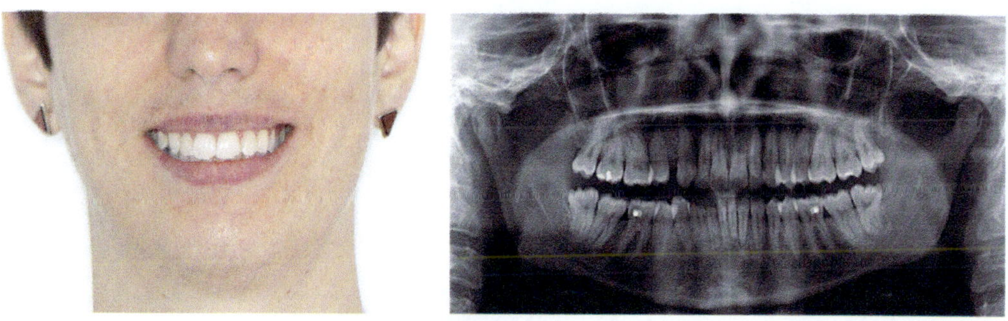

Fig. 23.90 Refinement: the midline has been centred and exposure increased; roots are parallel.

ClinCheck 2: Requirements for the Technician

- Lose anchorage by mesializing 15–17, use 18 as anchorage and open space between this and 17
- Class II + class III elastics right side, 12 + 12 hours
- Vertical and space closure control
- Rectangular vertical attachment on 15 to control root tipping
- Second quadrant as anchorage

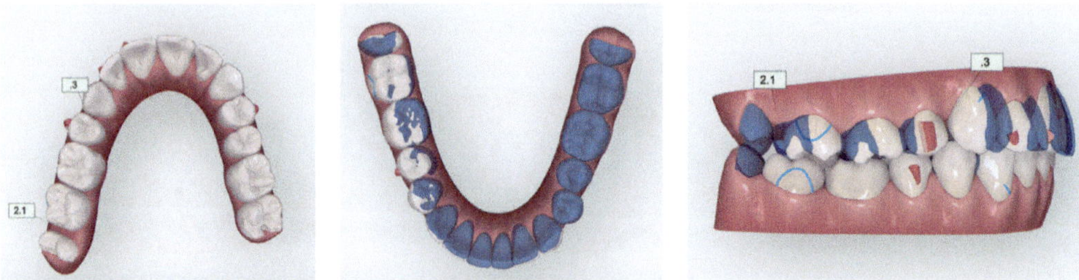

Fig. 23.91 Refinement ClinChecks.

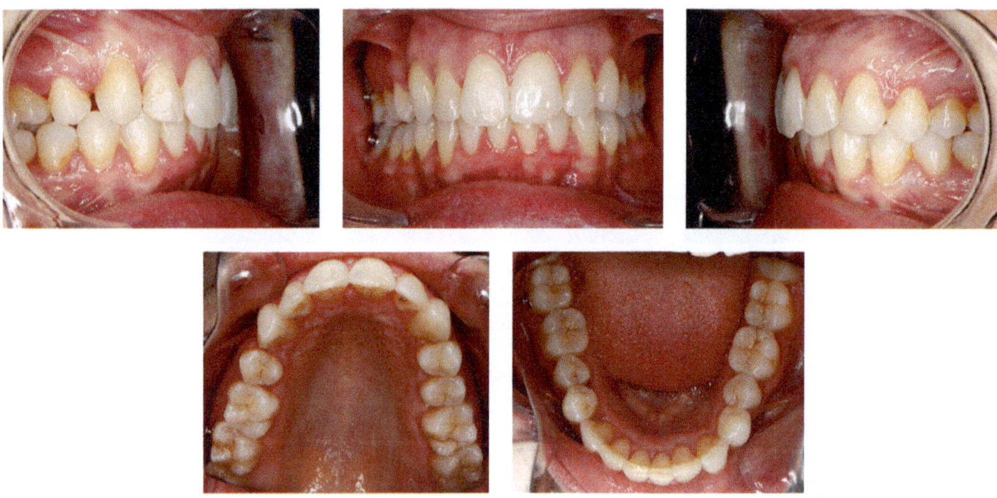

Fig. 23.92 Second refinement: intraoral views.

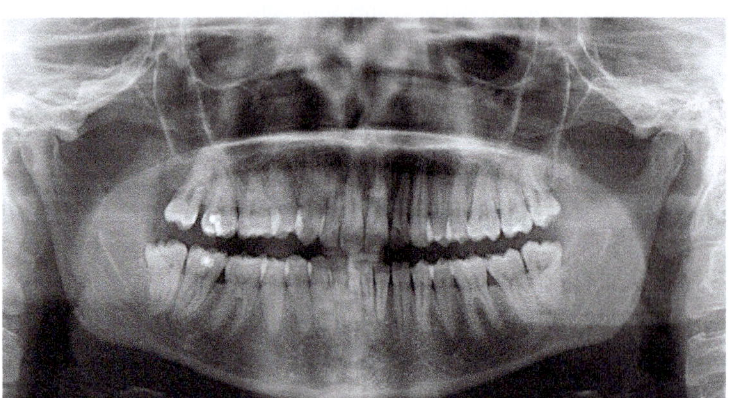

Fig. 23.93 Second refinement: space distal to 17 can be observed on the panoramic X-ray, as well as lack of parallelism between 13 and 15.

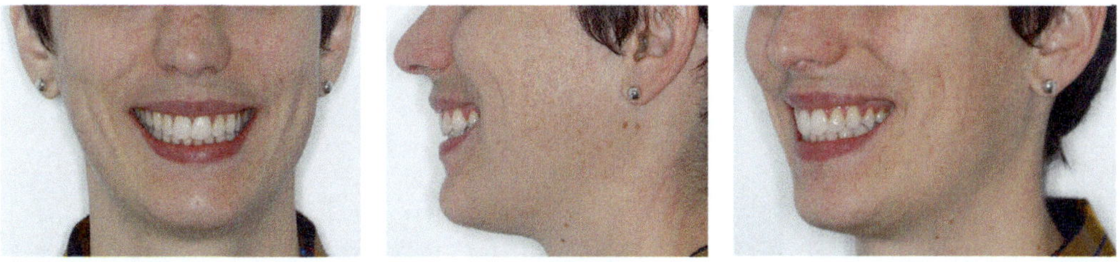

Fig. 23.94 Second refinement: space distal to 17 can be observed, as well as lack of parallelism between 13 and 15.

ClinCheck 3: Requirements for the Technician

- Lower fourth quadrant expansion anchored on the rest of the arch and 48
- Upper quadrant space closure on 14
- Precision cutouts on right side for buttons and elastics and bonded Powerarms

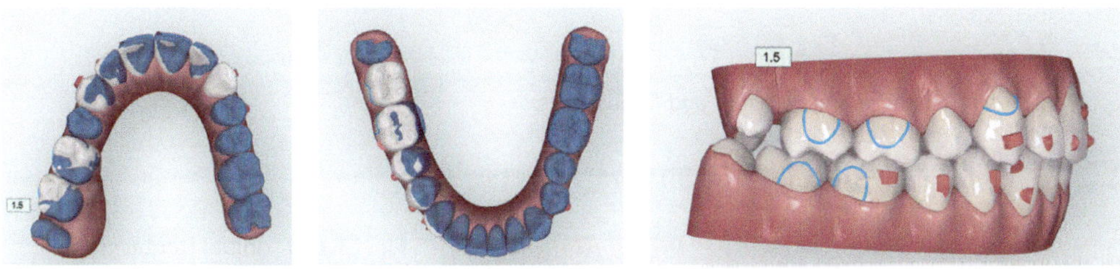

Fig. 23.95 Second refinement ClinChecks.

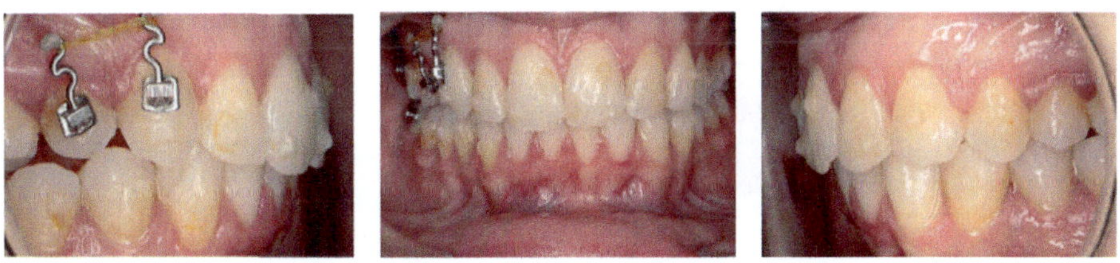

Fig. 23.96 Intraoral views with Powerarms to straighten roots for 13 and 15 after space closure at 14.

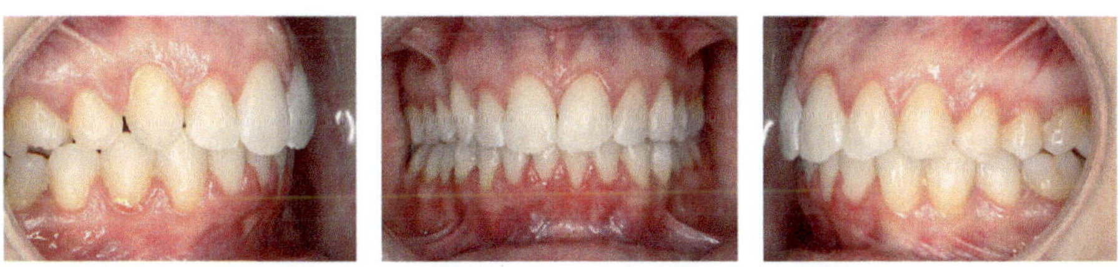

Fig. 23.97 Current intraoral views pending 5 aligners to the end of treatment.

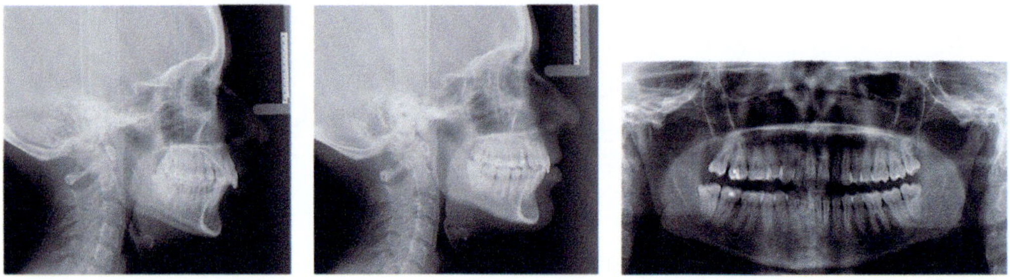

Fig. 23.98 Initial and final lateral and panoramic X-ray showing profile changes and root parallelism.

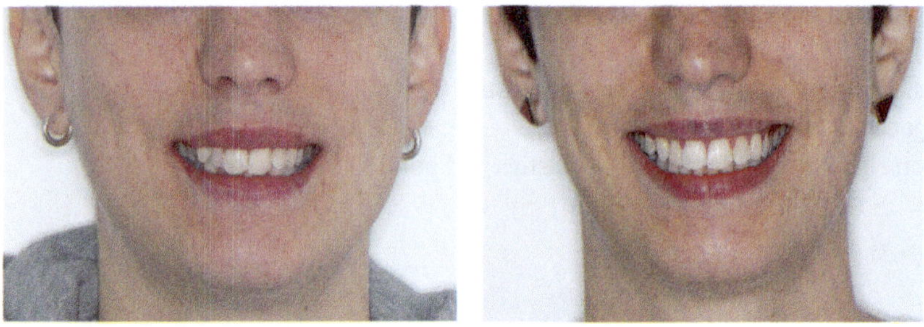

Fig. 23.99 Comparison of pretreatment and final smiles.

23.2.7 Extraction of 14 and 24 on Bilateral Full Class II

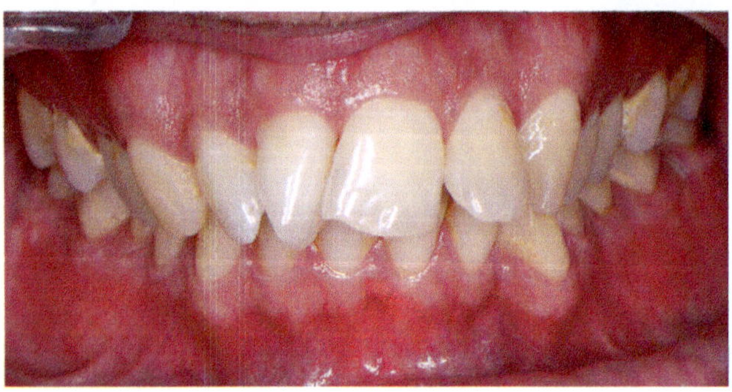

Fig. 23.100 Initial frontal view.

Diagnosis

- Anterior deep bite 80%
- Proper display
- Posterior compression
- Dentoskeletal discrepancy
- Bilateral full Class II
- Irregular 11 shape and size

Treatment Plan

- Extract 14–24
- Retract 13–23 avoiding any anchorage loss

- Expand posterior sectors
- Intrude lower incisors to flatten curve of Spee
- Leave anterior spacing for veneers for 14–24 to improve smile aesthetics

ClinCheck 1: Requirements for the Technician

- 14 and 24 extraction: G6 protocol
  - 1/3 Canine movement
  - Anterior retraction after this
- Class II elastics for anchorage and retraction
- Expand both arches
- Set second molars as unmovable so as to increase posterior anchorage

Treatment Summary

- First set had 56 aligners, but the patient was rescanned on number 36 owing to fitting issues in the anterior sector, after a 7-day change. Second set had 43 aligners changed every 7 days
- Patient wore Class II elastics at night during the whole treatment
- Extractions were accomplished between aligners two and three
- After treatment, patient is expecting veneers
- Severe 11 rotation needed from auxiliary buttons and Powerchain to be solved

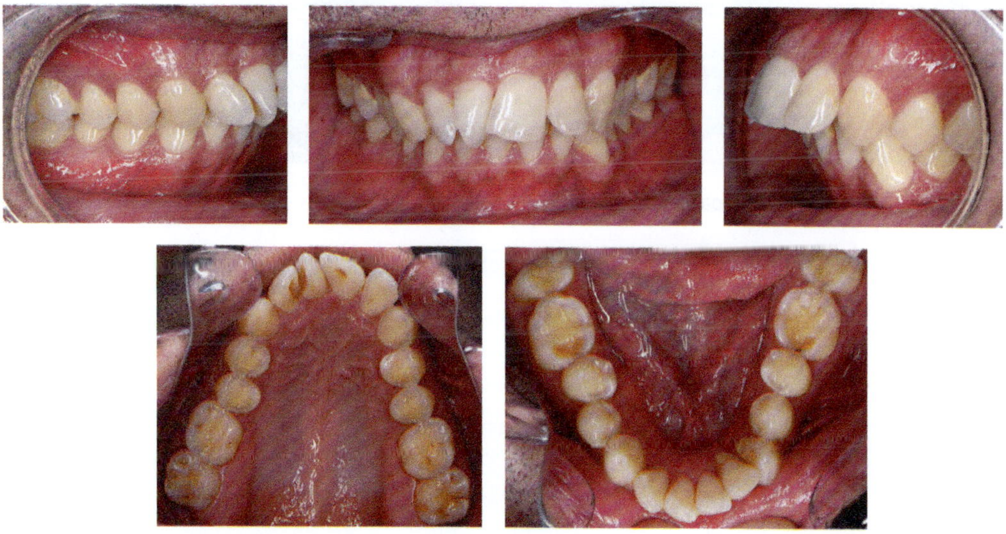

Fig. 23.101 Initial intraoral situation.

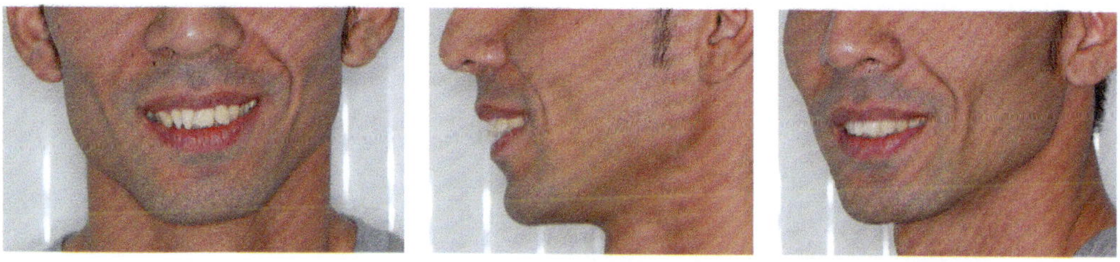

Fig. 23.102 Initial extraoral views.

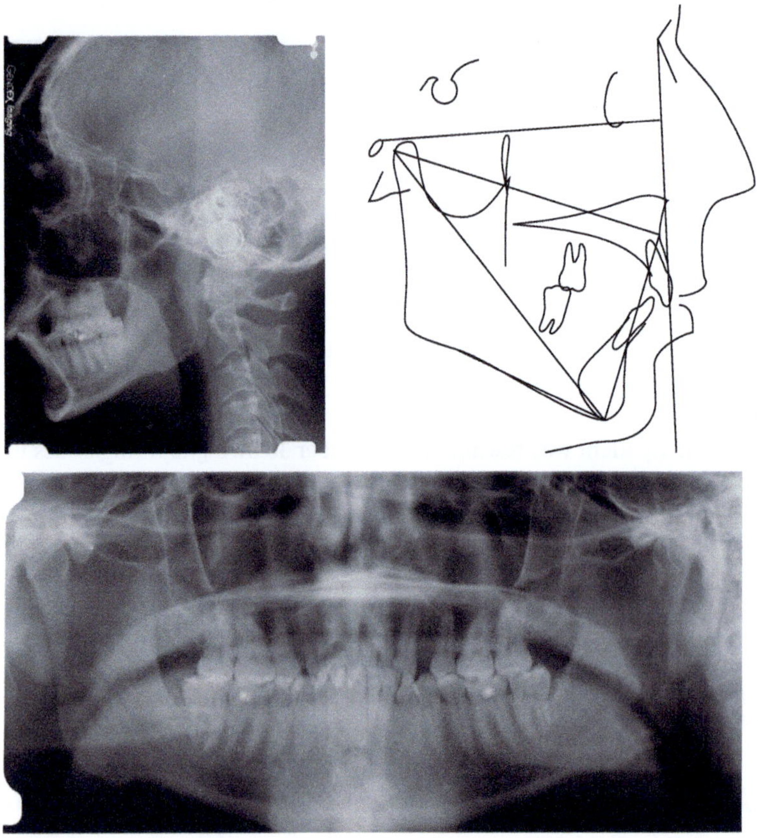

Fig. 23.103 Initial lateral and panoramic X-rays and cephalometric analysis.

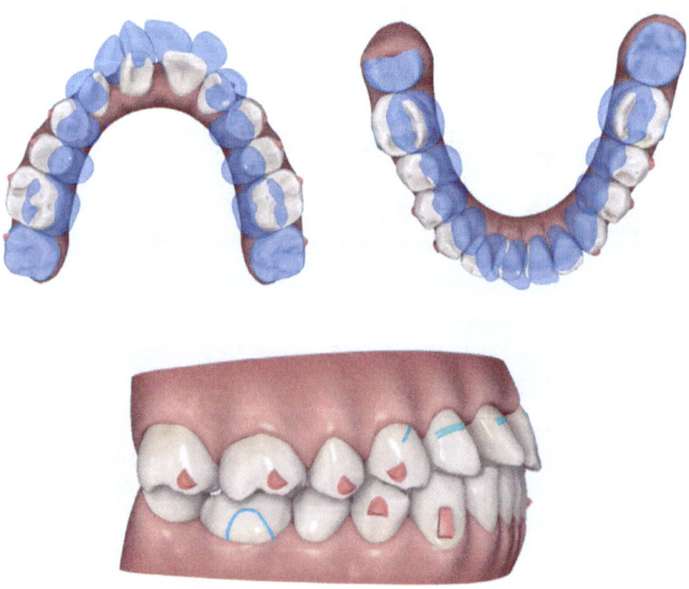

Fig. 23.104 Initial ClinChecks.

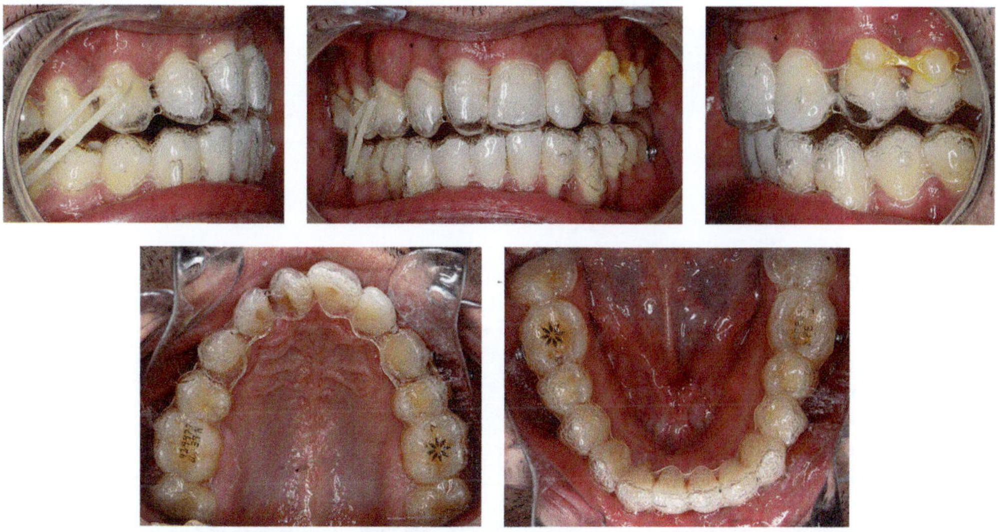

Fig. 23.105 Intraoral views when anterior misfitting was detected.

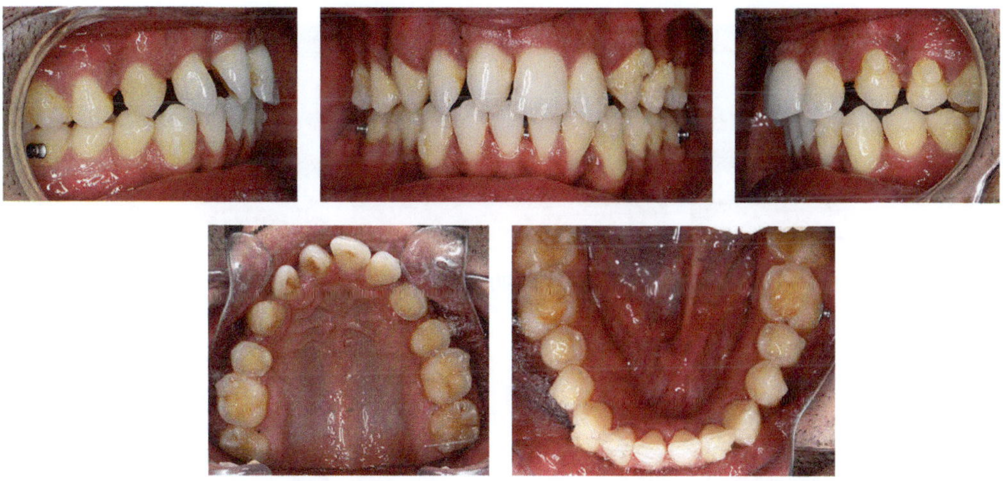

Fig. 23.106 Refinement: intraoral views.

ClinCheck 2: Requirements for the Technician

- Precision cuts on lingual surface of 23–13 to help with rotation while wearing Class II elastics
- Conventional vertical attachments on 11, bevelled to a position opposed to rotation on both buccal and lingual surfaces. During treatment, manual precision cuts for buttons and powerchain 11–15 to be made to help with its rotation
- Leave spaces on anterior sectors, as agreed with cosmetic dentist
- Sequential distalization on second quadrant, as a result of loss of anchorage on the first set of aligners

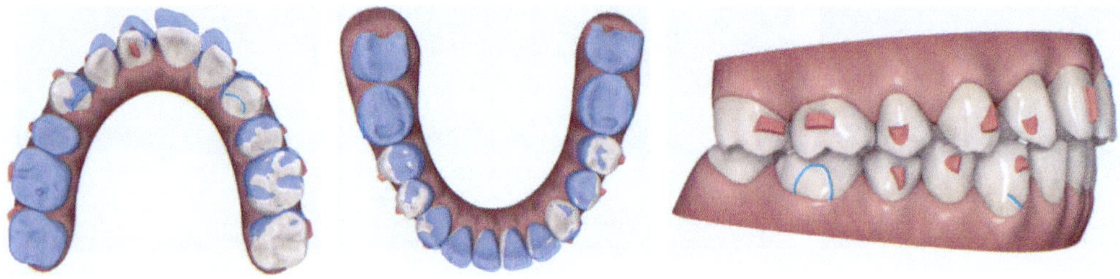

Fig. 23.107 Refinement ClinCheck.

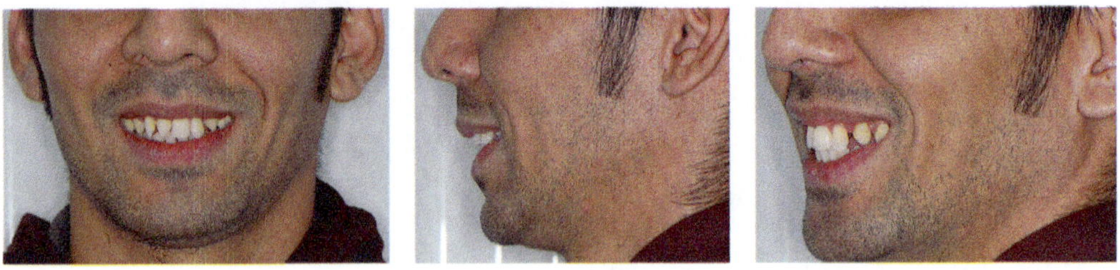

Fig. 23.108 Refinement: extraoral views.

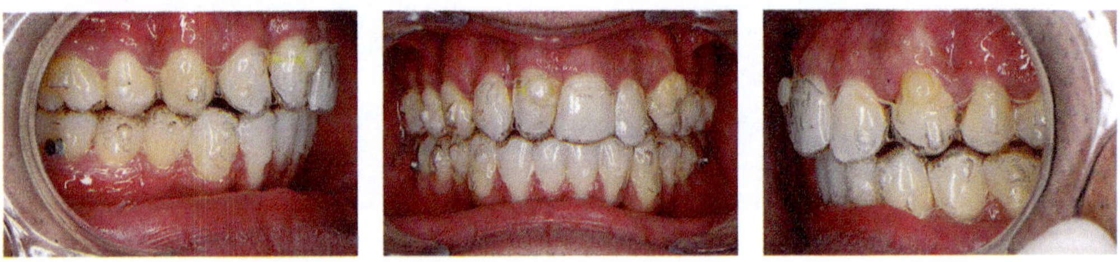

Fig. 23.109 A Powerchain was used to reduce rotations resulting from a lack of fit.

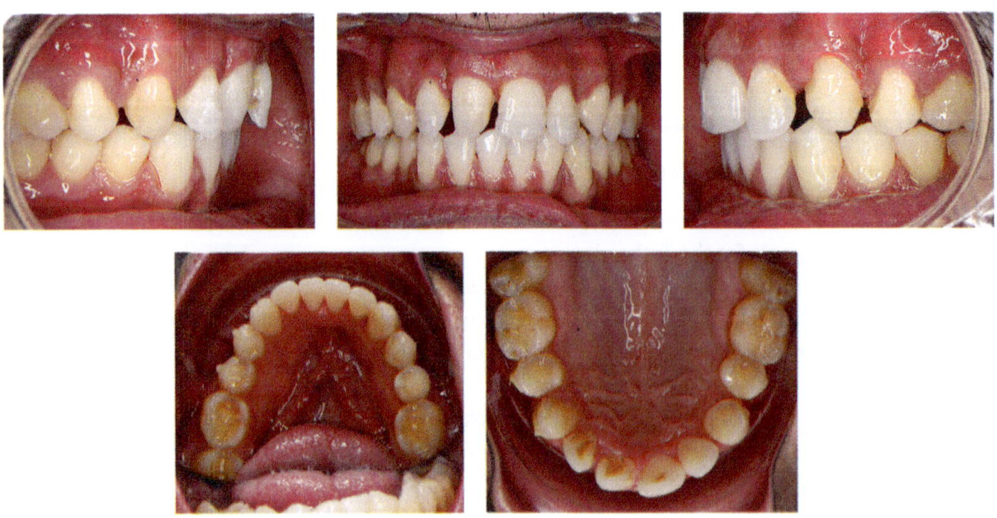

Fig. 23.110 Space distribution equal to final ClinCheck position, and patient is almost ready for veneers after treatment for 22 months.

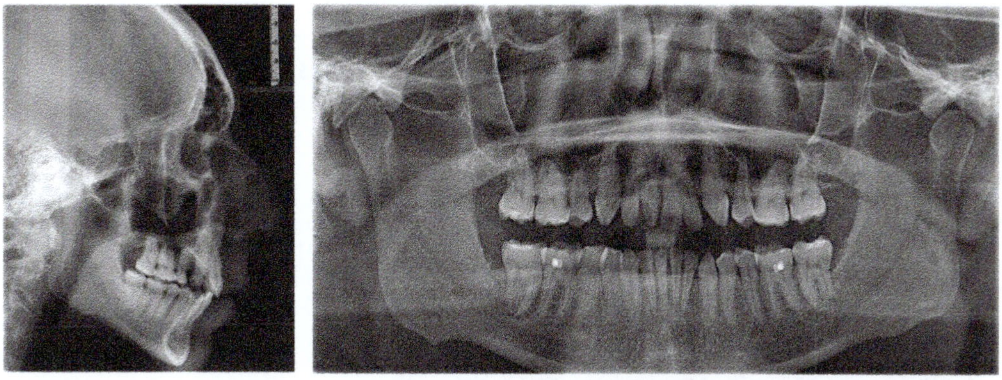

Fig. 23.111 Lateral and panoramic X-rays taken before aesthetic restoration.

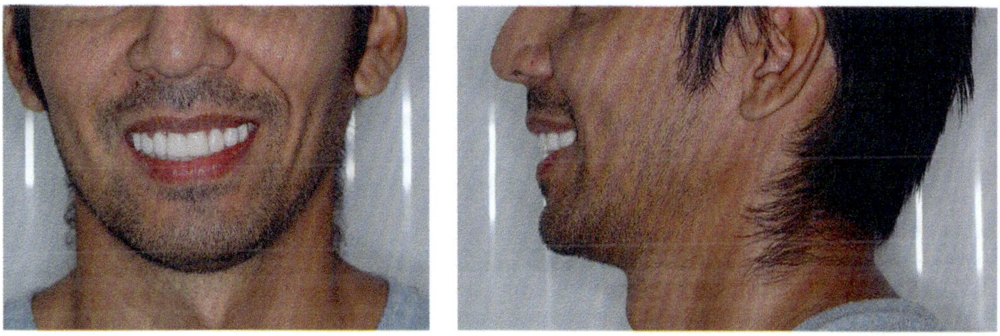

Fig. 23.112 Current extraoral views.

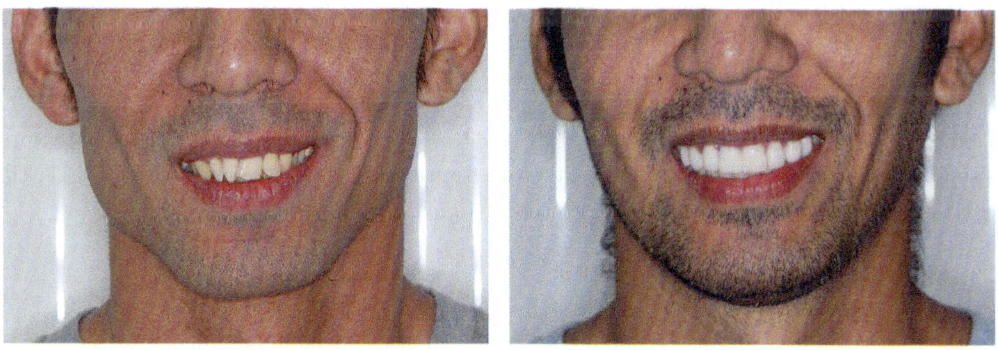

Fig. 23.113 Smile before and after treatment.

23.2.8 Lower Space Closure for Class III Patient

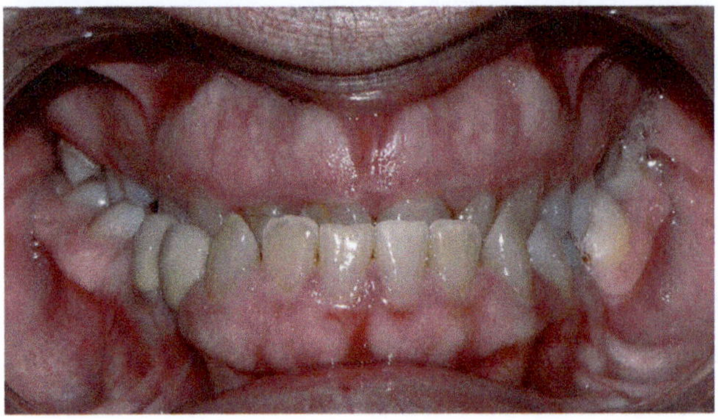

Fig. 23.114 Initial frontal view.

Diagnosis

The patient presented with an anterior deep bite of 100%, anterior crossbite, short display, posterior compression, a dentoskeletal discrepancy and bilateral Class III. This case had several key factors that need to be addressed for successful treatment:

- Upper arch compression
- Lower absence on 36
- Cantilever bridge on 44
- Lower incisors, severe extrusion and gummy smile

Treatment Plan

- Intrude both upper and lower incisors to solve anterior deep bite and gummy smile, at the same time as posterior extrusion is created with button and elastics, anterorotating the mandible and reducing the Class III component
- Develop upper arch by planning a Class II mechanics without elastics: this would procline anterior incisors by upper wisdom tooth distalization, which would then create enough space for transversal development
- Make molars on third quadrant unmovable, by closing mesial space to them by anterior retrusion and consider a cantilever bridge as the space from a previously extracted tooth will be closed using a regular protocol

ClinCheck 1: Requirements for the Technician

- Lower intrusion: 33–43, helping with posterior attachments.
- Lower retrusion to close spacing, adding IPR with extra LRT to maintain proper crown torque.
- Upper intrusion: 13–23, helping with posterior attachments.
- Upper distalization, in order to produce anterior proclination to resolve the anterior crossbite. First and second molar should be expanded after wisdom tooth distalization and space creation.

Treatment Summary

- The total number of aligners is distributed in two sets changed every 7 days
- Both first and second set of aligners had to be followed by posterior buttons and elastics to help close posterior open bite
- Extraction (cantilever bridge drilling) was accomplished between aligners two and three
- After treatment, patient had veneers fitted

ClinCheck 2: Requirements for the Technician

- Buttons and elastics on posterior sectors
- Closure of anterior space
- Additional expansion

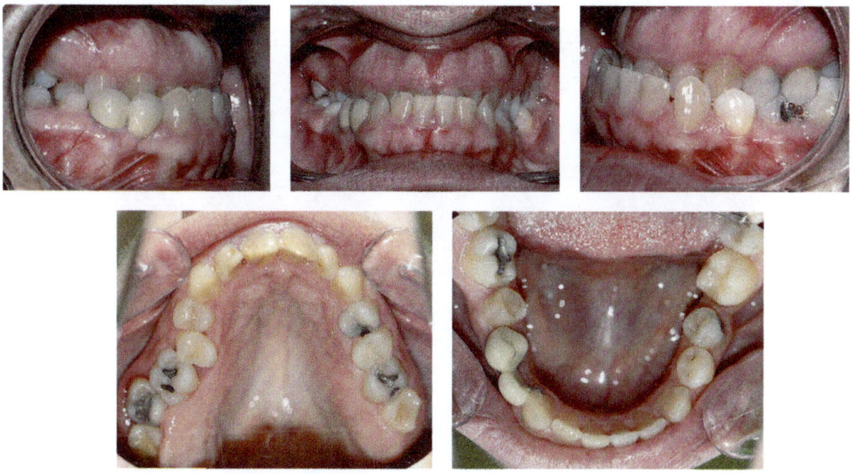

Fig. 23.115 Initial intraoral views.

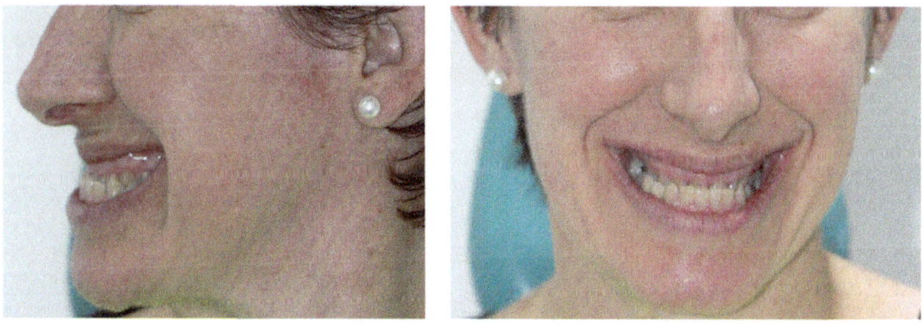

Fig. 23.116 Initial extraoral views.

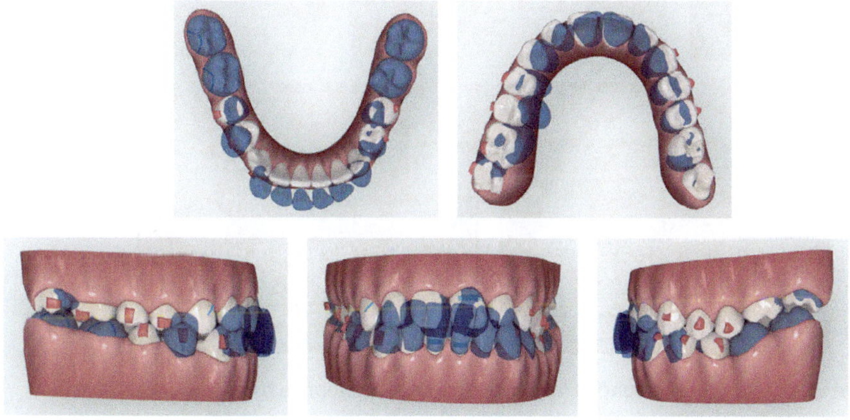

Fig. 23.117 Initial ClinChecks.

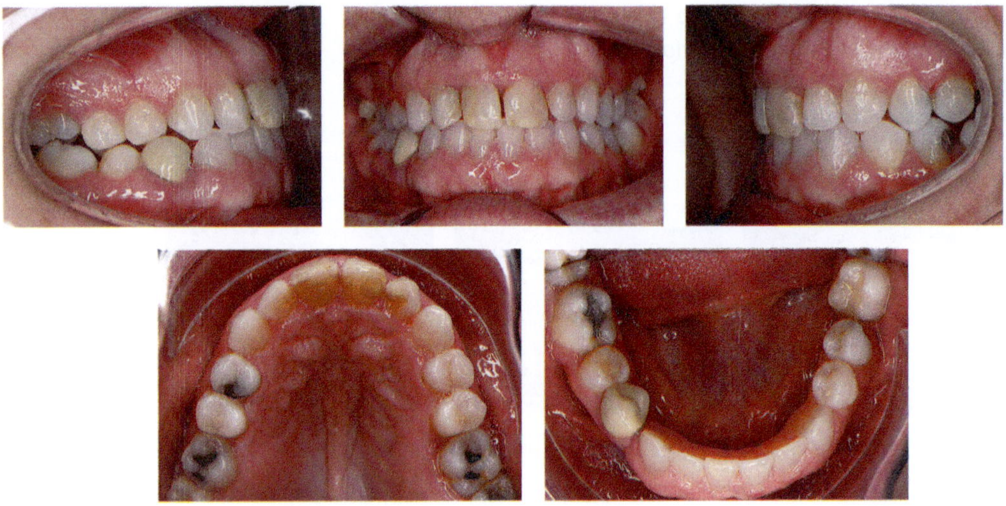

Fig. 23.118 Refinement: intraoral situation after first set of aligners.

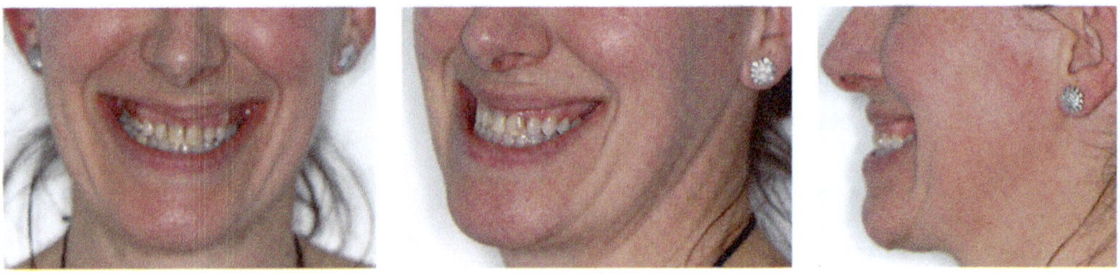

Fig. 23.119 Refinement: initial extraoral views.

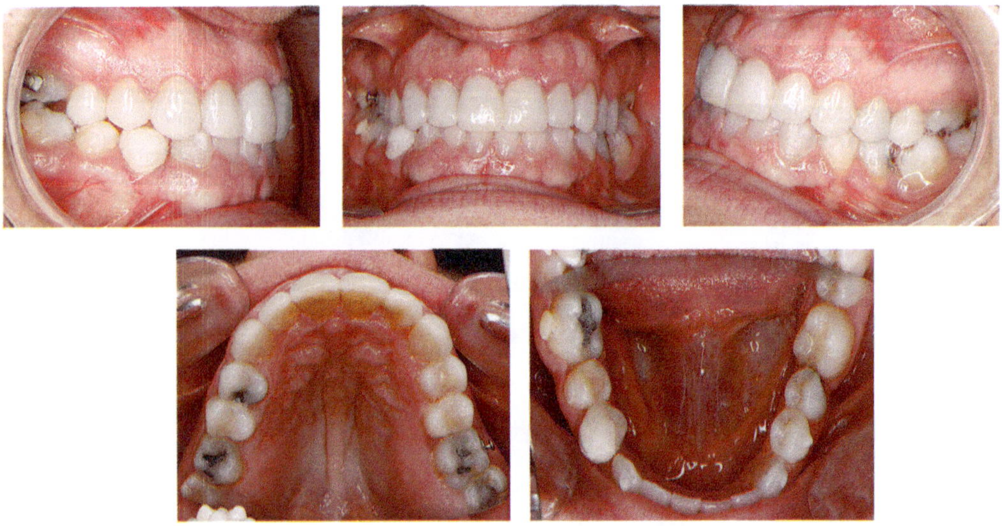

Fig. 23.120 Final views with veneers bonded (aesthetic treatment performed by Dr Ignacio Vázquez Natividad).

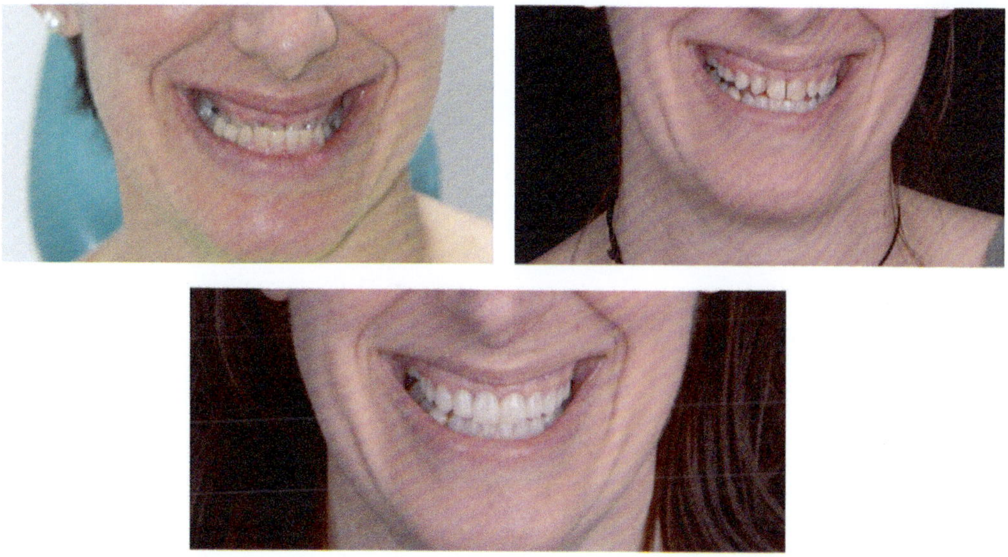

Fig. 23.121 Views at start and after refinement with veneers.

Fig. 23.122 Final cephalometric measurements.

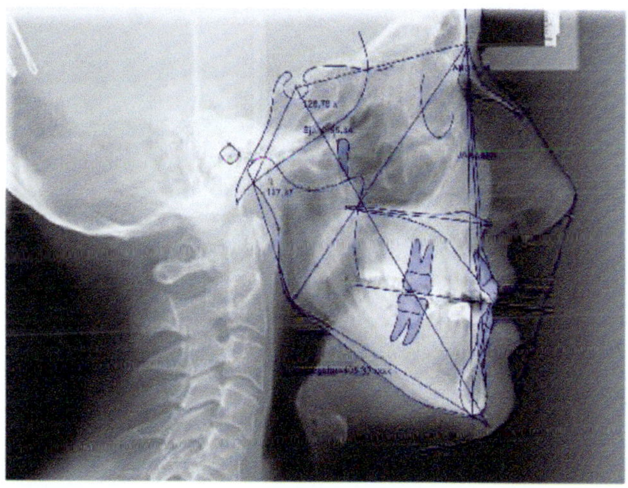

24

Multidisciplinary Cases: Implants

24.1 TADs to Intrude Upper Molars

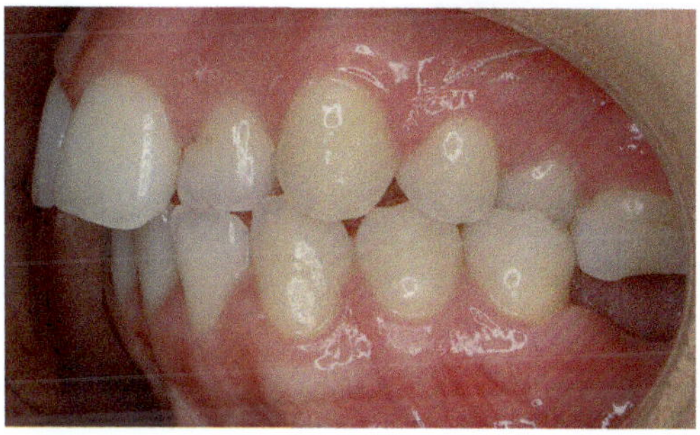

Fig. 24.1 Initial intraoral view.

Diagnosis

A 27-year-old woman with hyperdivergent skeletal Class II presented with constricted dental arches, Class II division 1, posterior crossbite of 25, severely extruded 26, and missing 36 and 46. They had a left-side deviation of the lower midline, slight labial incompetence, retruded chin and a gummy anterior smile of 3 mm.

Treatment Plan

Maxilla:

- Symmetrical expansion and intrusion of 26 using TADs: one labial, one in mesial and another distal to the tooth
- During the refinement, once the implant for 46 could be placed the TADs could be removed and the intrusion of 26 assisted by a provisional crown at 46

Mandible:

- Expansion and arch form coordination
- Centre lower midline with upper midline

Aligner Techniques in Orthodontics, First Edition. Susana Palma Moya and Javier Lozano Zafra.

Companion website: www.wiley.com/go/lozano-zafra/aligner-techniques

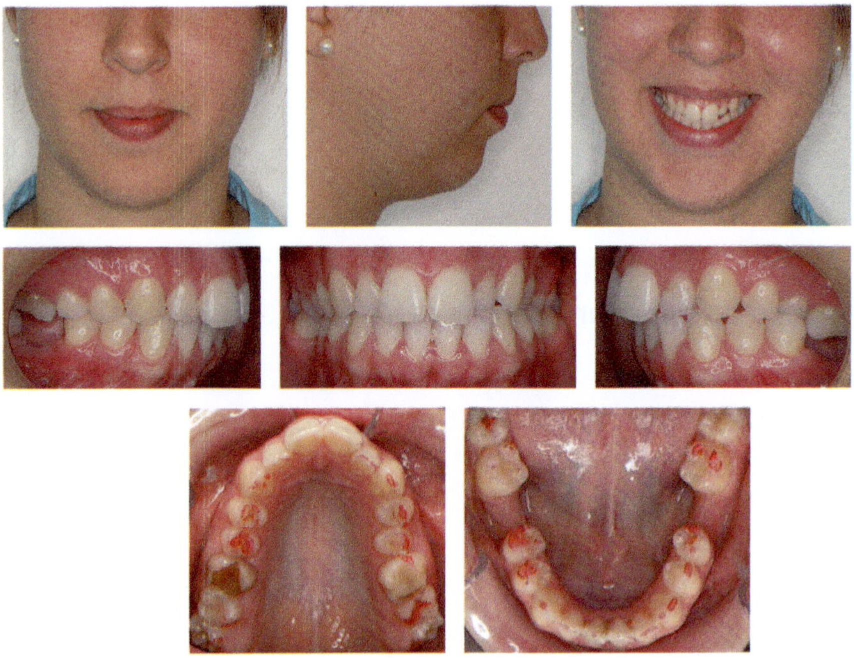

Fig. 24.2 Pretreatment extraoral and intraoral views.

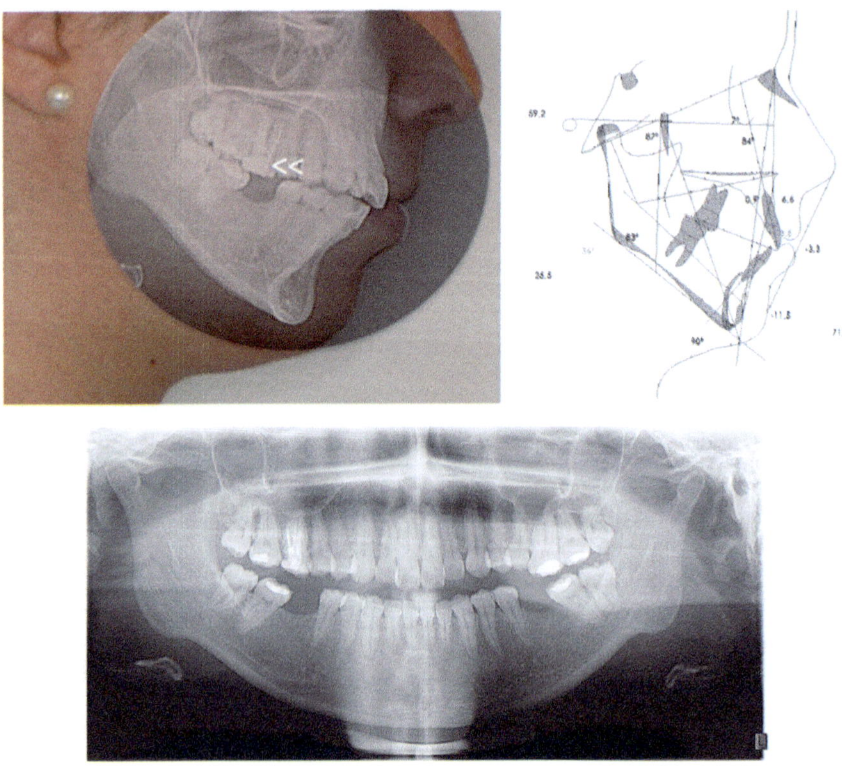

Fig. 24.3 Initial: teleradiograph, cephalometry and panoramic X-rays.

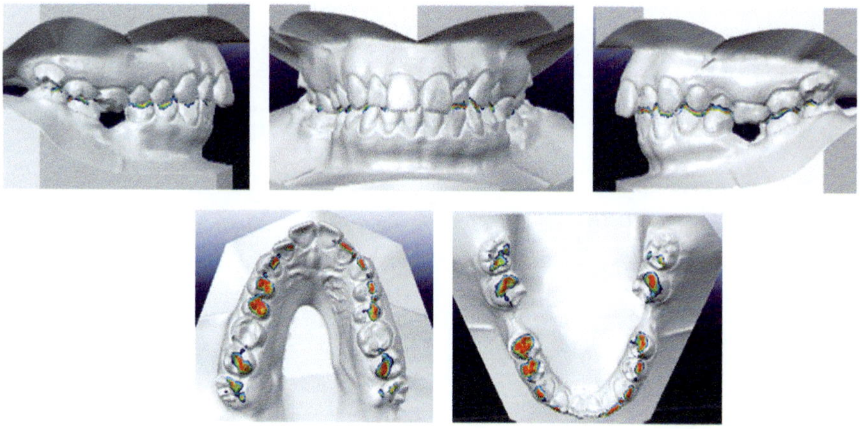

Fig. 24.4 Initial occlusal contact point.

Requirements for the Technician

Maxilla

- Symmetrical expansion of the upper arch with attachments to control the molar torque in the first premolar and first molars during expansion.
- For 26 intrusion, an attachment is not necessary but attachments on adjacent teeth (25 and 27) will assist the intrusion, helped by the occlusal contact between 27 and 47.
- In order to be able to intrude, the 26 space is opened between the molar and the premolar and between the first and second molar of 0.25 mm so that the first molar would have enough room for the intrusion.

Mandible:

- Use the expansion to open 10 mm of space for future implants of 36 and 46
- Use the expansion space to centre the lower midline with the upper midline

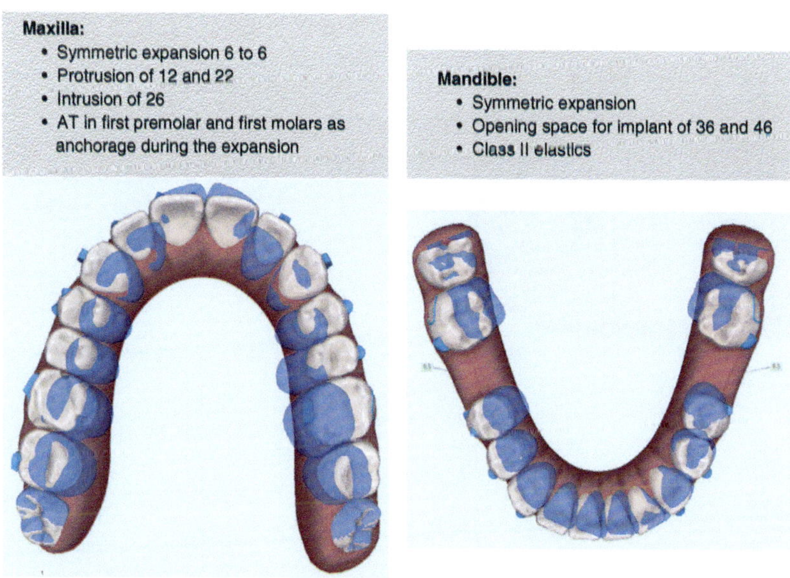

Fig. 24.5 Occlusal ClinCheck views.

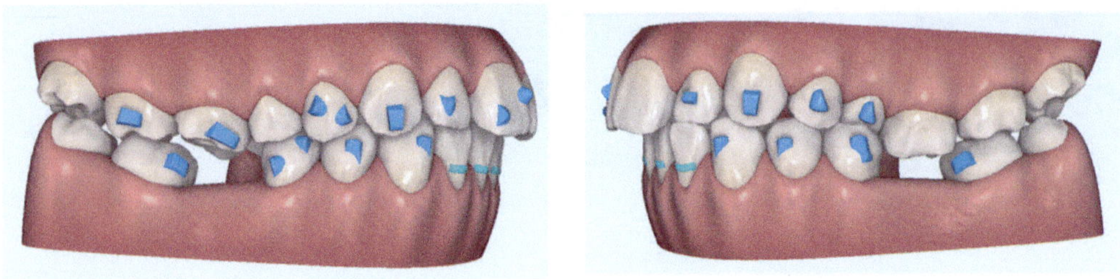

Fig. 24.6 Lateral ClinCheck views.

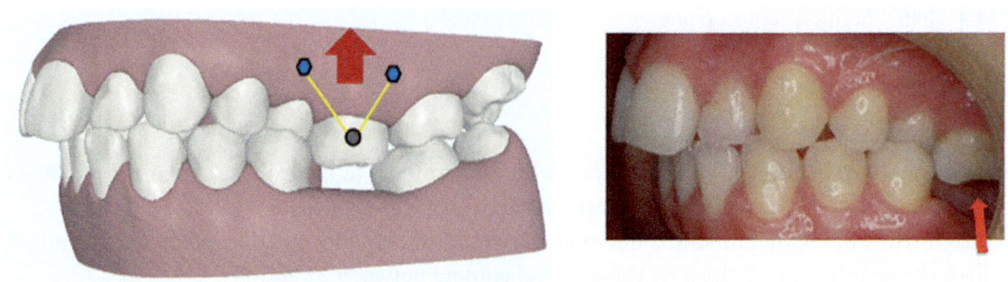

Fig. 24.7 Interproximal reduction was not planned in the ClinCheck, but was made mesial and distal to 26 during the intrusion to provide space for the movement.

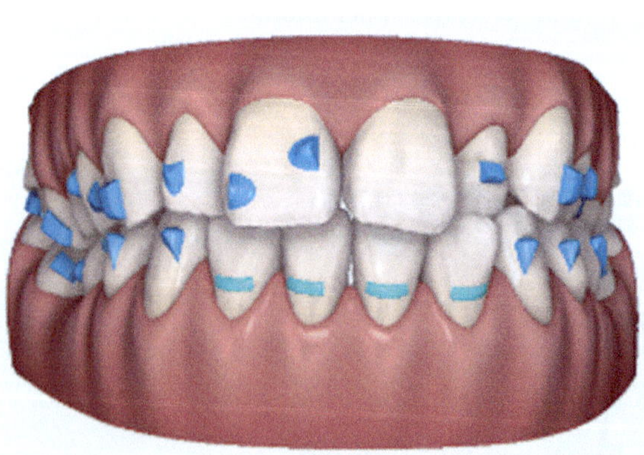

Fig. 24.8 Initial frontal ClinCheck view.

Treatment Summary

- Total treatment time was 13 months.
- The patient wore 27 aligners in the first phase with 10-day change intervals; during that phase she used criss-cross elastic on the left-side with a class II component, and class II elastic on the right, both with full-time wear.
- Two microscrews placed mesial and distal of the 26 and a Powerchain from a button in 26 were used to assist the 26 intrusion.
- After these 27 aligners, a set of additional aligners were requested to complete the intrusion of 26, in that moment the implant of 36 and 46 had already been placed with provisional crowns.
- Occlusal contact between the provisional crown in 46 and the extruded 26 completed the correction.
- The TADs and the final provisional crown in the 46 over the implant were critical to the success of the intrusion of the 26.
- The smile of the patient improved considerably as a result of the transversal development of the arches, a bilateral class I was achieved with normal overjet and overbite and with both midlines centred.

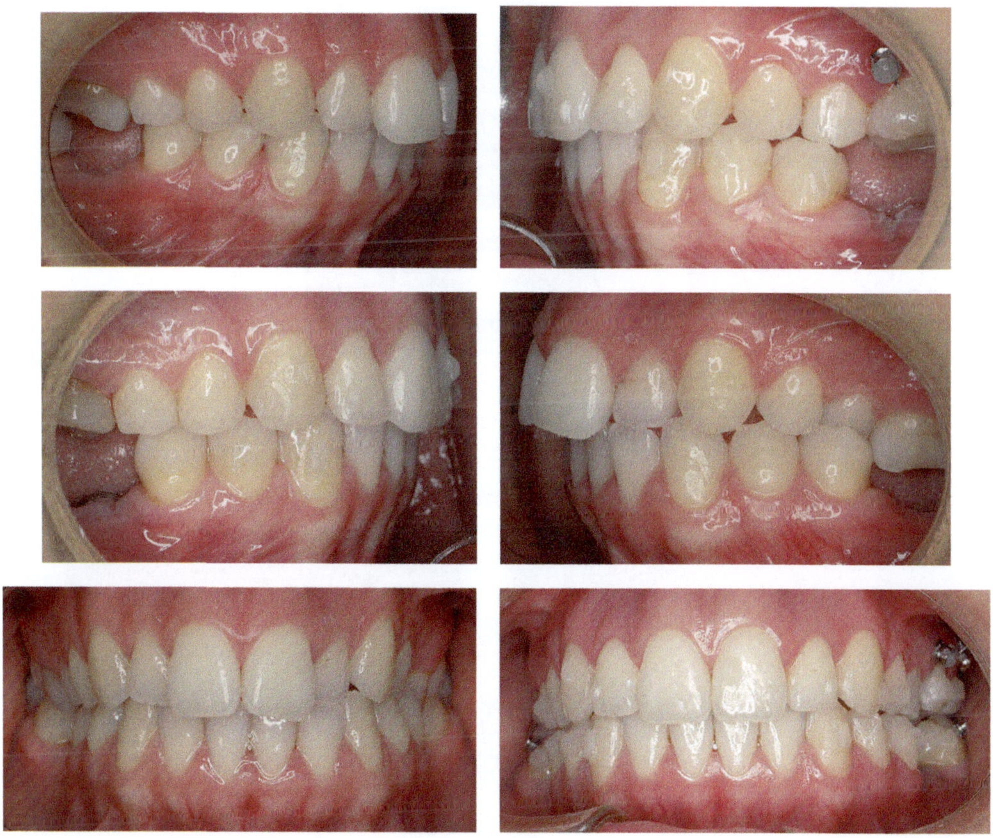

Fig. 24.9 Situation before additional aligners. Results after the first set of 27 aligners and the use of two microscrews to intrude 26.

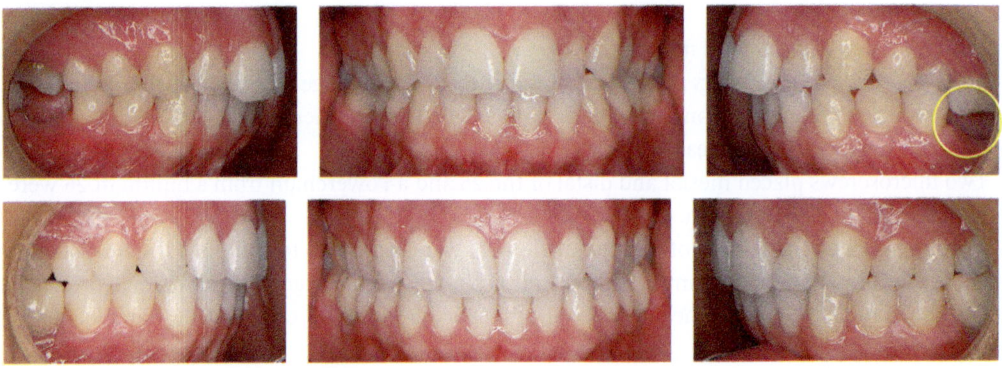

Fig. 24.10 Initial (upper) and final (lower) occlusion. Final result after refinement and provisional crowns on 36 and 46 implants.

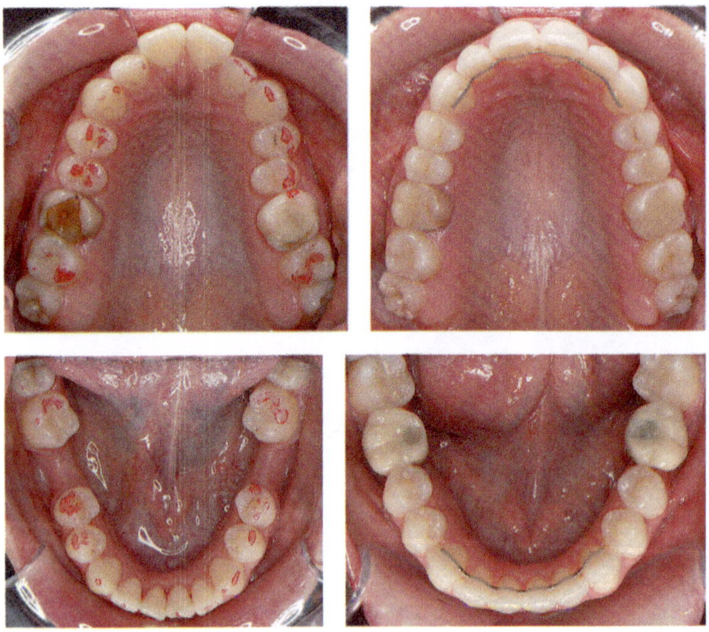

Fig. 24.11 Initial (left) and final (right) occlusals.

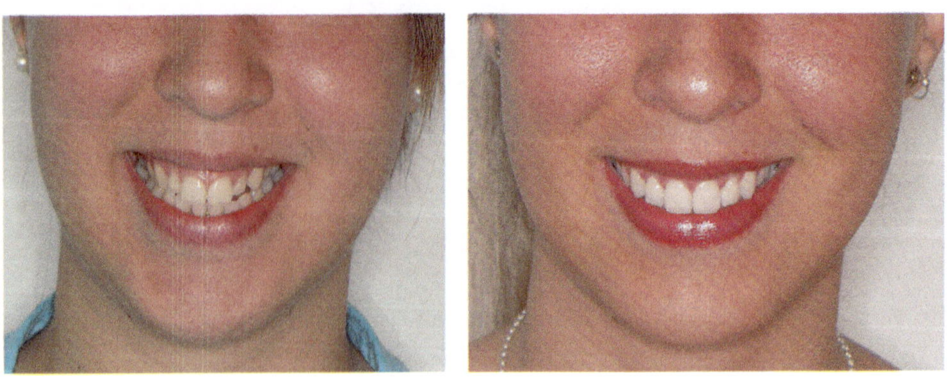

Fig. 24.12 Initial and final smile.

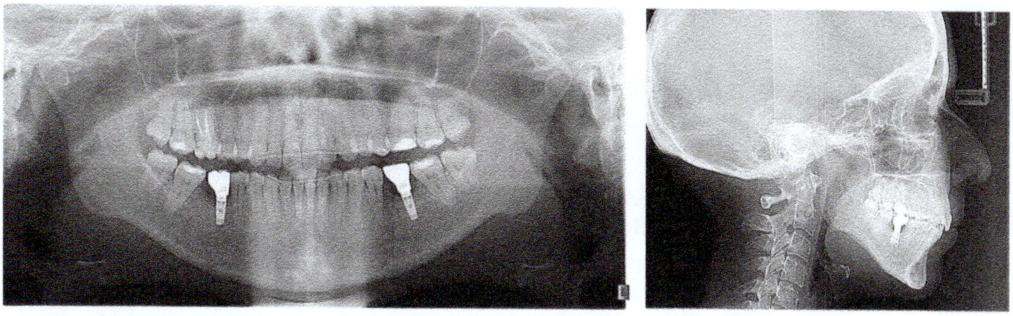

Fig. 24.13 Final panoramic and lateral X-rays.

24.2 Upper Midline Shift

24.2.1 Opening Space for Implant of 23

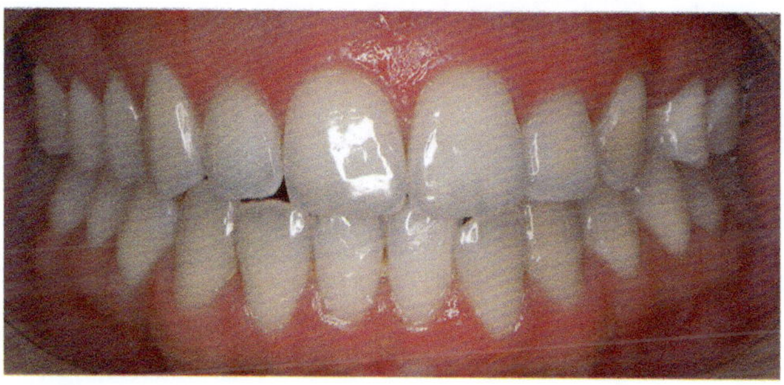

Fig. 24.14 Initial intraoral view.

Diagnosis

A 31-year-old woman with a normodivergent skeletal Class III presented with constricted upper arch, unilateral Class III on left side, a missing 23 and left-side deviation of the upper midline.

Treatment Plan

Maxilla:

- Symmetrical expansion 5–5
- Opening space for implant of 23
- Crown of 24 and 25 were separated in a previous orthodontic treatment when she was a child. However, as the roots of 24 and 25 were convergent, it was decided to open a space for the missing 23 instead and distalize 24 to place it in its normal position

Mandible:

- Expansion and arch form coordination

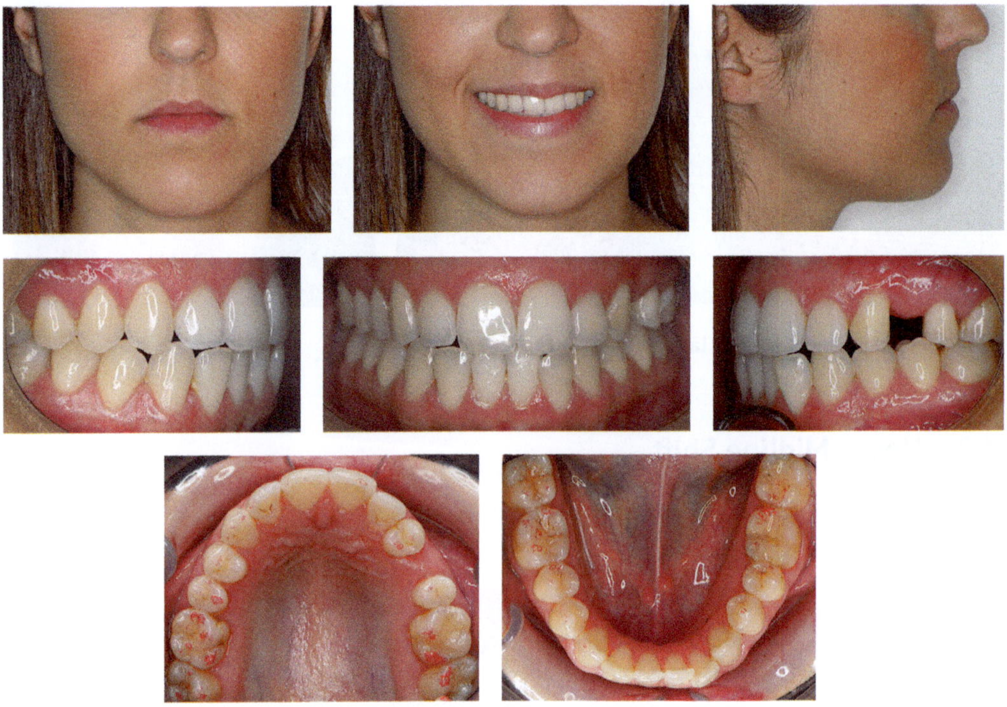

Fig. 24.15 Pretreatment extraoral and intraoral views.

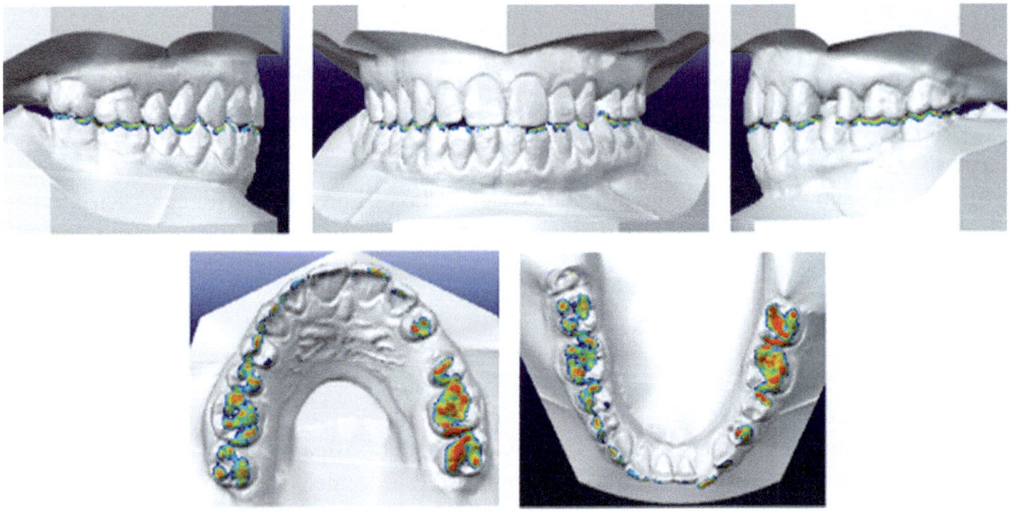

Fig. 24.16 Initial occlusal contact.

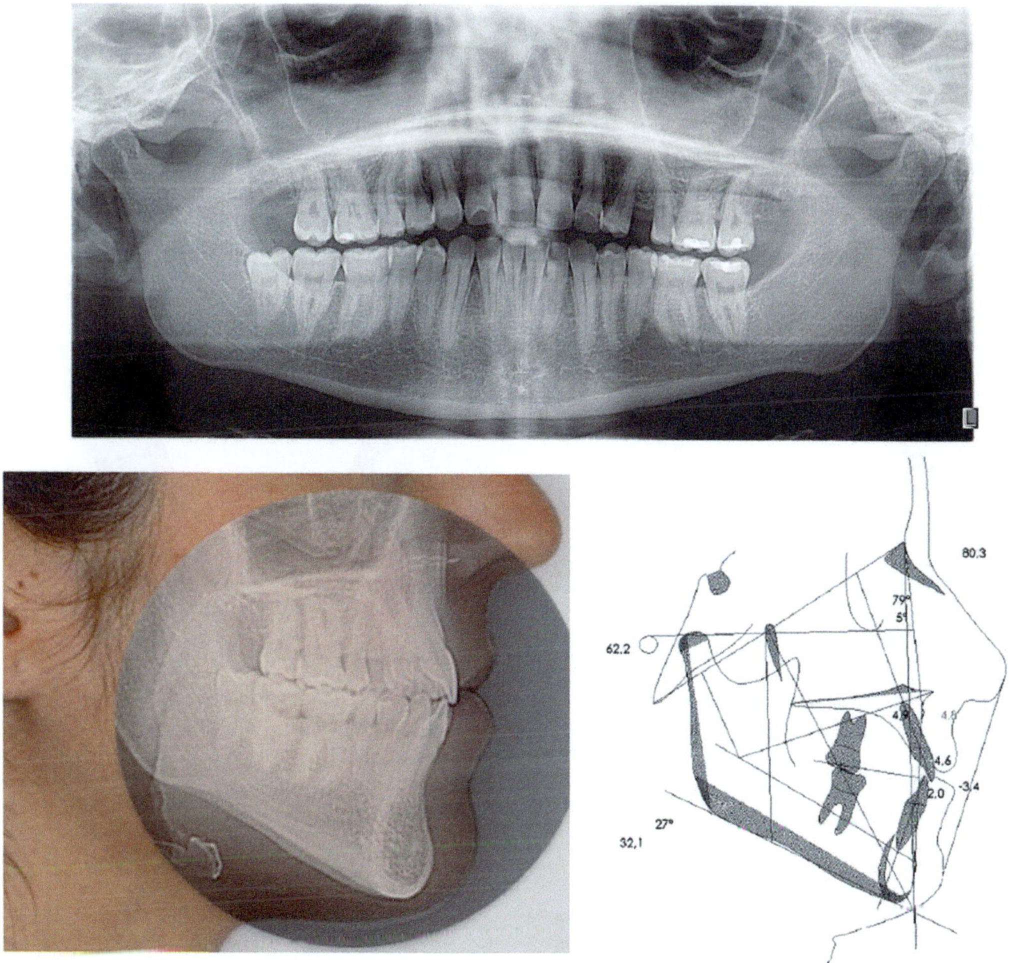

Fig. 24.17 Panoramic and lateral X-rays. Cephalometric analysis.

Requirements for the Technician

Maxilla:

- Symmetrical expansion of the upper arch with attachments to control molar torque in first premolar and first molars during the expansion
- Open a space of 8 mm for the missing 23 and provide mesial-tipping to the root of 22 and distal-tipping to the root of 24 to ensure space for the future implanting of the canine

Mandible:

- Coordinate arches and make IPR 3–3 to provide a final overjet of 1.5 mm

Staging maxillary:
- Do not move molars, they are in Class I
- Expansion 5 to 5
- Centre upper midline during proclination of upper incisors
- Open space for implant of 23 by distalization of 24

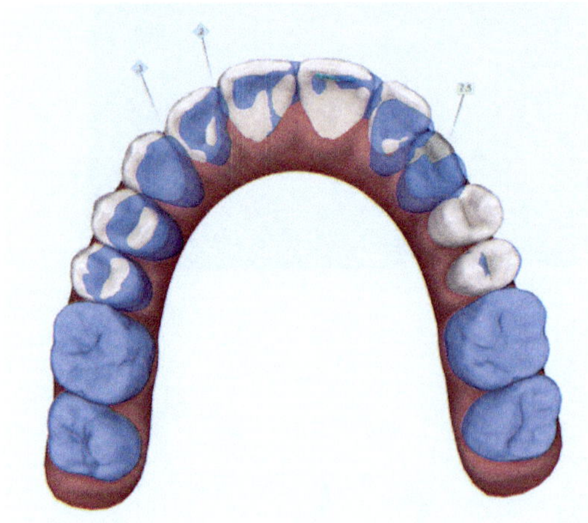

Fig. 24.18 Opening space for missing 23.

Staging mandible:
- Expansion + lower incisors IPR + retraction of lower incisors

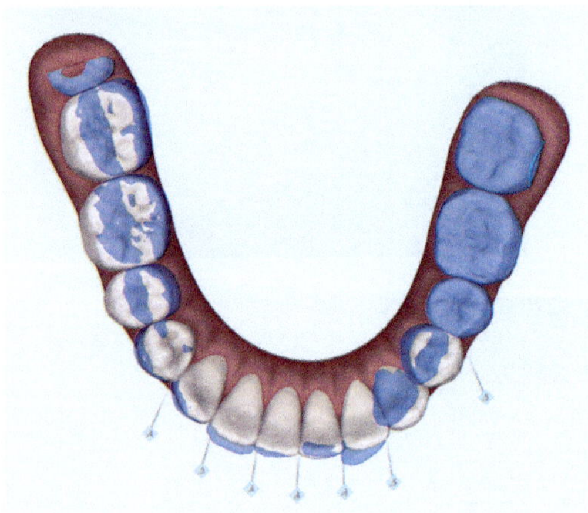

Fig. 24.19 Interproximal reduction 3 to 3 to allow retraction of lower incisors and create positive overjet.

Open space for missing 23 → Procline upper incisors + distalize 2.4

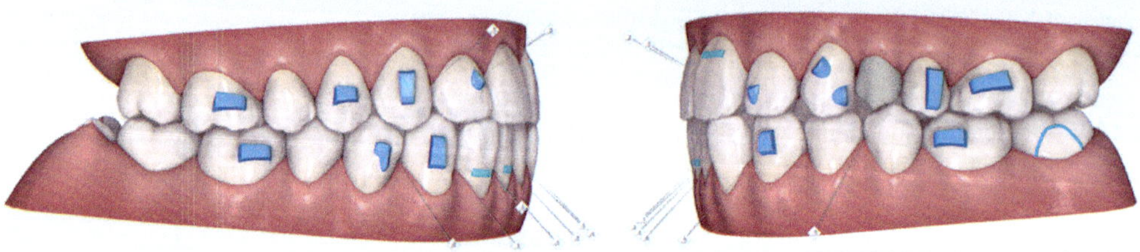

Fig. 24.20 Initial lateral ClinCheck views.

Treatment Summary
- Total treatment time was 16 months.
- The patient wore 34 aligners in the first phase with 7-day change intervals; during that phase she used class II elastic on the left-side to move 24 to distal, and triangular elastics on right side.
- After these 34 aligners, a set of 16 additional aligners were requested to complete opening space for implant of 23.
- The smile of the patient improved considerably as a result of the transversal development of the arches; a bilateral class I with normal overjet and overbite, and with both midlines centred was achieved and the surgeon was able to place the implant for 24.
- Retention was provided by fix retainers and Vivera retainers for night use.

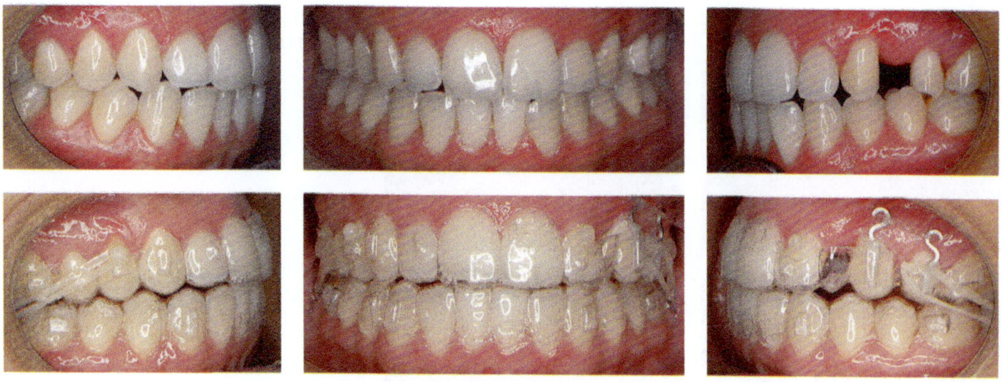

Fig. 24.21 Powerarm to make roots of 25 and 24 closer.

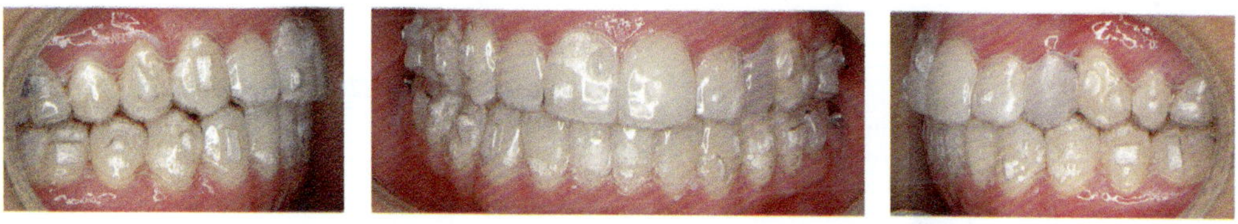

Fig. 24.22 Evolution at 12 months.

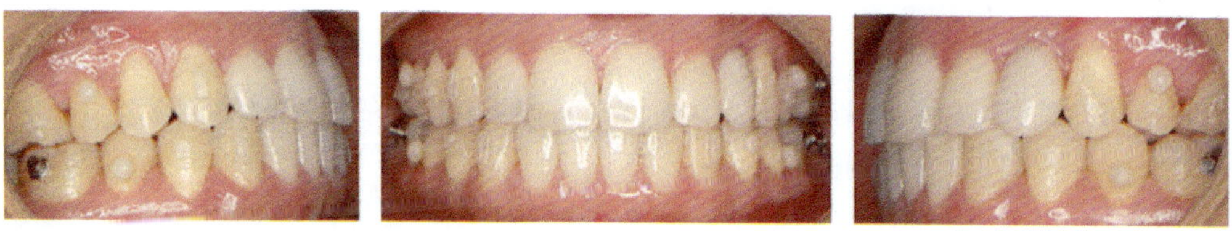

Fig. 24.23 Evolution after using additional aligners.

Fig. 24.24 Final views with implant for 13.

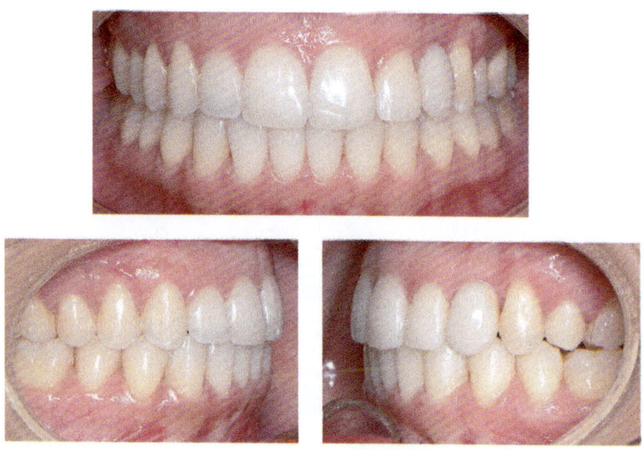

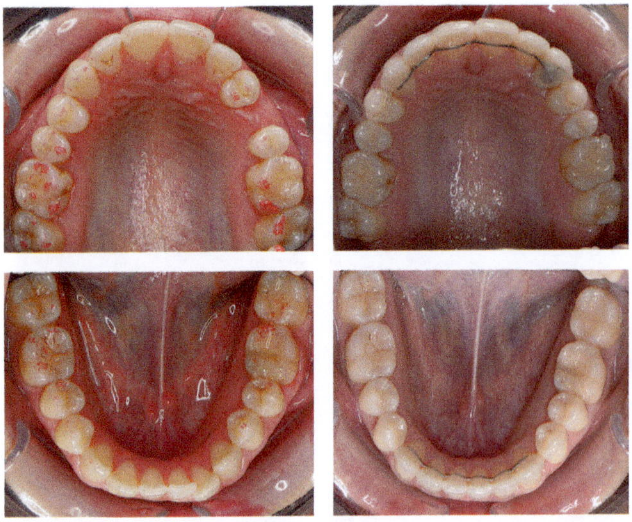

Fig. 24.25 Initial (left) and final (right) occlusal.

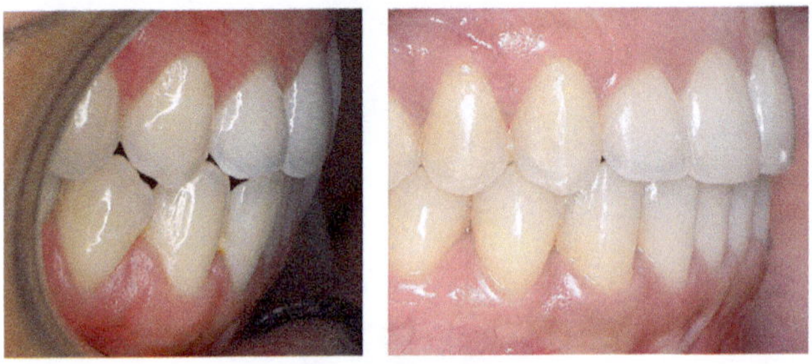

Fig. 24.26 Initial and final overjet.

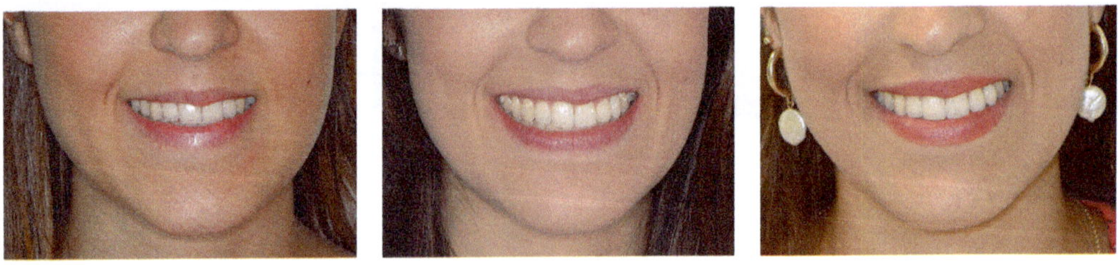

Fig. 24.27 Evolution of the patient's smile (from left): initial, before additional aligners and final result.

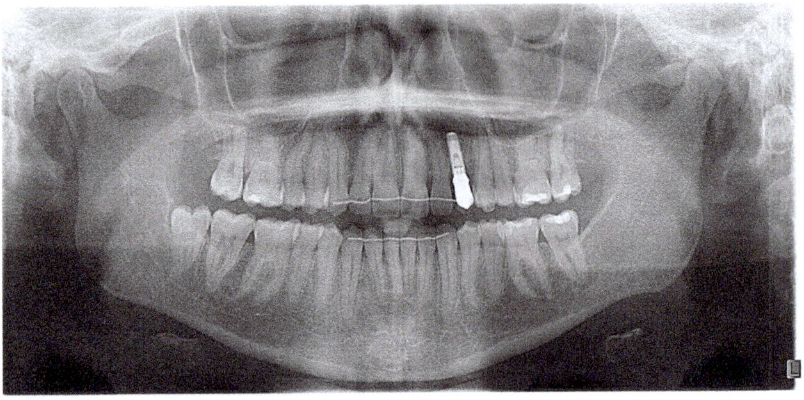

Fig. 24.28 Final panoramic X-ray with implant for 23.

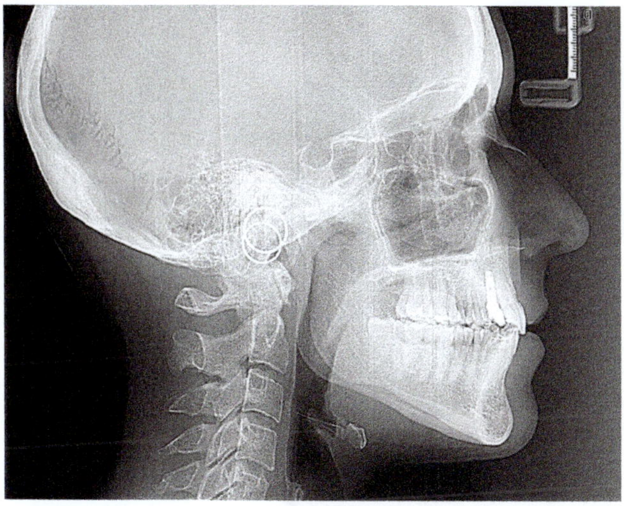

Fig. 24.29 Final teleradiograph with overjet corrected.

24.3 Posterior Bite Collapse

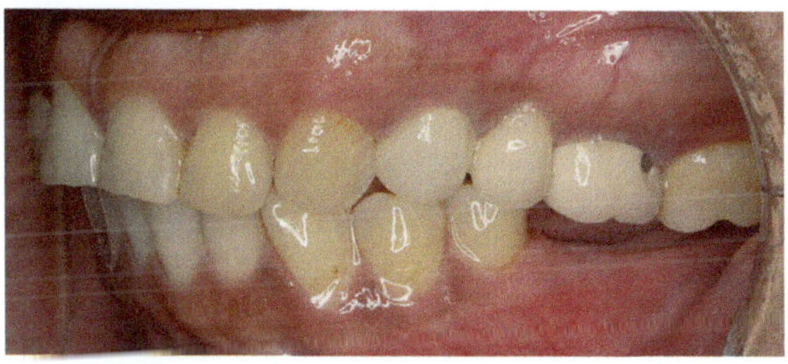

Fig. 24.30 Initial left intraoral view.

Diagnosis

A 39-year-old woman with skeletal class I presented with dentoalveolar protrusion, posterior bite collapse owing to missing lower molars, severe extrusion of the upper molars with posterior gummy smile and TMJ disorder; her upper midline was centred. She had attrition of the edges of upper and lower incisors (occlusal wear) as a result of the anticlockwise mandible rotation that happened when she lost her lower molars, with a consequent edge to edge situation in the anterior incisors.

Treatment Plan

- The oral surgeon made a mock-up to estimate the vertical dimension needed
- In order to have anchorage to intrude the upper molars and to retract the proclined incisors, the surgeon placed the implants on the lower arch with temporary crowns. With the occlusal contacts, the aligners would be able to provide an effective intrusive force
- With the help of lower arch implants and provisional crowns, the plan was to intrude upper molars, level the upper occlusal plane and provide anchorage to retrude the lower incisors and create positive overjet

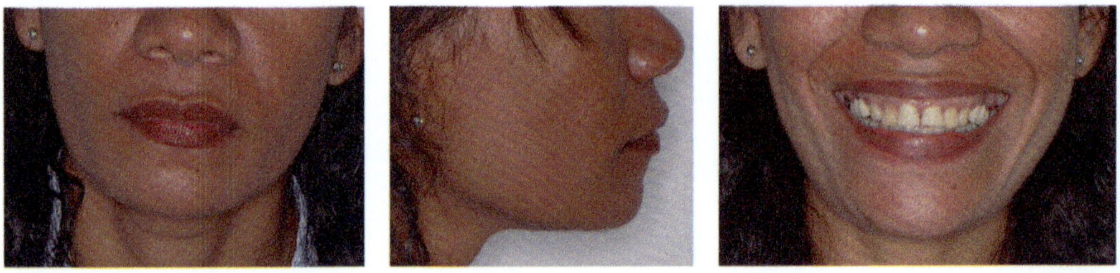

Fig. 24.31 Pretreatment extraoral views.

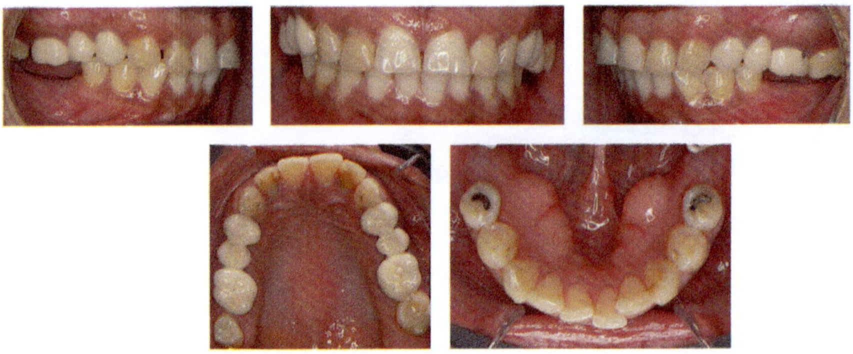

Fig. 24.32 Pretreatment intraoral views.

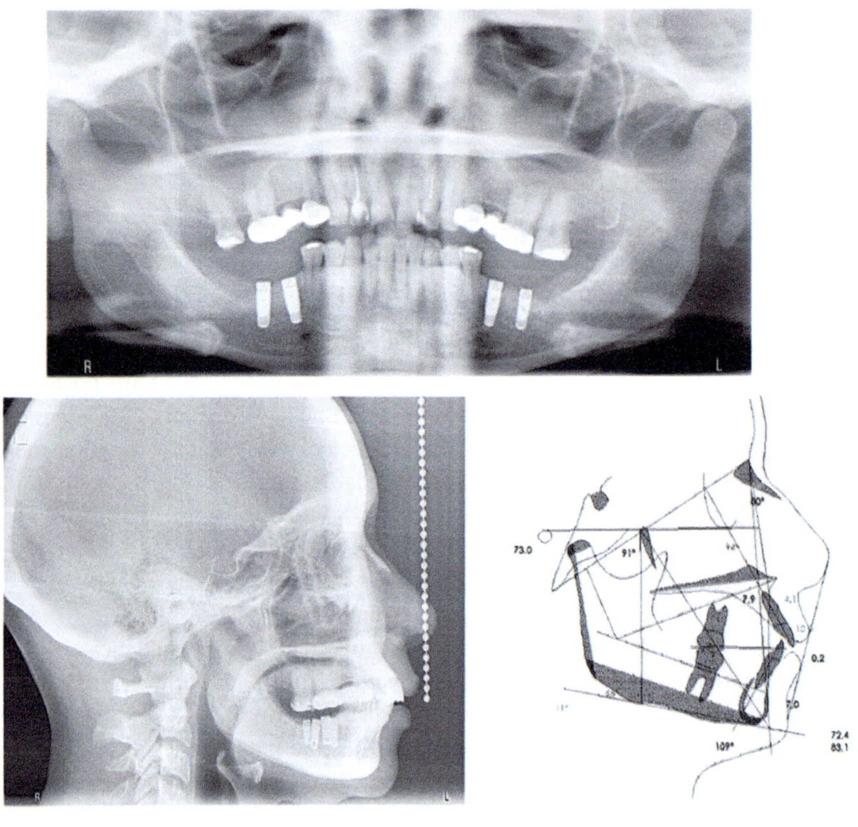

Fig. 24.33 Initial panoramic X-ray, teleradiograph and cephalometry.

Requirements for the Technician
- Distalize and intrude upper molars to create space for 15 and 25
- IPR 3 to 3 in the lower arch and retrude the lower incisors to create positive overjet in order to retrocline the upper incisors without ending in an edge to edge position

Treatment Summary
- Total treatment time was 19 months+
- The patient had a first phase with 29 aligners, with 2-week change intervals and night use class II elastic to provide anchorage for retrusion of upper incisors
- A set of additional aligners was requested to settle the posterior occlusion
- The incisal edges were repaired after a bleaching treatment and the final prosthesis was placed
- A final class I was achieved, the upper occlusal plane was levelled and occlusal clearance created for the final restorative treatment. The patient's smile improved considerably

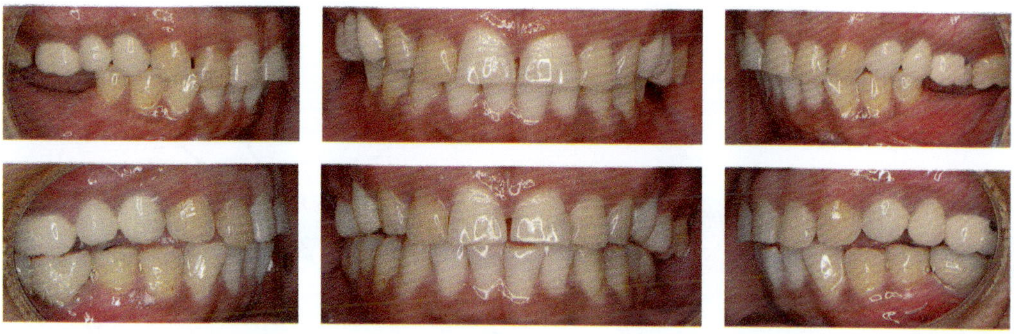

Fig. 24.34 Initial views and views after placing provisional crowns over the implants.

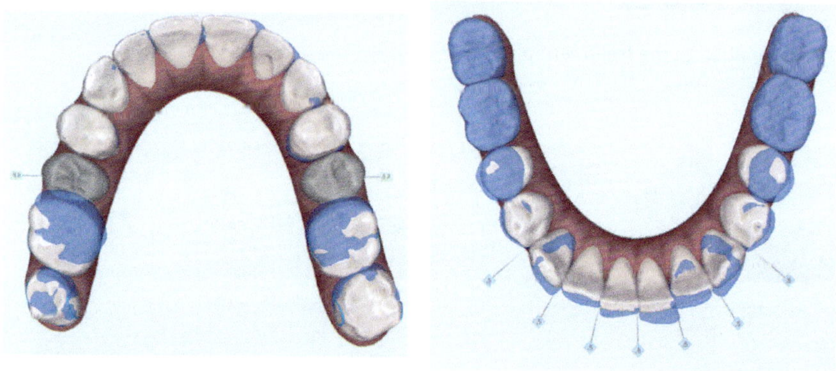

Fig. 24.35 Initial occlusal ClinCheck views.

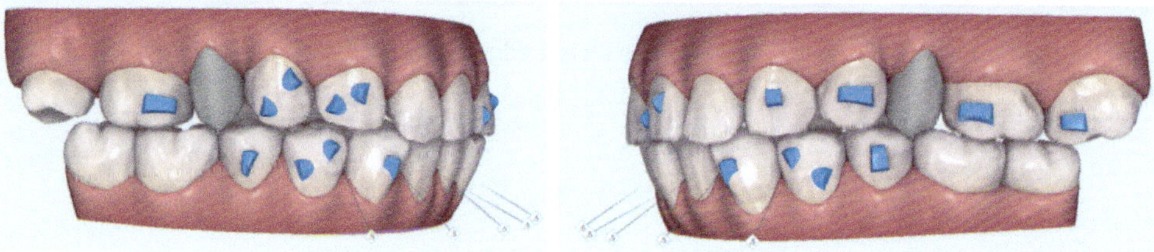

Fig. 24.36 Initial lateral ClinCheck views.

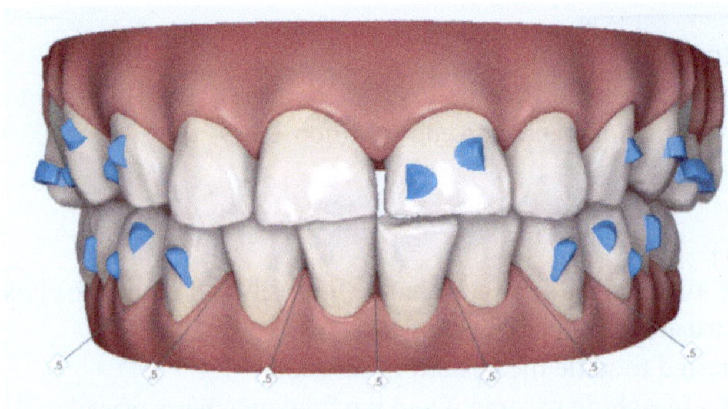

Fig. 24.37 Initial front ClinCheck view.

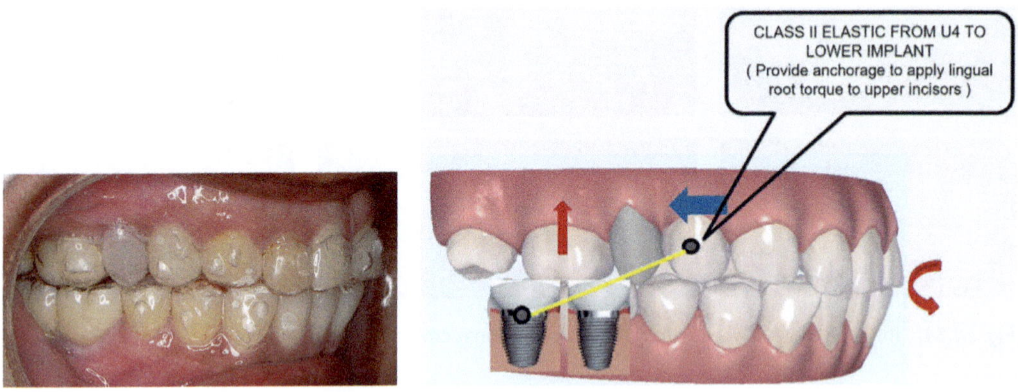

Fig. 24.38 Biomechanics applied to the treatment plan.

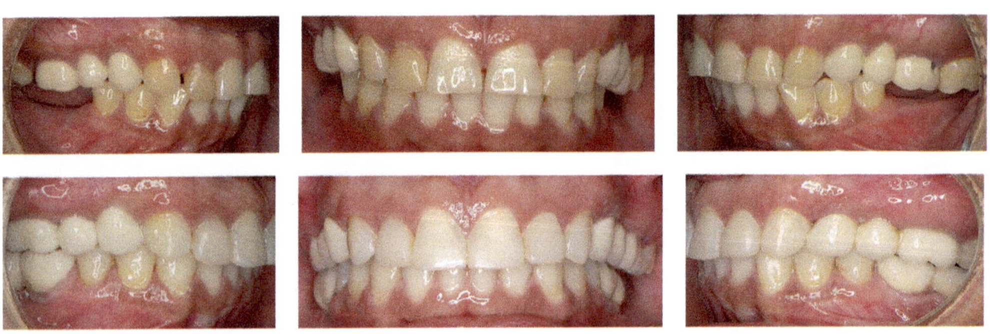

Fig. 24.39 Initial (upper) and final (lower) views: the incisal edges were repaired after a bleaching treatment and the final prosthesis was placed.

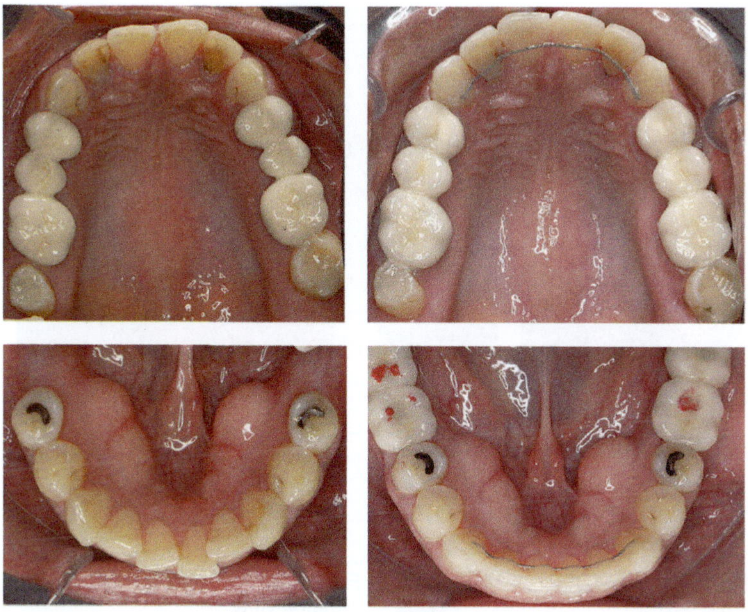

Fig. 24.40 Initial (left) and final occlusal (right).

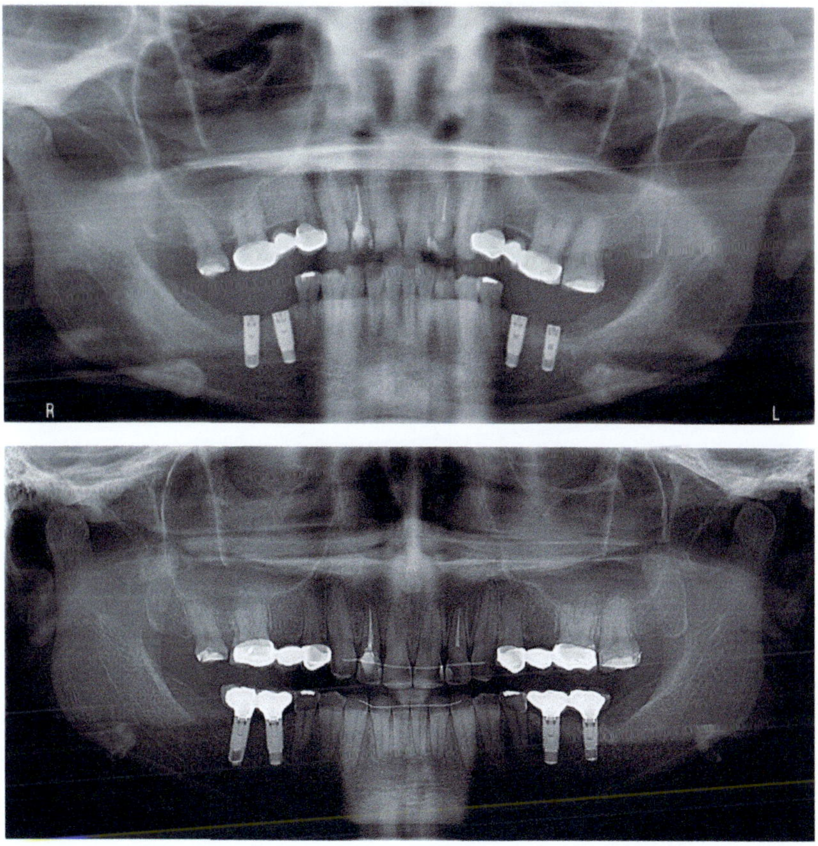

Fig. 24.41 Initial and final panoramic X-rays: levelling of the occlusal plane.

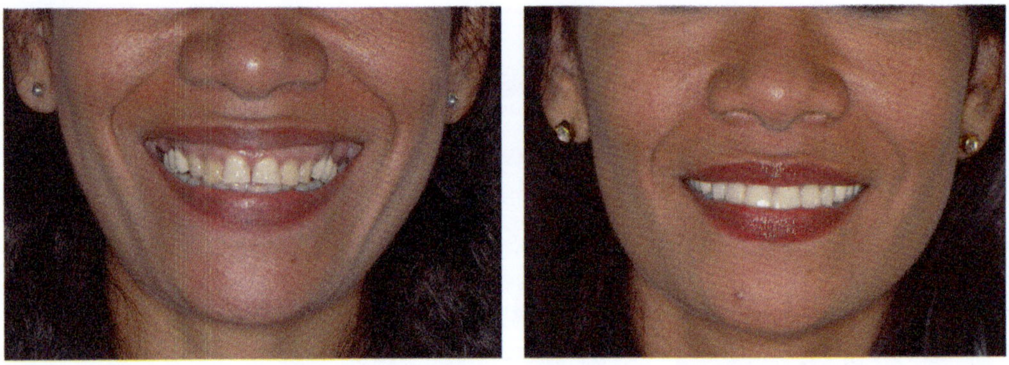

Fig. 24.42 Initial and final smile.

24.4 Posterior Bite Collapse with Deep Bite

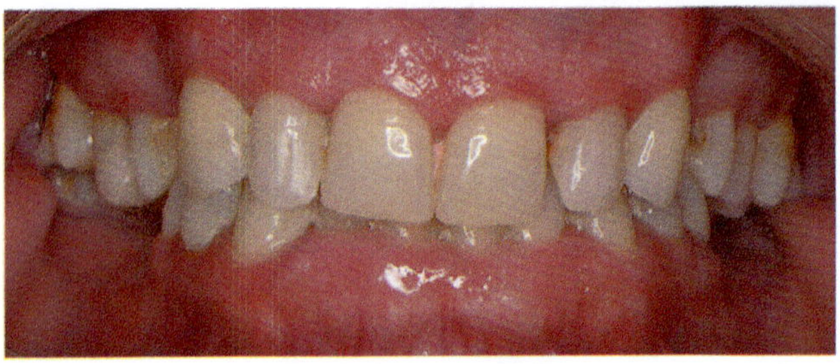

Fig. 24.43 Initial frontal intraoral view.

Diagnosis

A 55-year-old woman with hypodivergent skeletal Class I presented with a 90% deep bite and posterior bite collapse with extrusion of upper molars and missing lower molars. In the panoramic X-ray, cavities were found in 16 and 17 and the upper and lower incisors were severely retroclined and presented a steep lower curve of Spee. In the periodontal examination, the upper molars showed severe movement with insertion bone loss and deep periodontal pockets.

Treatment Plan

- The treatment plan included extractions of 16 and 17
- Place lower implants with temporary crowns
- Lower implants were critical to have the necessary anchorage to level the steep curve of Spee
- A mock-up to be made to estimate the vertical dimension needed for the provisional crowns of the implants
- With the implants placed, there would be an absolute anchorage to correct the upper incisors torque and level the curve of Spee

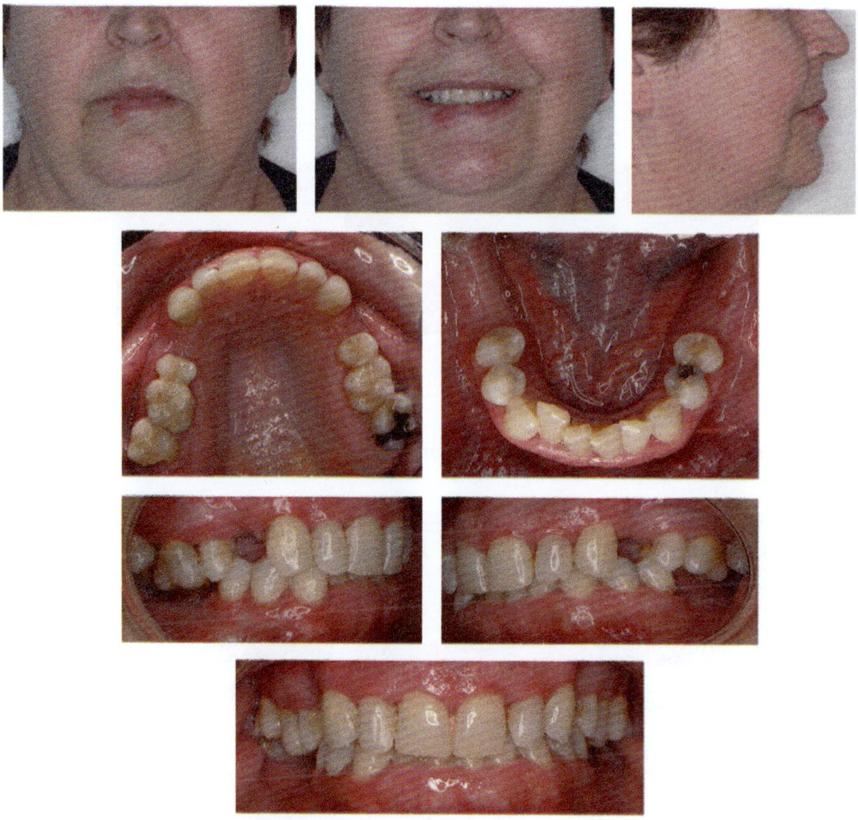

Fig. 24.44 Initial extraoral and intraoral views.

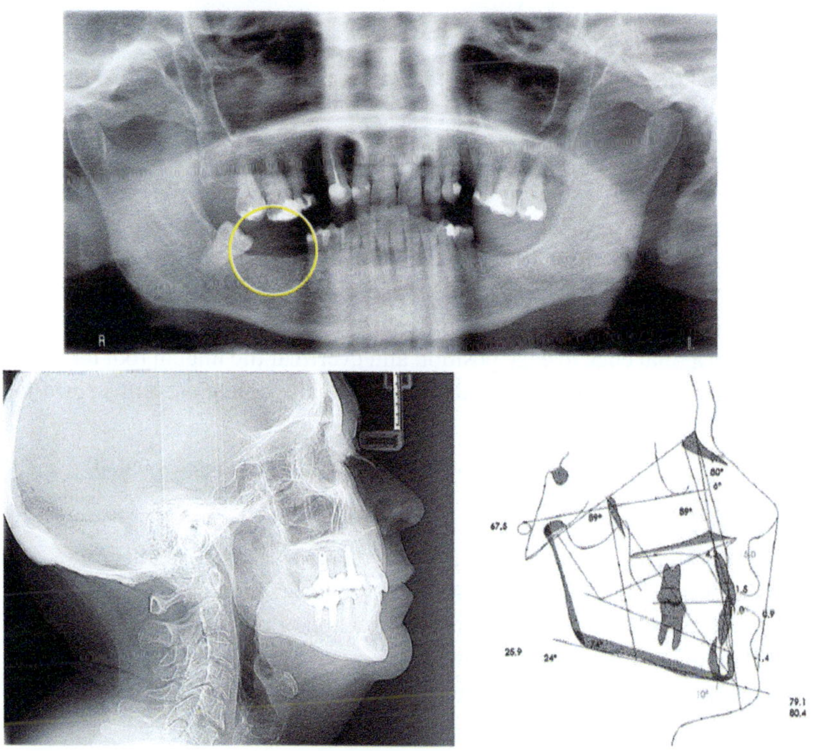

Fig. 24.45 Initial panoramic X-ray, teleradiograph and cephalometry: upper molars extrusion; missing 14/24/36/37/46/47; periodontal bone loss; cavities in 16/17.

Mock-up to Estimate Vertical Dimension

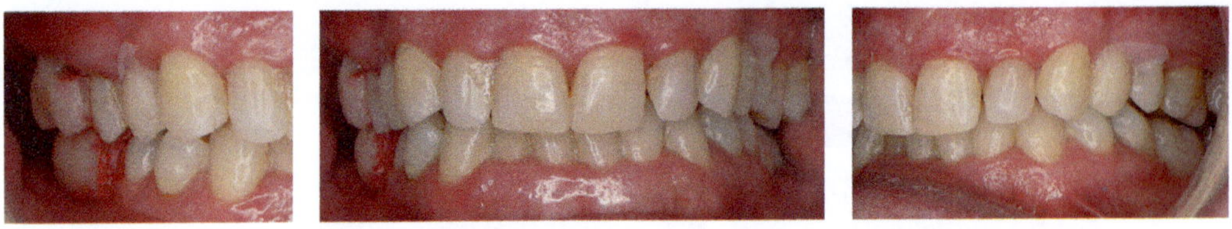

Fig. 24.46 Mock-up to estimate vertical dimension.

Implants and Provisional Crowns Were Placed Before Treatment Started

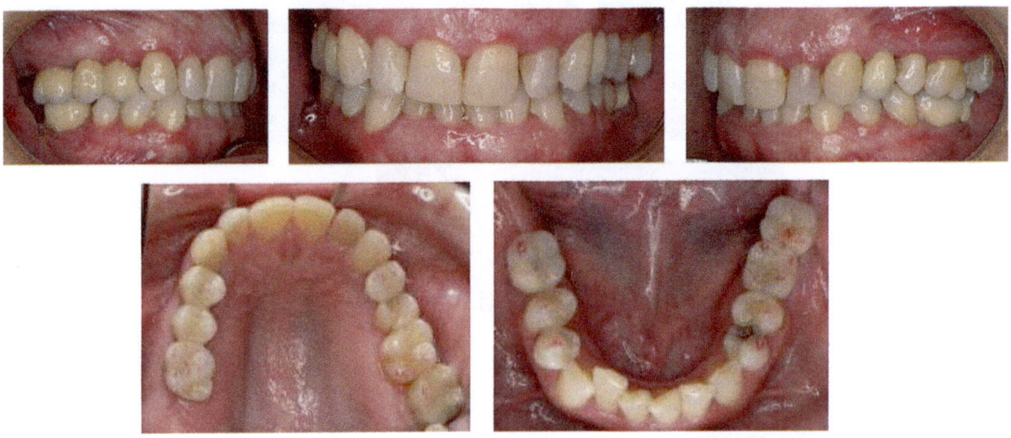

Fig. 24.47 These are the intraoral views when the case was sent to Align Technology.

Requirements for the Technician

- Apply labial crown torque and lingual root torque to the upper incisors
- After removing the roots from the cortical bone, apply a simultaneous movement of intrusion, retrusion and lingual root torque
- In the lower arch, the implants provide absolute anchorage to level the curve of Spee through lower proclination (relative intrusion) and absolute intrusion of the lower incisors
- Overtreat the deep bite into a final edge to edge position and overtreat the lingual root torque of the upper incisor at the end of the treatment to create occlusal clearance and prevent a posterior open bite

Treatment Summary

- Total treatment time was 14 months
- The patient used 14 aligners and a set of additional aligners on a 2-week change interval
- The patient used class II elastic from the upper canine to the lower implants (night wear) to avoid loss of anchorage in the upper arch during torque correction of the incisors
- The implants and the temporary crowns on the lower arch provided the anchorage needed to resolve the deep bite successfully through incisor proclination and intrusion of lower incisors

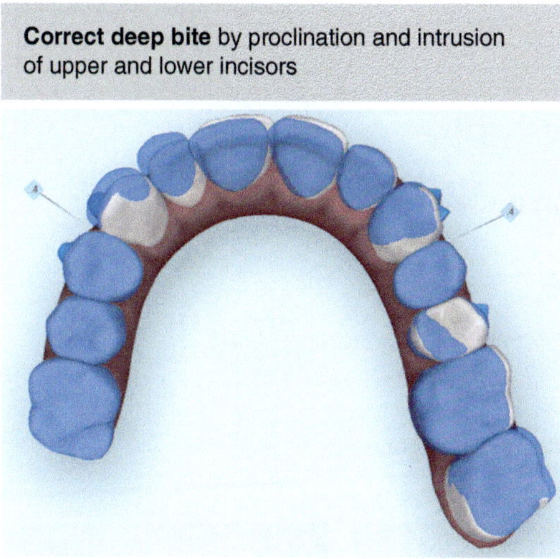

Fig. 24.48 Initial upper ClinCheck.

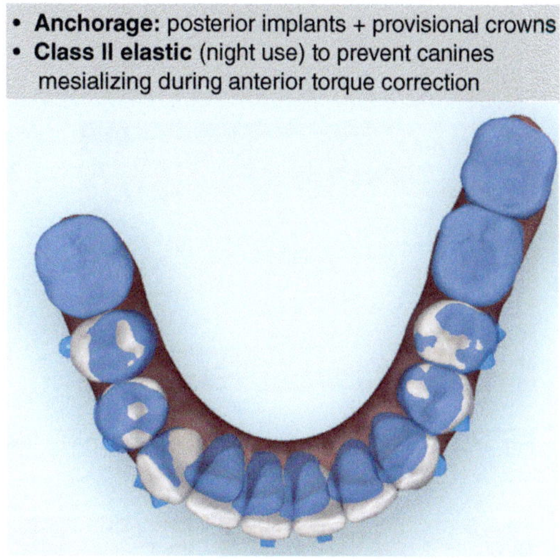

Fig. 24.49 Initial lower ClinCheck.

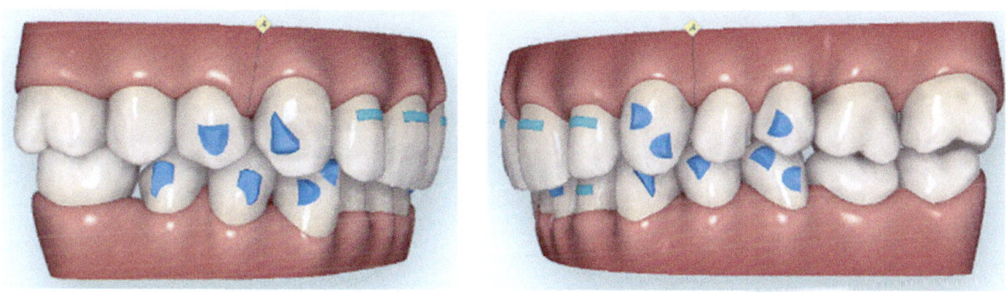

Fig. 24.50 Initial lateral ClinChecks.

Fig. 24.51 Initial frontal ClinCheck.

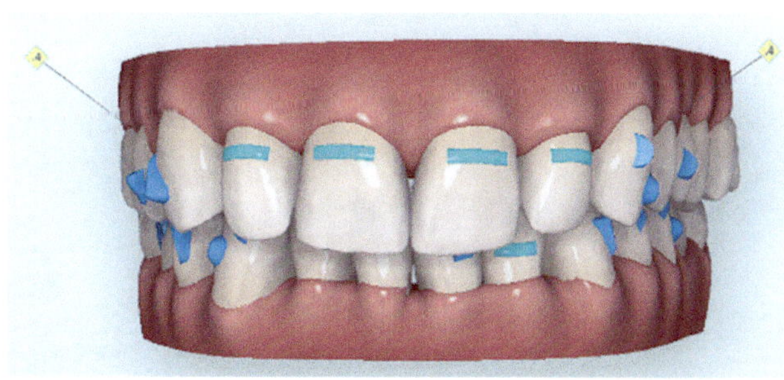

Treatment goals: correct deep bite by relative intrusion of incisors, apply lingual root torque to upper incisors, using as anchorage posterior implants + Class II elastic (night use).

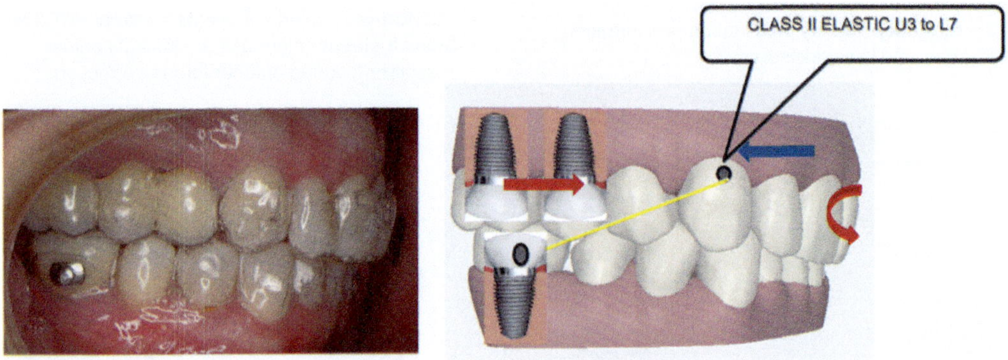

Fig. 24.52 Class II elastic from upper canine to lower first molar (night use).

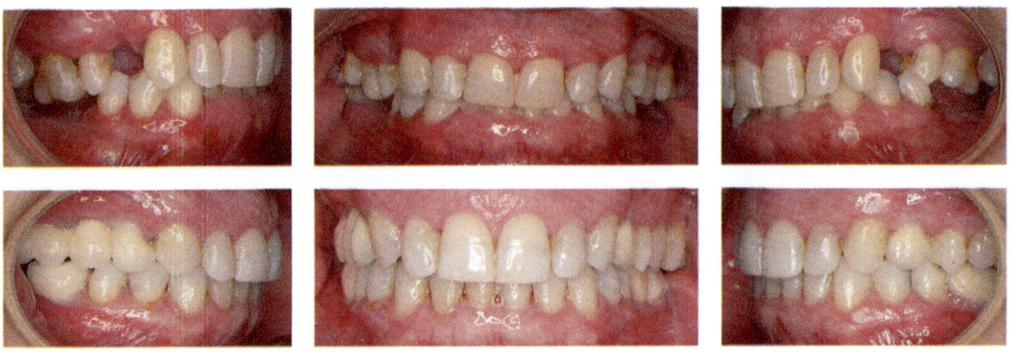

Fig. 24.53 Initial and final occlusion.

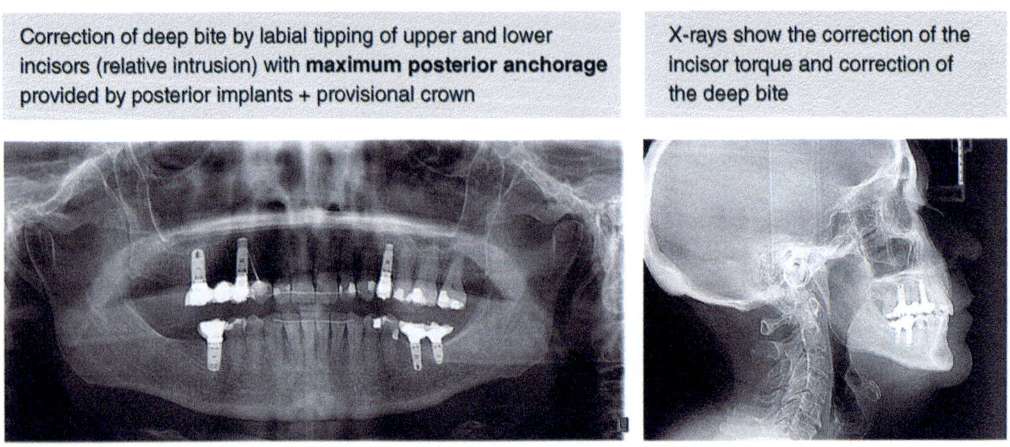

Fig. 24.54 Final panoramic and lateral X-rays.

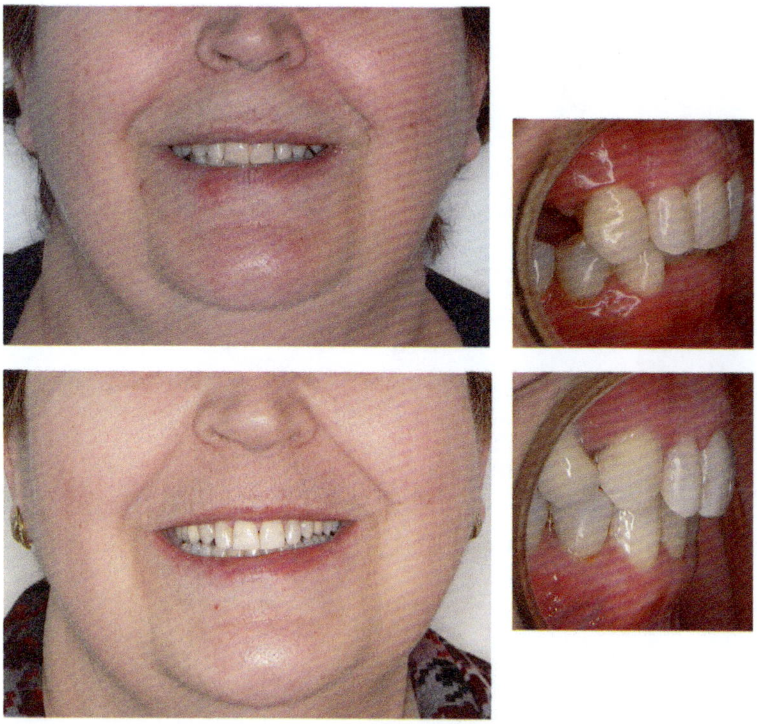

Fig. 24.55 Comparison of initial and final smile and overjet.

24.5 Biomechanics of the Locatelli for Mesialization of the Lower Dental Arch Opening Space for Implants

Locatelli is especially indicated when premolars are tipped to distal and molars are tipped to mesial. The Locatelli force pushes the molar crown to distal and the premolar to mesial. As the wisdom teeth are present in the mouth, the Locatelli generates a stronger force of mesialization on the lower arch. This force, when combined with expansion will guide the lower arch to mesial.

To avoid second premolar rotation, the technician should place a vertical attachment on the lingual surface of the second premolars.

Fig. 24.56 Simulation of force vectors applied by a Locatelli spring.

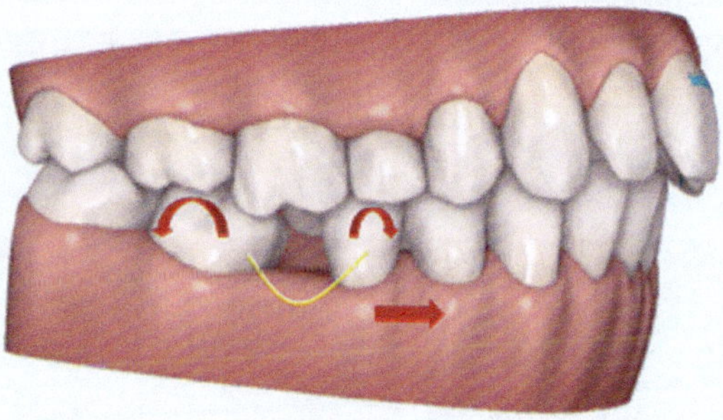

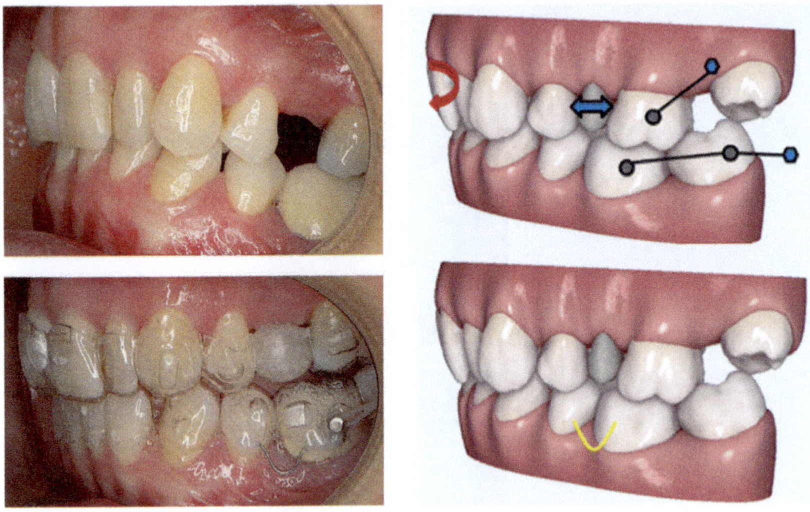

Fig. 24.57 Locatelli to open space for implanting 35 and 45.

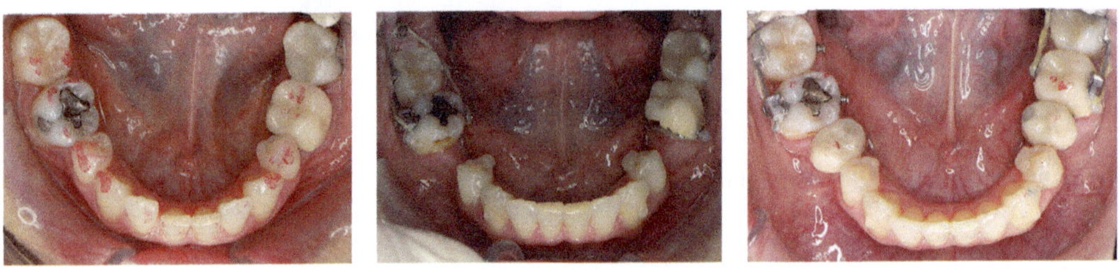

Fig. 24.58 Distalization of molars from temporary anchorage devices and mesialization from 4 to 4 with Locatelli.

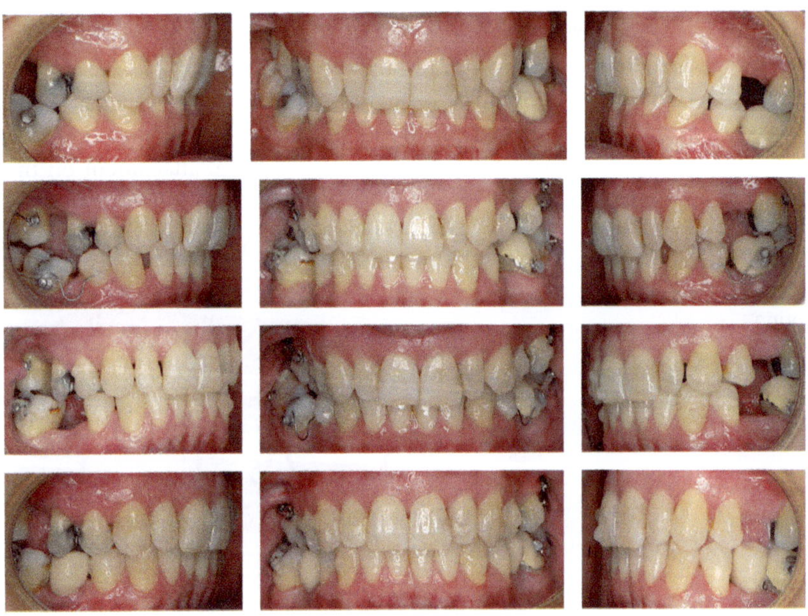

Fig. 24.59 The sequence of opening space for implants of 35 and 45, helping to level the curve of Spee and assisting in the correction of the full Class II.

24.5.1 Locatelli to Open Space for Single Tooth Posterior Implant Side

Simultaneous Lower Mesialization

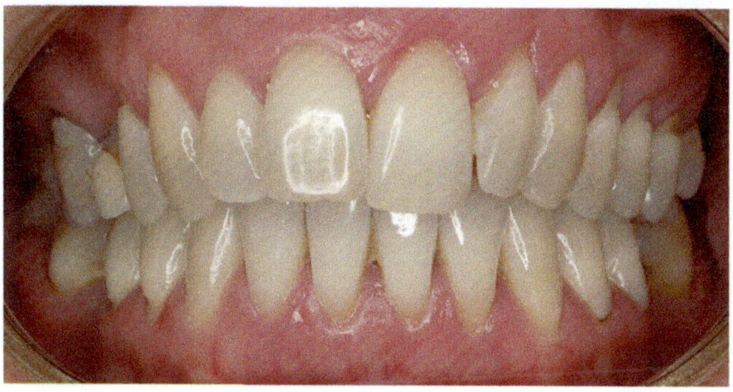

Fig. 24.60 Initial intraoral view.

Diagnosis

A 51-year-old woman with a normodivergent skeletal Class II pattern presented with constricted dental arches and a narrow smile with posterior gummy smile caused by negative lateral torque. They had wide buccal corridors, prominent nasolabial fold and labial incompetence with contraction of the perioral muscles. The intraoral view revealed full Class II division 1 with lingual tipping of posterior teeth, missing 36 and 46 and labial tipping of lower incisors, periodontal tissue and bone loss because of the negative lateral torque; 18 and 28 were present in the mouth.

Treatment Plan

- Correct the Class II by lower simultaneous mesialization, avoiding extraction of upper premolars or upper distalization so as not to flatten the profile
- Expand the arches, changing torque in order to upright the posterior zone and leave premolars and molars perpendicular to the bone to reduce the gum recessions
- In the lower arch, simultaneous mesialization using a Locatelli from second molar to second premolars opening the space for missing 36 and 46

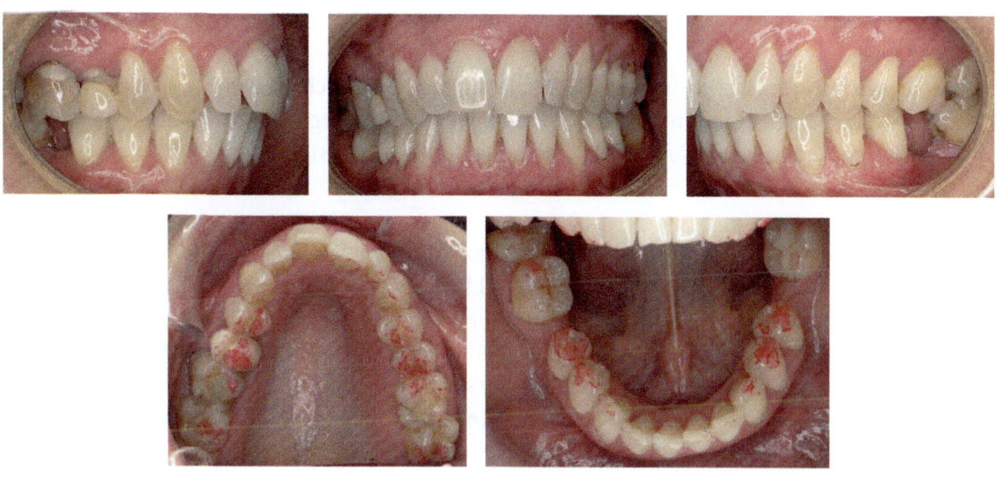

Fig. 24.61 Pretreatment intraoral views.

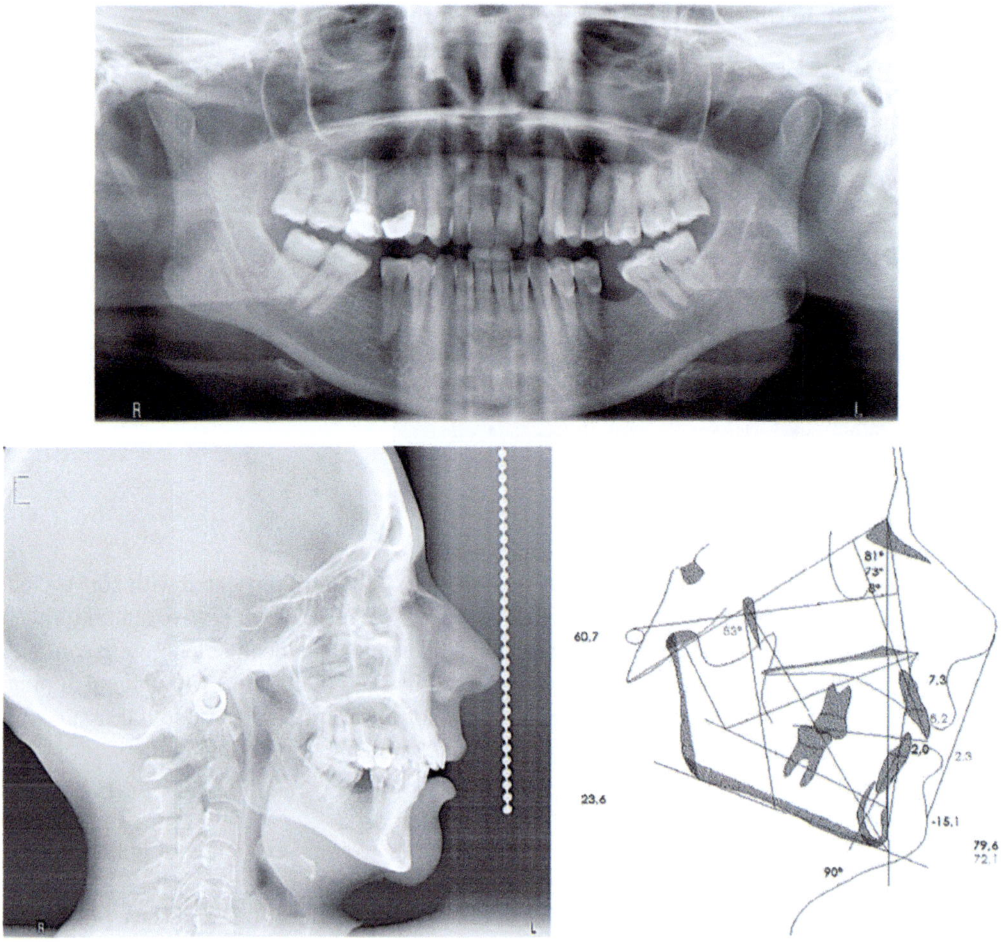

Fig. 24.62 X-ray analysis (panoramic, teleradiograph and cephalometry): normodivergent class II with labial tipping lower incisors and narrow symphysis.

Requirements for the Technician

Maxilla:

- Make a symmetric expansion with simultaneous retraction of incisors
- Use the space gained through the expansion to move the upper teeth to distal and not move second and third molars to use them as anchorage for the expansion

Mandible:

- Make a reciprocal movement of lower expansion and mesialization 5 to 5 and reciprocal retrusion of the lower incisors. This movement would be assisted by the Locatelli, for that reason button cutouts are planned on labial surface of second molars and second premolars
- In order to avoid the side-effect of the Locatelli of intrusion and rotation of the second premolars, a vertical attachment is placed lingual to the second premolars
- A virtual jump is required at the end of the treatment to simulate the effect of the Locatelli and the class II elastics

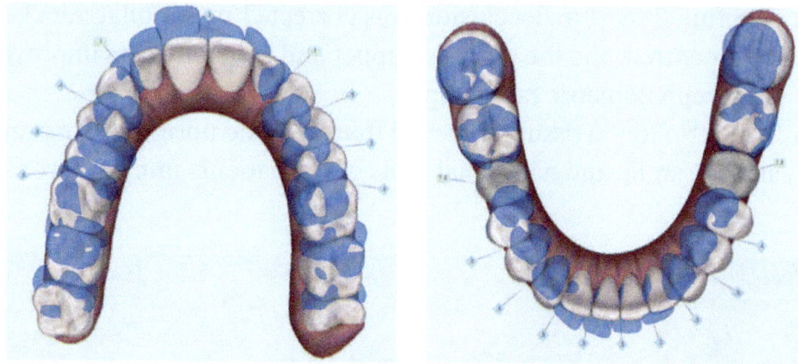

Fig. 24.63 Initial occlusal, upper and lower ClinCheck views.

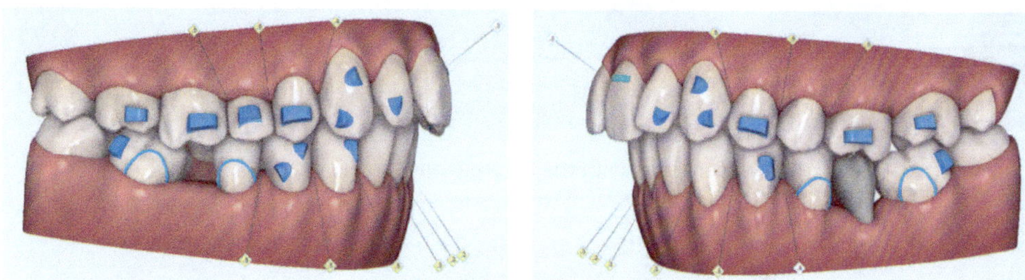

Fig. 24.64 Initial left and right ClinCheck views.

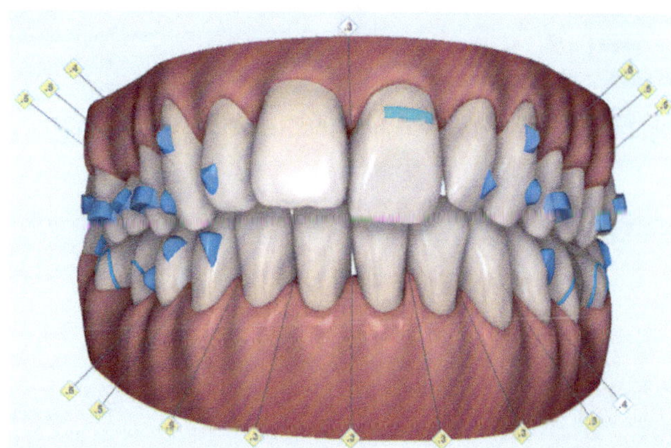

Fig. 24.65 Initial front ClinCheck view.

Treatment Summary

- Total treatment time was 21 months.
- The patient had a first phase with 29 aligners with 2-week change intervals; during that phase the patient used full-time class II elastic.
- The Locatelli was placed at the point in the ClinCheck that the technician started the simultaneous movements of expansion, lower mesialization and anterior incisor retrusion.
- After these 29 aligners, the patient needed an additional set of aligners to complete the class II correction and to complete opening space for implants of 36 and 46.
- The class II elastics were interrupted 6 weeks before finishing the treatment.
- The push force provided by the Locatelli was critical to achieving the amount of lower mesialization planned.

- The full class II malocclusion was corrected into a bilateral class I relationship, both midlines were centred, and the torque of upper and lower incisors improved considerably, as shown in the final cephalometric radiographs.
- The periodontal tissue improved thanks to the uprighting of premolars and canines on the bone and the smile and nasolabial folds of the patients improved considerably.

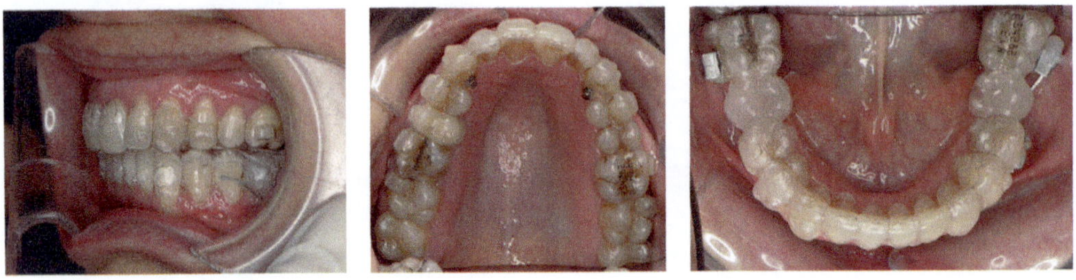

Fig. 24.66 Intraoral views: right, upper, lower with the Locatelli and the aligner.

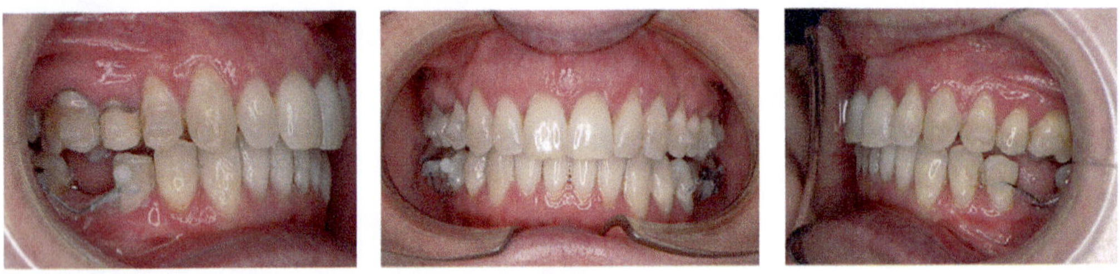

Fig. 24.67 Intraoral views: right, front, left with the Locatelli.

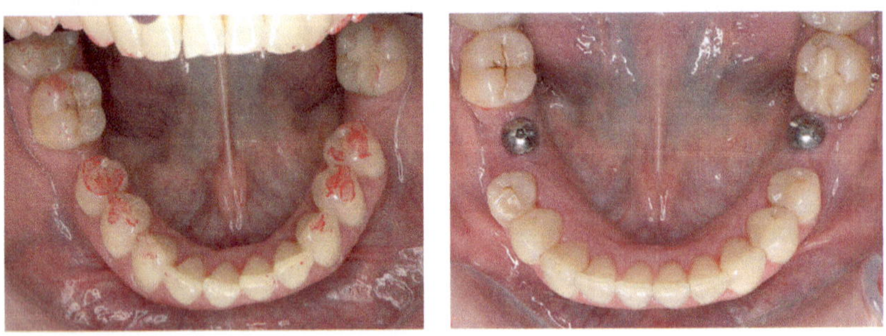

Fig. 24.68 Intraoral views at the beginning and after placing the implants.

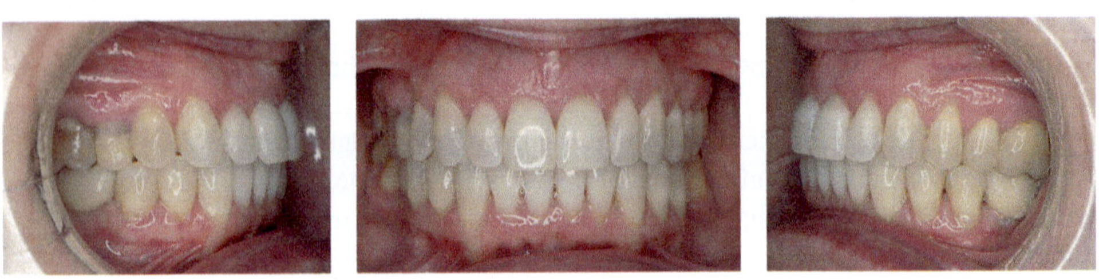

Fig. 24.69 Intraoral views after loading implants.

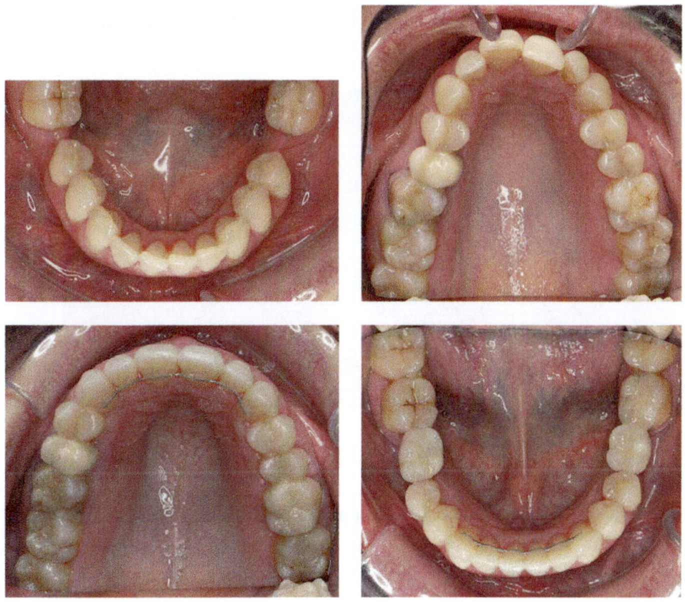

Fig. 24.70 Intraoral views before and after treatment (upper and lower occlusal).

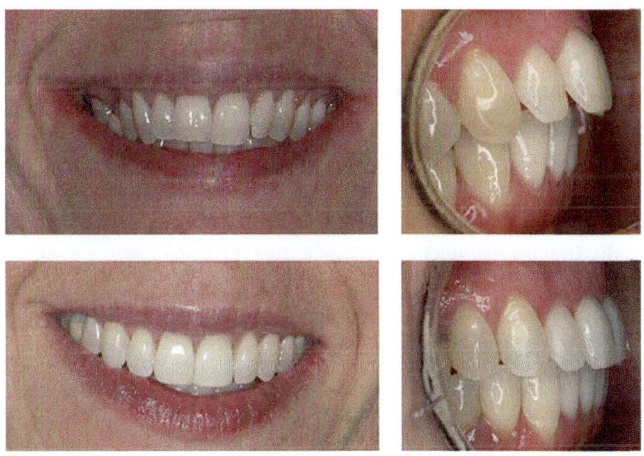

Fig. 24.71 Comparison of smile and overjet before and after treatment.

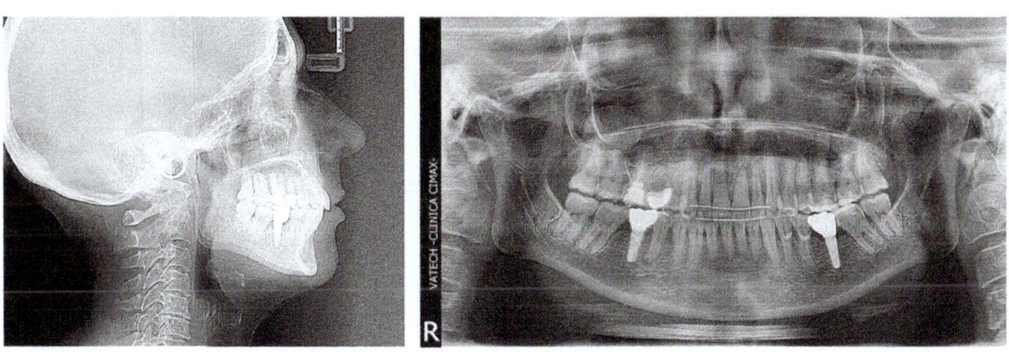

Fig. 24.72 Final panoramic and lateral X-ray.

24.6 Gingivectomy, Passive Eruption Case

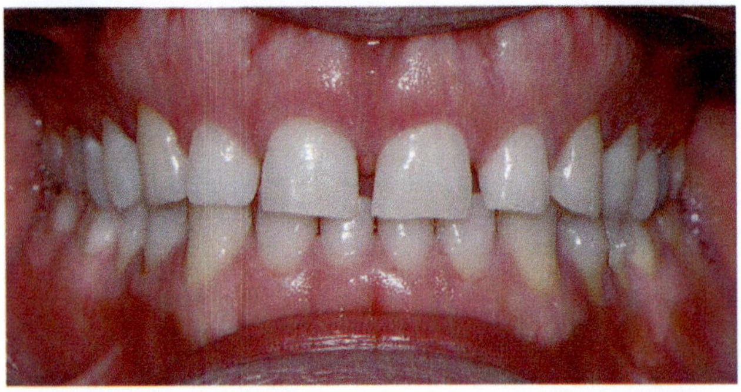

Fig. 24.73 Skeletal Class I with spacing.

Diagnosis

A 35-year-old patient, symmetrically presented with dental Class I with proper display. The patient had upper and lower diastemas, bigger in the upper arch with abrasion on the incisal edges of upper and lower incisors. There were short clinical crowns on upper incisors.

Treatment Plan

- Close spaces and maintain anterior torque
- Perform a gingivectomy at the initial stage in order to increase the size of clinical crowns (however, patient refused and postponed this to second set of aligners)

Requirements for the Technician

- In order to correct upper spacing add ClinCheck PRO 10 degrees extra of palatal root torque to upper incisors, as well as the lower ones with ClinCheck
- To increase anchorage, set molars and second premolars as unmovable, helping to improve posterior retention to anterior space closure by retraction
- Finally, lower IPR to create overjet, as spacing was bigger in the lower arch and it is desirable to avoid anterior interferences

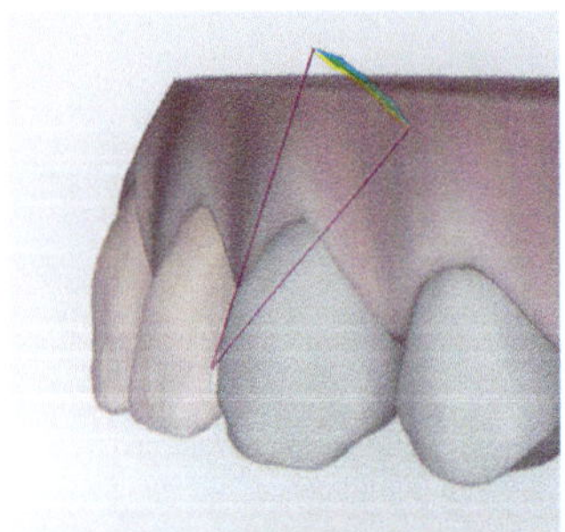

Fig. 24.74 Extra palatal root torque to anterior sector, selecting multiple teeth with ClinCheck PRO.

Treatment Summary

- Treatment was completed in 16 months
- Upper and lower diastemas were successfully closed, thanks to the gingivectomy performed before the second set of aligners, with bigger clinical crowns
- Class I occlusion was maintained
- Patient did not use intermaxillary elastics during treatment

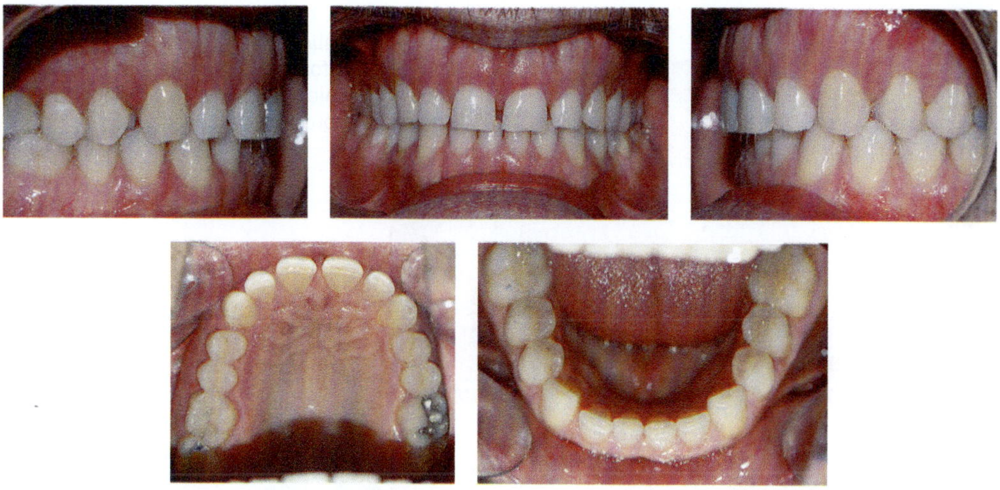

Fig. 24.75 Initial intraoral views.

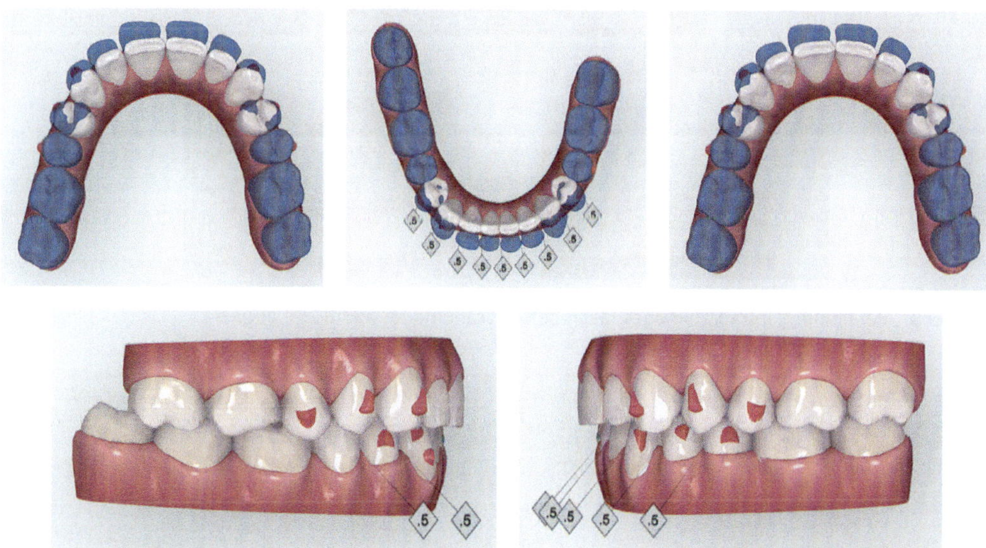

Fig. 24.76 Initial ClinChecks.

ClinCheck 1: Communication with Technician

- Set molars as unmovable on both upper and lower arch
- Add extra LRT to 12–22 and 32–32. Solve rotations of premolars at the same time as retrusion, creating a reciprocal movement
- Use optimized deep bite attachments on premolars to help with anterior intrusion and avoid deep bite causing interferences

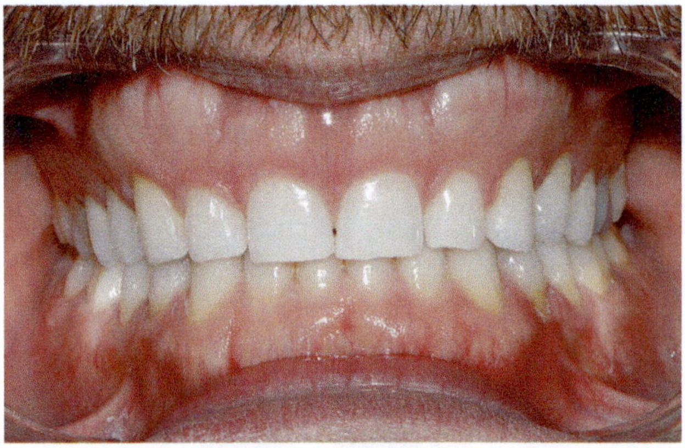

Fig. 24.77 Refinement: after first set of aligners, gingivectomy was performed in order to increase clinical crown contact surface and improve patient aesthetics.

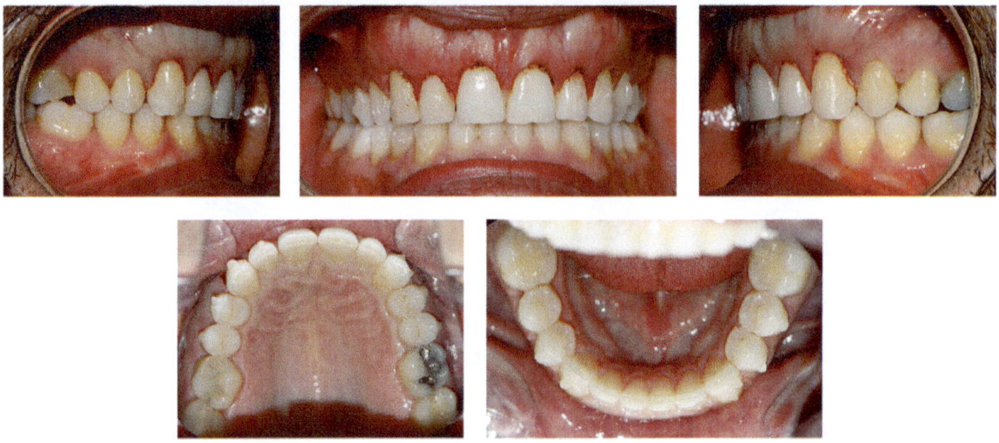

Fig. 24.78 Refinement: intraoral images taken before scanning for additional aligners.

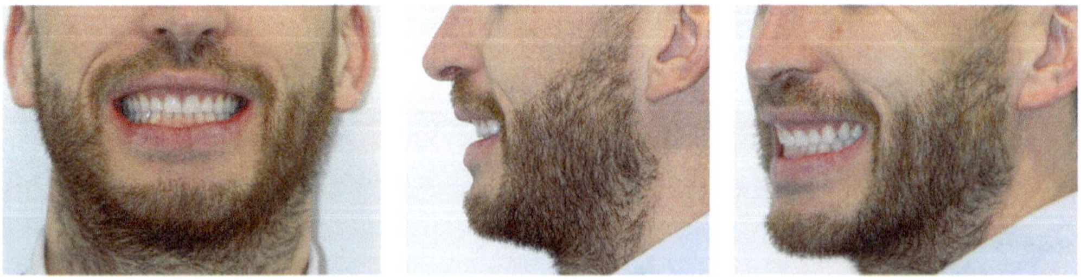

Fig. 24.79 Refinement: extraoral views.

ClinCheck: Communication with Technician

- After closing most of the spacing, anterior torque was not as good as predicted, so a second set of aligners was ordered in order to create more anterior torque and avoid posterior open bite
- The current attachments were left on for anchorage, as the rotations were resolved
- A gingivectomy was performed before scanning the patient so there were bigger clinical crowns to allow for the addition of Power ridges
- Finally overcorrection aligners (3, at the end of the treatment stage) were ordered to be used only if residual spacing was present

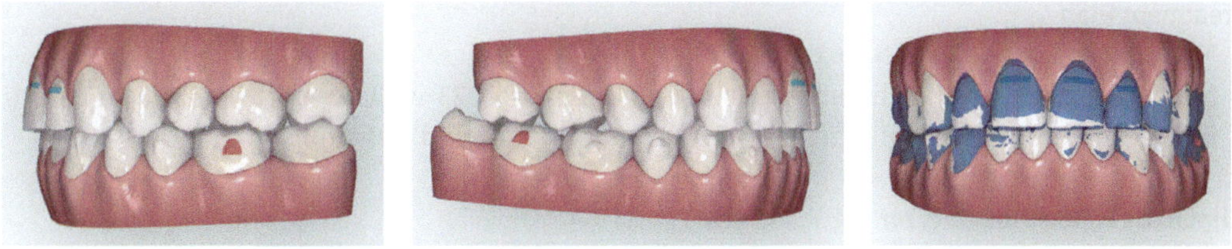

Fig. 24.80 Refinement ClinChecks.

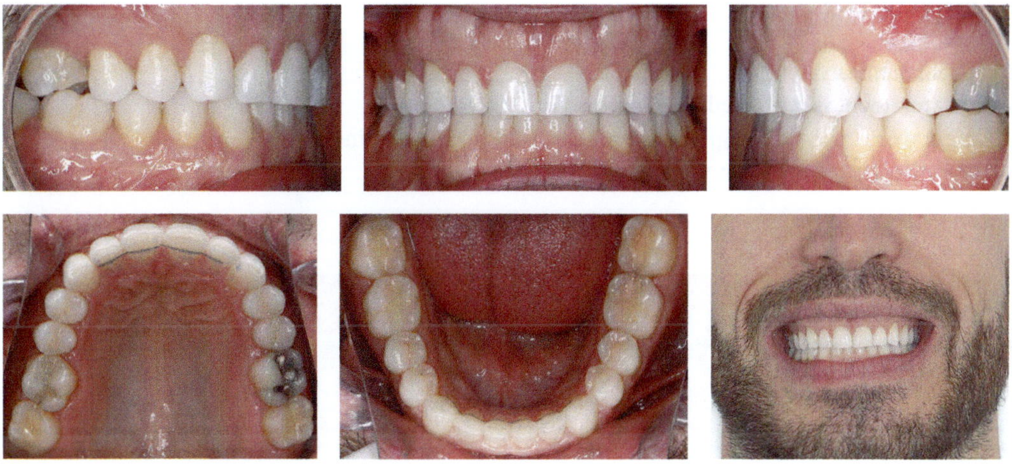

Fig. 24.81 Intraoral views and smile at the end of treatment.

24.7 Anterior Intrusion Anchored on Dental Implant

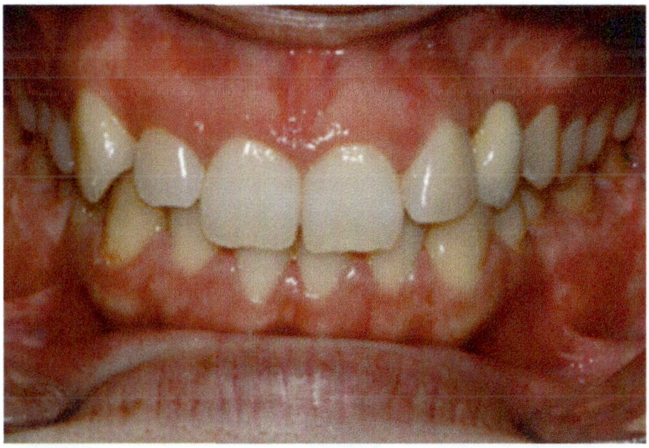

Fig. 24.82 Intraoral view.

Diagnosis

A 34-year-old woman with a hypodivergent skeletal Class I pattern presented with constricted dental arches, an implant on 23 and a narrow, anterior gummy smile.

Treatment Plan

- Mandible: align and level Spee curve
- Maxilla: use absolute anchorage on temporary crown on 23 with an extrusion attachment to intrude anterior incisors and help in solving gummy smile while aligning.

ClinCheck 1: Requirements for the Technician

- Level gingival edges to 23
- Extrusion attachments on 12–22
- Central incisors intrusion
- Attachment on 23

Treatment Summary

- Total treatment is estimated at 4 months
- Patient wore one set of aligners to help in intruding anterior incisors
- Ceramic permanent crown was placed

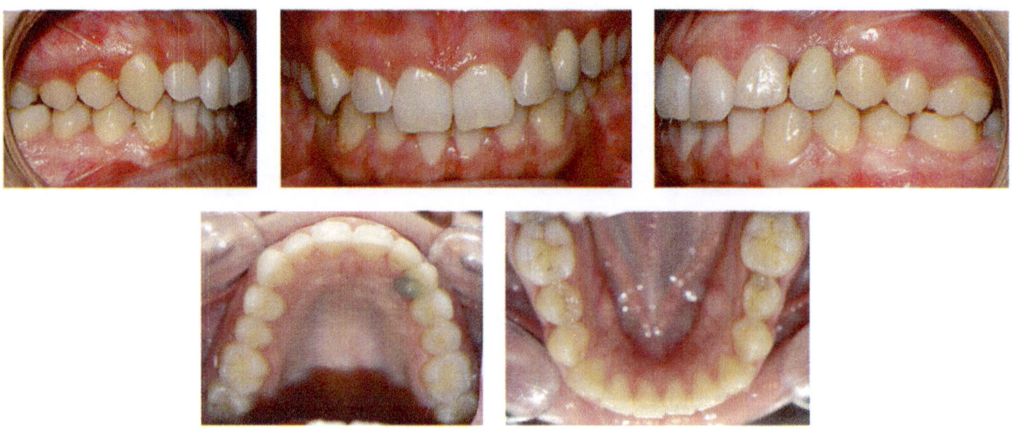

Fig. 24.83 Initial intraoral views.

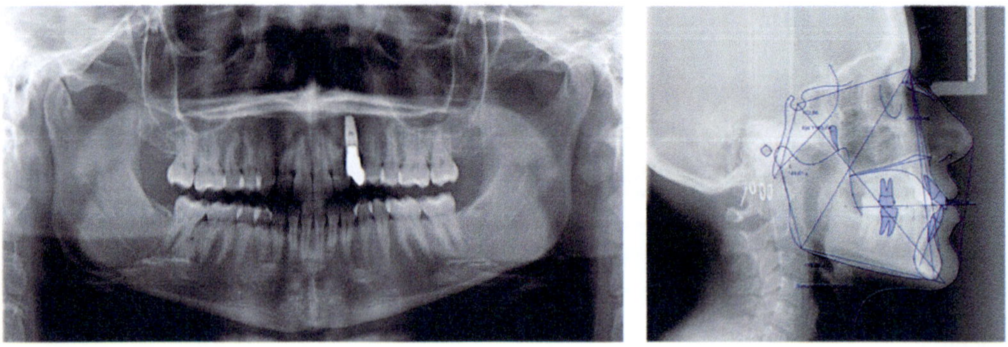

Fig. 24.84 Initial panoramic and lateral X-rays.

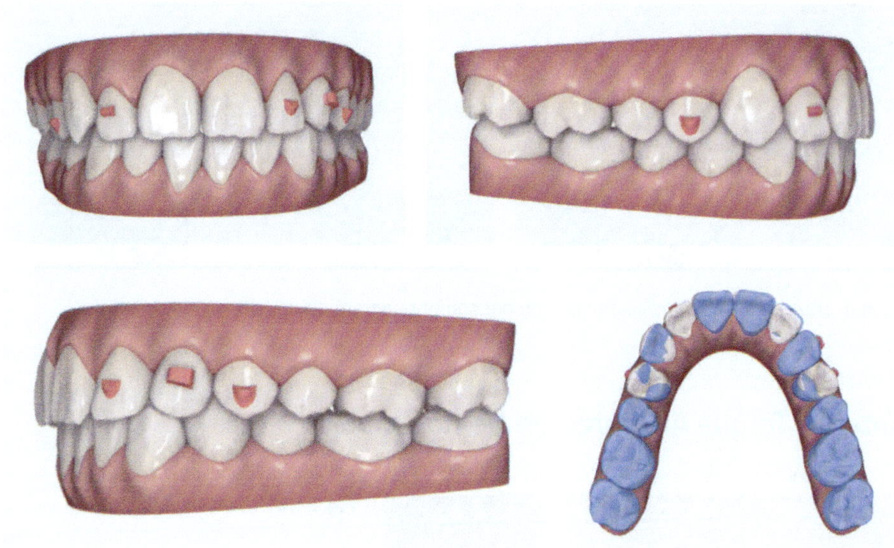

Fig. 24.85 Initial ClinChecks.

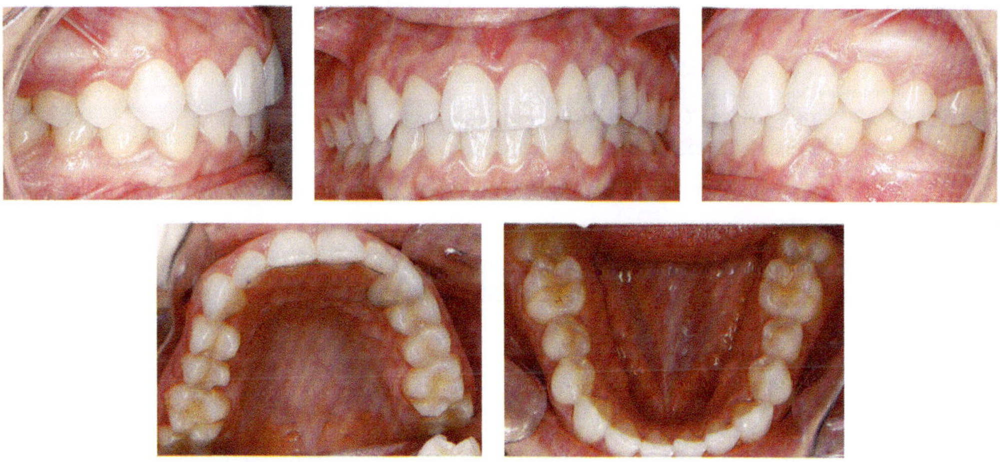

Fig. 24.86 Final Intraoral views.

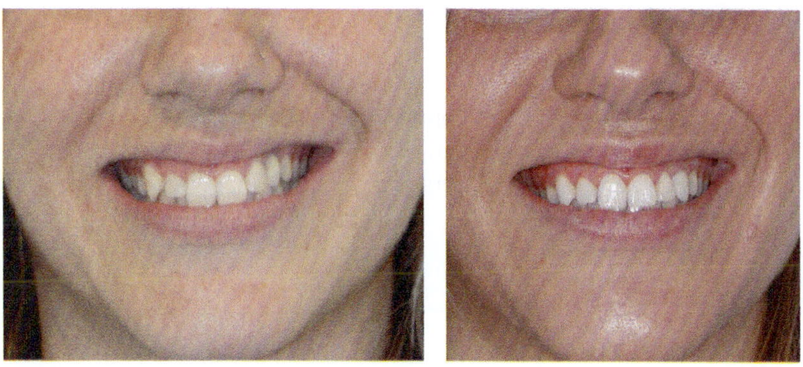

Fig. 24.87 Pretreatment and final smile.

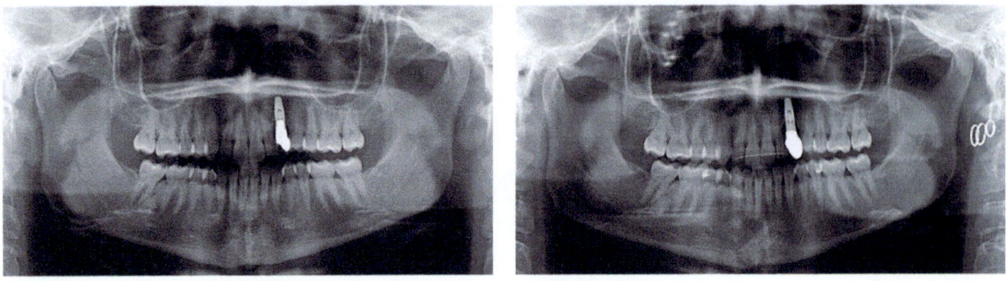

Fig. 24.88 Final: anterior intrusion is visible on comparison of panoramic X-rays.

24.8 Anterior Torque Anchored on Dental Implant

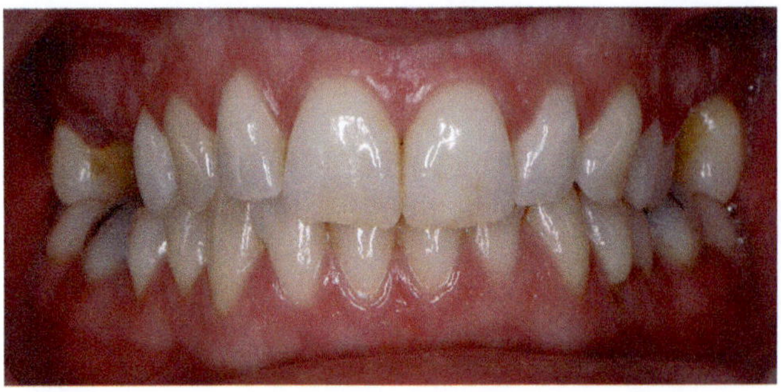

Fig. 24.89 Intraoral view.

Diagnosis

A 32-year-old woman with a hypodivergent skeletal Class I pattern presented with constricted dental arches and implants on the upper molars. She had a narrow smile with anterior short incisor display.

Treatment Plan

- Mandible: align and level curve of Spee.
- Maxilla: correct anterior torque and expand posterior sectors to improve the smile aesthetics.

ClinCheck 1: Requirements for the Technician

- Improve anterior torque 12 to 22 with Power ridges
- Posterior expansion, anchoring on distal molars
- Leave space for abutments (pontics)
- Extrude 12 to level gingival architecture (place an optimized extrusion attachment)
- Open space for molar crowns to help create overjet after lower alignment
- Set molars as unmovable to increase posterior anchorage

Treatment Summary

- Total treatment is estimated at 10 months
- The patient wore two sets of aligners to improve anterior torque, align and coordinate arches
- The patient had the extractions done in a different clinic before the treatment started, and therefore was expecting implant abutments as had been planned with her oral surgeon
- Before second treatment phase started the patient had her ceramic crowns done, so these were included in the scan in order to increase posterior anchorage
- Smile aesthetics were improved during implants procedure with clear aligners therapy correcting anterior torque and deep bite (but not fully, in order not to reduce incisors display) as well as aligning, while night bleaching was performed with the aligners

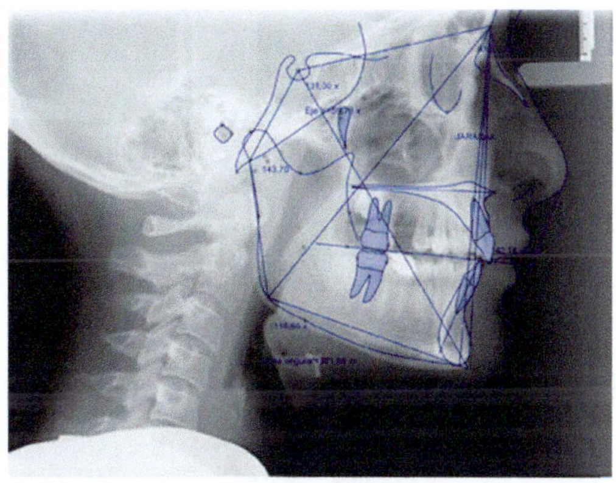

Fig. 24.90 Initial cephalometric measurements.

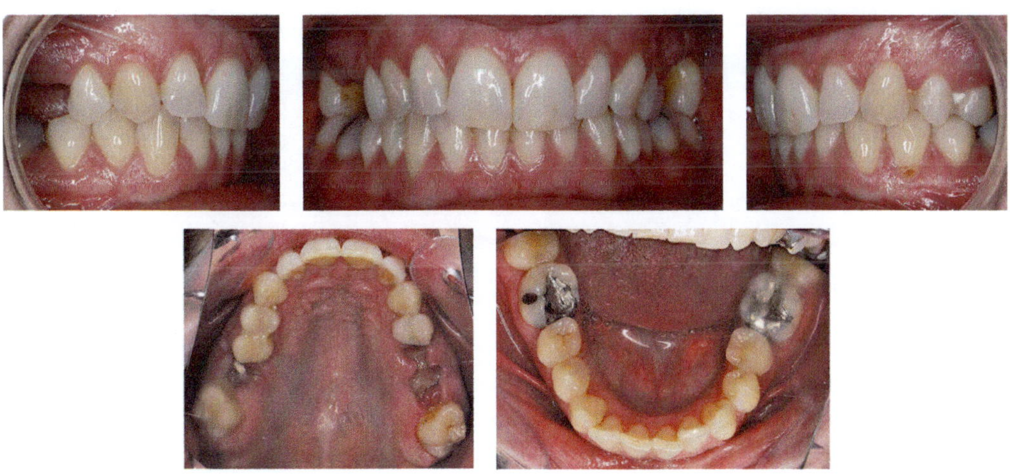

Fig. 24.91 Initial intraoral views.

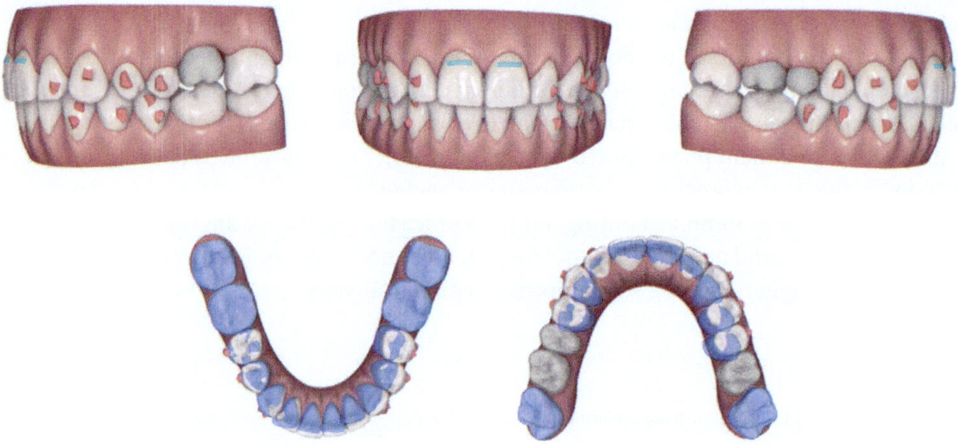

Fig. 24.92 Initial ClinChecks.

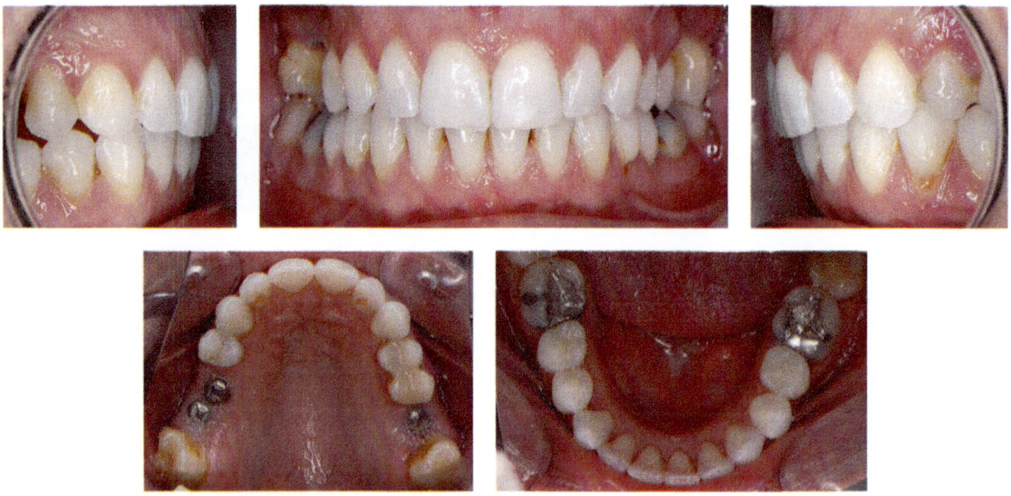

Fig. 24.93 Refinement: intraoral views.

ClinCheck 2: Requirements for the Technician

- Improve anterior torque of 12 to 22 with Power ridges, to help resolve the posterior open bite that is creating a Class II as a result of excessive anterior contact
- Posterior expansion, anchoring on implants
- Rescan after crown placement to obtain full posterior anchorage
- Intrude 33 to 43 to make sure that curve of Spee is totally flattened

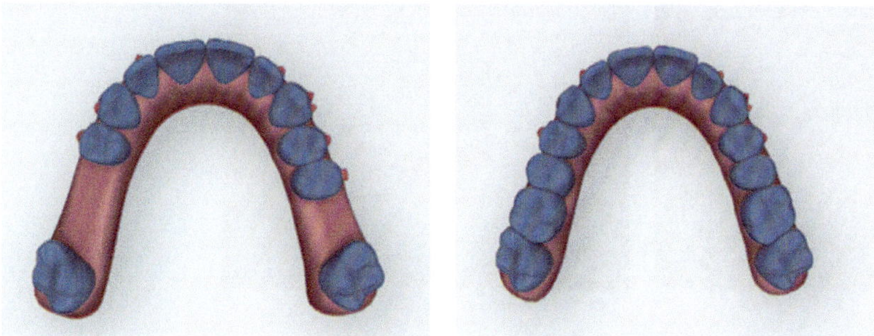

Fig. 24.94 Refinement: change of scan to include molars and increased anchorage.

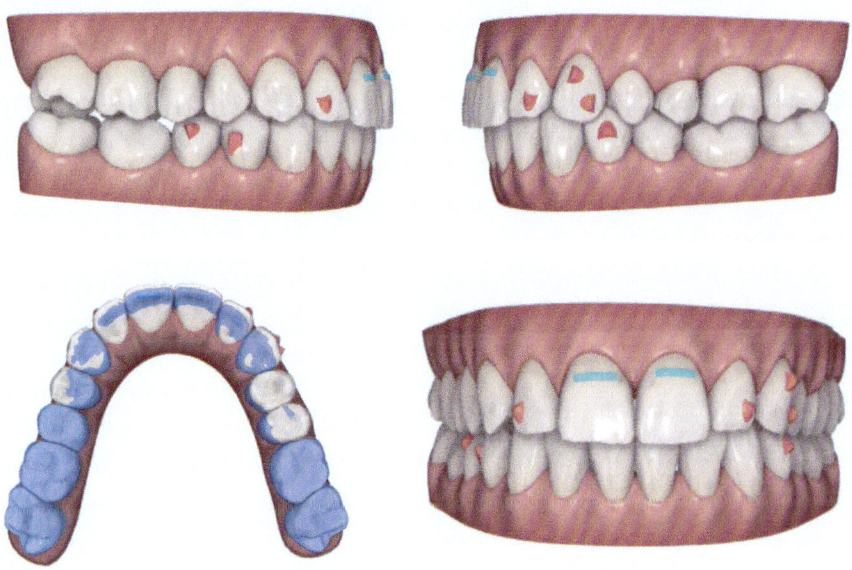

Fig. 24.95 Refinement ClinChecks.

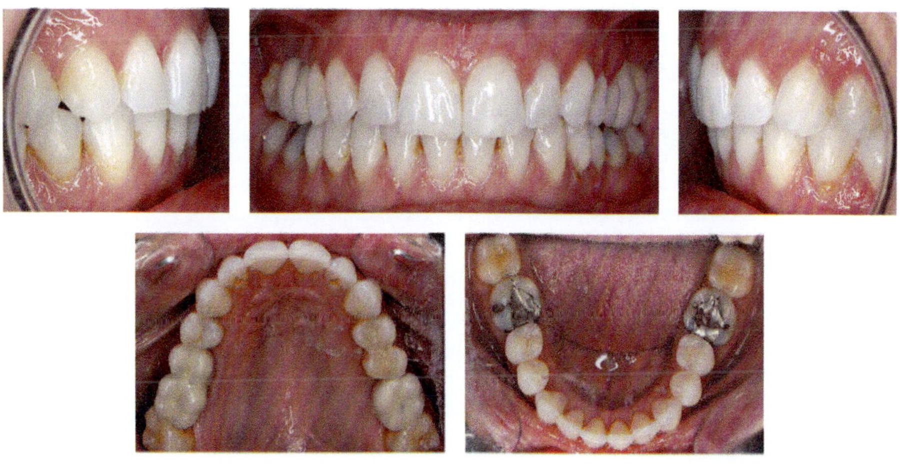

Fig. 24.96 Final intraoral views.

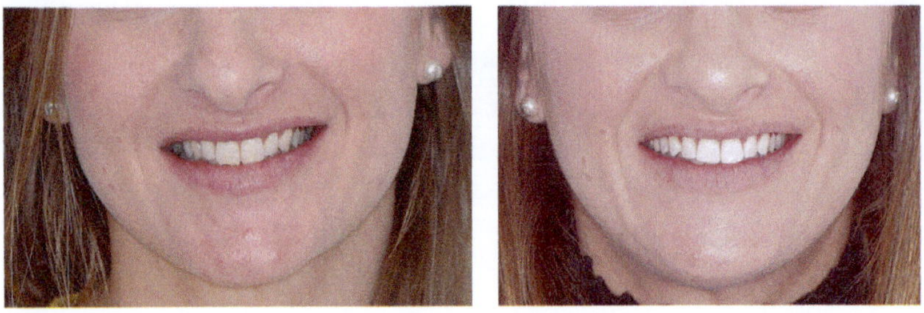

Fig. 24.97 Final smile.

25

Prerestorative Orthodontics: Veneers

Orthodontics is one of the key drivers of success in cosmetic dentistry, as space is needed for prosthetic restorations and cosmetic dentists require orthodontic collaboration to minimize tooth preparation in these patients. Clear aligners have been a really powerful tool in these situations, as many adults would refuse cosmetic dentistry in the past because they had to wear fixed appliances, which, in many circumstances, were viewed as incompatible with their professional and personal life.

That said, some patients do allow full comprehensive aligner treatment whereas some will just require a previous orthodontic preparation for the cosmetic procedure (mostly veneers) for which we again focus on three planes of space: transverse, sagittal and vertical.

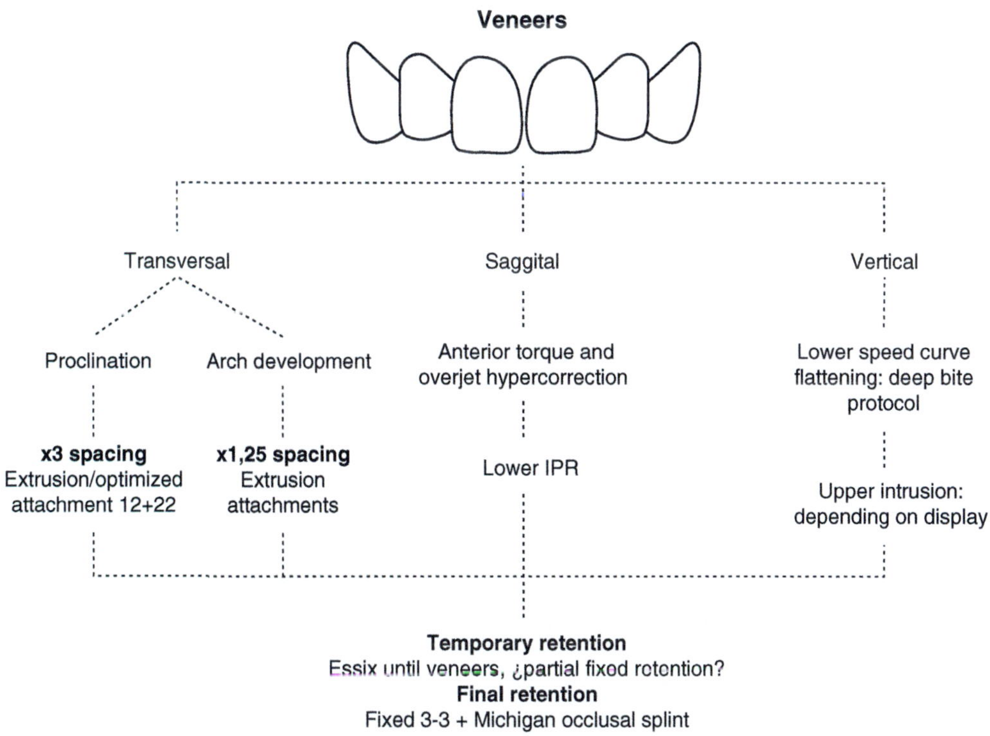

Fig. 25.1 Aesthetic protocol for veneers preparation with aligners.

Aligner Techniques in Orthodontics, First Edition. Susana Palma Moya and Javier Lozano Zafra.

Companion website: www.wiley.com/go/lozano-zafra/aligner-techniques

Transversally, it is known that the golden proportion for teeth requires very concrete spacing in order to get the most natural result, which might already be ideal from the beginning or may require orthodontic intervention.

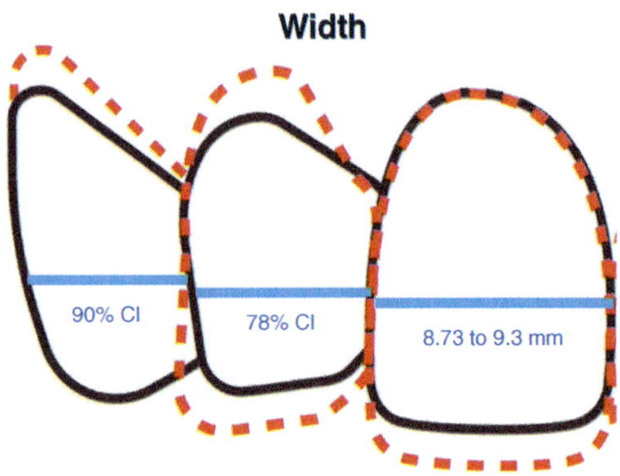

Fig. 25.2 Anterior teeth width has to be determined carefully in order to end in an aesthetic position.

The most common intervention is Bolton discrepancy, which affects upper lateral incisors. This is sometimes resolved by reducing the width of the lower incisors by performing interproximal reductions. Another alternative is leaving space distal to laterals and bond veneers to them. Whichever is used, every space is related to the upper central incisor, as long as it has a regular size, as both laterals and canines have to adapt to this.

The only exception to this is abnormal size or shape of the upper central incisors, in which we can refer to the contralateral central incisor or set a proportion according to most frequent sizes and shapes both in the smile of a man or woman.

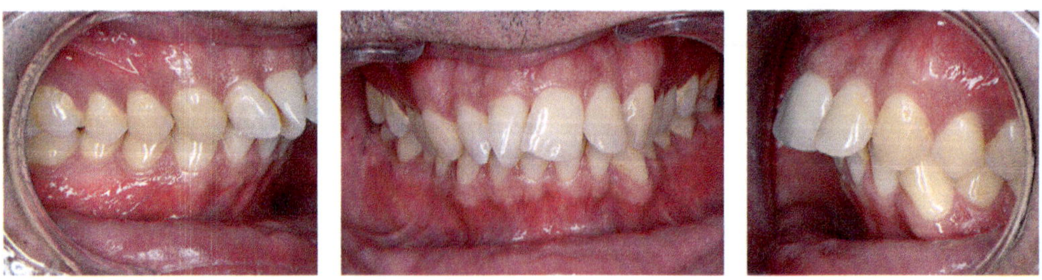

Fig. 25.3 This bilateral full Class II case has an abnormal 11 size and shape, which requires planning spaces to distal and mesial, as agreed with the cosmetic dentist.

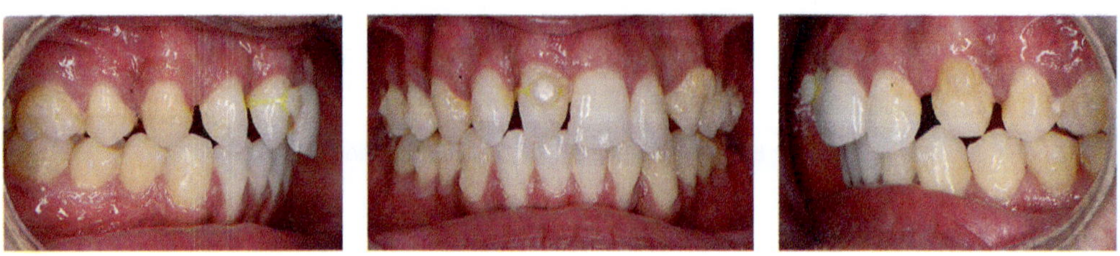

Fig. 25.4 Auxiliary buttons and Powerchains are used to help with a severe 90 degree rotation.

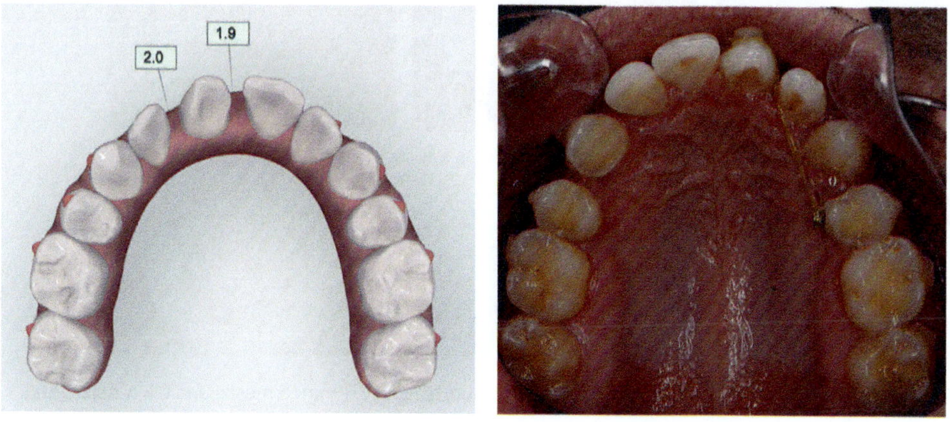

Fig. 25.5 Mesial and distal spacing is planned at the end of the case for a proper restoration of dental veneers with minimal preparation.

For this transverse spacing we might work in two different directions according to the protocol for protruding anterior incisors. Whenever there is a chance to procline, the result will be acceptable unless it comes from a retroclination of anterior incisors, as regular torque makes it difficult to create space because incisors are impacted into the cortical bone.

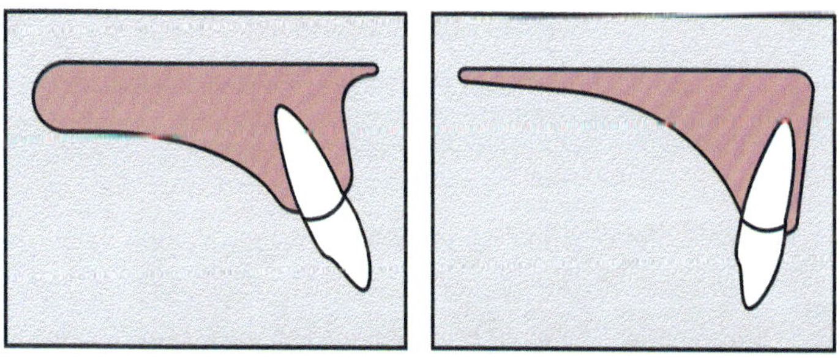

Fig. 25.6 The left image is complex if we have to create anterior spacing for veneers on a transverse dimension, but the right image is highly predictable, as we only need crown protrusion.

For this reason, a hypercorrection of this space opening is needed, together with attachments on lateral incisors, which, as mentioned before, affects the tooth more, together with a small crown size, thereby leading to misfitting. Otherwise, there is not usually enough space to place veneers/crowns (as can be seen in Figs 25.2 and 25.14, and in the Cases described in this chapter).

That said, transverse spacing might also be created by transverse development in patients with a compressed arch also needing an overcorrection from expected spacing, mainly because plastic amongst selected teeth has to be 'seen', therefore usually hypercorrecting the space by about 1.25 times.

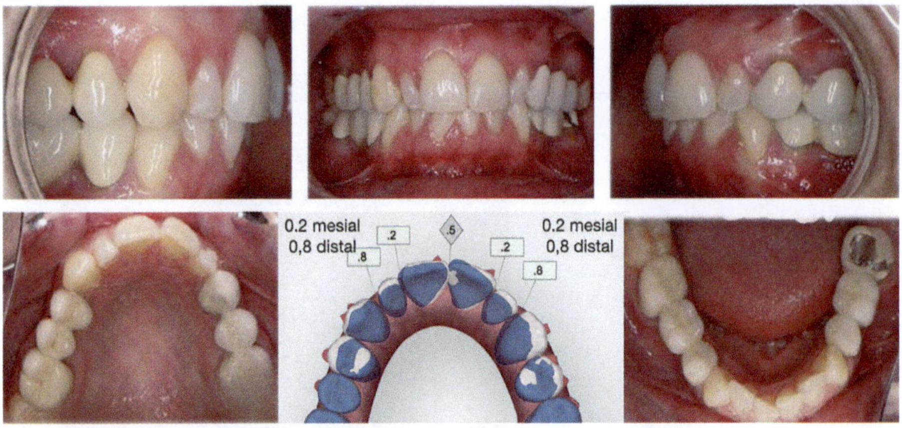

Fig. 25.7 Transverse space planning is made with protrusion, leaving 0.2 mm to mesial and 0.8 mm to distal.

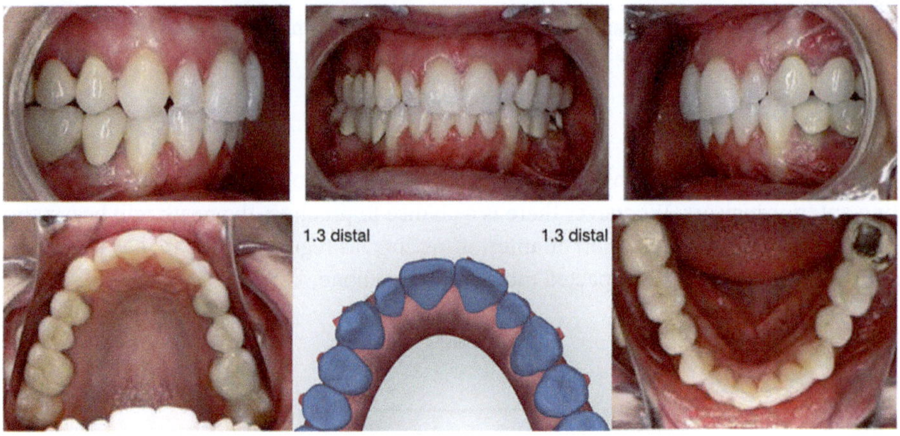

Fig. 25.8 After no space creation mesial or distal to affected tooth, transverse space planning is made with protrusion, leaving 0.2 mm to mesial and 1.3 mm to distal.

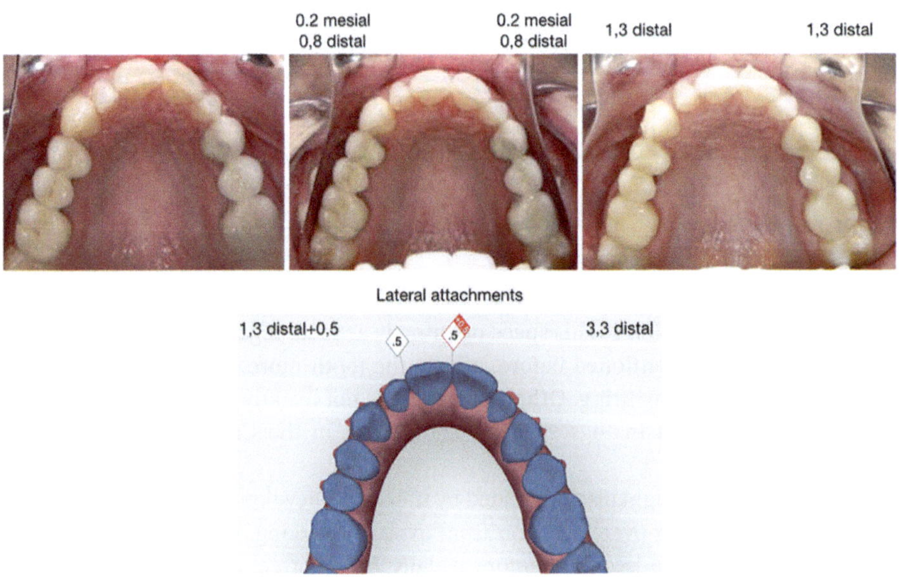

Fig. 25.9 After 1.3 mm space planning, this only happens in the lateral with a bigger crown, namely 12, thus creating the need to add an attachment on the refinement on 22 to increase tooth surface contact with the aligner.

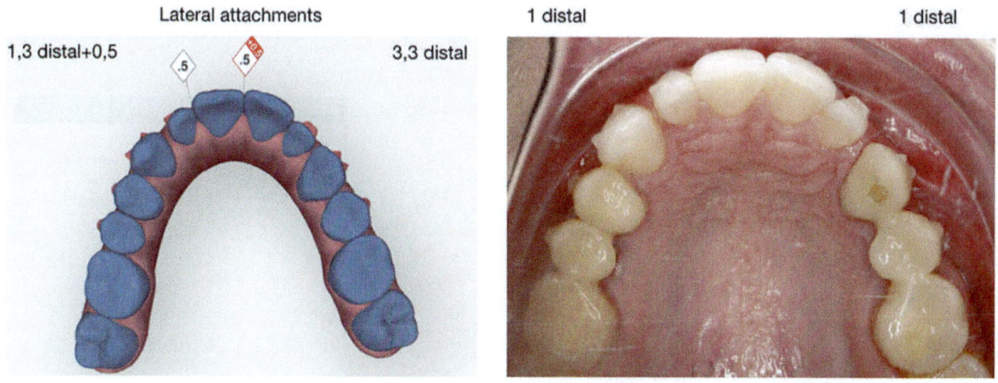

Fig. 25.10 After attachment and threefold overcorrection, non-predictable anterior protrusion leads to space creation for veneer bonding.

Sagittally, an overjet is needed and is achieved with anterior torque correction by protrusion, for which both buccal and palatal Power ridges are convenient, lowering IPR to retrude the lower incisors. That said, it is important to understand what is meant in Align Technology by 'overjet', which might differ from what clinicians consider, especially since the introduction of the overjet/overbite tool on ClinCheck PRO.

In this sense, Align technicians and software measure overjet as the distance between the buccal surface of the lower incisor and half the crown of the upper incisor, instead of its palatal surface, therefore not being exactly the same concept you might be using. For this, it is essential to add 0.5 mm (considering 1 mm as upper incisor average thickness) to the desired overjet agreed with the cosmetic dentist.

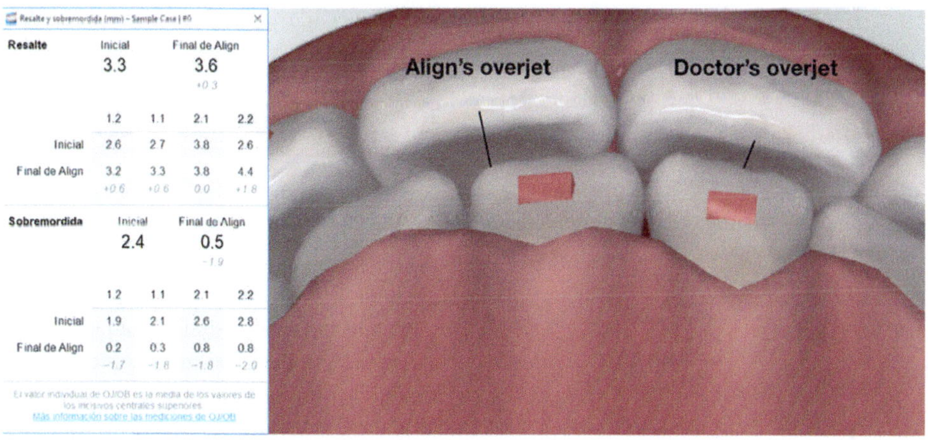

Fig. 25.11 Align's overjet concept might be different from the one the practitioner is using, so it is essential to fully understand the difference in order to avoid a lack of space for posterior restorations.

With regard to this, whenever there is a large posterior expansion, as a result of the 'pearl necklace effect' we have seen previously, in order to avoid additional aligners sets, natural arch depth loss will be considered again: for example an estimate of 1 mm would add an additional 1 mm overjet to achieve the desired result. Taking into account the CAD designers, measure the overjet in a different way including the thickness of the upper incisor. In order to communicate effectively with the CAD designer order a final virtual space of 1.5 mm between the palatal surface of upper incisors and the labial surface of lower incisors.

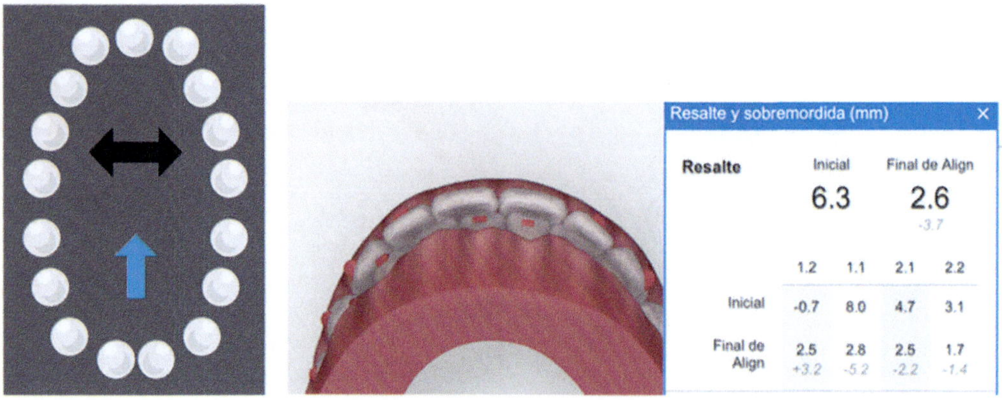

Fig. 25.12 Natural arch depth loss owing to large posterior expansions has to be estimated in the ClinCheck plan to ensure final result is ideal for ceramic restorations.

Finally, from a vertical perspective, anterior teeth have to be considered both from gingival and incisal perspectives in order to decide which is the priority for final aesthetics in the patient. In this, the clinical conversations with the patient have a special importance with regard to the use of composite or ceramic final restorations after orthodontic treatment.

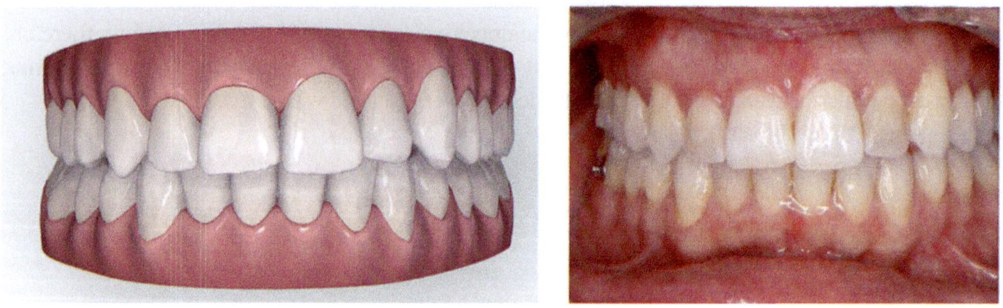

Fig. 25.13 In this patient, if 11 is in a proper incisal position we might perform a gingivectomy on it or, if 21 is in a good gingival situation and it is decided to intrude 11, add an incisal restoration, as both cases increase its final clinical length.

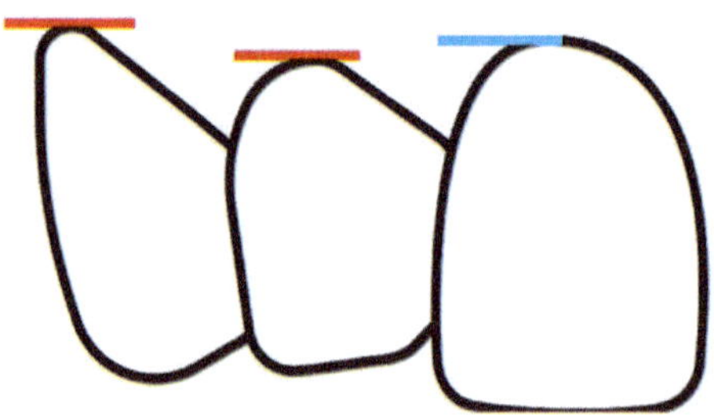

Fig. 25.14 Incisors and canines have usually higher gingival margins than laterals, with 'zeniths' in different positions, depending on several patient factors.

Cosmetic dentists will usually manage 'pink aesthetics', levelling incisors and canines at the same height, and laterals slightly lower (around 0.5 mm). There are several variations around this topic according to gender, ethnicity or even practitioners' preferences, which might change the treatment plan, as used to happen with brackets bonding closer or distal to the incisal edge.

With regard to incisal edges, it is also commonly accepted that, as happened with width, central incisors are the reference to define the height of both laterals and canines, using these as a gold standard for length (as seen in Fig. 25.16).

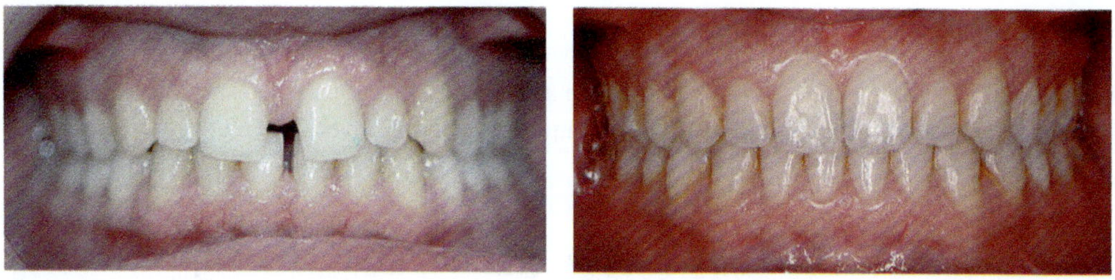

Fig. 25.15 This spacing is an example of how final gingivectomy might help improve teeth aesthetics without final restoration, when an altered passive eruption is detected.

Incisal edges are usually 0.5 mm 'higher' for laterals than central incisors and canines, which again might vary considerably depending on tooth wear, especially for canines, or any other aesthetic preference of the practitioner and patient.

From a vertical perspective, overbite again has to be clearly stablished from the very beginning of the treatment with the cosmetic dentist. This, if deep bite protocols are followed from the beginning, should not be overcorrected as results are highly predictable but, in order to facilitate cosmetic dentist work, can be magnified by slightly overcorrecting the lower curve of Spee by 0.5–1 mm lower intrusion from 33 to 43, with an open bite tendency to leave enough space for restorations to be naturally bonded.

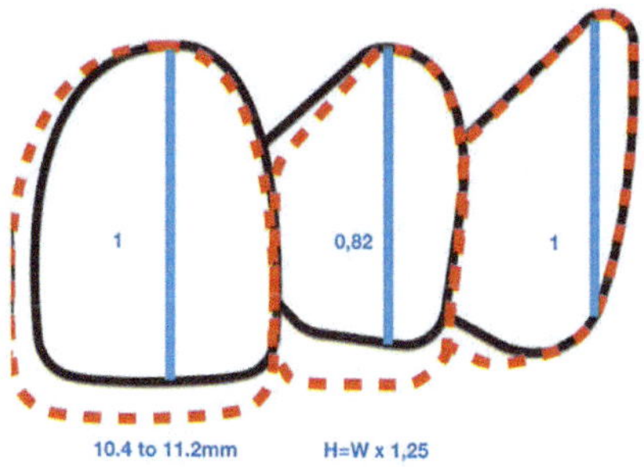

Fig. 25.16 Incisors and usually canines have higher gingival margins than laterals, with 'zeniths' in different positions, depending on several patient factors.

Independently on what restoration is better for the patient, temporary retention is performed during the cosmetic procedure, as cosmetic dentists usually cannot work accurately with upper fixed retentions.

There are several options for this, such as partial fixed retainers on non-affected teeth, but possibly the most common and useful is having an 'essix' plastic retainer 24 hours a day while the wax-up and mock-up procedures are performed. As soon as final restorations are placed, another 'plastic' retainer has to be executed, until regular retention is performed, as seen previously.

25.1 Bleaching

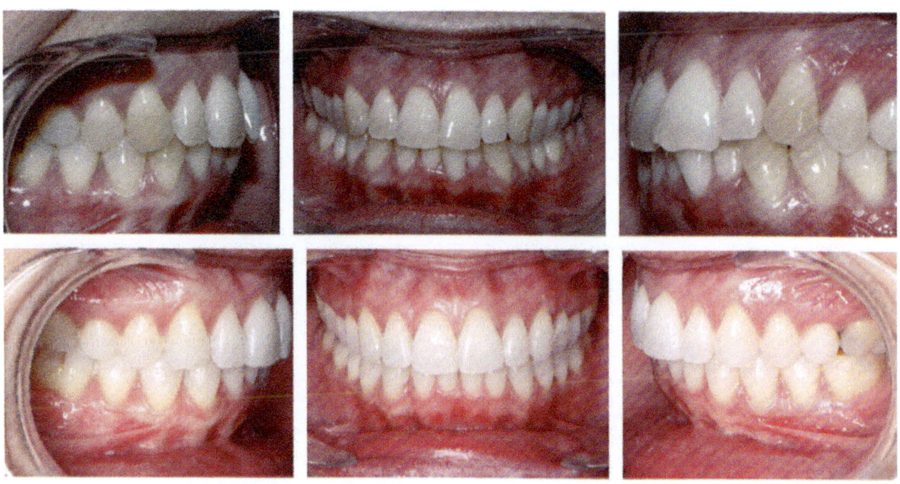

Fig. 25.17 This patient had a selective whitening treatment, focusing more on upper and lower canines to help create a white smile at the end of the treatment.

Bleaching helps with veeners as having the teeth an ideal white colour at the start of the aesthetic treatment, allows the use of ceramics free of opaquers needed to cover dark teeth.

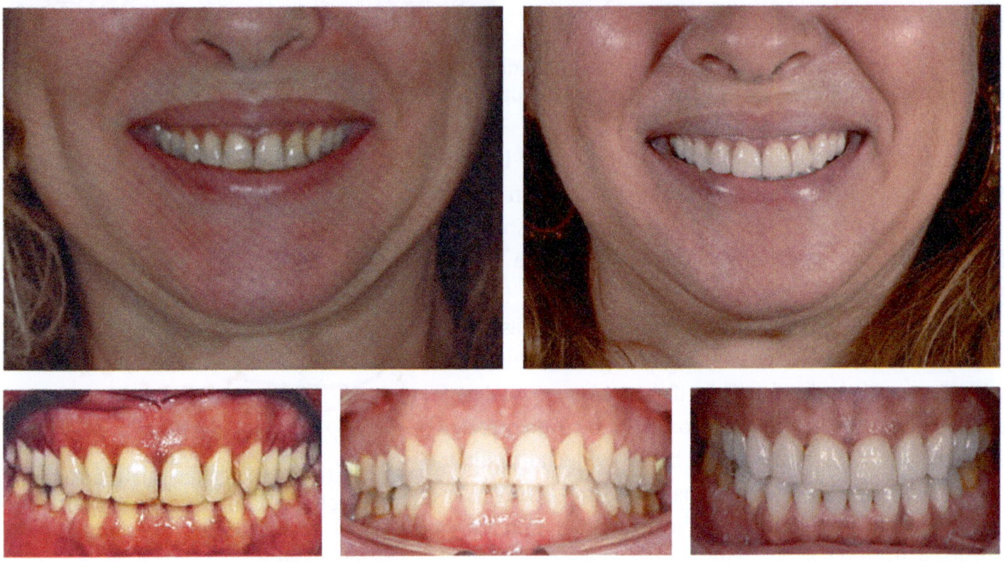

Fig. 25.18 Patient's habits included smoking and drinking coffee on a daily basis, creating the need for whitening teeth before the veneers procedure, which was performed during an orthodontic treatment with 14 + 14 aligners (veneers by Dr Ignacio Vázquez Natividad).

25.2 Veneers to Solve Lateral Bolton Discrepancy in a Class III Patient

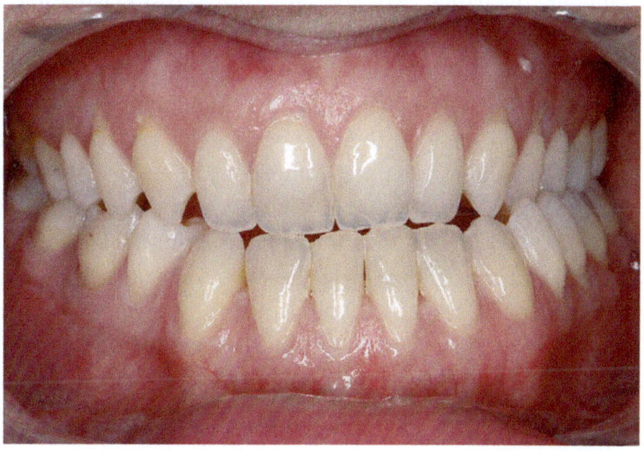

Fig. 25.19 Bolton discrepancy in upper incisors as well as a maxillary skeletal compression.

Diagnosis

A 36-year-old woman with a hypodivergent skeletal class III pattern presented with a relapse from a previous extraction of 44. She had a skeletally constricted upper arch, mandibular asymmetry and a short display with an open bite tendency. Intraorally, there were negative anterior torques and anterior crossbite. There was left crossbite 3 to 5, with recessions resulting from a thin periodontal biotype and a lower midline shift to the left.

Treatment Plan

- Miniscrew assisted rapid palatal expansion (MARPE) was placed at the beginning of the treatment, together with the aligners, manually cutting upper aligners distal to second premolars to allow metal bands
- This reduced posterior anchorage in order to improve anterior upper torque in the first set of aligners but helped to avoid anterior gap between central incisors, as seen previously in two MARPE patients (see cases in Chapters 19 and 20), as the patient refused to have an anterior diastema because of its aesthetic implications
- The upper arch was developed by a torque change both in anterior and posterior, which was also planned in the lower arch, moving the roots to a better position inside the bone

Requirements for the Technician

- 33 to 43: lingual root torque and IPR to reduce teeth with close spacing with an 'en masse' movement
- 13 to 23: open space for upper lateral reconstruction by proclination and extrusion with the Align Technology protocol
- Posterior: upper aligners trimmed distal to 5s to allow presence of maxillary skeletal expander (MSE) and lower precision cuts on buccal molars side to allow future criss-cross elastics
- Arches: expand upper, centring midline with spaces distal to laterals. Compress lower by IPR + LRT to both anterior and posterior teeth, improving occlusion without expanding crowns

Treatment Summary

- Total treatment time was 21 months
- The patient had a first phase with 44 aligners with weekly change. For the duration of this set of aligners the patient wore posterior criss-cross elastics to compress the lower arch
- Space distal to laterals did not ‘appear’ at the end of this set of aligners because of the MARPE planning, which included cutting aligners on upper molars, thereby losing anchorage for anterior torque and spacing, despite the threefold hypercorrection applied
- On a second set of 38 aligners the MARPE was removed and upper molars were engaged in the aligners, helping to improve anterior torque in night use Class III elastics with hand trimmed upper button cutouts and lower hooks. In this case no overcorrection for anterior spacing was needed, as posterior anchorage and anterior negative torque were successful
- Anterior and posterior crossbite were corrected, the arches were properly developed and midlines were improved, although not fully resolved. Aesthetics improved both from posterior expansion and increased display, thanks to anterior pure extrusion and larger upper laterals

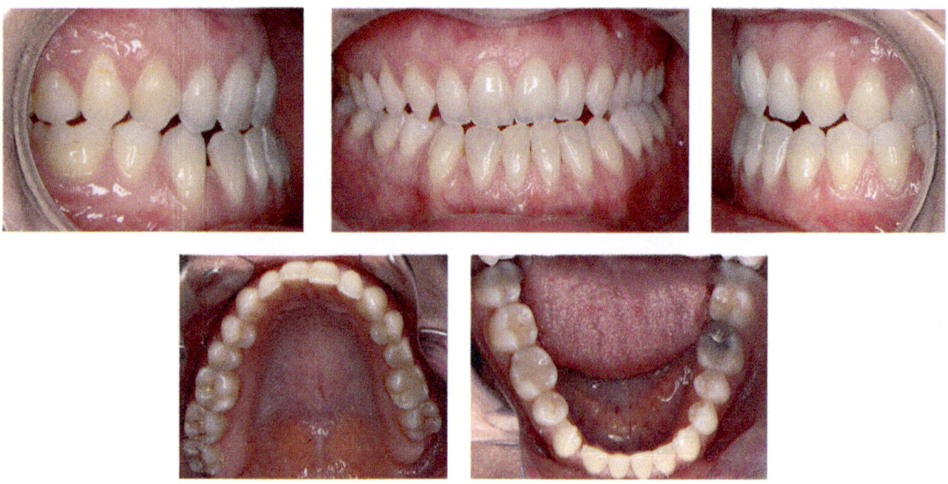

Fig. 25.20 Initial intraoral views.

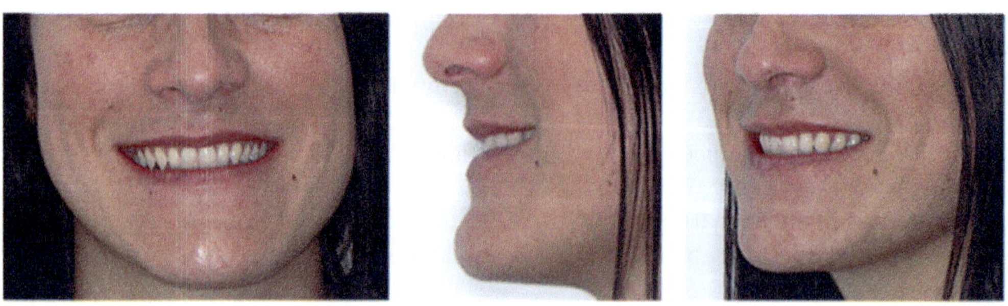

Fig. 25.21 Initial extraoral pictures.

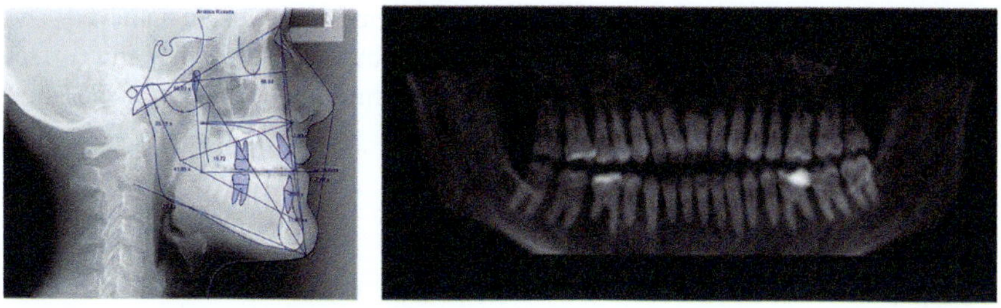

Fig. 25.22 Initial lateral and panoramic X-rays.

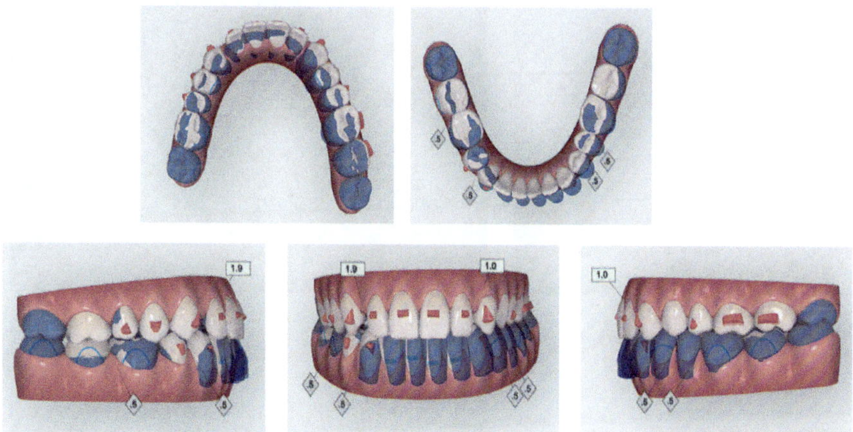

Fig. 25.23 Initial ClinChecks.

The MARPE design was made based on published papers,[1] and by sending the laboratory a scan of the patient together with a drawing of where the screw should be placed and so mini-implants (usually as distally as possible, before the soft palate starts, when soft tissue changes from pink to red).

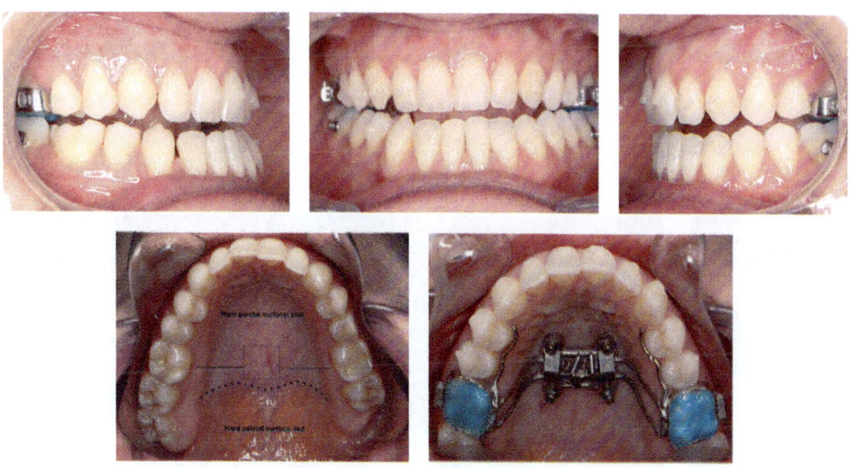

Fig. 25.24 MARPE: the design was made considering that aligners would be trimmed on upper molars, which would have posterior bite blocks to help resolve the crossbite when patient was not wearing aligners.

---

1 Suzuki *et al*. Miniscrew-assisted rapid palatal expander (MARPE): the quest for pure orthopedic movement. *Dental Press J Orthod*. 2016;21(4):17–23.

After using MARPE, the patient was scanned to check the amount of expansion achieved. The result was around 2 mm transversal increase, which would lead to better final stability and correct the relationship between tooth and bone, bearing in mind that thin biotype should avoid large dental expansions.

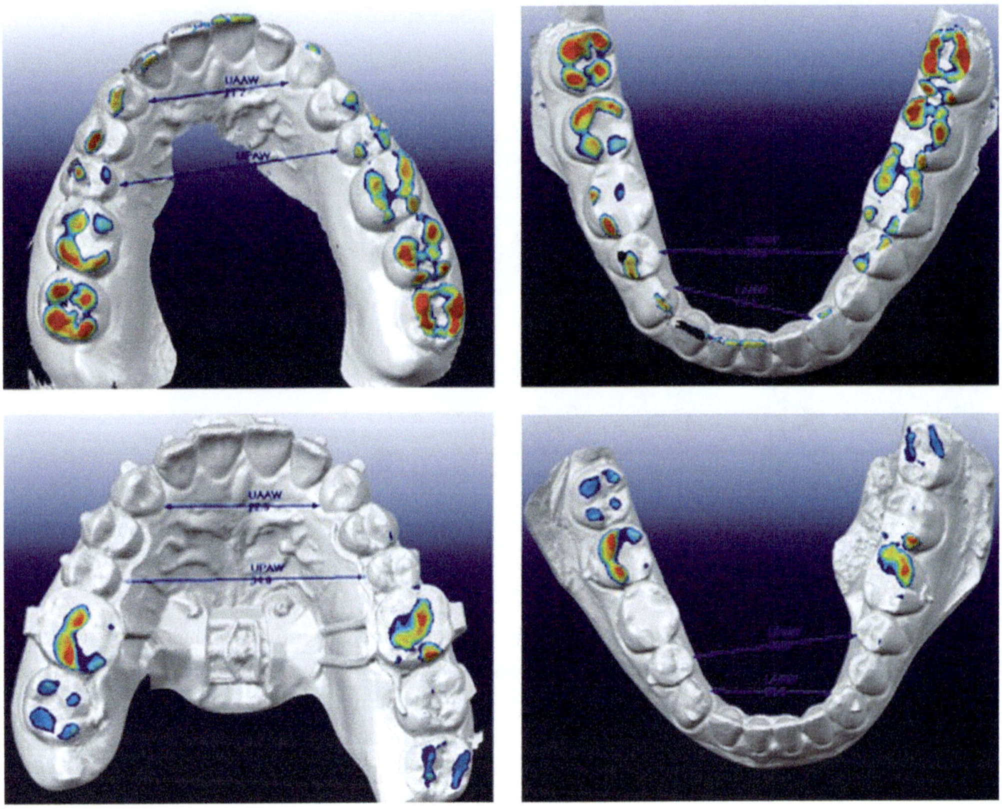

Fig. 25.25 MARPE: iTero software occlusal analysis.

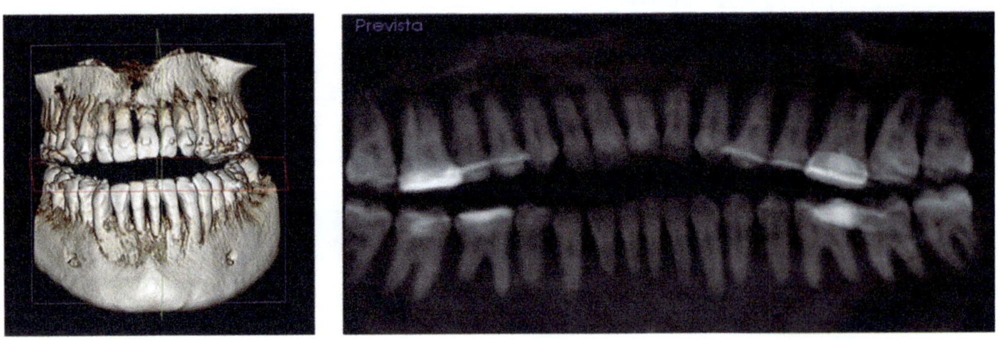

Fig. 25.26 Cone beam computed tomography and panoramic X-ray and after MARPE expansion.

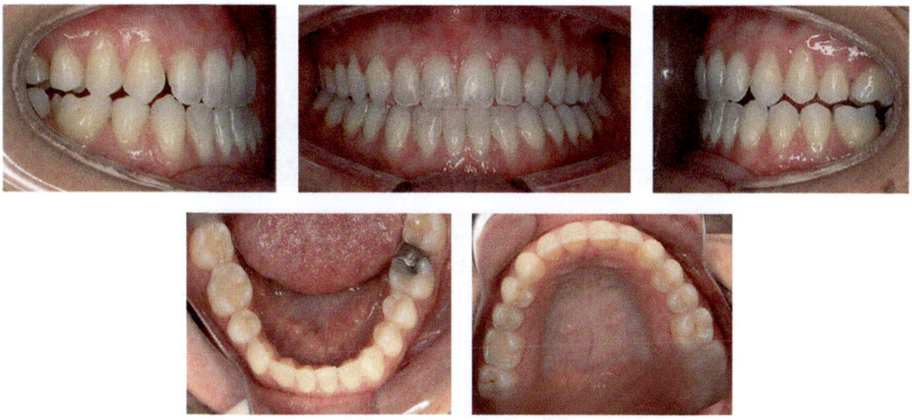

Fig. 25.27 Refinement: after 11 months the patient had the MARPE removed. The scars caused by the miniscrews can be seen on the upper occlusal picture. Space was not created distal to lateral as planned because of the lack of posterior anchorage for anterior overjet.

Requirements for the Technician

- Lower arch lingual root torque
- Upper expansion: centre midline to the left at the same time
- Open more space distal to centrals and have patient ready for veneers
- Manual cutouts for Class III elastics for upper mesialization + vertical component
- Distal molars set as unmovable to increase anchorage

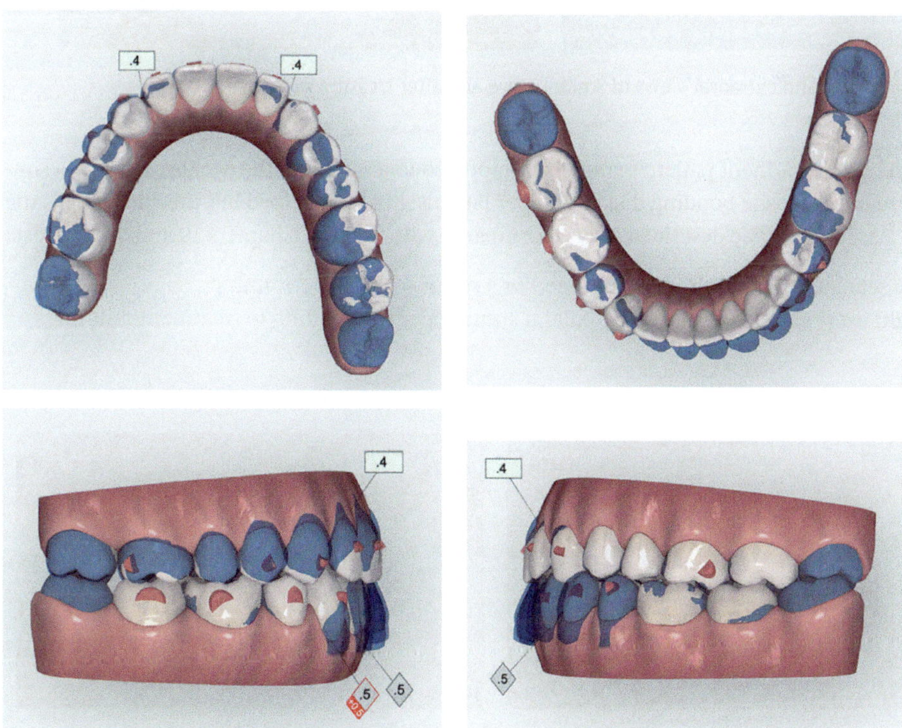

Fig. 25.28 Refinement ClinChecks.

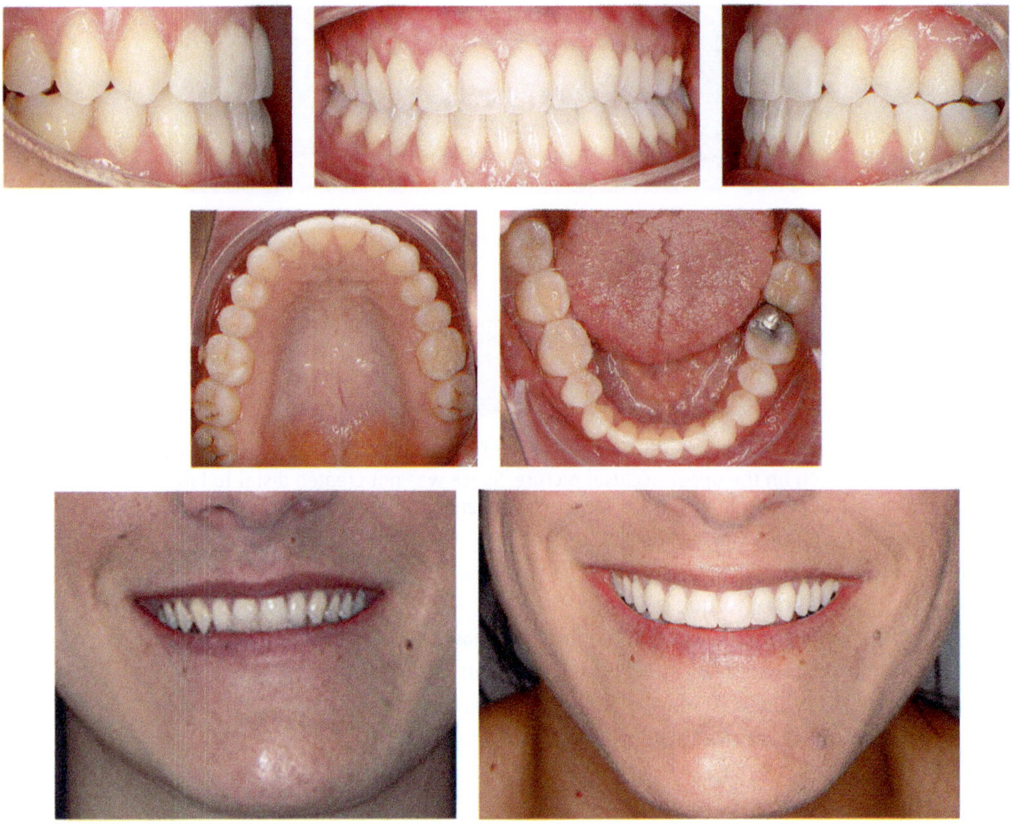

Fig. 25.29 Intraoral and extraoral views of smile before and after treatment.

At the end of the treatment patient's smile had improved together with the occlusion, using a simple procedure of composite bonding distal to upper laterals. MARPE helped but this planning is the one we like least of the three described earlier (compared with cases in Chapters 19 and 20) because:

- As can be seen, anterior anchorage is missed as a result of aligner trimming
- They might exert an opposed force for palatal suture opening, leading to treatment failure

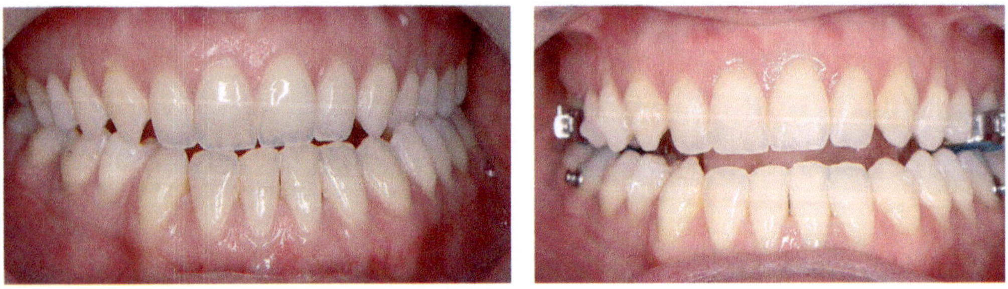

Fig. 25.30 Intraoral views before and after treatment.

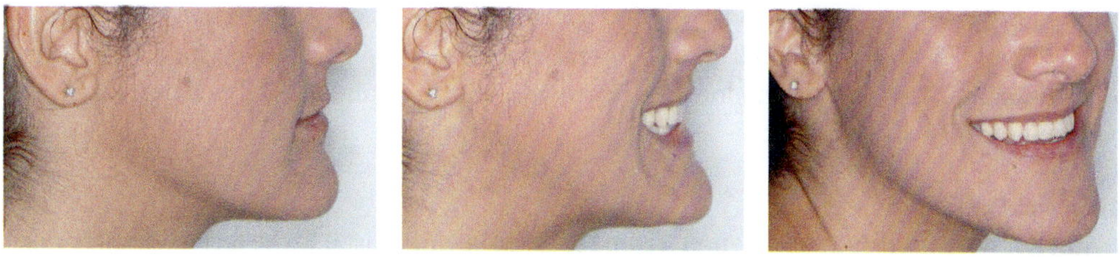

Fig. 25.31 Final extraoral views.

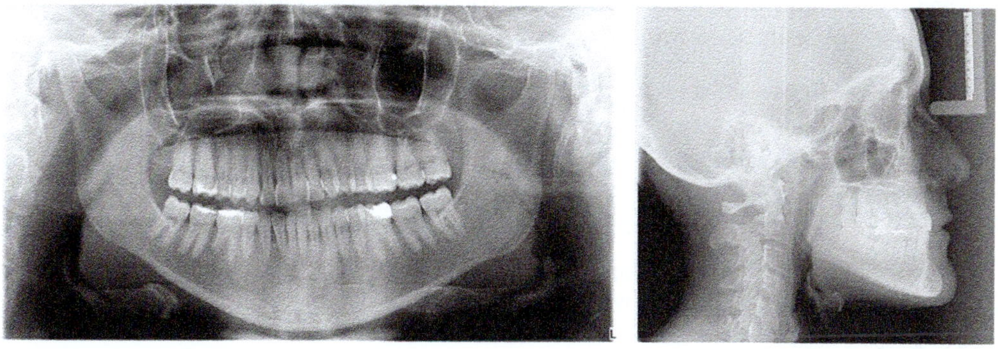

Fig. 25.32 Final panoramic and lateral X-rays.

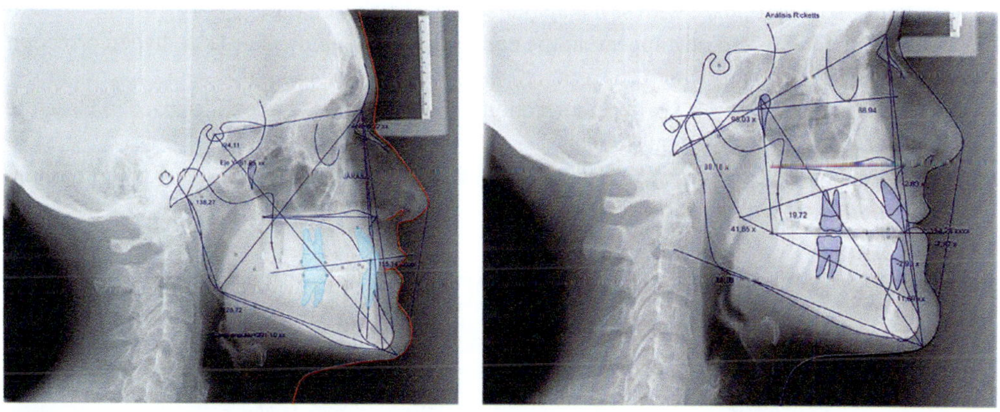

Fig. 25.33 Initial and final cephalometric analysis.

25.3 Space Opening for Anterior Crowns and Implants

Fig. 25.34 Previous cantilever bridge provided smile aesthetics that were unsatisfactory to the patient.

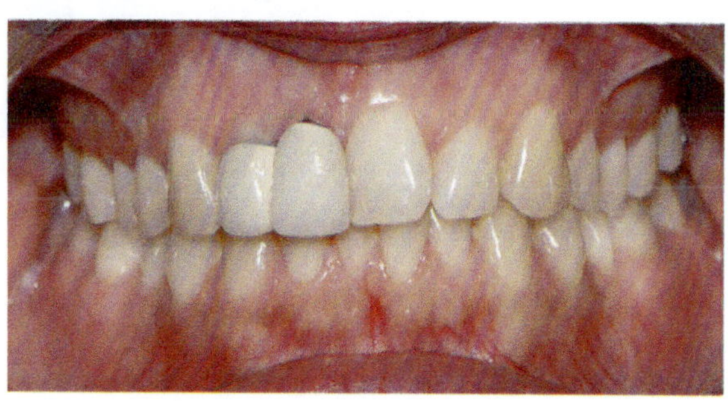

Diagnosis

A 26-year-old woman presented with bilateral class II and constricted arches. The patient refused comprehensive orthodontic treatment and demanded only anterior crown replacement.

Treatment Plan

- Anterior expansion and proclination leading to space opening distal to the metal ceramic bridge the patient was wearing, with a cantilever extension on 11
- As the patient refused comprehensive orthodontic treatment, she was persuaded to have an express anterior treatment to the previous crown replacement so as to have enough space for the implant and its aesthetic crown

1.1	7.24 mm	7.24 mm	2.1
1.2	6.08 mm	6.08 mm	2.2
1.3	7.04 mm	7.04 mm	2.3
1.4	6.32 mm	6.32 mm	2.4
1.5	6.19 mm	6.19 mm	2.5
1.6	9.32 mm	9.32 mm	2.6

Fig. 25.35 The Bolton tool was used to set space needed

ClinCheck 1: Requirements for the Technician

- 33 to 43: correct torque and align: intrusion was not feasible in 7 aligners
- 13 to 23: expand and procline, leaving 11 to 12 as unmovable, as well as the molars to increase anchorage
- Space opening was omitted on the first set of aligners so there was not enough space at the end of the treatment

Treatment Summary

- Total treatment time was 4 months
- The patient had a first phase with seven aligners with a weekly change
- Space distal to laterals did not 'appear' at the end of this set of aligners because hypercorrection was not added
- On a second set of seven a 1.25x hypercorrection factor was added to provide space to place the implant, as requested by the oral surgeon
- Space was made and crown was changed with satisfactory aesthetic results for the patient, although occlusion did not improve

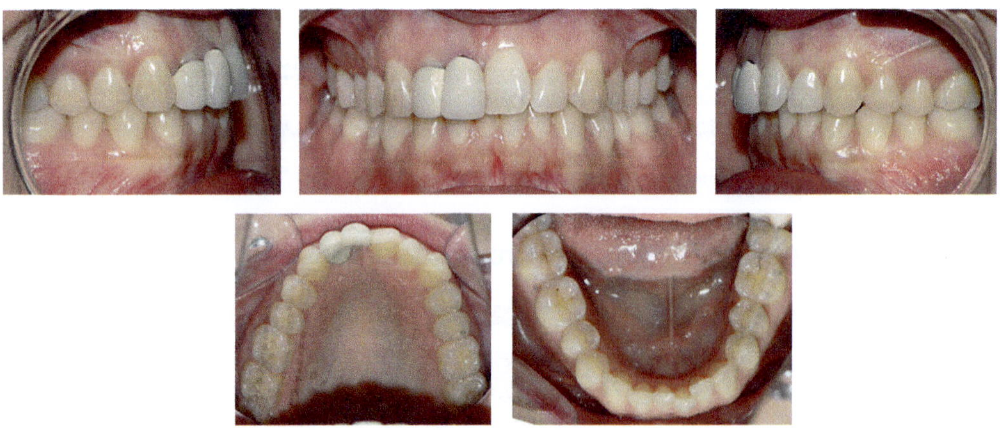

Fig. 25.36 Initial intraoral views.

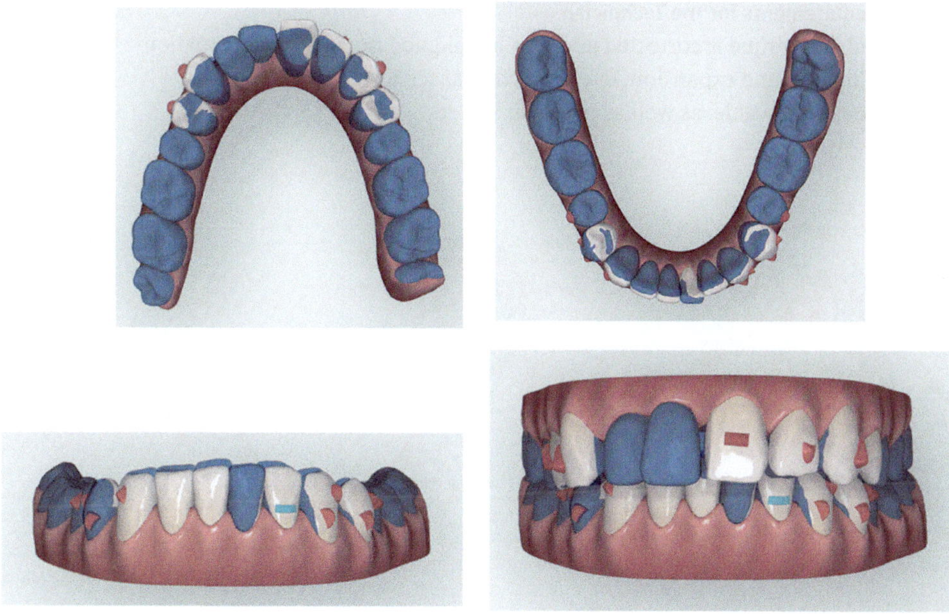

Fig. 25.37 Initial ClinChecks.

Fig. 25.38 Initial smile.

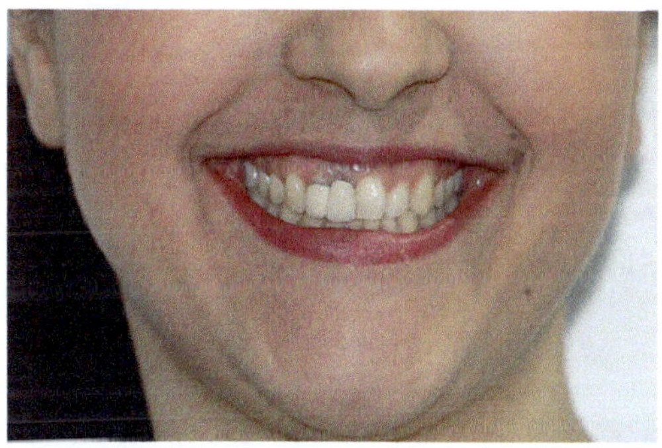

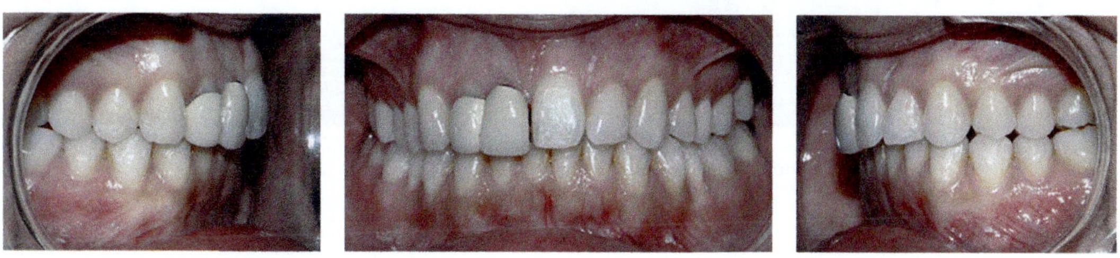

Fig. 25.39 Refinement: intraoral views.

ClinCheck 2: Requirements for the Technician

- 33–43: intrude, as torque is corrected and they are aligned from previous situation
- 13–23: proclination and expansion, overcorrecting space opening
- 11 and 12 kept unmovable, as well as posterior sectors

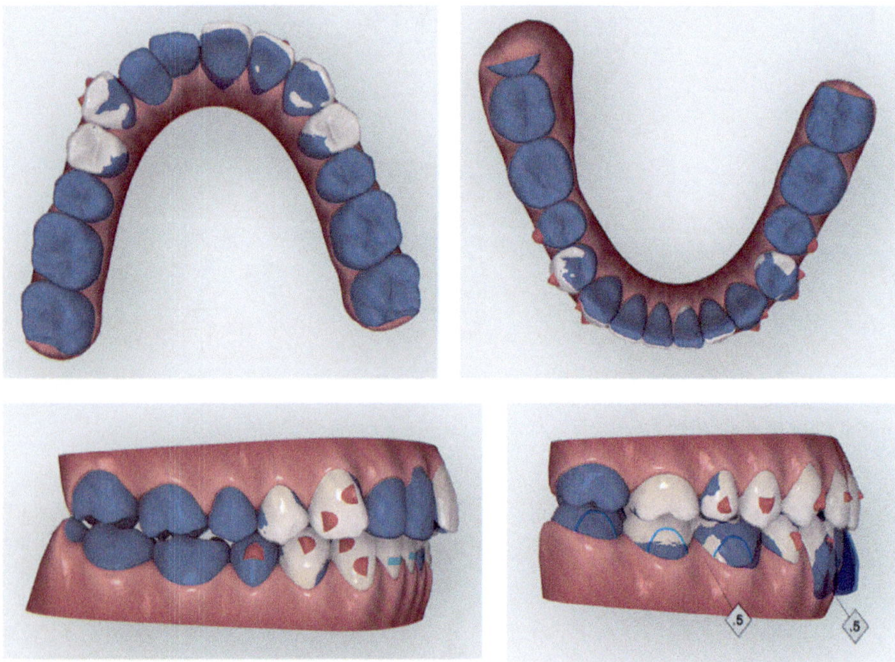

Fig. 25.40 Refinement ClinChecks.

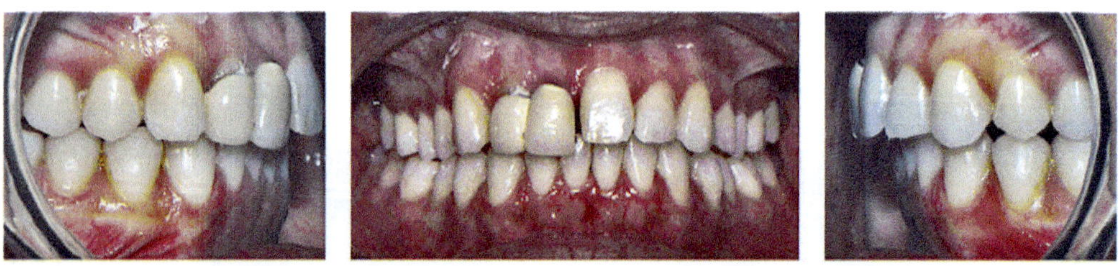

Fig. 25.41 Final intraoral views before fitting veneers.

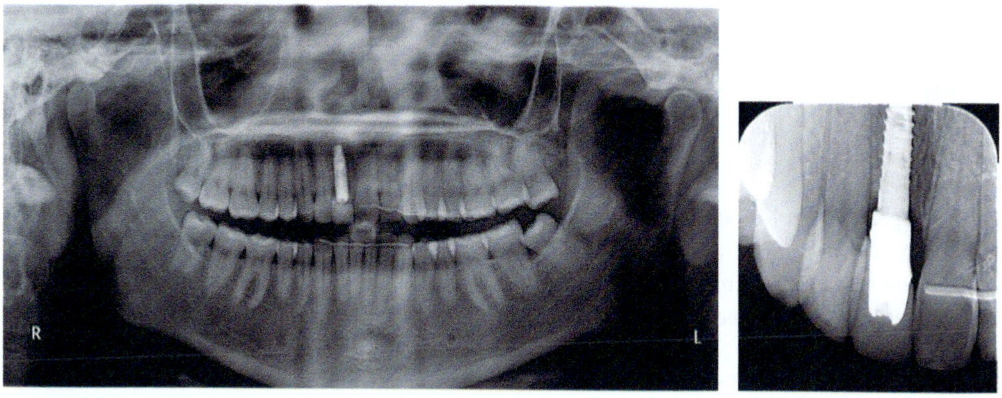

Fig. 25.42 Final X-ray views.

Fig. 25.43 Change in smile after ceramic restoration (Dr Ignacio Vázquez Natividad).

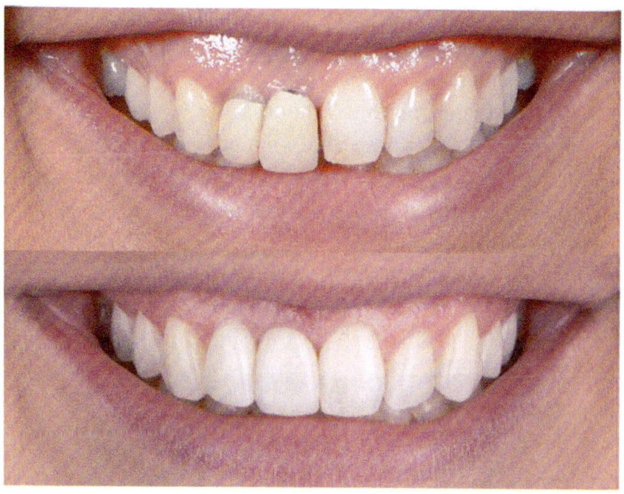

25.4 Anterior Intrusion for Two Central Incisor Veneers

Fig. 25.44 Tooth wear on anterior teeth led to severe attrition of 11–21.

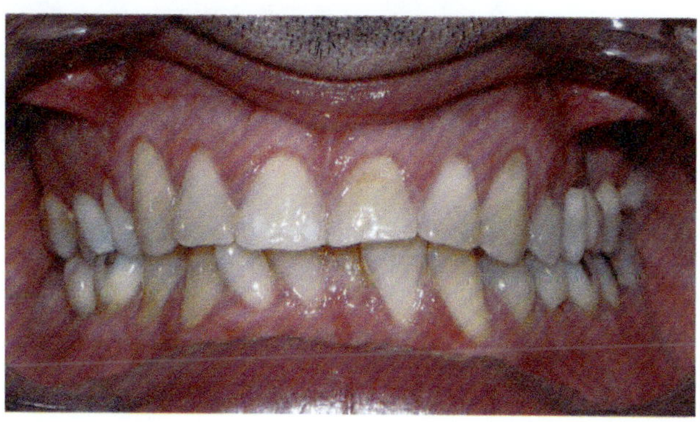

Diagnosis

42-year-old normodivergent man presented with a bilateral Class I. He refused fixed appliances but was disposed to clear aligners. He had constricted arches, anterior extrusion of 11–21 and implants on 26 and 47.

Treatment Plan

- Arch expansion and proclination, together with 11–21 intrusion, left the patient in a suitable position to have ceramic veneers
- One set of aligners were made with dental implants set as unmovable to increase anchorage, and aligning the rest of the teeth to this would create a good arch shape

ClinCheck 1: Requirements for the Technician

- 11–21: correct torque and intrude, use extrusion attachments on adjacent teeth and upper laterals to create a counterforce
- 33–43: expand and procline, intrude anterior to level the curve of Spee and increase both overbite and overjet

Treatment Summary

- Total treatment time was 7 months
- The patient had a phase of 21 aligners with weekly change
- Anterior intrusion hypercorrection was performed, after satisfactory torque had been achieved
- Finally overjet and overbite were created and veneers were bonded with satisfactory aesthetic results for the patient

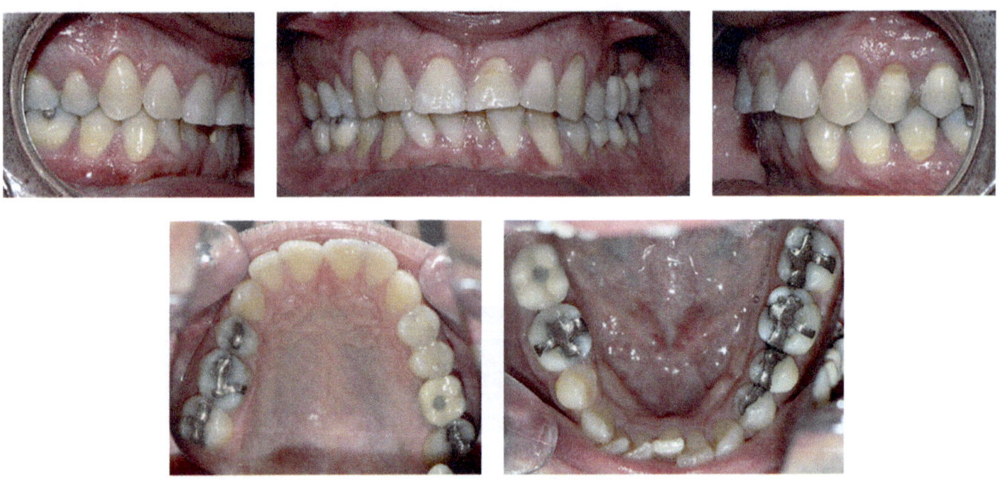

Fig. 25.45 Initial intraoral views.

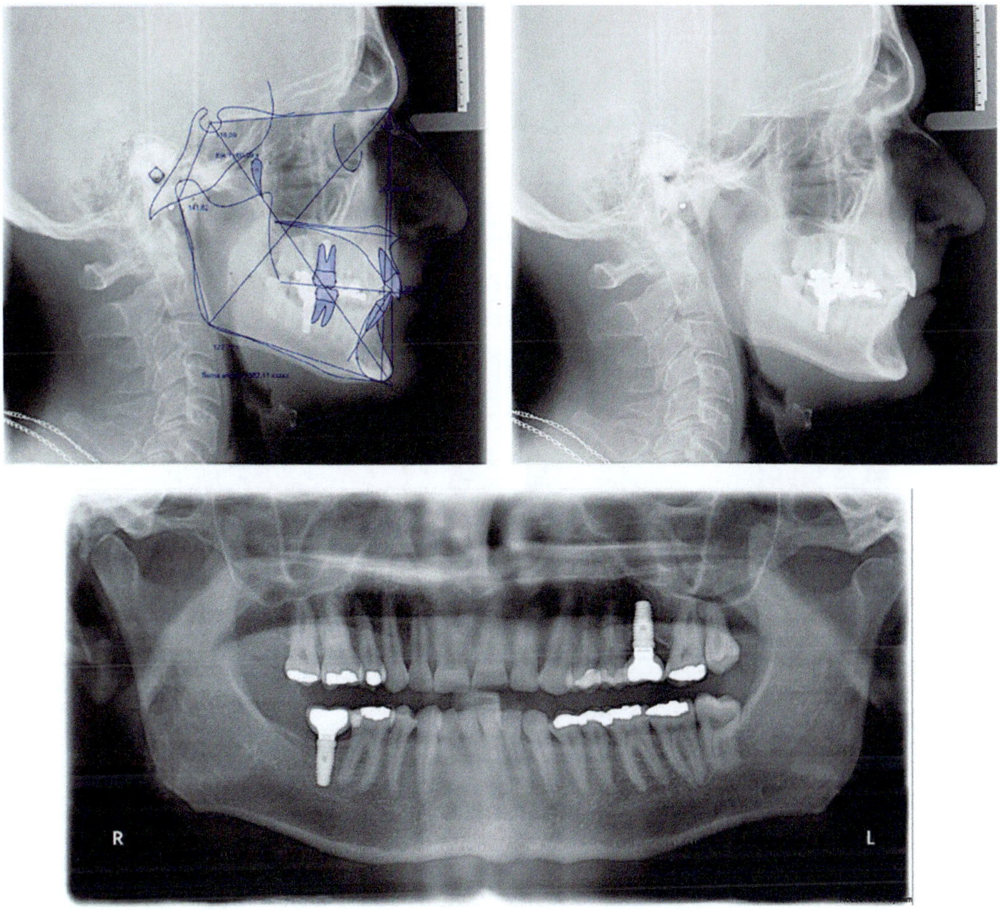

Fig. 25.46 Initial lateral and panoramic X-rays and cephalometric analysis.

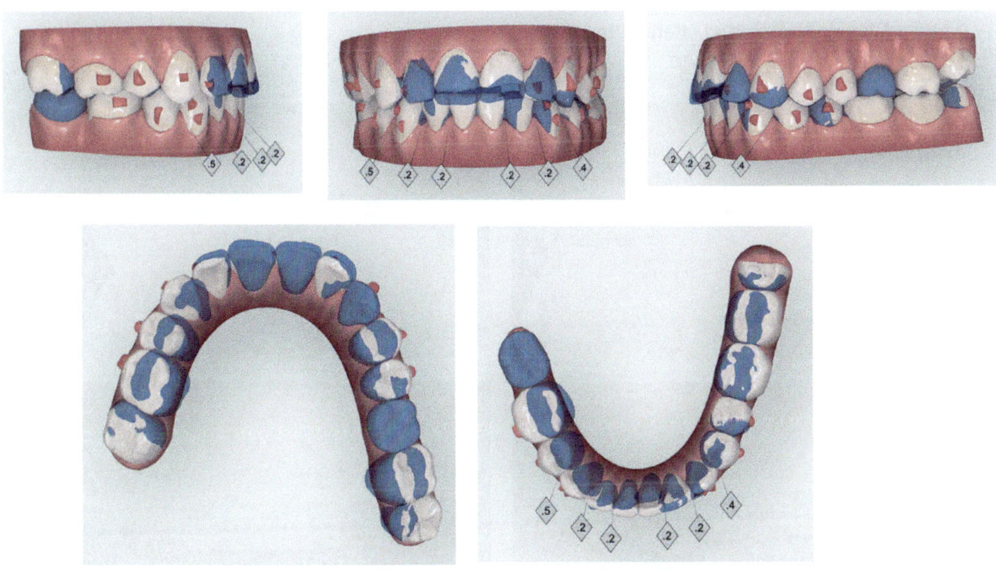

Fig. 25.47 Initial ClinChecks.

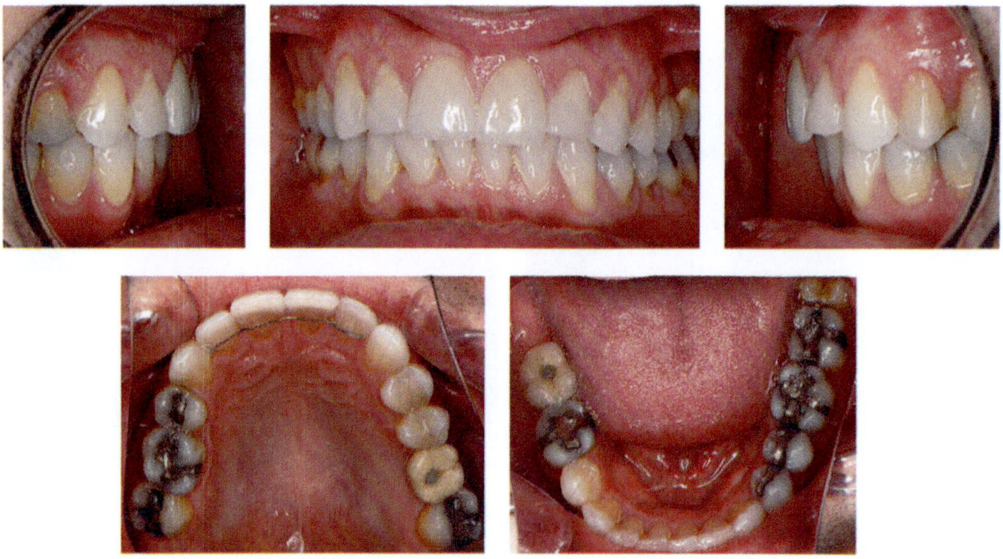

Fig. 25.48 Final intraoral views.

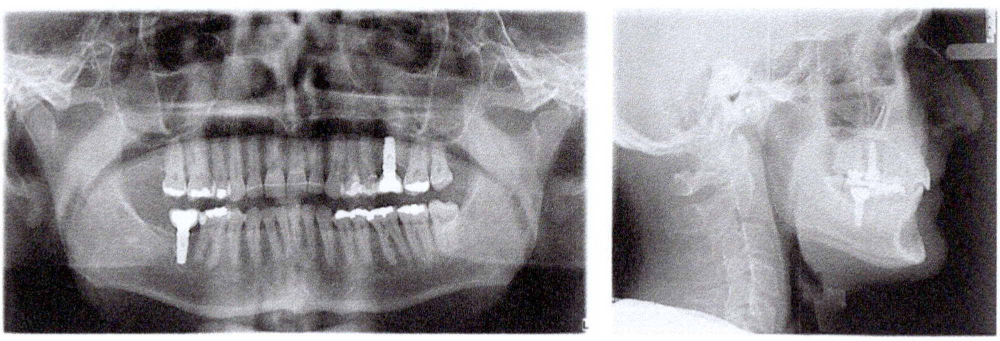

Fig. 25.49 Final panoramic and lateral X-rays.

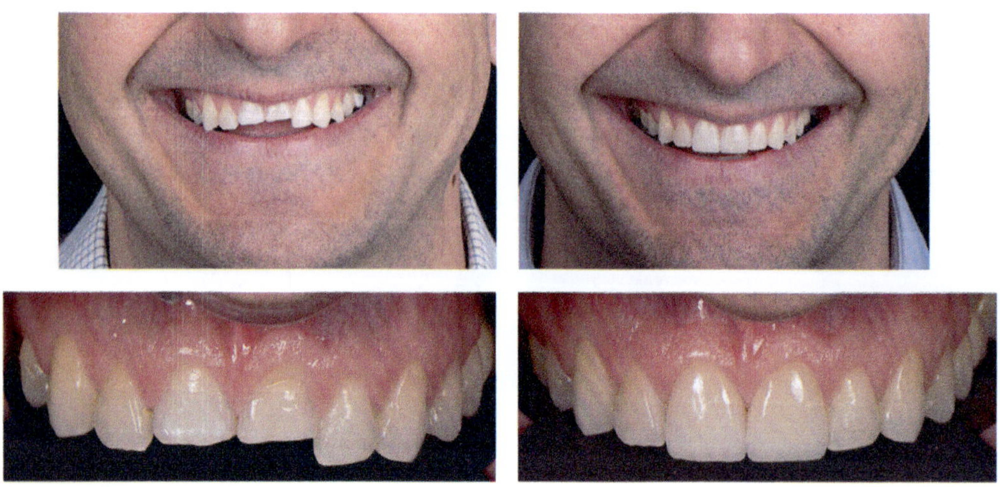

Fig. 25.50 Final smile after veneer bonding (work performed by Dr Ignacio Vázquez Natividad).

25.5 Edge-to-Edge Bite Preparation for Veneers

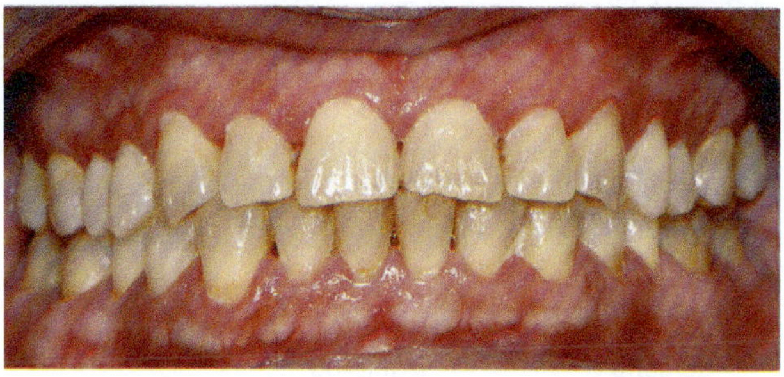

Fig. 25.51 Patient wanted to improve smile aesthetics with veneers, for which overjet was needed.

Diagnosis

A 42-year-old normodivergent woman presented with bilateral dental Class I, constricted arches, a deep bite and lack of overjet. She had appropriate posterior torques, limiting expansion.

Treatment Plan

- Lower retrusion by performing IPR and providing posterior extrusion attachments to help with anterior intrusion
- Two sets of 14 aligners were made for this, improving overjet and overbite with no expansion or protrusion (just IPR and arch coordination)
- Cephalometric analysis showed that incisors should be carefully managed, as they were protruded in relation to bone, so CBCT was done and teeth proclined carefully according to that

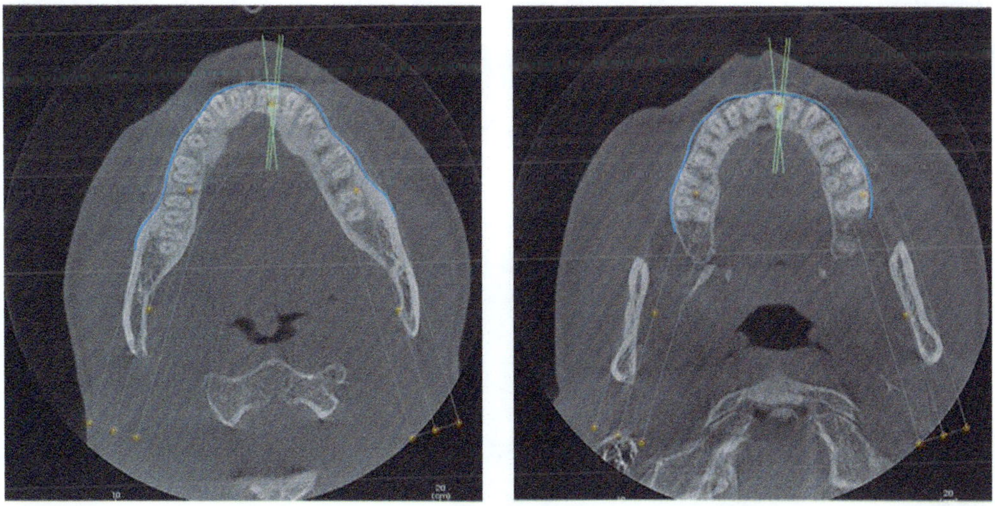

Inf Sup

Fig. 25.52 Lower/upper cone beam computed tomography.

1.1	8.32 mm	7.92 mm	2.1
1.2	5.98 mm	5.77 mm	2.2
1.3	7.13 mm	7.02 mm	2.3
1.4	6.27 mm	6.56 mm	2.4
1.5	5.54 mm	5.81 mm	2.5
1.6	9.70 mm	9.57 mm	2.6

Inferior derecho		Inferior izquierdo	
4.1	5.13 mm	5.04 mm	3.1
4.2	5.78 mm	5.77 mm	3.2
4.3	6.39 mm	6.46 mm	3.3
4.4	6.89 mm	6.71 mm	3.4
4.5	6.54 mm	6.44 mm	3.5
4.6	9.90 mm	10.33 mm	3.6

Fig. 25.53 Bolton analysis showed possibility for lower premolar interproximal reduction.

Treatment Summary

- Total treatment time was 10 months
- The patient had a phase of 14 + 14 aligners with weekly change
- Lower retrusion was achieved with IPR on premolars after a Bolton discrepancy was detected
- Overjet and overbite were created and veneers were bonded with satisfactory aesthetic results for the patient

ClinCheck 1: Requirements for the Technician

- Slight anterior expansion based on CBCT (this is only achievable because of a totally individualized archform design and only possible with aligners, as conventional wires for fixed appliances are usually preformed)
- IPR to reduce arch width and improve anterior overbite by retruding lower incisors
- Lingual attachments for minor anterior movement with additional anchorage

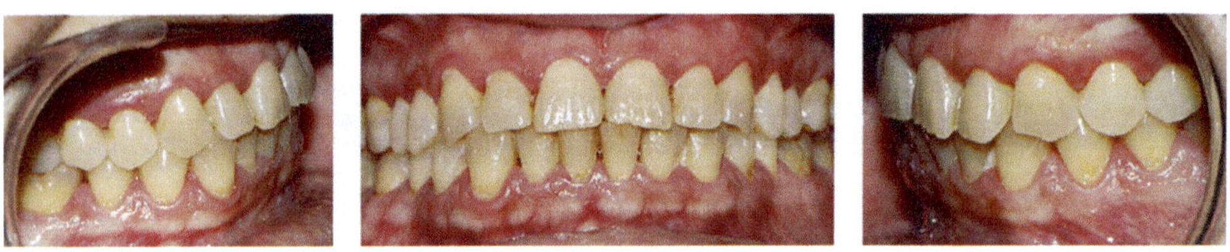

Fig. 25.54 Initial intraoral views.

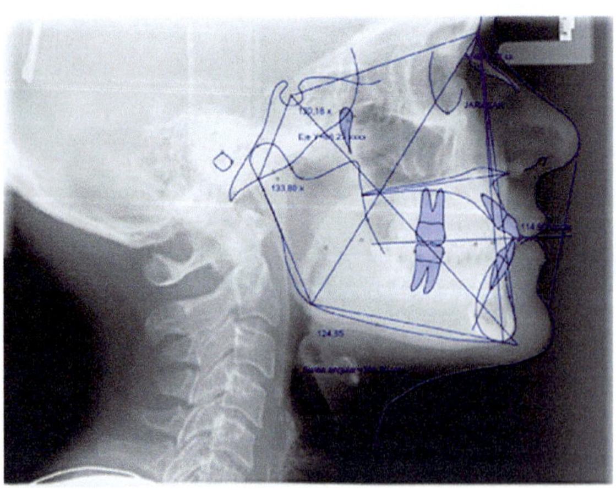

Fig. 25.55 Initial cephalometric analysis.

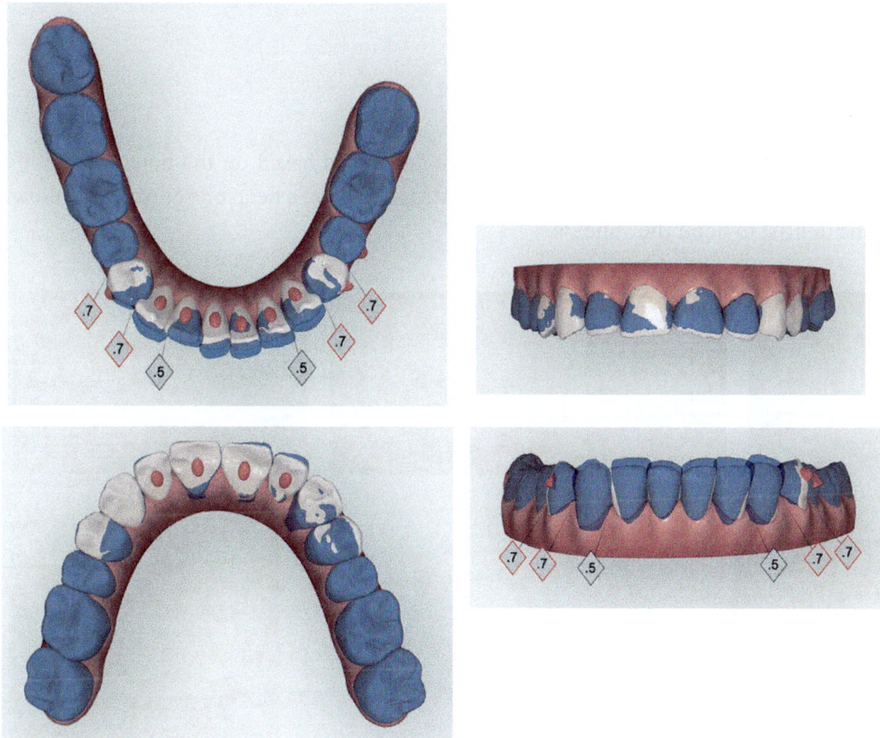

Fig. 25.56 Initial ClinChecks.

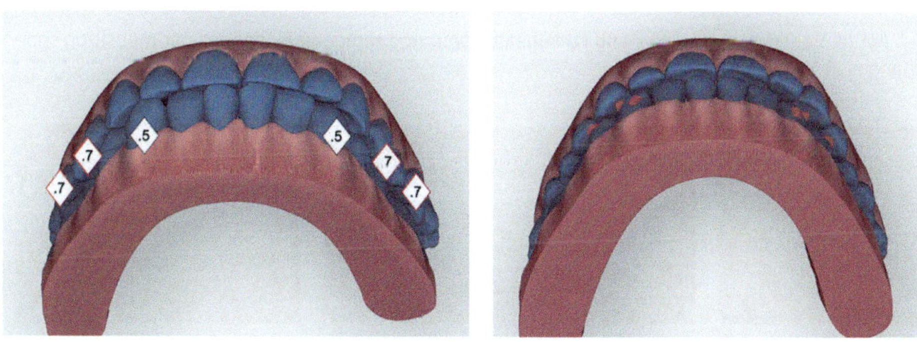

Fig. 25.57 Refinement: the second ClinCheck showed change from edge-to-edge to overjet.

ClinCheck 2: Requirements for the Technician

- Only lower arch treatment
- Virtual C-chain for spaces and LRT on 32–42
- Final settlement and aligning

After refinement, both upper and lower arches were developed based on the bone availability seen on the CBCT; overjet was achieved and anterior intrusion drove a deep bite correction, allowing the cosmetic dentist to bond the veneers.

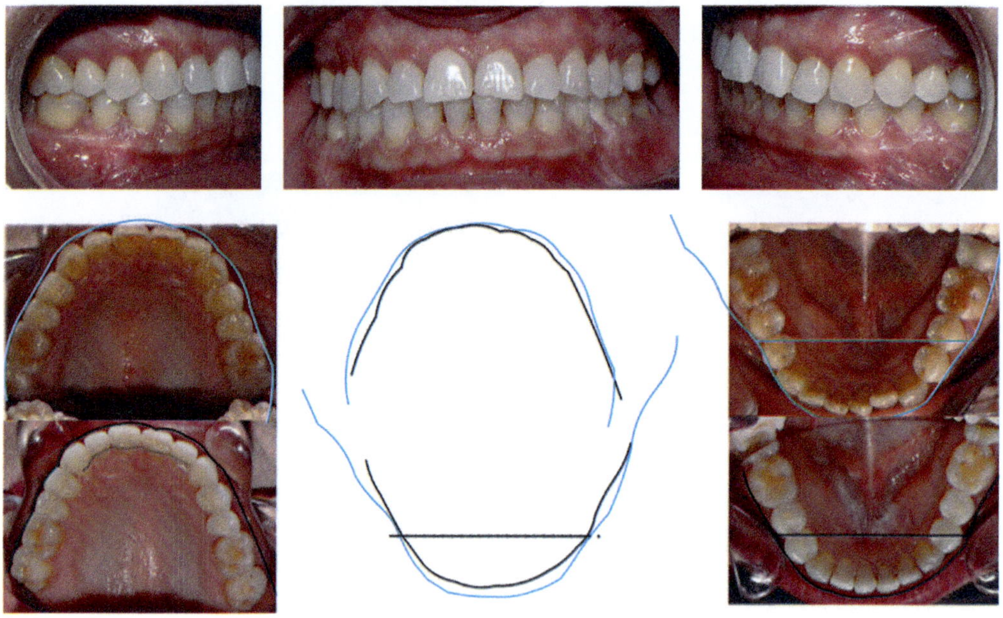

Fig. 25.58 Refinement: intraoral views and cone beam computed tomography bone superimposition show suitable changes at the end.

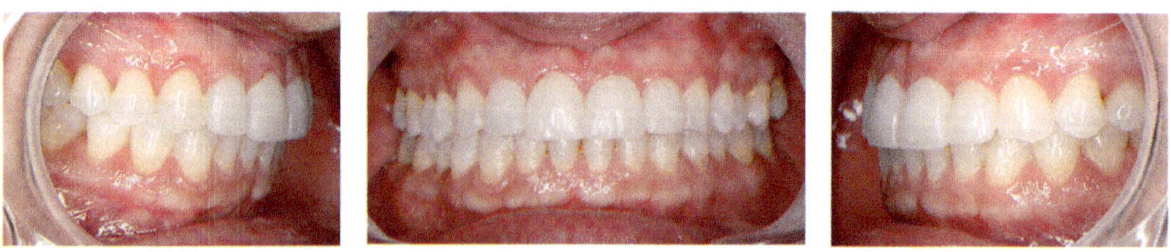

Fig. 25.59 Good final results were achieved thanks to detailed multidisciplinary work (veneers by Dr Ignacio Vázquez Natividad).

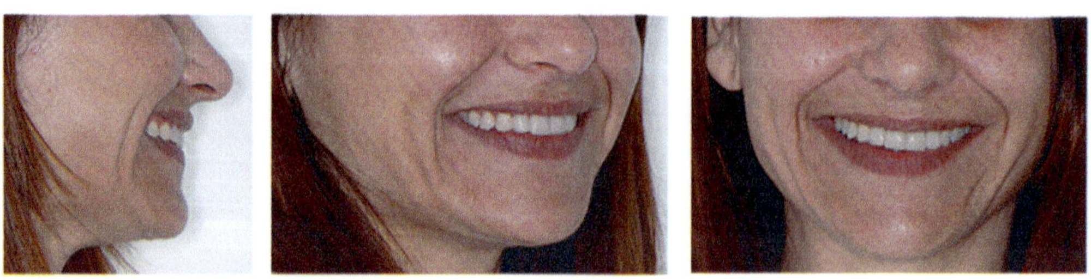

Fig. 25.60 Final extraoral views.

Index

Aligner Techniques in Orthodontics, First Edition. Susana Palma Moya and Javier Lozano Zafra.

Companion website: www.wiley.com/go/lozano-zafra/aligner-techniques